# Clinical Management
# of Intestinal Failure

# Clinical Management of Intestinal Failure

Edited by
Christopher P. Duggan
Tom Jaksic
Kathleen M. Gura

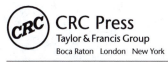

CRC Press
Taylor & Francis Group
Boca Raton  London  New York

CRC Press is an imprint of the
Taylor & Francis Group, an **informa** business

Photographs on companion CD courtesy of Debora Duro, MD, MS, Medical Director, Intestinal Rehabilitation and Nutrition Program, Attending Physician in Pediatric Gastroenterology, Hepatology, and Nutrition, Assistant Professor of Clinical Pediatrics, University of Miami School of Medicine, Miami, Florida

CRC Press
Taylor & Francis Group
6000 Broken Sound Parkway NW, Suite 300
Boca Raton, FL 33487-2742

Printed in the United States of America on acid-free paper
Version Date: 20111103

International Standard Book Number: 978-1-4398-1390-4 (Hardback)

---

**Library of Congress Cataloging-in-Publication Data**

---

Clinical management of intestinal failure / editors, Christopher P. Duggan, Kathleen Gura, Tom Jaksic.
    p. cm.
  Includes bibliographical references and index.
  ISBN 978-1-4398-1390-4 (hardback)
  1. Malabsorption syndromes. 2. Pediatric gastroenterology. I. Duggan, Christopher, MD II. Gura, Kathleen. III. Jaksic, Tom.

RC862.M3C65 2011
616.3'99--dc23                                            2011038753

---

**Visit the Taylor & Francis Web site at**
**http://www.taylorandfrancis.com**

**and the CRC Press Web site at**
**http://www.crcpress.com**

# Contents

## Part I    Intestinal Failure

## Part II    Medical and Surgical Management

## Part III  Prevention and Treatment of Complications of Intestinal Failure

## Part IV   Nursing Management

## Part V   Emerging Diagnostic and Therapeutic Methods

## Part VI   Long-Term Care

# Editors

**Christopher P. Duggan, MD, MPH**, has been performing clinical studies in the fields of pediatric nutrition, gastroenterology, and global health for over 20 years. He is an attending pediatric gastroenterologist and nutrition physician at Children's Hospital Boston where he directs the Clinical Nutrition Service. He is the medical director of the Center for Advanced Intestinal Rehabilitation, one of the largest centers in the United States for the care of children with intestinal failure/chronic diarrhea syndromes. His funded research efforts include trials of nutrient supplementation in women and children susceptible to infectious diseases in Tanzania, India, and other countries. He is the codirector of the Harvard College course, "Nutrition and Global Health" and mentors undergraduate, graduate, and postdoctoral students at Harvard. He is an associate professor of pediatrics at Harvard Medical School and an associate professor in the Department of Nutrition at Harvard School of Public Health.

**Tom Jaksic, MD, PhD**, is the surgical director of the Center for Advanced Intestinal Rehabilitation (CAIR) at Children's Hospital Boston, Vice-Chairman of Pediatric General Surgery at Children's Hospital Boston and the W. Hardy Hendren Professor of Surgery at Harvard Medical School. In addition to being a practicing pediatric surgeon he has a Ph.D in Nutritional Biochemistry from the Massachusetts Institute of Technology (M.I.T.) and has had a career-long research interest regarding the metabolic requirements of critically ill infants as well as the surgical and nutritional management of children with intestinal failure. He is the President-elect of the American Society of Parenteral and Enteral Nutrition (A.S.P.E.N.).

**Kathleen M. Gura, PharmD, BCNSP, FASHP**, is the team leader with Surgical Programs and a clinical pharmacist with the Clinical Nutrition Service in the Division of Gastroenterology and Nutrition at Children's Hospital Boston. She is also an associate professor of pharmacy practice at the Massachusetts College of Pharmacy in Boston. Her professional focus is on academic clinical pharmacy and research, and her areas of expertise include nutritional support for critically ill pediatric patients, nutritional support in intestinal failure, sterile products preparation, aluminum toxicity, and drug–nutrient interactions. She is a member of numerous professional organizations, including the American Society for Parenteral and Enteral Nutrition and the European Society for Parenteral and Enteral Nutrition. She was the recipient of the 2008 ASPEN Serlick Award for safe practices in the field of parenteral nutrition and the 2009 Drug Therapy Research Award of the American Society of Health Systems Pharmacists. Her research in the area of parenteral nutrition–associated liver injury is currently funded by the March of Dimes with additional funding coming from the FDA's Orphan Drug Development Program.

# Contributors

**Steven A. Abrams**
USDA/ARS Children's Nutrition Research
   Center
Texas Children's Hospital
and
Department of Pediatrics
Baylor College of Medicine
Houston, Texas

**Julie E. Bines**
The University of Melbourne
and
Department of Gastroenterology and
   Clinical Nutrition
Royal Children's Hospital
Murdoch Childrens Research Institute
Victoria, Australia

**Joan Bishop**
Oley Foundation
Albany Medical Center
Albany, New York

**George Blackburn**
Beth Israel Deaconess Medical Center
Boston, Massachusetts

**Dana Boctor**
Department of Pediatrics
Alberta Children's Hospital and University
   of Calgary
Calgary, Alberta, Canada

**Megan Brenn**
Center for Advanced Intestinal
   Rehabilitation
Children's Hospital Boston
Boston, Massachusetts

**Carlo Buonomo**
Department of Radiology
Children's Hospital Boston
and
Harvard Medical School
Boston, Massachusetts

**David L. Burns**
Division of Gastroenterology
Lahey Clinic
Tufts University School of Medicine
Burlington, Massachusetts

**Indraneel Chakrabarty**
Division of Gastroenterology
Tufts University School of Medicine
Burlington, Massachusetts

**Mary Petrea Cober**
Department of Pharmacy
Akron Children's Hospital
Akron, Ohio
and
Department of Pharmacy Practice
Northeast Ohio Medical University
College of Pharmacy
Rootstown, Ohio

**Conrad R. Cole**
Division of Gastroenterology, Hepatology, and
   Nutrition
Cincinnati Children's Hospital Medical
   Center
and
Department of Pediatrics
University of Cincinnati College of
   Medicine
Cincinnati, Ohio

**Sharon Collier**
Clinical Nutrition Service
Division of GI/Nutrition
Children's Hospital Boston
Boston, Massachusetts

**Virginie Colomb**
Faculté René Descartes
Pediatric Home Parenteral Nutrition Centre
Reference Centre for Rare Digestive Diseases
Hôpital Necker-Enfants Malades
Paris, France

**Ivan R. Diamond**
Group for Improvement of Intestinal Function
    and Treatment
The Hospital for Sick Children
Toronto, Ontario, Canada

**John K. DiBaise**
Division of Gastroenterology and
    Hepatology
Mayo Clinic College of Medicine
Scottsdale, Arizona

**Stephanie DiPerna**
Department of Radiology
Children's Hospital Boston
and
Harvard Medical School
Boston, Massachusetts

**Christopher P. Duggan**
Center for Advanced Intestinal
    Rehabilitation
Children's Hospital Boston
and
Harvard Medical School
Boston, Massachusetts

**Debora Duro**
Department of Pediatrics
University of Miami Miller School of
    Medicine
Miami, Florida

**Erica M. Fallon**
Department of Surgery and the Vascular
    Biology Program
Children's Hospital Boston
Boston, Massachusetts

**Sara Gibbons**
Children's Hospital Boston
Boston, Massachusetts

**Tracy C. Grikscheit**
Division of Pediatric Surgery
Keck School of Medicine
and
Saban Research Institute
Los Angeles, California

**Kathleen M. Gura**
Clinical Pharmacy Gastroenterology and
    Nutrition
Center for Advanced Intestinal
    Rehabilitation
Children's Hospital Boston
Boston, Massachusetts

**Ivan M. Gutierrez**
Center for Advanced Intestinal
    Rehabilitation
Children's Hospital Boston
Boston, Massachusetts

**Gil Hardy**
Institute of Food, Nutrition and
    Human Health
Massey University
Auckland, New Zealand

**Sanjiv Harpavat**
Department of Pediatrics
Baylor College of Medicine
Texas Children's Hospital
Houston, Texas

**Sara N. Horst**
Division of Gastroenterology, Hepatology, and
    Nutrition
Vanderbilt University Medical Center
Nashville, Tennessee

**Lyn Howard**
The Oley Foundation
Albany Medical Center
Albany, New York

**Melissa A. Hull**
Department of Surgery
Children's Hospital Boston
and
Harvard Medical School
Boston, Massachusetts

**Julie Iglesias**
Center for Advanced Intestinal
    Rehabilitation
Children's Hospital Boston
Boston, Massachusetts

**Tom Jaksic**
Center for Advanced Intestinal
    Rehabilitation
Children's Hospital Boston
and
Harvard Medical School
Boston, Massachusetts

**Brian A. Jones**
Department of Surgery
Children's Hospital Boston
and
Harvard Medical School
Boston, Massachusetts

**Daniel S. Kamin**
Center for Advanced Intestinal
    Rehabilitation
Children's Hospital Boston
and
Harvard Medical School
Boston, Massachusetts

**Kuang Horng (Jamie) Kang**
Center for Advanced Intestinal
    Rehabilitation
Children's Hospital Boston
Boston, Massachusetts

**Darlene G. Kelly**
Division of Gastroenterology and
    Hepatology
Mayo Clinic College of Medicine
and
Mayo Clinic
Rochester, Minnesota

**Heung Bae Kim**
Department of Surgery
Pediatric Transplant Center
Children's Hospital Boston
and
Harvard Medical School
Boston, Massachusetts

**Mark G. Klang**
Research Pharmacy
Memorial Sloan-Kettering Cancer Center
New York, New York

**Samuel Kocoshis**
Division of Gastroenterology
    and Nutrition
Cincinnati Children's Hospital
Cincinnati, Ohio

**Esi S. N. Lamousé-Smith**
Division of Gastroenterology and
    Nutrition
Children's Hospital Boston
and
Harvard Medical School
Boston, Massachusetts

**Jonathan Lockwood**
Tight Lines Fishing Service
Wilmont, New Hampshire

**Margaret McGuire**
Department of Surgery
University of Massachusetts Medical
    Center
Worcester Massachusetts

**Milissa A. McKee**
Department of Pediatric Surgery
Yale University School of Medicine
Yale–New Haven Children's Hospital
New Haven, Connecticut

**M. Molly McMahon**
Division of Endocrinology, Diabetes,
    Metabolism, Nutrition, and Internal
    Medicine
Mayo Clinic
Rochester, Minnesota

**Nilesh M. Mehta**
Division of Critical Care Medicine
Department of Anesthesia
Children's Hospital Boston
and
Harvard Medical School
Boston, Massachusetts

**Lisa Crosby Metzger**
The Oley Foundation
Albany Medical Center
Albany, New York

**John M. Miles**
Division of Endocrinology, Diabetes,
    Metabolism, Nutrition, and
    Internal Medicine
Mayo Clinic
Rochester, Minnesota

**Eva S. Nagy**
Murdoch Childrens Research
    Institute
and
Department of Gastroenterology
    and Clinical Nutrition
The University of Melbourne
Victoria, Australia

**Khiet D. Ngo**
Loma Linda University Children's Hospital
Gastroenterology, Hepatology, and Nutrition
Loma Linda University School of Medicine
Loma Linda, California

**Samuel Nurko**
Center for Motility and Functional
    Gastrointestinal Disorders
Children's Hospital Boston
Boston, Massachusetts

**Erin M. Nystrom**
Department of Hospital Pharmacy
    Services
Mayo Clinic
Rochester, Minnesota

**Ellen A. O'Donnell**
Department of Surgery
Children's Hospital Boston
Boston, Massachusetts

**Horacio Padua**
Department of Radiology
Children's Hospital Boston
and
Harvard Medical School
Boston, Massachusetts

**Stephanie Petruzzi**
Center for Advanced Intestinal
    Rehabilitation
Children's Hospital Boston
Boston, Massachusetts

**Kristina M. Potanos**
Department of Surgery
Children's Hospital Boston
and
Harvard Medical School
Boston, Massachusetts

**Mark Puder**
Department of Surgery and the Vascular
    Biology Program
Children's Hospital Boston
and
Harvard Medical School
Boston, Massachusetts

**Sandy Quigley**
Department of Surgery
Children's Hospital Boston
Boston, Massachusetts

**Denise S. Richardson**
Center for Advanced Intestinal
    Rehabilitation
Children's Hospital Boston
Boston, Massachusetts

**Leonel Rodriguez**
Center for Motility and Functional
    Gastrointestinal Disorders
Children's Hospital Boston
Boston, Massachusetts

**Douglas L. Seidner**
Division of Gastroenterology, Hepatology,
    and Nutrition
Vanderbilt University Medical Center
Nashville, Tennessee

**Robert J. Shulman**
Department of Pediatrics
Baylor College of Medicine
and
Children's Nutrition Research Center
Texas Children's Hospital
Houston, Texas

**David L. Sigalet**
Department of Surgery
Alberta Children's Hospital and University
    of Calgary
Calgary, Alberta, Canada

**Jason S. Soden**
Section of Pediatric Gastroenterology,
    Hepatology, and Nutrition
University of Colorado School of Medicine
and
Children's Hospital Colorado
Aurora, Colorado

**Daniel H. Teitelbaum**
Department of Pediatric Surgery
University of Michigan
Ann Arbor, Michigan

**Clarivet Torres**
Children's National Medical Center
George Washington University
Georgetown University
Washington, District of Columbia

**Robert S. Venick**
Division of Gastroenterology, Hepatology and
    Nutrition
Mattel Children's Hospital at UCLA
Los Angeles, California

**Paul W. Wales**
Division of General Surgery
The Hospital for Sick Children
Toronto, Ontario, Canada

**Vivian M. Zhao**
Nutrition and Metabolic Support
    Service
Emory University Hospital
Emory University School of Medicine
Atlanta, Georgia

**Thomas R. Ziegler**
Department of Medicine
Emory University School of Medicine
and
Division of Biological and
    Biomedical Sciences
Emory University
Atlanta, Georgia

# Introduction

## A Multidisciplinary Approach to Intestinal Failure

The syndrome of intestinal failure (IF) has been increasingly appreciated as a complex disease entity afflicting tens of thousands of patients and costing hundreds of thousands of dollars per year per patient [1]. Owing to improvements across a wide range of disciplines (medicine, surgery, nursing, pharmacy, and nutrition), the outlook for improved survival and quality of life in IF patients has increased steadily. After the classic paper by Wilmore in 1968 noted an overall survival rate of 54% among infants with short bowel syndrome (SBS), the advent of parenteral nutrition (PN) immediately reduced deaths due to dehydration and malnutrition. More recent advances in survival have been attributed to improved catheter composition and care, increased awareness of the importance of aggressive treatment and prevention of bloodstream infections, newer surgical approaches to shortened bowel, modifications to the composition of parenteral nutrition, including fat emulsions, and the

**TABLE I.1**

**Progressive Improvement in Mortality Rates in the IF Literature**

| Site and Date Reference | Dates | N | Definition of IF | Survival (%) |
|---|---|---|---|---|
| Reports in the English literature [2] | Before 1972 | 50 | Infants <2 months of age with residual small bowel length <75 cm | 54% |
| Los Angeles, CA [3] | 1977–1984 | 13 | Residual small bowel length <38 cm | 69% |
| Paris, France [4] | 1975–1991 | 87 | Extensive SB resection in neonatal period | 89.7% |
| Los Angeles, CA [5] | 1977–2000 | 78 | Children with residual small bowel length <75 cm who required PN for >3 months | 73% |
| Paris, France [6] | 1980–2000 | 141 | Neonates with SBS | 93% |
| Boston, MA [7] | 1986–1998 | 30 | PN >90 days; neonates | 70% |
| Pittsburgh, PA [8] | 1996–2006 | 338 | Children cared for in the intestinal rehabilitation center and/or referred for transplantation evaluation who were on PN | 68% |
| Toronto, Canada [9] | 1997–2001 | 40 | PN >6 weeks or residual small bowel length <25% expected (n = 40) | 63% |
| Ann Arbor, Michigan [10] | 1997–2003 | 80 | PN >60 days or residual small bowel length <50% expected | 73% |
| Boston, MA [11] | 1999–2006 | 54 | PN >90 days; neonates | 89% |
| Omaha, Nebraska [12] | 2000–not stated | 50 | Adults and children who underwent surgical therapy of SBS | 86% |
| Omaha, Nebraska [13] | 2001–2005 | 51 | PN-dependent patients referred for transplantation evaluation | 90% |
| Calgary, Canada [14] | 1998–2006 2006–2009 | 33 22 | Children with residual small bowel <40 cm or PN >60 days | 73% (early cohort) 100% (later cohort) |
| 14 centers across the United States and Canada [15] | 2000–2004 | 272 | Infants <12 months receiving PN for >60 days | 74% |

advent of intestinal and multivisceral transplantation. Table I.1 lists several representative papers in the literature confirming continual improvements in survival rates in IF over the past decades.

Several authors have noted that a multidisciplinary approach to the care of these patients is instrumental in achieving optimal patient outcomes. Advantages of the multidisciplinary approach include more efficient lines of communication, improved monitoring of medications and their effects, more detailed evaluation of growth parameters, and facilitation of the creative process that can lead to research breakthroughs. As students and practitioners in the field, we believed that the time had come for a textbook on IF whose editors and authors reflected the diverse and multidisciplinary aspects of clinical care and research that have been demonstrated to be so effective in the literature. We therefore assembled a broad range of clinician scientists in the field of IF, including gastroenterologists, surgeons, nurses, pharmacists, dietitians, social workers, and patients, to author state-of-the-art summaries of the field. Both pediatric and adult specialists have contributed to the text, since the etiology and management of IF in these groups are often so different.

As patient survival continues to improve, a focus on quality of life and other new challenges undoubtedly will emerge that require us to rethink our current approaches. We believe that this textbook will help advance the discipline of IF by summarizing the current state of the "art" of patient management, as well as the state of the "science" of new research discoveries in tissue engineering, advances in the medical and surgical therapy of IF, transplantation science, and other aspects of the field. We thank all of the authors of the chapters, Randy Brehm of CRC Press, and Carlotta Hayes for diligently and expertly guiding the process to completion.

## REFERENCES

1. Spencer AU, Kovacevich D, McKinney-Barnett M, Hair D, Canham J, Maksym C, et al. Pediatric short-bowel syndrome: The cost of comprehensive care. *Am J Clin Nutr.* 2008;88(6):1552–9.
2. Wilmore DW. Factors correlating with a successful outcome following extensive intestinal resection in newborn infants. *J Pediatr.* 1972;80(1):88–95.
3. Dorney SF, Ament ME, Berquist WE, Vargas JH, Hassall E. Improved survival in very short small bowel of infancy with use of long-term parenteral nutrition. *J Pediatr.* 1985;107(4):521–5.
4. Goulet O, Baglin-Gobet S, Talbotec C, Fourcade L, Colomb V, Sauvat F, et al. Outcome and long-term growth after extensive small bowel resection in the neonatal period: A survey of 87 children. *Eur J Pediatr Surg.* 2005;15(2):95–101.
5. Quiros-Tejeira RE, Ament ME, Reyen L, Herzog F, Merjanian M, Olivares-Serrano N, et al. Long-term parenteral nutritional support and intestinal adaptation in children with short bowel syndrome: A 25-year experience. *J Pediatr.* 2004;145(2):157–63.
6. Colomb V, Dabbas-Tyan M, Taupin P, Talbotec C, Revillon Y, Jan D, et al. Long-term outcome of children receiving home parenteral nutrition: A 20-year single-center experience in 302 patients. *J Pediatr Gastroenterol Nutr.* 2007 Mar;44(3):347–53.
7. Andorsky DJ, Lund DP, Lillehei CW, Jaksic T, Dicanzio J, Richardson DS, et al. Nutritional and other postoperative management of neonates with short bowel syndrome correlates with clinical outcomes. *J Pediatr.* 2001;139(1):27–33.
8. Nucci A, Burns RC, Armah T, Lowery K, Yaworski JA, Strohm S, et al. Interdisciplinary management of pediatric intestinal failure: A 10-year review of rehabilitation and transplantation. *J Gastrointest Surg.* 2008;12(3):429–35; discussion 35–6.
9. Wales PW, de Silva N, Kim JH, Lecce L, Sandhu A, Moore AM. Neonatal short bowel syndrome: A cohort study. *J Pediatr Surg.* 2005;40(5):755–62.
10. Spencer AU, Neaga A, West B, Safran J, Brown P, Btaiche I, et al. Pediatric short bowel syndrome: Redefining predictors of success. *Ann Surg.* 2005;242(3):403–9; discussion 9–12.
11. Modi BP, Langer M, Ching YA, Valim C, Waterford SD, Iglesias J, et al. Improved survival in a multidisciplinary short bowel syndrome program. *J Pediatr Surg.* 2008;43(1):20–4.
12. Sudan D, DiBaise J, Torres C, Thompson J, Raynor S, Gilroy R, et al. A multidisciplinary approach to the treatment of intestinal failure. *J Gastrointest Surg.* 2005;9(2):165–76; discussion 76–7.

13. Torres C, Sudan D, Vanderhoof J, Grant W, Botha J, Raynor S, et al. Role of an intestinal rehabilitation program in the treatment of advanced intestinal failure. *J Pediatr Gastroenterol Nutr.* 2007;45(2):204–12.

14. Sigalet D, Boctor D, Robertson M, Lam V, Brindle M, Sarkhosh K, et al. Improved outcomes in paediatric intestinal failure with aggressive prevention of liver disease. *Eur J Pediatr Surg.* 2009;19(6):348–53.

15. Squires R, Duggan C, Teitelbaum DH, Wales PW, Balint J, Venick R, Rhee S et al. Pediatric intestinal failure in the intestinal transplant era: A retrospective review of 272 infants. *Gastroenterology* 2011;140(5) (Supp 1): S-79.

# Part I

Intestinal Failure

# 1 Etiology and Epidemiology of Intestinal Failure

*Conrad R. Cole and Thomas R. Ziegler*

## CONTENTS

## 1.1 DEFINITIONS OF INTESTINAL FAILURE

The term intestinal failure was initially coined by Milewski et al. [1]. In an initial attempt to standardize the definition of intestinal failure, both anatomical (length of residual small intestine) and functional measures were proposed as diagnostic criteria for this disorder. Intestinal failure has more recently been defined as the presence of functional gut mass less than the minimal amount necessary for adequate absorption to meet nutrient and fluid requirements for maintenance in adults and growth in children [2,3]. Intestinal failure can be due to anatomical or functional loss of gut mucosal absorptive surface area, as seen in short bowel syndrome (SBS) following massive small bowel ± colonic resection, the most common cause of intestinal failure in multiple series [4–9]. Intestinal failure can also be due to a variety of congenital anomalies (e.g., microvillus inclusion disease, intestinal epithelial dysplasia, intestinal atresia), mucosal diseases (e.g., inflammatory bowel disease, severe villous atrophy), dysmotility disorders (e.g., pseudo-obstruction), severe maldigestive disorders, and a variety of other conditions, independent of bowel resection or length of residual bowel [1–9].

In patients with intestinal failure due to SBS, it has been assumed that bowel length and anatomy had the greatest impact on nutritional independence (i.e., ability to be weaned from parenteral nutrition [PN]); thus, bowel length was assessed in the definition of severity of SBS-induced intestinal failure in two of the largest series [4,5]. Carbonel et al. [4] studied 103 adults with residual small bowel length 17–150 cm, of whom 24 lost nutritional autonomy (i.e., required chronic PN), suggesting that longer residual small bowel length and presence of a jejunoileal anastomosis promoted autonomy, whereas end jejunostomy increased the risk of losing nutritional autonomy. High-risk patients for loss of nutritional autonomy were: those with jejunoileal anastomosis and remaining small bowel length <35 cm, patients with jejunocolic anastomosis and remaining small bowel length <60 cm, and patients with an end jejunostomy and remaining small bowel length <115 cm [4]. In 124 adults with nonmalignant SBS, Messing et al. [5] found that survival and PN-dependence probabilities were 86% and 49%; and 75% and 45%; at 2 and 5 years, respectively. Others have proposed functional measures based on energy losses measured in adults dependent on PN after significant intestinal resection as measures for defining intestinal failure [10].

In children, some investigators have defined intestinal failure, based on durations of PN dependence ranging from 27 days to 90 days [11–14]. However, when the duration of PN is included as part of the criteria for diagnosing intestinal failure, patients, especially children, who die early due to complications of the primary disorder or complications of therapy are excluded, which has an impact on the true incidence/prevalence of the disorder.

The currently accepted consensus definition states that *Intestinal failure results from obstruction, dysmotility, surgical resection, congenital defect, or disease-associated loss of absorption and is characterized by the inability to maintain protein-energy, fluid, electrolyte, or micronutrient balance when on a conventionally accepted, normal diet* [15]. Intestinal failure in children is defined as "insufficient functional intestinal mass needed to adequately digest and absorb nutrients and fluids required for appropriate growth and development" [16]. Nutrient and fluid requirements of individuals with intestinal failure can be met by either complete or partial dependence on PN or intravenous fluids and/or electrolytes, typically in combination with highly individualized enteral diets, tube feedings, or enteral/oral nutrient supplements as indicated.

## 1.2   EPIDEMIOLOGY

The precise epidemiology and incidence rate of intestinal failure in adults and children are unknown. The rarity of the disease, the multifactorial etiologies, and varying definitions used for patient inclusion make it difficult to obtain and compare data across studies [17]. However, there are a few national studies that provide insight to the potential magnitude of the problem. In the United States, the Oley Foundation estimated that there were 40,000 patients with PN-dependent intestinal failure in 1992 based on home PN use [7,15]. Evaluation of the underlying diagnosis available on 5000 home PN-dependent individuals revealed that approximately 40% had cancer and the remainder mainly SBS due to Crohn's disease, mesenteric ischemia, radiation enteritis, severe motility disorders, and congenital abnormalities [7]. Data from Europe revealed the prevalence of intestinal failure in older children (>16 years of age) through adulthood, as defined by use of home PN (HPN), in terms of patients/million inhabitants/year to be 12.7 in Denmark, 3.7 in the United Kingdom and Netherlands, 3.6 in France, 3 in Belgium, 1.1 in Portugal, and 0.65 in Spain

---

**TABLE 1.1**

**Underlying Etiology for Intestinal Failure Requiring Home Parenteral Nutrition for Short Bowel Syndrome in Adults**

| | Carbonnel et al. [4] | Messing et al. [5] | Bakker et al. [6] | Howard et al. [7] | Wilmore and Robinson [20] | Lloyd et al. [8] | Raman et al. [9] |
|---|---|---|---|---|---|---|---|
| *N* | 135 | 124 | 494 | 5000 | 87 | 188 | 150 |
| Location | France | France | Europe (9 countries) | USA | USA | UK | Canada |
| Period | 1972–1995 | 1980–1992 | 1997 | 1985–1992 | 1990–1996 | 1979–2003 | 2004–2006 |
| Type of intestinal failure | SBS | SBS | HPN required | HPN required | SBS | HPN required | HPN required |
| **Underlying Etiology (%)** | | | | | | | |
| Crohn's disease | 16% | 9% | 19% | 12% | 24% | 32% | 51% |
| Mesenteric infarction | 30% | 40% | 15% | 7% | 31% | 16% | 24% |
| Radiation enteritis | 23% | 23% | 7% | 3% | 8% | 11% | NR |
| Intestinal volvulus | 13% | 7% | NR | NR | 12% | NR | NR |
| Other causes | 18% | 21% | 20% | 38% | 25% | 23% | 18% |
| Cancer | NR | NR | 39% | 40% | — | 4% | 7% |

*Note:*  HPN, home parenteral nutrition required (with or without short bowel syndrome); NR, not reported; SBS, short bowel syndrome.

[18]. A questionnaire-based survey conducted across European referral centers (23 centers in 6 countries), revealed that in the year 2000, there were 882 new adult patients referred to these centers for the management of intestinal failure [19]. The incidence and prevalence of SBS in adults in the United States is unknown. The estimate from Europe is about 2 per million adults [18].

The underlying proportions of specific etiologies for intestinal failure overall and SBS in particular in adults vary depending on the particular study [20]. Major findings summarizing underlying etiologies in patients with HPN dependence or SBS are shown in Table 1.1. In a series of HPN patients, who may or may not have an element of SBS, bowel obstruction due to cancer appears to be a major cause of intestinal failure (≈40%) (Table 1.1) [6,7]. Clearly, the medical center referral base, patient care mix, and location of the center plays a major role in these percentages. For example, our unpublished data from Emory University Hospital in Atlanta, which receives a large number of complex intestinal surgical and fistula cases from outside hospitals, show the underlying reason for the need for HPN in 101 consecutive discharged adult patients as intestinal fistula (29%), postoperative bowel dysmotility (15%), chronic pancreatitis (14%), SBS (10%), miscellaneous causes of bowel obstruction (10%), cancer (5%), and a variety of malabsorptive conditions and miscellaneous causes (17%).

In children, the precise incidence of intestinal failure is also uncertain. However, multicenter networks and individual center reports indicate that SBS is the most common cause of intestinal failure in children in developed countries. The distribution of the etiology of intestinal failure based on a network of centers in Italy and single-center data from the United States, Canada, and Finland is shown in Figure 1.1 [21–24]. The average incidence rate reported from Neonatal Intensive Care Unit (NICU) admissions was 7/1000 [25]. SBS has the broadest age of presentation as it depends on the primary cause for surgery (Table 1.1) and makes up for the largest group of children with intestinal failure (Figure 1.1). The proportion of infants with NEC is significantly higher in preterm (delivered before 37 completed weeks of gestation) babies and those with low birth weight (<1500 g) [25,26]. A recent multicenter analysis of children with intestinal failure identified: birth weight <750 g, the use of parenteral antibiotics and mechanical ventilation on the

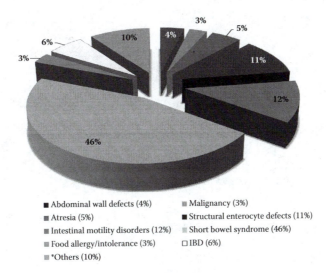

- ■ Abdominal wall defects (4%)
- ■ Atresia (5%)
- ■ Intestinal motility disorders (12%)
- ■ Food allergy/intolerance (3%)
- ■ *Others (10%)
- ■ Malignancy (3%)
- ■ Structural enterocyte defects (11%)
- ■ Short bowel syndrome (46%)
- ☐ IBD (6%)

**FIGURE 1.1** Distribution of the causes of pediatric intestinal failure. $N = 303$. (*Disorders included in the other category are spontaneous intestinal perforation, autoimmune enteropathy, enterocolitis, lymphangiectasia, and bile malabsorption syndromes.) Data from Europe and North America. (Adapted from Casey, L., *Nutr Clin Pract* 2008;23(4):436–442; Guarino, A. and De Marco, G., *J Pediatr Gastroenterol Nutr* 2003;37(2):136–141; Pakarinen, M.P., Koivusalo, A.I., and Rintala, R.J., *J Pediatr Surg* 2009;44(11):2139–2144; Vargas, J.H., Ament, M.E., and Berquist, W.E., *J Pediatr Gastroenterol Nutr* 1987;6(1):24–32.)

**TABLE 1.2**

**Etiology of Pediatric Short Bowel Syndrome as Reported from North America**

| Causes of Short Bowel Syndrome in Children | Wales et al. [12] $n = 40$ | Cole et al. [25] $n = 89$ | Quiros-Tejeira [29] $n = 78$ |
|---|---|---|---|
| Necrotizing enterocolitis | 35% | 96% | 22% |
| Congenital intestinal atresia (jejuna, ileal, apple peel) | 10% | 1% | 24% |
| Abdominal wall defects (gastroschisis, omphalocele) | 12.5% | 1% | 24% |
| Volvulus | 10% | 2% | 20% |
| Hirschsprung's disease | 2.5% | NR | NR |
| Meconium ileus | 20% | NR | NR |
| Others | 10% | NR | 10% |

*Note:* NR, not reported.

day of NEC diagnosis, and the percentage of small bowel resected as significant factors associated with increased risk for developing intestinal failure in infants with NEC [27].

Infants with abdominal wall defects (gastroschisis and omphalocele) and motility disorders also form a significant proportion of the infants with intestinal failure and SBS (Table 1.2). The incidence of abdominal wall defects and motility disorders as the predisposing disease for intestinal failure increases with term deliveries (delivery after 37 completed weeks of gestation) [26].

## 1.3 SHORT BOWEL SYNDROME

Surgical SBS is characterized by insufficient bowel length to digest and absorb adequate nutrients needed to maintain protein and energy balance which are required for growth and development [25]. The incidence of SBS due to massive intestinal resection in the U.S.-born infants with birth weights less than 1500 g (very low birth weight [VLBW] infants) admitted to the neonatal intensive care units enrolled in the neonatal research network of the *Eunice Kennedy Shriver* National Institute of Child health and Human Development (NICHD) was reported as 7/1000. The risk for developing this syndrome increases with decreasing gestational age and decreasing birth weight. The incidence increases to 11/1000 in infants with birth weight less than 1000 g (extremely low birth weight [ELBW] infants). Male infants have an increased risk of developing surgical SBS (unadjusted relative risk = 1.7; confidence interval: 1.1–2.6) compared to females [25]. Initial case reports had implicated that infants born to younger mothers of African descent (Black race) were at increased risk for developing necrotizing enterocolitis (NEC) and subsequently SBS [28,29]. However, in a larger multicenter data set, maternal age or race were not associated with increased risk of developing SBS [25]. The incidence of SBS reported from the neonatal research network of the NICHD is only for VLBW infants with surgical SBS that leads to some degree of intestinal failure. This report excluded nonsurgical causes of intestinal failure [25].

The Canadian SBS incidence rate, which included non-surgical causes of intestinal failure, is based on data from a single center and is higher at 22.1/1000 neonatal intensive care admissions and 24.5/100,000 live births [12]. This report was a retrospective single-center cohort study, the results of which cannot be generalized to other large centers with a different population. The primary disorders associated with SBS reported from the Canadian data and the NICHD data are shown in Table 1.2. The most frequently associated cause of resection leading to SBS in children is NEC [11,12,25,30].

In adults, as noted above, extensive small bowel resection ± colonic resection is related to inflammatory bowel disease (typically Crohn's disease), mesenteric vascular disease, malignancies, intestinal volvulus and postoperative adhesions and other complications [31]. As the management of these patients improves, the prevalence of adult SBS patients is increasing. It is also presumed that as the children with SBS will continue to survive and become adults, this would contribute to the increased prevalence in adults [32]. As can be seen in Table 1.1, in studies of intestinal failure due to SBS alone [4,5,20], different series report underlying SBS etiology as being due to Crohn's disease in 9–24% of cases; mesenteric infarction (which itself could have a variety of underlying causes) in 30–40% of cases; radiation enteritis requiring partial bowel resection in 3–23% of cases, intestinal volvulus in 7–13% of cases; and other/miscellaneous causes (e.g., trauma, postoperative complications requiring multiple abdominal surgeries and bowel resections due to intestinal tumors/malignancy) in 18–25% of cases (Table 1.1).

## 1.4 OUTCOME OF PATIENTS WITH INTESTINAL FAILURE

Morbidity and mortality associated with the diagnosis of intestinal failure is high and the overall mortality rates reported by centers who manage these children range between 25% and 40% [25,32–35]. However, with multidisciplinary approach to managing these children, the overall morbidity and mortality rates have decreased [36,37]. The primary goal of managing these patients is to achieve intestinal autonomy.

In early publications, survival following small bowel resection in infants was reported to be unlikely if remnant small bowel length measured <40 cm without an ileocecal valve (Figure 1.2). However, with an ileocecal valve present, survival was possible with remnant bowel lengths <40 cm but unlikely with lengths less than 15 cm [38]. The other factors which correlated with survival in these early studies included birth weight and lack of associated anomalies. Studies carried out 30 years later also confirmed these findings that survival was better with bowel lengths >38–40 cm [21,30]. However, the remnant small bowel as a percentage of normal bowel length has been shown to be a stronger predictor of mortality (if < 10% of normal length, relative risk [RR] of death = 5.7,

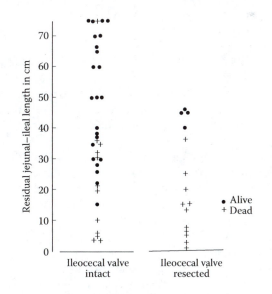

**FIGURE 1.2** Relationship between survival in infants following massive intestinal resection to the length of the residual bowel and presence of the ileocecal valve. (Reprinted from *J Pediatr*, 80(1), Wilmore, D.W., Factors correlating with a successful outcome following extensive intestinal resection in newborn infants, 88–95, Copyright 1972, with permission from Elsevier.)

$P = 0.003$) [35]. The use of the percentage of expected bowel length rather than absolute bowel length in children is due to the potential for the small bowel to continue to grow in newborn infants through childhood [39,40].

Other anatomical factors associated with improved survival include: intact ileocecal valve and colon, takedown surgery after ostomy, and primary anastomosis [30]. Absence of the ileocecal valve causes small bowel bacterial overgrowth and mucosal inflammation, thus impairing intestinal function and prolonging the duration of PN dependence [41,42]. Liver failure is a relatively common complication in children with intestinal failure. In children with intestinal failure as a result of surgical SBS, direct bilirubin levels >4 mg/dL for more than 6 months was identified as a significant predictor of liver failure [43]. In a more recent cohort review of SBS infants with PN-associated liver disease; a serum total bilirubin level of >11 mg/dL, platelet count $\leq 168 \times 10^3/\mu L$ (thrombocytopenia), and serum albumin level $\leq 3$ g/dL increases the odds for irreversible liver failure [44,45]. Early closure of diverting ileostomy/colostomy and enteral feeding with a protein hydrolysate formula were associated with decreased severity of liver disease in these children [33].

Some children with intestinal failure adapt over time. The presence of an ileocecal valve (RR: 11.8, $P = 0.001$) and small bowel length $\geq 10\%$ of normal (RR: 3.9, $P = 0.0005$) are associated with increased probability of weaning off PN [35]. Enteral feeding with breast milk or an amino acid-based formula, longer residual bowel length, and the percentage of calories delivered enterally at 6 weeks after surgery are associated with a shorter duration of PN [33]. Sondheimer et al. [13] have shown that the proportion of enteral feeds tolerated at 12 weeks of age and the length of residual small bowel length after the initial surgery are associated with the probability of attaining enteral independence. Serum citrulline has been shown in children to be predictive of children with intestinal failure who are likely to be weaned off PN [46]. Serum citrulline levels $\geq 19$ µmol/L had 94% sensitivity and 67% specificity for predicting children who can be weaned off PN [46]. Patients with surgical SBS were more likely to achieve intestinal competence and be weaned off PN than patients with motility disorders or structural enterocyte disorders [11,22,23]. The proportion of children eventually been weaned off PN varies between 40% and 85% with improved outcomes reported from centers with multidisciplinary teams [11,22,36,47]. In VLBW (birth weight <1500 g) infants with SBS as the cause of intestinal failure, the mortality is high (20%) in the initial hospital (perinatal) period [25]. Among the ELBW (birth weight <1000 g) infants with SBS who survive to 18–22 months, the rate of hospital admissions during the first year of life is high (79%) [25]. Hospital admissions are usually due to central line infections, dehydration, and poor growth. The cost of care for these children averages $500,000 (2005 estimate) in the first year of life [48]. Despite such a high cost of care and receiving adequate calories, these children were more likely to be shorter and have small head circumferences compared to similar gestational age and birth weight children who do not have SBS [25]. In order for these children to achieve comparable growth when on PN or after weaning, careful monitoring of growth and nutrient status and sometimes additional nutritional support is required [47].

In adults diagnosed with intestinal failure, PN was terminated in 19–38% of those followed over a period of 5 years owing to intestinal adaptation [49–51]. Predictors of intestinal adaptation and weaning off PN include greater bowel length, lower body weight, and greater length–body weight ratio [52]. Unlike in children, serum citrulline has not been shown in a study of PN-dependent SBS adults to be predictive of the potential to wean off PN [53]. However, a "citrulline generation test" was used to distinguish between nonadapted and adapted adults with SBS when making a decision to wean the patient off PN [54]. Mortality is usually due to the primary disease although some mortality can be accounted for by the complications associated with chronic PN use and newly occurring disorders. Mortality rate is higher in cancer patients than in noncancer patients (including patients with inflammatory bowel disease) [49]. Morbidity associated with the prolonged use of venous catheters for HPN includes sepsis, catheter displacement and breakage, and thrombosis. For adults with SBS, survival is related to the length of bowel and age, as those with bowel length <50 cm and age >45 years of age when PN was initiated had higher mortality compared to others [50]. Duration of PN dependence is negatively related to remnant postduodenal bowel length, absence of terminal ileum, and colon incontinuity [5]. Small bowel bacterial overgrowth also may negatively impact the need for PN as this condition itself contributes to maldigestion and malabsorption [55].

In the comprehensive study of Messing et al. in adults with SBS and no history of cancer, multivariate analysis showed that patient survival was related negatively to end-enterostomy, to small bowel length of <50 cm, and to arterial infarction as the cause of SBS [5]. PN dependence was negatively related to postduodenal small bowel lengths of <50 and between 50 and 99 cm and to the absence of terminal ileum and/or colon incontinuity. Residual small bowel lengths separating transient from permanent intestinal failure (partial or complete PN dependence) were 100, 65, and 30 cm in end-enterostomy, jejunocolic, and jejunoileocolic types of anastomosis, respectively [5].

Intestinal failure and the subcategory SBS in adults and children are complex disorders which pose complex management challenges and are responsible for significant health care costs, morbidity, and mortality. Intestinal failure can be classified as reversible or irreversible depending on whether intestinal adaptation occurs for the patient to meet all nutrient and fluid needs. Management in multidisciplinary teams improves survival and decreases morbidity in adults and children with intestinal failure. Intestinal failure patients should be referred early in an optimum nutritional state to multidisciplinary teams with expertise in transplantation in order to improve outcomes [12]. Larger multicenter studies are needed to identify the estimate of the true disease burden especially in adults. These larger studies will be useful for evaluating and identifying risk factors associated with poor outcomes so that transplantation can be done earlier and also improve the posttransplant survival and quality of life.

## REFERENCES

1. Milewski, P.J., Gross, E., Holbrook, I., Clarke, C., Turnberg, L.A., and Irving, M.H. Parenteral nutrition at home in management of intestinal failure. *Br Med J* 1980;280(6228):1356–1357.
2. Goulet, O., Ruemmele, F., Lacaille, F., and Colomb, V. Irreversible intestinal failure. *J Pediatr Gastroenterol Nutr* 2004;38:250–269.
3. Ziegler, T.R. and Leader, L.M. Parenteral nutrition: Transient or permanent therapy in intestinal failure? *Gastroenterology* 2006;130(2 Suppl 1):S37–S42.
4. Carbonnel, F., Cosnes, J., Chevret, S., Beaugeri, L., Ngo, Y., Malafosse, M., Parc, R., Le Quintrec, Y., and Gendre, J.P. The role of anatomic factors in nutritional autonomy after extensive small bowel resection. *JPEN* 1996;20(4):275–280.
5. Messing, B., Crenn, P., Beau, P., Boutron-Ruault, M.C., Rambaud, J.C., and Matuchansky, C. Long-term survival and parenteral nutrition dependence in adult patients with the short bowel syndrome. *Gastroenterology* 1999;117(5):1043–1050.
6. Bakker, H., Bozzetti, F., Staun, M., Leon-Sanz, M., Hebuterne, X., Pertkiewicz, M., Shaffer, J., and Thul, P. Home parenteral nutrition in adults: A European multicentre survey in 1997. ESPEN-home artificial nutrition working group. *Clin Nutr* 1999;18(3):135–140.
7. Howard, L. and Ashley, C. Management of complications in patients receiving home parenteral nutrition. *Gastroenterology* 2003;124(6):1651–1661.
8. Lloyd, D.A., Vega, R., Bassett, P., Forbes, A., and Gabe, S.M. Survival and dependence on home parenteral nutrition: Experience over a 25-year period in a UK referral centre. *Aliment Pharmacol Ther* 2006;15(24):1231–1240.
9. Raman, M., Gramlich, L., Whittaker, S., and Allard, J.P. Canadian home total parenteral nutrition registry: Preliminary data on the patient population. *Can J Gastroenterol* 2007;21(10):643–648.
10. Jeppesen, P.B. and Mortensen, P.B. Intestinal failure defined by measurements of intestinal energy and wet weight absorption. *Gut* 2000;46(5):701–706.
11. Salvia, G., Guarino, A., Terrin, G., Salvia, G., Guarino, A., Terrin, G., Cascioli, C. et al. Neonatal onset intestinal failure: An Italian multicenter study. *J Pediatr* 2008;153(5):674–676.
12. Wales, P.W., de Silva, N., Kim, J., Lecce, L., To, T., and Moore, A. Neonatal short bowel syndrome: Population-based estimates of incidence and mortality rates. *J Pediatr Surg* 2004;39(5):690–695.
13. Sondheimer, J.M., Asturias, E., and Cadnapaphornchai, M. Infection and cholestasis in neonates with intestinal resection and long-term parenteral nutrition. *J Pediatr Gastroenterol Nutr* 1998;27(2):131–137.

14. Sondheimer, J.M., Cadnapaphornchai, M., Sontag, M., and Zerbe, G.O. Predicting the duration of dependence on parenteral nutrition after neonatal intestinal resection. *J Pediatr* 1998;132(1):80–84.

15. O'Keefe, S.J., Buchman, A.L., Fishbein, T.M., Jeejeebhoy, K.N., Jeppesen, P.B., and Shaffer, J. Short bowel syndrome and intestinal failure: Consensus definitions and overview. *Clin Gastroenterol Hepatol* 2006;4(1):6–10.

16. Goulet, O., Ruemmele, F., Lacaille, F., and Colomb, V. Irreversible intestinal failure. *J Pediatr Gastroenterol Nutr* 2004;38(3):250–269.

17. Koffeman, G.I., van Gemert, W.G., George, E.K., and Veenendaal, R.A. Classification, epidemiology and aetiology. *Best Pract Res Clin Gastroenterol* 2003;17(6):879–893.

18. Bakker, H., Bozzetti, F., Staun, M., Leon-Sanz, M., Hebuterne, X., Pertkiewicz, M., Shaffer, J., and Thul, P. Home parenteral nutrition in adults: A European multicentre survey in 1997. ESPEN-home artificial nutrition working roup. *Clin Nutr* 1999;18(3):135–140.

19. Staun, M., Hebuterne, X., Shaffer, J., Haderslev, K.V., Bozzetti, F., Pertkiewicz, M., Micklewright, A., Moreno, J., Thul, P., and Pironi, L. Management of intestinal failure in Europe. A questionnaire based study on the incidence and management. *Dynamic Medicine* 2007;6(1):7.

20. Wilmore, D.W. and Robinson, M.K. Short bowel syndrome. *World J Surg* 2000;24:1486–1492.

21. Casey, L., Lee, K.H., Rosychuk, R., Turner, J., and Huynh, H.Q. 10-year review of pediatric intestinal failure: Clinical factors associated with outcome. *Nutr Clin Pract* 2008;23(4):436–442.

22. Guarino, A. and De Marco, G. Natural history of intestinal failure, investigated through a national network-based approach. *J Pediatr Gastroenterol Nutr* 2003;37(2):136–141.

23. Pakarinen, M.P., Koivusalo, A.I., and Rintala, R.J. Outcomes of intestinal failure—a comparison between children with short bowel and dysmotile intestine. *J Pediatr Surg* 2009;44(11):2139–2144.

24. Vargas, J.H., Ament, M.E., and Berquist, W.E. Long-term home parenteral nutrition in pediatrics: Ten years of experience in 102 patients. *J Pediatr Gastroenterol Nutr* 1987;6(1):24–32.

25. Cole, C.R., Hansen, N.I., Higgins, R.D., Ziegler, T.R., Stoll, B.J., and for the Eunice Kennedy Shriver, National Institute of Child health and Human Development neonatal research network. Very low birth weight preterm infants with surgical short bowel syndrome: Incidence, morbidity and mortality, and growth outcomes at 18 to 22 months. *Pediatrics* 2008;122(3):e573–e582.

26. Navarro, F., Gleason, W.A., Rhoads, J.M., and Quiros-Tejeira, R.E. Short bowel syndrome: Epidemiology, pathophysiology and adaptation. *Neoreviews* 2009;10(7):e330–e338.

27. Duro, D., Mitchell, P.D., Kalish, L.A., Martin, C., McCarthy, M., Jaksic, T., Dunn, J. et al. Risk factors for parenteral nutrition-associated liver disease following surgical therapy for necrotizing enterocolitis. *J Pediatr Gastroenerolo Nutr* 2011;52(5):595–600.

28. Holman, R.C., Stoll, B.J., Curns, A.T., Yorita, K.L., Steiner, C.A., and Schonberger, L.B. Necrotising enterocolitis hospitalisations among neonates in the United States. *Paediatr Perinat Epidemiol* 2006;20(6):498–506.

29. Stoll, B.J. Epidemiology of necrotizing enterocolitis. *Clin Perinatol* 1994;21(2):205–218.

30. Quiros-Tejeira, R.E., Ament, M.E., Reyen, L., Herzog, F., Merjanian, M., Olivares-Serrano, N., and Vargas, J.H. Long-term parenteral nutritional support and intestinal adaptation in children with short bowel syndrome: A 25-year experience. *J Pediatr* 2004;145(2):157–163.

31. Thompson, J.S. Inflammatory disease and outcome of short bowel syndrome. *Am J Surg* 2000;180(6):551–554; discussion 554–555.

32. Thompson, J.S. Overview of etiology and management of intestinal failure. *Gastroenterology* 2006;130(2 Suppl 1):S3–S4.

33. Andorsky, D.J., Lund, D.P., Lillehei, C.W., Jaksic, T., Dicanzio, J., Richardson, D.S., Collier, S.B., Lo, C., and Duggan, C. Nutritional and other postoperative management of neonates with short bowel syndrome correlates with clinical outcomes. *J Pediatr* 2001;139(1):27–33.

34. Diamond, I.R., de Silva, N., Pencharz, P.B., Kim, J.H., and Wales, P.W. Neonatal short bowel syndrome outcomes after the establishment of the first Canadian multidisciplinary intestinal rehabilitation program: preliminary experience. *J Pediatr Surg* 2007;42(5):806–811.

35. Spencer, A.U., Neaga, A., West, B., Safran, J., Brown, P., Btaiche, I., Kuzma-O'Reilly, B., and Teitelbaum, D.H. Pediatric short bowel syndrome: Redefining predictors of success. *Ann Surg* 2005;242(3):403–409; discussion 409–412.

36. Modi, B.P., Langer, M., Ching, Y.A., Valim, C., Waterford, S.D., Iglesias, J., Duro, D., Lo, C., Jaksic, T., and Duggan, C. Improved survival in a multidisciplinary short bowel syndrome program. *J Pediatr Surg* 2008;43(1):20–24.

37. Sudan, D., DiBaise, J., Torres, C., Thompson, J., Raynor, S., Gilroy, R., Horslen, S., Grant, W., Bitha, J., and Langnas, A. A multidisciplinary approach to the treatment of intestinal failure. *J Gastrointest Surg* 2005;9(2):165–176; discussion 176–177.

38. Wilmore, D.W. Factors correlating with a successful outcome following extensive intestinal resection in newborn infants. *J Pediatr* 1972;80(1):88–95.

39. Touloukian, R.J. and Smith, G.J. Normal intestinal length in preterm infants. *J Pediatr Surg* 1983;18(6):720–723.

40. Struijs, M.C., Diamond, I.R., de Silva, N., and Wales, P.W. Establishing norms for intestinal length in children. *J Pediatr Surg* 2009;44(5):933–938.

41. Kaufman, S.S., Loseke, C.A., Lupo, J.V., Young, R.J., Murray, N.D., Pinch, L.W., and Vanderhoof, J.A. Influence of bacterial overgrowth and intestinal inflammation on duration of parenteral nutrition in children with short bowel syndrome. *J Pediatr* 1997;131(3):356–361.

42. Cole, C.R., Frem, J.C., Schmotzer, B., Gerwirtz, A.T., Meddings, J.B., Gold, B.D., and Ziegler, T.R. The rate of bloodstream infection is high in infants with short bowel syndrome: Relationship with small bowel bacterial overgrowth, enteral feeding, and inflammatory and immune responses. *J Pediatr* 2010;156(6):941–947.e1.

43. Coran, A.G., Spivak, D., and Teitelbaum, D.H. An analysis of the morbidity and mortality of short-bowel syndrome in the pediatric age group. *Eur J Pediatr Surg* 1999;9(4):228–230.

44. Kaufman, S.S., Pehlivanova, M., Fennelly, E.M., Rekhtman, Y.M., Gondolesi, G.E., Little, C.A., Matsumoto, C.S., and Fishbein, T.M. Predicting liver failure in parenteral nutrition-dependent short bowel syndrome of infancy. *J Pediatr* 2010;156(4):580–585 e1.

45. Kaufman, S.S., Atkinson, J.B., Bianchi, A., Goulet, O.J., Grant, D., Lannas, A.N., McDiamond, S.V., Mittal, N., Reyes, J., and Tzakis, A.G. Indications for pediatric intestinal transplantation: A position paper of the American Society of Transplantation. *Pediatr Transplant* 2001;5(2):80–87.

46. Rhoads, J.M., Plunkett, E., Galanko, J., Lichtman, S., Taylor, L., Maynor, A., Weiner, T., Freeman, K., Guarisco, J.L., and Wu, G.Y. Serum citrulline levels correlate with enteral tolerance and bowel length in infants with short bowel syndrome. *J Pediatr* 2005;146(4):542–547.

47. Goulet, O., Baglin-Gobet, S., Talbotec, C., Fourcade, L., Colomb, V., Sauvat, F., Jais, J.P., Michel, J.L., Jan, D., and Ricour, C. Outcome and long-term growth after extensive small bowel resection in the neonatal period: A survey of 87 children. *Eur J Pediatr Surg* 2005;15(2):95–101.

48. Spencer, A.U., Kovacevich, D., McKinney-Barnett, M., Hair, D., Canham, J., Maksym, C., and Teitelbaum, D.H. Pediatric short-bowel syndrome: The cost of comprehensive care. *Am J Clin Nutr* 2008;88(6):1552–1559.

49. Jeppesen, P.B., Staun, M., and Mortensen, P.B. Adult patients receiving home parenteral nutrition in Denmark from 1991 to 1996: Who will benefit from intestinal transplantation? *Scand J Gastroenterol* 1998;33(8):839–846.

50. Vantini, I., Benini, L., Bonfante, F., Talamini, G., Sembenini, C., Chiarioni, G., Maragnolli, O., Benini, F., and Capra, F. Survival rate and prognostic factors in patients with intestinal failure. *Dig Liver Dis* 2004;36(1):46–55.

51. Messing, B., Lemann, M., Landais, P., Gouttebel, M.C., Gerard-Boncompain, M., Saudin, F., Vangossum, A., Beau, P., Guedon, C., and Bamoud, D. Prognosis of patients with nonmalignant chronic intestinal failure receiving long-term home parenteral nutrition. *Gastroenterology* 1995;108(4):1005–1010.

52. Wilmore, D.W., Lacey, J.M., Soultanakis, R.P., Bosch, R.L., and Byrne, T.A. Factors predicting a successful outcome after pharmacologic bowel compensation. *Ann Surg* 1997;226(3):288–292; discussion 292–293.

53. Luo, M., Fernandez-Estivariz, C., Manatunga, A.K., Bazargan, N., Gu, L.H., Jones, D.P., Klapproth J.M. et al. Are plasma citrulline and glutamine biomarkers of intestinal absorptive function in patients with short bowel syndrome? *JPEN* 2007;31(1):1–7.

54. Peters, J.H.C., Wiersdma, N.J., Teerlink, T., Leeuwen, P.A.M.V., Mulder, C.J.J., and Bodegraven, A.A.V. The citrulline generation test: Proposal for a new enterocyte function test. *Aliment Pharmacol Ther* 2008;27(12):1300–1310.

55. Ziegler, T.R. and Cole, C.R. Small bowel bacterial overgrowth in adults: A potential contributor to intestinal failure. *Curr Gastroenterol Rep* 2007;9(6):463–467.

# 2 Pathophysiology of Intestinal Failure

*Indraneel Chakrabarty and David L. Burns*

## CONTENTS

## 2.1 INTESTINAL FAILURE

Intestinal failure (IF) or short bowel syndrome (SBS) is defined as a malabsorptive state that results from insufficient intestinal surface area, resulting in inadequate nutritional and fluid absorption leading to long-term total parenteral nutrition (PN). As discussed in Chapter 1 (Etiology and Epidemiology of Intestinal Failure), in adults, this most commonly occurs from surgical resection of a large portion of the small bowel and/or the colon. SBS in children or infants may be postsurgical from congenital malformations, necrotizing enterocolitis, inflammatory bowel disease, or vascular thromboses. In adults, this syndrome often occurs when <200 cm of the intestine remains in an affected individual. However, there is significant variation as the syndrome largely depends on the extent of resection, location of resection(s), and eventual compensatory intestinal adaptation of the remaining intact bowel. Examples range from patients with limited ileocolonic resection, where mild-to-moderate nutritional decline can be seen, to those with severe malabsorption such as in individuals with extensive ileal and colonic resection who may have a duodenostomy, proximal jejunostomy, or a jejunocolonic anastomosis.[1-3]

Understanding the underlying pathophysiology of IF is critical in evaluating patient symptoms, designing rationale treatment regimens, as well as planning novel medical and surgical therapies. We review normal gastrointestinal (GI) physiology as well as the pathophysiological aspects of IF.

## 2.2  HISTOLOGY

The human GI tract can be divided into four layers: mucosa, submucosa, muscularis externa (or muscularis propria), and adventitia (or serosa). The mucosa comprises of epithelium, lamina propria, and muscularis mucosa. The epithelium lines the lumen of the intestine and exhibits several special functions, including immunity, secretion of various enzymes and fluids (water and electrolytes), and nutrient absorption. The muscularis mucosa contracts and relaxes contributing to a change in the surface area of the epithelium in the GI lumen thereby contributing to digestion and absorption. The submucosa contains a dense layer of connective tissue, blood vessels, lymphatics, and the submucosal or Meissner's plexus branching into the mucosa and muscularis externa. The muscularis externa consists of an inner circular layer and an outer longitudinal muscular layer. Contraction of the inner circular layer decreases the diameter of the GI tract lumen, while the longitudinal layer shortens the GI tract. The myenteric plexus or Auerbach's plexus lies between the two muscle layers. The coordinated contractions of these two smooth muscle layers create peristalsis. The serosa is the outermost layer of the GI tract and consists of several layers of epithelia and connective tissue.[4–7] Enterocyte function is depicted in Figure 2.1.

## 2.3  GI MOTILITY

Coordinated contractions regulated by the extrinsic and intrinsic nervous systems occur in the esophagus, gastric antrum, and small intestine. Extrinsic innervation of the GI tract is by the parasympathetic and sympathetic systems. The sympathetic nervous system has an inhibitory role on the GI tract and the parasympathetic nervous system, carried by the vagus and pelvic nerves, has a stimulatory role on the GI tract. The vagus nerve innervates the esophagus, stomach, pancreas, and proximal large intestine. Consequently, patients who have had esophagectomies or gastric resections with truncal vagotomies often exhibit gastroparesis. The intrinsic nervous system (myenteric or Auerbach's plexus, and submucosal or Meissner's plexus) coordinates and relays information between the parasympathetic and sympathetic nervous systems. These local reflexes relay information within the GI tract and control functions such as motility, secretions, and blood flow even when the extrinsic nervous system has been compromised by surgical resection including transplantation.[1,6,7]

Oscillating membrane potentials, or slow waves, are inherent to smooth muscle cells in the GI tract and regulate contraction. The distal gastric body and antrum are set at 3 slow waves/min and the duodenum is the fastest at 12 slow waves/min, with the frequency of the contractions decreasing distally towards the colon. Contraction occurs behind the bolus and relaxation occurs in front of the bolus, propelling chyme forward. In addition, segmental contractions also occur propelling chyme backward and forward, however, net movement is forward. These peristaltic reflexes are coordinated by the enteric nervous system. Parasympathetic stimulation increases the frequency of smooth muscle contractions, while sympathetic stimulation decreases it. These coordinated movements promote mixing and increases nutrient exposure to intestinal villi for improved efficiency in absorption.[1,6,7]

## 2.4  OROPHARYNX AND ESOPHAGUS

The process of digestion begins in the mouth prior to initiating chewing. As one sees food, a parasympathetic response initiates salivary gland secretion in the mouth and gastric acid secretion in the stomach. The food bolus is broken down to smaller particles by chewing and lubricated by saliva. Then, the food bolus moves down the esophagus via peristalsis to the stomach. The

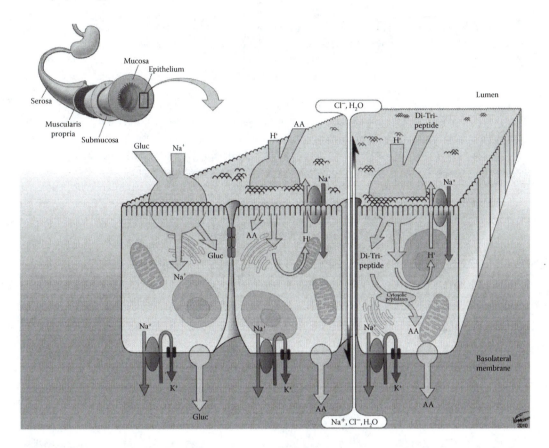

**FIGURE 2.1**   Intestinal histology and enterocyte carbohydrate and protein absorption. The GI tract can be divided into four layers: mucosa, submucosa, muscularis externa, and serosa. The mucosa comprises of epithelium, lamina propria, and muscularis mucosa. The epithelium lines the lumen of the intestine and predominantly specializes in absorption of nutrients, secretion of various enzymes, and water. The mechanisms of carbohydrate and protein absorption are shown at the cellular level. (AA, amino acids; Cl⁻, chloride; Fruc, fructose; Glu, glucose; H⁺, hydrogen; $H_2O$, water; K⁺, potassium; Na⁺, sodium.)

proximal stomach relaxes to allow the food bolus to enter the stomach, a process termed receptive relaxation.[1,6,7]

## 2.5   STOMACH

A significant role of the stomach is immunological, as it kills pathogens present within a food bolus by exposing it to a highly acidic environment. Gastric acid is released through several pathways. The initial stimulation comes by way of parasympathetic innervation (triggered by seeing food, chewing, etc.). This causes acetylcholine and the neuropeptide gastrin-releasing peptide (GRP) to be released from the vagus nerve. The vagus nerve directly innervates gastrin (G) cells and parietal cells. G cells are predominantly, located in the antrum, while parietal cells are predominantly located in the body and fundus. Acetylcholine acts on parietal cell M1 receptors and stimulates hydrochloric acid (HCl) secretion, while GRP stimulates G cells to release gastrin, which in turn stimulates parietal cells to secrete more acid. In addition, to parasympathetic stimulation, gastrin is secreted by other stimuli such as small peptides and amino acids (especially phenylalanine and tryptophan) entering the stomach and gastric distention. Amino acids are the most potent stimulators of gastrin release and gastrin is the most potent stimulator of parietal cell acid secretion. Gastrin is also a trophic stimulator of gastric, small intestine, and colonic mucosa. Gastrin also stimulates enterochromaffin cells (ECL) to release histamine, which directly stimulate $H_2$ receptors on parietal cells to further secrete acid (see Table 2.1). Thus, histamine potentiates the direct gastrin and vagal stimulation of parietal cell acid secretion. Histamine is also secreted by mast cells in the gastric mucosa but their role still remains to be elucidated.[1,4–7]

Acid secretion is inhibited by several pathways. For instance, $H^+$ inhibits gastrin secretion directly via negative feedback. Fatty acids and amino acids entering the duodenum stimulate cholecystokinin (CCK) release from duodenal endocrine cells. CCK indirectly inhibits acid secretion by stimulating D cells in the gastric mucosa to release somatostatin which further inhibits histamine and gastrin release by ECL and G cells, respectively[1,4–7] (see Table 2.1).

Another significant role of the stomach is the breakdown of food for digestion and absorption by chemical and mechanical means. Chemical breakdown begins through pepsinogen. Pepsinogen is a protease secreted by the chief cells of the stomach and is activated to pepsin when the gastric pH reaches 1–3. Pepsin begins to break down proteins into peptides but is not essential for protein digestion. Once activated, it converts additional pepsinogen into pepsin. Pepsin is denatured when the pH is >5 as occurs in the duodenum when pancreatic juices containing $HCO_3^-$ enter the duodenum and increases the pH. Parietal cells secrete HCl which contributes to protein denaturing and intrinsic factor (the latter of which complexes with B12 for absorption in the ileum). As for mechanical breakdown of food in the stomach, a wave of contraction closes onto the distal antrum churning food and slowly moving chyme into the duodenum through the pylorus. However, the majority of

## TABLE 2.1
## Key Anabolic Hormones in Intestinal Failure

|  | Site of Production | Stimulus for Release | Actions | Anabolic Properties |
|---|---|---|---|---|
| Gastrin | G cells in the gastric mucosa | Vagus stimulation, amino acid, gastric wall distention | Gastric acid secretion, histamine release by gastric enterochromaffin and mast cells | Gastric, intestinal, and colonic mucosa |
| Ghrelin | P/D1 endocrine cells in gastric fundus and duodenum, epsilon cells in the pancreas, neurons in the arcuate nucleus | Fasting | Stimulates growth hormone secretion, increases appetite and weight gain, promotes gastric emptying | Intestinal cell proliferation |
| GLP1 and GLP2 | Ileum and proximal colon | Intraluminal carbohydrates and fats | Ileal brake, inhibits gastric acid secretion | Small bowel |
| PYY | Ileum and proximal colon | Intraluminal carbohydrates and fats | Ileal brake, inhibits gastric acid secretion | Small bowel |
| GH | Somatotroph cells in the anterior pituitary gland | Growth hormone releasing hormone, ghrelin, androgens, estrogen, hypoglycemia, fasting, arginine, vigorous exercise, deep sleep | Stimulates insulin-like growth factor 1, gluconeogenesis in the liver, lipolysis, maintenance and function of pancreatic islet cells and immune system | Growth of all organs including small bowel, except the brain |

*Note:* GH, growth hormone; GLP1 and GLP2, glucagon like peptide 1 and 2; PYY, peptide YY.

food bolus is retropulsed back into the body of the stomach during churning, only to be churned again, eventually breaking the food bolus into smaller pieces. This repetitive motion breaks food particles into smaller pieces or chyme. Gastric contractions are increased by vagal stimulation and inhibited by sympathetic stimulation. As chyme enters the duodenum, gastric emptying is inhibited or slowed by the presence of fatty acids, amino acids and a low pH in the proximal duodenum creating a negative feedback loop. Fatty acids and amino acids entering the duodenum stimulate CCK release, which inhibits gastric emptying. Hydrogen ions entering the duodenum also slow down gastric emptying via stimulation of direct interneural reflexes in the GI plexuses. During fasting states, the hormone motilin mediates gastric contractions every 90 min to clear the stomach of residual food. Gastric emptying is fastest when stomach contents are isotonic and slower when they are hypo- or hypertonic. Finally, the presence of food in the stomach regulates motility and local reflexes throughout the distal gut, promoting relaxation of the ileocecal valve, and the gastro-colonic reflex that mediates a bowel movement.[1,4–7]

The discovery of the hormone ghrelin has also given more insight into the role of the stomach. Ghrelin is secreted by endocrine cells known as P/D1 cells that are predominantly located in the gastric fundus and the duodenum. It stimulates growth hormone (GH) secretion and increases appetite by stimulating the arcuate nucleus and hypothalamus. It also promotes gastric contraction and emptying. Circulating ghrelin levels increase during fasting and starvation (negative energy balances) but the exact mechanism of stimulation and inhibition is still unclear. Levels have been shown to be low after eating and in patients with obesity. Gastric bypass patients do not demonstrate the premeal increase in plasma ghrelin levels that is seen in normal individuals and is thought to be one of the mechanisms by which gastric bypass promotes weight loss.[8–10] The role of ghrelin in patients with IF remains to be characterized as it may have a role in intestinal adaptation.

## 2.6 DUODENUM

The mucosa of the duodenum is characterized by villi and mucosal folds. Villi are finger-like projections that increase mucosal surface area and are the primary site for absorption of nutrients. Once food or chyme enters the duodenum, several GI hormones are activated and cause a cascade of events that contribute to digestion and the absorption of nutrients. The primary hormones include CCK, secretin, gastric inhibitory peptide (GIP), somatostatin, vasoactive intestinal peptide (VIP), GRP, enkephalins, and ghrelin.

CCK is secreted by the duodenal and jejunal mucosa in response to amino acids, small peptides, fatty acids, and monoglycerides entering the duodenum from the stomach. CCK stimulates contraction of the gall bladder, relaxes the sphincter of Oddi, stimulates pancreatic enzyme secretion, stimulates growth of the exocrine pancreas, and inhibits gastric emptying. Acidification of the duodenum causes secretin release which stimulates bile, bicarbonate, and water secretion from the gall bladder and liver, pancreatic bicarbonate secretion, and inhibits hydrogen secretion by gastric parietal cells. GIP, a new class of hormones called incretins, is secreted by the duodenal and jejunal mucosa in response to the presence of fatty acids, amino acids, carbohydrates, and glucose hyperosmolarity in the duodenal lumen. GIP stimulates insulin release, promotes fatty acid metabolism or triglyceride synthesis in adipocytes, and inhibits gastric acid secretion. VIP is released from neurons within the mucosa and smooth muscle of the GI tract. It promotes relaxation of the smooth muscle, stimulates pancreatic bicarbonate secretion, stimulates water and electrolyte secretion into the small intestine, and inhibits gastric acid secretion and intestinal absorption. $H^+$ also stimulates the release of somatostatin, which is released by neuroendocrine cells in the GI mucosa. It inhibits the secretion of all GI hormones and inhibits gastric acid secretion. Vagus stimulation inhibits somatostatin release. The combination of all of these hormones promote the mixing of pancreatic enzymes and bile with chyme entering the duodenum, resulting in the neutralization of gastric acid and the initiation of protein and carbohydrate digestion and mixing of bile with lipids for absorption. Thus, chyme entering the duodenum autoregulates the rate at which food passes from the stomach into the small intestine for proper and timely absorption of nutrients, fluids, electrolytes, and glycemic control.[1,4–7]

## 2.7  JEJUNUM

The jejunum has very long villi creating a large absorptive surface area with highly concentrated digestive enzymes and many transport carrier proteins. Consequently, it is the primary digestive and absorptive site of most nutrients. It is also a very leaky organ, permitting the rapid movement of water and electrolytes through the mucosa from the plasma to the lumen, thus adequately diluting luminal contents. As a result, marked fluid secretion in the jejunum occurs in response to hypertonic feeding. Most of the fluid is reabsorbed in the ileum and in the colon.[1,4–7] When the jejunum is resected, a reduction in absorption of most nutrients occurs. The remaining jejunum may adapt functionally by promoting hypertrophy of remaining villi, but less significant changes in length and diameter are observed, compared to the ileum.[1–3,11,12]

## 2.8  ILEUM

The ileum is the site of primary absorption of fluids and is the specific site of absorption of vitamin B12 and bile acids. The mucosa is characterized by finger-like villi and Peyer's patches which are lymphoid tissue in the submucosa. The ileum exhibits tighter junctions than the jejunum, resulting in less water moving back into the intestinal lumen. Thus, there is net absorption of fluid within the ileum. When significant ileal resection occurs, site-specific receptors for bile acids and the B12-intrinsic factor complex are lost, leading to bile acid and B12 malabsorption.[1–7] Glucagon-like peptide 1 and 2 (GLP-1, GLP-2), neurotensin, and peptide YY (PYY) are also produced in the ileum and proximal colon. They are secreted in response to intraluminal carbohydrates and fats. These hormones cause a delay in gastric emptying, inhibit gastric acid secretion, and slow intestinal transit, that is, "the ileal brake." GLP-1, GLP-2, and PYY (see Table 2.1) have also been shown to promote intestinal growth in animal models.[1,13–17] GLP-1 is also an incretin and has shown to augment insulin secretion after ingesting a meal. The ileocecal valve assists in regulating the passage of fluid and nutrients from the ileum into the colon and is a major barrier to reflux of colonic material thereby preventing colonic bacteria from entering the small bowel. Some studies have identified the presence of the ileocecal valve as a key prognostic factor, since it prevents bacterial colonization of the small intestine and prolongs intestinal transit time. The ileum has shorter villi and, therefore, less surface area than the jejunum, but is capable of undergoing marked adaptation in structure, with significant increments in length and diameter, in contrast to the jejunum.[1–3,11,12]

## 2.9  LARGE INTESTINE

The large bowel or colon predominantly functions to absorb water and some nutrients, thereby concentrating chyme into semisolid stool. Chyme enters the cecum through the ileocecal valve. As in the small bowel, segmented contractions occur in the colon as well. Mass movements occur 1–3 times/day. Most colonic water absorption occurs in the proximal colon and fecal material becomes more solid as it moves into the distal colon and rectum. The colonic mucosa is characterized by the presence of crypts of Lieberkuhn, associated predominantly with goblet cells intermixed with a few absorptive and enteroendocrine cells. The colon is impermeable secondary to tight junctions and consequently does not allow solutes to reenter the lumen and thereby prevents water from reentering the lumen. Dietary fiber is broken down in the colon by enteric bacteria into short-chain fatty acids which are readily absorbed in the colon. This represents a caloric salvage pathway allowing for calorie absorption from the colon from short-chain fatty acids.[1,4–7]

As the rectum fills with fecal material, it contracts and the internal sphincter relaxes (rectosphincteric reflex). When filled to ~25% of its capacity, there is an urge to defecate. Finally, the gastrocolic reflex is a response to food in the stomach and duodenum where colonic motility is increased causing mass movement through rapid parasympathetic innervation and a slower response to CCK and gastrin.[1,4–7]

## 2.10   DIGESTION AND ABSORPTION

The small intestine functions in the digestion and absorption of nutrients. Nutrients in the duodenum are mixed with pancreatic digestive enzymes and bile secreted by the gall bladder and liver, initiating the digestion of chyme into optimal building blocks suited for absorption. The remainder of nonabsorbable material is eventually propelled to the large intestine. Carbohydrates, protein, and lipids are digested and absorbed in the small intestine. The surface area in the small intestine is greatly increased by the presence of the brush border where absorption occurs. Enterocytes appear uniform from the duodenum to the ileocecal valve but villi are taller and crypts are deeper in the jejunum than in the ileum. In addition, the activity of microvillus enzymes and nutrient absorptive capacity per unit length of intestine are several-fold higher in the brush border of the proximal intestine compared to distally.[1,4–7]

## 2.11   CARBOHYDRATES

Carbohydrates are predominantly absorbed in the duodenum and jejunum, decreasing in absorptive capacity per unit length of intestine in a proximal to distal gradient. Carbohydrates must be digested to glucose, galactose, and fructose for absorption to proceed as only monosaccharides are absorbed. Carbohydrate digestion begins with α-amylase which is secreted in salivary and pancreatic secretions. It hydrolyzes 1,4 glycosidic bonds to oligosaccharides forming maltose, maltotriose, and α-limit dextrins. These starches are further hydrolyzed to glucose by maltase, α-dextrinase, and sucrase, which are located on the brush border. Other disaccharides are hydrolyzed to monosaccharides by lactase, trehalase, and sucrase, which are also located on the brush border. Lactase hydrolyzes lactose to glucose and galactose; trehalase hydrolyzes trehalose to glucose; and sucrase hydrolyzes sucrose to glucose and fructose. Glucose and galactose are transported from the intestinal lumen into enterocytes via secondary active $Na^+$-dependent co-transporters located on the luminal membrane where $Na^+$ is transported down its gradient into the cell dragging monosaccharides along with it against its gradient. These sugars are then transported into the blood by facilitated diffusion (see Figure 2.1). Lactose intolerance results from the absence of lactase in the brush border, which commonly develops as people age. The nonabsorbed lactose prevents water from being absorbed secondary to a hyperosmotic gradient and leads to osmotic diarrhea.[1,4–7]

## 2.12   PROTEIN

Pancreatic proteases are the primary enzymes, that break down protein and include both endopeptidases (hydrolyze interior peptide bonds) and exopeptidases (hydrolyze one amino acid at a time from the C-terminus of proteins and peptides). Trypsin, chymotrypsin, elastase, carboxypeptidase A, and carboxypeptidase B are the primary enzymes. All of these enzymes are secreted in their inactive form or zymogen into the duodenum. Once trypsin enters the duodenum, the brush border enzyme enterokinase will activate trypsinogen to its active form, trypsin. Trypsin then converts trypsinogen, proelastase, chymotrypsinogen, carboxypeptidase A and B, and other pancreatic proteases into their active forms. In contrast to carbohydrates which are only absorbed as monosaccharides, proteins can be absorbed as free amino acids, dipeptides, and tripeptides. Similar to carbohydrate absorption, secondary active $H^+$-dependent amino cotransporters are present on the brush border, however, there are separate carriers for free neutral, acidic, basic, and imino amino acids. The free amino acids are transported into the cell via downhill $H^+$ gradient and then from cell to blood by facilitated diffusion. However, absorption of dipeptides and tripeptides are faster than absorption of free amino acids. Like free amino acids, there are H$^+$-dependent co-transporters for dipeptides and tripeptides on villi (see Figure 2.1). Once absorbed into the cell, cytoplasmic peptidases hydrolyze them to individual amino acids which are then subsequently transported into plasma by the same facilitated diffusion as in free amino acid absorption. Like carbohydrate absorption, proteins are predominantly absorbed in the duodenum and jejunum, decreasing in absorptive capacity per unit length of intestine in a proximal to distal gradient.[1,4–7]

## 2.13   LIPIDS

Approximately 30–40% of adult energy requirements is supplied by lipids, the major portion of which is triglycerides. In the stomach, churning breaks lipids into crude droplets or emulsification thereby increasing the surface area for digestion by pancreatic enzymes. Lingual lipase digests some of the ingested triglycerides to monoglycerides and fatty acids, but most of the ingested lipids are digested in the intestine by pancreatic lipases. As chyme enters the duodenum, pancreatic lipases (pancreatic lipase, cholesterol ester hydrolase, and phospholipase A$_2$) are released and hydrolyze lipids to fatty acids, monoglycerides, cholesterol, and lysolecithin. Bile salts are also released from the liver and gall bladder, emulsifying these lipids and further increasing their surface area for absorption. This is done when bile acids interact with lipids to create micelles, where the hydrophobic portion of lipids are internalized and hydrophilic portion of lipids are placed on the outer rim of a micelle droplet, allowing lipids to become soluble in a aqueous layer. Micelles bring long-chain fatty acids (LCFAs), cholesterol, and phospholipids (i.e., the products of lipid digestion), into contact with the absorptive surface of the brush border. The majority of lipids are absorbed in the jejunum.[18] It was commonly believed that the fatty acids, monoglycerides, and cholesterol diffuse passively across the luminal membrane into the cells. However, it has been determined that some fatty acids are actively transported across the apical brush border via fatty acid transport proteins and cholesterol is actively absorbed by proteins such as the Niemann-Pick C1 like 1 transporter.[18,19,20] Within the enterocyte, LCFAs are reesterified to triglycerides, cholesterol ester, and phospholipids and complex with apo proteins to form chylomicrons. Chylomicrons are exocytosed from enterocytes and into lymph as they are too large to enter capillaries. They finally enter the blood stream via the thoracic duct. However, medium-chain fatty acids and some polyunsaturated fatty acids diffuse freely into the cell and across the basolateral membrane into plasma and the portal vein. Finally, the colon has the ability to absorb short-chain fatty acids passively.[1,4–7] Lipid absorption and metabolism has proven to be complex and many investigations are underway to further characterize it.

## 2.14   WATER, ELECTROLYTES, MINERALS, VITAMINS, AND TRACE ELEMENTS

On average, the adult daily luminal fluid load of the gut is composed of oral intake and secretions and is ~7–9 L/day. Oral intake is estimated to be 2 L/day on average and salivary secretion is 1.5 L/day. Gastric secretion is ~2.5 L/day. Gall bladder secretion is 500 mL/day and pancreatic secretion is 1 L/day. Intestinal secretion is ~1 L/day on average. Approximately 8–9 L/day or more is reabsorbed in the GI tract of which 7–8 L (max 12 L) in the small intestine, and 1.5–2.0 L (maximum 5 L) in the colon. Approximately 100–200 mL are excreted in stool[1] (see Table 2.2).

Electrolytes and water may cross intestinal epithelial cells by either cellular or paracellular routes. Tight junctions secure enterocytes to one another and contribute to the permeability of intestinal mucosa. The permeability of tight junctions to solutes and fluids varies with intestinal location but essentially decreases from proximal-to-distal bowel as tight junctions become more concentrated in the epithelium. The GI tract secretes electrolytes and water from plasma to the lumen when hypertonic chyme is present to maintain isosmolarity. Chloride channels located in the crypts are the primary secretory mechanism. As Cl$^-$ is actively secreted into the lumen, Na$^+$ passively follows Cl$^-$, and water follows NaCl to maintain isosmolarity. However, as nutrient absorption begins to occur, Na$^+$ moves back across the mucosa and down its electrochemical gradient by several mechanisms located

## TABLE 2.2
## Fluid Intake and Losses

| Location | Average Liters/Day |
|---|---|
| Oral intake | 2 |
| Salivary secretions | 1.5 |
| Gastric secretions | 2.5 |
| Biliary secretions | 0.5 |
| Pancreatic secretions | 1 |
| Intestinal secretions | 1 |
| Intestinal reabsorption | 7–8 (12 max) |
| Colonic reabsorption | 1.5–2 (5 max) |
| Stool losses | 0.1–0.2 |

on the brush border: passive diffusion through $Na^+$ channels, secondary active $Na^+$-glucose or $Na^+$-amino acid co-transporters, $Na^+$–$Cl^-$ co-transport, and $Na^+$–$H^+$ cation exchange (see Figure 2.1). As a result, water is reabsorbed passively, secondary to solute drag or sodium absorption. In the colon, water permeability is much lower than in the small intestine and feces become hypertonic. In the colon, passive diffusion via $Na^+$–$K^+$ or $Na^+$–$H^+$ cation exchange channels is the primary means of $Na^+$ absorption into the enterocyte and is similar to those in the distal renal tubule. It is also stimulated by aldosterone. Dietary $K^+$ is absorbed in the small intestine by passive diffusion via a paracellular route but can be actively secreted in exchange for $Na^+$ by the colon as mentioned above. Hence, in diarrhea, $K^+$ secretion by the colon is increased because of increased delivery of sodium in stool to the colon leading to hypokalemia.[1,4–7]

In adults, most minerals (calcium, magnesium, phosphorous, iron, zinc, copper, folate, etc.) are predominantly absorbed in the duodenum and proximal jejunum.[1,4–7] Dietary calcium is absorbed throughout the small intestine by active and passive transport. The biochemical rate-limiting step for calcium absorption is the required presence of active vitamin D (1,25-dihydroxycholecalciferol) which requires adequate sun exposure and functioning kidneys. Vitamin D deficiency or chronic renal failure thus can lead to inadequate calcium absorption causing rickets in children and osteomalacia in adults. The colon can also absorb calcium. Magnesium absorption appears to be greater in the ileum than the jejunum.[1,4–6]

Iron is absorbed in the duodenum and jejunum by two pathways: as iron bound to hemoglobin or myoglobin (heme iron) or as free ferrous iron. Heme iron is transported into duodenal and jejunal enterocytes where it is degraded and $Fe^{2+}$ is released. However, free luminal ferrous iron is absorbed into the enterocyte via a transporter called divalent metal transporter 1 (DMT1). Other divalent metals have been shown to compete with iron absorption for transport into the enterocyte via the DMT1 pathway.[21,22] From within the enterocyte, $Fe^{2+}$ is subsequently transported into the blood where it is bound to transferrin and is soon delivered to the liver for storage and eventually transported to bone marrow for the production of hemoglobin. On average, only 10% of dietary iron is absorbed although this can increase by 20% during pregnancy and severe iron deficiency. Iron absorption is tightly regulated at the mucosal level to avoid iron overload. Because iron is absorbed proximally, surgical bypass or resection commonly results in iron deficiency. Examples include gastric bypass and Billroth II procedures.[1,4–6]

Zinc transporters of various forms are located throughout the small intestine, which secrete and reabsorb zinc as part of a known enterohepatic circulation. Reabsorption appears to be the greatest in the distal jejunum. Copper is absorbed in the proximal small intestine and is competitively absorbed with zinc at the same receptor site. Dedicated copper transporters in the brush border have been discovered in addition to DMT1 transporters.[23] This can be used therapeutically for Wilson's

**TABLE 2.3**

**Site-Specific Nutrient Absorption in Normal Intact Bowel**

| Location | Carbohydrates | Proteins | LCFAs and FSV | SCFA's | Bile Salts | Iron | Calcium | Magnesium | WSV | B12 |
|---|---|---|---|---|---|---|---|---|---|---|
| Duodenum | ++++ | ++++ | ++ | +++ | ++ | ++++ | ++++ | ++ | ++++ | N/A |
| Jejunum | +++ | +++ | ++++ | ++++ | ++ | ++++ | +++ | +++ | ++++ | N/A |
| Ileum | + | + | +++ | + | ++++ | ++ | ++ | ++++ | ++ | ++++ |
| Colon | N/A | N/A | N/A | +++ | N/A | N/A | ++ | ++ | N/A | N/A |

*Note:* FSV, fat-soluble vitamins; LFCAs, long-chain fatty acids; SCFA's, short-chain fatty acids; WSV water-soluble vitamins.

Disease, a copper overload syndrome, where therapy can include oral zinc supplementation to hinder copper absorption.[1,4–7]

Dietary folate is predominantly absorbed in the proximal jejunum after it is broken down into its monoglutamate forms by brush border enzymes. Uptake is achieved by a specific sodium-dependent carrier-mediated pH-sensitive process. In addition to dietary folate, microflora in the colon can synthesize folate which can also be absorbed by the colon.[1,4–7]

Vitamin B12 is only absorbed selectively in the ileum. Intrinsic factor is secreted by the parietal cells in the stomach and combines with B12 to form a B12-intrinsic factor complex which binds to receptors in the terminal ileum for absorption. Hence, gastrectomy results in the loss of gastric parietal cells and consequently intrinsic factor, resulting in B12 deficiency. B12 deficiency can also result from pernicious anemia where antibodies against parietal cells and intrinsic factor result in their destruction and, consequently, the B12-intrinsic factor complex is never formed. Ileal resection and the above mechanisms commonly results in B12 deficiency and requires long-term supplementation by parenteral, intranasal, or sublingual routes.[1,4–7]

In adults, most water-soluble vitamins are absorbed in the duodenum and proximal jejunum by secondary active Na$^+$-dependent cotransport mechanisms. Fat-soluble vitamins (vitamins A, D, E, and K) are incorporated into micelles similar to lipids and was previously thought to be absorbed passively along with other lipids into the proximal jejunum.[1,4–7,18] However, like lipid absorption, newer data suggest that some fat-soluble vitamins such as vitamin A is absorbed by saturable carrier-mediated and nonsaturable diffusion-dependent processes from micelles predominantly in the jejunum. Vitamin E has also been shown to be absorbed from micelles by a saturable, temperature-dependent process.[18] Consequently, if one loses a significant portion of ileum and becomes severely bile salt depleted, micelle formation does not occur, and fat-soluble vitamin deficiency and fat malabsorption occurs (see Section 2.18 for more details). See Table 2.3 for a general overview of site-specific nutrient absorption in the GI tract in adults.

## 2.15  PATHOPHYSIOLOGY

The degree of malabsorption in IF depends on the location of bowel resected, the extent of intestinal resection, the degree of intestinal surface area lost, the loss of site-specific transport processes, and the degree of adaptation possible in the residual bowel over time. There are three predominant types of intestinal resection encountered among adults in the United States: (1) limited ileal–cecal resection often with terminal ileal-cecectomy or terminal ileal resection with a right hemicolectomy; (2) Extensive ileal resection with or without partial colectomy or with a jejunocolonic reanastomosis; and (3) Extensive small bowel resection and total colectomy resulting in proximal jejunostomy. In adults, the latter two groups can suffer from either Crohn's disease or mesenteric infarction, whereas the first group almost exclusively suffers from Crohn's disease. As outlined in Chapter 1, children suffer from a wider variety of congenital and acquired diseases of the GI tract that can lead to more substantial bowel loss, including multiple intestinal atresias, midgut vovulus, and necrotizing enterocolitis.

## 2.16   INTESTINAL ADAPTATION

Intestinal adaptation refers to the gross, microscopic, and functional changes in the residual small bowel after massive resection or loss of the gut. These have generally included lengthening of the intestine, dilatation of the bowel (presumably to increase mucosal surface area), increased concentrations of digestive enzymes, and different expressions of numerous genes. Over the past 50 years, numerous factors have been found to affect intestinal adaptation and mucosal hypertrophy in normal intact intestines. Adaptive response to dietary load has been well characterized. Increased activity and upregulation of brush border transporters have been described as the dietary load of sugars (except lactose), peptides, and nonessential amino acids increase. The reverse is seen with a number of vitamins and trace elements in order to avoid toxicity. Pancreatic secretions are also known to adapt to dietary influence. A high protein diet enhances proteolytic enzyme production, whereas a high carbohydrate diet enhances amylase secretion. In addition, long-term stimulation by a dedicated diet (such as a high protein diet) has shown to commit the pancreas to continue secreting the respective pancreatic enzymes for the diet, even after the dedicated diet has been changed. Other causes of intestinal mucosal hypertrophy have been found in experimental animals such as lactation, pregnancy, diabetes, and extreme cold. However, intestinal adaptation is best characterized in animal models and humans with intestinal resection.[24,25]

Resection of greater than half of small bowel results in IF, malabsorption, and in net loss of fecal nitrogen. However, observation over time has found that fecal nitrogen loss slowly returns toward normal suggesting that an adaptative process is occurring and that the gut is compensating for a net loss in surface area. This has largely been explained by hypertrophy of the remaining intestinal mucosa as characterized by increased number of villus enterocytes, villus height, intestinal length, and variable increases in absorptive capacity of nutrients. With upregulation of digestive enzymes, mucosal co-transporters, and their activity, the process of adaptation can take from months to years to achieve, depending on the extent and location of resection. Adaptive absorption increases for all nutrients except for site-specific nutrient absorption such as B12 and bile acids which are selectively absorbed in the terminal ileum.[24,25] However, as mentioned previously, intestinal adaptation appears to be less effective in the duodenum and jejunum than in the ileum.[11,12] The reasons for this difference is unclear. Thus, the ileum has the best reserve for adaptation or mucosal hypertrophy. The colon can also undergo adaptive dilation, lengthening, and mucosal hypertrophy and can acquire the ability to absorb glucose and amino acids to a very limited degree.

As a general rule, if only proximal sections of small bowel are resected, it is less likely that permanent PN will be required since the ileum can readily adapt to function like the jejunum. In experimental animals, the ileum undergoes an adaptive response characterized by epithelial hyperplasia within 24–48 h after bowel resection. The length of villi and intestinal absorptive area have been shown to increase, and digestive and absorptive function gradually improve.[24,25] The key to this process in animal models is the provision of enteral nutrition immediately postsurgical resection which stimulates gut function and release of gut hormones. Studies in animals have identified a variety of genes known for mediating intestinal growth whose expressions are altered after intestinal resection.[9,14,15,17,26] The mechanism of increased expression of these genes is still being clarified.

In humans, after significant bowel resection and depending on which portions of bowel are removed, the remainder of the reconnected bowel will begin to adapt or compensate over time. Enteral feeding should be resumed as soon as possible when safe to stimulate adaptation as the process of digestion stimulates various hormones that when combined likely have a trophic effect on the remaining bowel. Furthermore, the signals that regulate the adaptive process may be different in duodenum, jejunum, and ileum. Luminal nutrition and pancreaticobiliary secretions are still thought to be the major stimuli for growth. For example, disaccharides and highly saturated fats appear to be more potent stimulants for adaptation than monosaccharides and less saturated fats. However, a variety of signals have been described to play a role in intestinal adaptation. These include GH, epidermal growth factor (EGF), EGF receptor, transforming growth factor-α, prostanoids, uncoupling proteins, peroxisome proliferator-activated receptor-α, insulin-like growth factor-1 (IGF-1) receptors and IGF-1 binding proteins, endothelin-1, Bcl-2, erythropoietin, enteroglucagon, GLP, gastrin, CCK, GLP-1, GLP-2, PYY, L-glutamine, and certain prostaglandins all have shown to have some role in intestinal adapation.[9,14,15,17,26,27] Other trophic factors have been identified and are being studied. Polyamines are also thought to be important local mediators of mucosal hypertrophy as epithelial production of polyamines following intestinal resection is increased and inhibition of their production prevents hypertrophy of the remaining bowel. They also appear to have a daily role on mucosal adaption as animal models have shown decreased levels after a 24 h fast and increased levels a few hours after a meal.[28]

Of the above discussed hormones, L-glutamine, GH, and GLP-2 are the only agents that have been evaluated in clinical trials in patients with SBS. L-Glutamine has been shown to promote intestinal growth in animals, although studies in humans have been inconclusive.[27] In hypophysectomized rats, mucosal hypoplasia of the small bowel develops but is subsequently reversed with the administration of GH. Transgenic mice expressing high levels of GH have been shown to develop hypertrophy of the small intestines. Consequently, GH has been shown to increase small bowel intestinal length and function per unit length in animals. However, in humans with SBS on PN, variable results have been obtained with the administration of high dose GH in uncontrolled trials. However, a prospective double-blinded randomized controlled trial performed by Byrne and colleagues, administering GH (0.1 mg/kg/day) combined with glutamine (30 g/day) revealed a reduction in weekly PN requirements.[29] Currently, GH is Food and Drug Administration approved for SBS necessitating PN use, however, anecdotally its use and benefits are limited.

Finally, GLP-2 has been shown to increase the adaptive response in rats with massive intestinal resection. In several controlled trials, Jeppesen and colleagues have shown significant increase in the percentage of absorption in energy and nitrogen and improvement in fluid balance with the use of a GLP-2 analogue, Teduglutide, in patients with SBS.[30–33] Additional studies need to be done to elucidate if L-glutamine, GH, or GLP-2 analogues or combinations of these agents will be of any long-term benefit to patients with IF. Overall, the process of adaptation in humans is not well characterized, and likely multiple growth factors are involved in the process.

## 2.17 JEJUNAL RESECTION AND EXTENSIVE BOWEL RESECTION

Most macronutrients (carbohydrates, protein, fat, nitrogen) are absorbed in the proximal 100–150 cm of intestine. As previously mentioned, the activity of microvillus enzymes and nutrient absorptive capacity per unit length of intestine are several-fold higher in the brush border of the proximal versus distal intestine. Consequently, loss of a portion of jejunum initially will compromise absorption more than loss of a similar-sized ileal segment. However, for reasons that still remain to be elucidated, the ileum can eventually compensate for jejunal loss but the jejunum is unable to compensate for the site-specific ileal absorption of bile salts and vitamin B12.[11,12] Patients with a proximal jejunostomy (<100 cm of jejunum) often have rapid intestinal transit leading to insufficient time for mixing with biliary and pancreatic secretions, digestion, and enterocyte contact time with chyme, resulting in malabsorption (Table 2.4). In addition, the proximal small intestine receives 7–9 L of water and electrolytes daily from food and secretions and 6–8 L are reabsorbed in the small bowel. However, patients with <100 cm of jejunum with unrestricted diets cannot reabsorb these large volumes of fluid, which can be hyperosmolar further increasing gut losses. Thus, they excrete more fluid than absorb secondary to net secretion of salt and fluid not only due to loss of intestinal surface area but also secondary to loss of inhibitory feedback mechanisms resulting in large volume diarrhea. Gastrin, CCK, secretin, GIP, and motilin are produced by endocrine cells in

**TABLE 2.4**
**Overview of IF**

| Location of Resection | Malabsorption | Fluid Losses | Intestinal Transit | Adaptation of Remaining Bowel | Prognosis |
|---|---|---|---|---|---|
| Jejunum | Minimal[a] | Minimal | Normal | Good ileal adaptation | Good |
| Ileum > 60 cm | B12 | Mild | Rapid | Poor jejunal adaptation | Fair |
| Ileum > 100 cm | B12 and bile acids | Mild | Rapid | Poor jejunal adaptation | Fair |
| Extensive[b] (colon present) | Fair to severe | Moderate to severe | Rapid | Poor jejunal adaptation | Fair to poor |
| Extensive[b] (colon absent) | Severe | Severe | Rapid | Poor jejunal adaptation | Poor |

[a] Unless greater than 75% resected.
[b] Loss of ileum and less than 100 cm of jejunum remaining.

the proximal GI tract, and regulate many secretory processes and motility as previously discussed. Consequently, these hormones are usually intact as most patients with IF normally have a preserved proximal bowel. However, in those with extensive bowel resection in the early postoperative phase, ~50% of patients will have hypergastrinemia resulting in increased gastric acid, fluid, and electrolyte secretion. The cause of hypergastrinemia is not clearly defined but felt to be secondary to a loss of inhibitory gut hormones previously produced in the resected small intestine. Additionally, hypergastrinemia increases gastric acid production, and its delivery to the duodenum overwhelms the buffering capacity of pancreatic bicarbonate production. This results in acidification of the duodenum, which can damage mucosa and denature digestive enzymes further fueling malabsorption. $H_2$ blockers or proton pump inhibitors are often given to these patients to decrease gastric secretions.

In addition, GLP-1, GLP-2, neurotensin, and PYY are produced in the ileum and proximal colon and their secretion is stimulated by intraluminal carbohydrates and fat. These hormones cause a delay in gastric empting, inhibit gastric acid secretion, slow intestinal transit, that is, "the ileal brake," and have shown to promote intestinal growth (see Table 2.1). In patients with a jejunostomy with loss of the ileocecal valve and proximal colon, rapid gastric emptying and rapid intestinal transit often occur as the release of these hormones is often impaired. However, preservation of the proximal colon has demonstrated increased levels of GLP-1 and GLP-2 and normal gastric emptying in patients with IF.[34,35]

Fluid management is often challenging to manage in these patients due to hypovolemia, hyponatremia, and hypokalemia. Patients with a proximal jejunostomy lose ~90–100 mEq of sodium and 10–20 mEq of potassium/L in their stoma output. Additionally, fluid losses can overwhelm the remaining absorptive capacity of the gut, which results in large net negative fluid balances. Patients with proximal jejunostomy malabsorb macronutrients, especially fats, which require bile salts for assimilation. Bile salts are lost in large volume stool output, thereby depleting the bile salt pool. Consequently, most patients with a small bowel length <100 cm and no colon carry a poor prognosis and will likely require long-term PN.

Patients with more than 100 cm of remaining small bowel can maintain a positive fluid balance with dietary manipulation by taking advantage of gut physiology.[36] Sodium-glucose and $Na^+$-amino acid cotransporters in the remaining jejunum promotes $Na^+$ absorption which drives water movement into gut enterocytes down a concentration gradient via solvent drag. This ultimately facilitates net sodium and water absorption. Drinking an oral solution of glucose-saline is more effective for water absorption than drinking plain water or sugar based beverages such as juices or sports drinks. Many prepared drinks are hyperosmolar, causing water movement into the gut lumen and aggravating fluid losses, and/or do not contain enough $Na^+$ to take advantage of the co-transport facilitated absorption. Thus, patients who require supplemental parenteral fluids may benefit with the use of an appropriate oral rehydration solution (ORS).[36] Some of the commercially available solutions are Pedialyte™, Ceralyte™, and World Health Organization Solution ORS. A recipe that contains the appropriate amounts of $Na^+$ and glucose is a liter of Gatorade™ with 1/2 teaspoon of salt added. This is relatively inexpensive compared to commercial brands since patients may require 2–3 L of oral electrolyte solution per day.

The absorption of some nutrients is restricted to certain areas of the intestine as previously discussed. Calcium, magnesium, phosphorous, iron, and water-soluble vitamins are predominantly absorbed in the duodenum and proximal jejunum. Most patients with IF have a preserved duodenum and some jejunum and consequently, the absorption of these nutrients is relatively preserved (Table 2.3). However, loss of calcium and magnesium is usually a consequence of fat malabsorption secondary to precipitation by unabsorbed LCFAs. Both calcium and magnesium absorption usually improve when these patients are placed on a low-fat diet.

Fat malabsorption results in impaired absorption of fat-soluble vitamins A, D, E, and K. Generally, most patients maintain adequate levels of these vitamins with an oral supplement daily. However, vitamin D deficiency is almost universal and requires aggressive repletion well beyond the Recommended Dietary Allowance of 400 IU. Patients may need loading and maintenance. Loading with vitamin D2 (ergocalciferol) is done with a 50,000 IU capsule weekly for 8 weeks followed by a required maintenance dose of 1000–2000 IU/day. Despite this, patients can frequently redevelop vitamin D deficiency and may require maintenance with 50,000 IU every other week or weekly. Serum vitamin D concentrations should be monitored serially.

## 2.18   ILEAL RESECTION

The absorption of vitamin B12 and bile acids is restricted to the ileum. In adults, if >60 cm of ileum is resected, B12 malabsorption occurs, requiring lifelong supplementation. Consequently, normal enteric absorption of B12 is bypassed in these patients and supplementation can be given via nasal, intramuscular, or sublingual routes.

Normally, the bile acid pool is well conserved and 80–90% is reabsorbed via enterohepatic recirculation. The liver has limited capacity to increase bile salt synthesis. Thus, the regulation of bile salt production is highly dependent on reabsorption, which predominantly occurs in the distal ileum. In ileal resection, there is increased delivery of unabsorbed bile acids and LCFAs to the colon, which leads to fluid and electrolyte secretion called bile salt or colorrheic diarrhea. LCFAs reaching the colon are hydroxylated by colonic bacteria and the hydroxylated LCFAs stimulate colonic electrolyte and water secretion, further exacerbating electrolyte–water losses. Moderate bile acid malabsorption can occur when <100 cm of ileum is removed causing bile salt diarrhea. However, >100 cm of ileal resection leads to disruption of the enterohepatic bile acid circulation resulting in severe bile acid depletion. Depleted bile acid pool size eventually leads to minimal micelle formation which in turn leads to fat malabsorption, fat-soluble vitamin deficiency, and steatorrhea.

Additionally, gallstone formation can occur in those with ileal resection and disruption of the enterohepatic bile circulation. Bile is a mixture of cholesterol, immunoglobulins, mucin, water, electrolytes, and bile salts. It is a viscous liquid produced by the liver and secreted into the gall bladder for storage and concentration. The gall bladder requires bile salts to maintain bile solubility and depletion of the bile salt pool results in precipitation of cholesterol. Cholesterol crystals in the gall bladder can form a nucleus resulting in gall stone formation. Patients with short gut syndrome or IF commonly develop gall stones and are at risk for biliary complications such as cholecystitis, cholangitis, biliary colic, and pancreatitis.

Bile salt-binding resins such as colestipol or cholestyramine have shown benefit in those with colorrheic diarrhea with limited ileal resections. However, bile-salt binders may exacerbate fat malabsorption in those with >100 cm of ileal resection contributing to further depletion of the bile salt pools. This was first shown by Hofmann and Poley where 13 patients with various lengths of ileal resection but retained ascending colon were given cholestyramine while fecal fat was measured. Figure 2.2 is an adaptation of their published findings revealing that patients with ileal resections >100 cm do not respond to cholestyramine and in fact this medication can potentially worsen fat malabsorption.[37] Finally, essential fatty acid (linoleic) deficiency is rare and medium chain fatty acids freely diffuse across the cell and into plasma and portal vein without requiring reesterification such as with LCFAs. Therefore, placing the affected patient on a low-fat diet with calcium and medium-chain fatty acid supplementation (such as coconut oil) often helps to reduce steatorrhea.

Free oxalate is readily absorbed in the colon but normally, free dietary oxalate complexes with dietary calcium to form an insoluble salt in the gut blocking free oxalate absorption. However, when fat malabsorption occurs, free fatty acids complex with gut calcium forming soap. This reduces available calcium to complex with oxalate. Thus, patients with extensive ileal resection with a colon in continuity can develop hyperoxaluria and nephrolithiasis. Clinically, this is commonly observed in patients with Crohn's disease with ileal resections.

Ileal resection often includes removal of the ileocecal valve, which is an anatomic barrier between the small and large intestine. This can lead to colonization of the small intestine with excessive colonic bacteria and anaerobic species a condition termed "small intestine bacterial overgrowth (SIBO)." In brief (the topic is considered in more depth in Chapter 24: Bacteral Overgrowth of the Small Intestine) clinical manifestations of SIBO can include diarrhea, steatorrhea, vitamin deficiencies, anemia, anorexia, weight loss, nausea, bloating, and abdominal discomfort. Biopsy of the small intestine mucosa in SIBO can demonstrate increase in intraepithelial inflammatory cells and villus atrophy similar to celiac disease. This results in malabsorption secondary to loss of surface area and decreased activity of mucosal digestive enzymes. In addition, bacteria from SIBO consume dietary B12 which leads to B12 deficiency and consequently, macrocytic anemia and neuropathy. They also synthesize abundant folate in the intestinal lumen, which are absorbed. Elevated folate levels are sometimes observed in patients with SIBO.

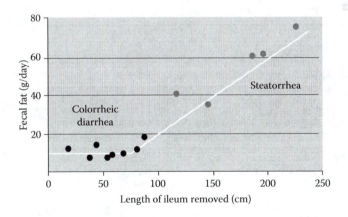

FIGURE 2.2   The relationship between length of ileal resection, degree of steatorrhea, and response to cholestyramine. Thirteen patients with various ileal resections with a retained ascending colon were given cholestyramine. Patients who responded are indicated by solid dots and nonresponders by gray dots. The break in the curve corresponds to the length of ileal resection (>100 cm) that is sufficiently great to impair bile acid reabsorption and where increased synthesis is no longer sufficient to restore bile acid pools. In patients with >100 cm of ileal resection, cholestyramine can further exacerbate fat malabsorption. [Adapted from Hofmann AF and Poley JR. *N Engl J Med* 1969;281(8):397–402.]

Bacteria from SIBO de-conjugate bile acids resulting in decreased bile acid reabsorption and decreased bile acid pools further fueling fat malabsorption and steatorrhea. When concerned, SIBO can be diagnosed with a radiolabeled breath test, a fasting hydrogen breath test, or quantitative culture of a duodenal aspirate demonstrating >$10^5$ bacteria or anaerobic bacteria and should be treated accordingly. However, these test are somewhat insensitive or invasive and if the pretest probability of SIBO is high, then empiric therapy with antibiotics is recommended. See Chapter 24 for further details on this topic.

## 2.19  COLONIC RESECTION

Preserving any portion of colon is beneficial in IF patients. The colon has a large reserve absorptive capacity for electrolytes and water, estimated to be 3–4 L of isotonic salt solution/day. Normally, only 100–200 $cm^3$ of water is lost in the stool each day (see Table 2.2). In addition, complex carbohydrates and fiber are fermented by bacterial enzymes in the colon to short-chain fatty acids and are absorbed by the colon. In adults the normal colon can absorb up to 500 kcal/day, which is a significant amount of calories for patients with SBS (see Table 2.3). Other benefits with colon preservation in SBS patients include the ability to slow intestinal transit and stimulate intestinal adaptation as demonstrated by colonic production of GLP-2. The presence of at least half of the colon is equivalent to about 50 cm of small bowel in the adult. Adults with no colon and <100 cm of jejunum are likely to require permanent PN and have a poor prognosis. Infants with <30 cm of small bowel and lacking the ileocecal valve are unlikely to be weaned from PN. In general, loss of the ileocecal valve in adults or children typically is associated with longer duration or higher likelihood of dependence on PN, and higher likelihood of bacterial overgrowth. Consequently, preservation of even a part of the colon and or ileocecal valve in patients with SBS can significantly reduce water and electrolyte losses, so patients should undergo reanastomosis as soon as is feasible.[1–3,36]

## 2.20  CONCLUSION

By understanding the normal physiology of the GI tract, the pathophysiology of various intestinal resections, and the intestinal adaptation potential of the remaining bowel, clinicians can predict the prognosis of patients with various intestinal resections. In general, with appropriate management of site-specific malabsorption, patients with limited small bowel resection have an excellent prognosis. Those with high permanent jejunostomies have severe malabsorption, are PN dependent, and are considered to have a poor nutritional and medical prognosis. However, the rate of survival, prognosis, and quality of life have been steadily improving over the last several years due to evolving experience with long-term home PN and improved management of nutritional needs. One study of 225 adult patients at the Mayo Clinic demonstrated a 5 year survival of 60% while on home PN. However, the probability of survival at 5 years appeared to be based on the primary disease and younger age of initiation of PN, 92% for IBD, 60% for ischemic bowel, 54% for radiation enteritis, 48% for motility disorder, and 38% for cancer.[38] Another study found similar results, with a survival rate of 86% at 2 years and 75% at 5 years in those with IF.[39] Similar improvements in survival rates have been demonstrated in the pediatric literature, and these rates may be improved further in the future with the implementation of medical, hormonal, and surgical advances.

## REFERENCES

1. Feldman M, Friedman LS, and Brandt LJ. Small and large intestine. In *Textbook: Sleisenger & Fordtran's Gastrointestinal and Liver Disease*, 8th Edition, Section X, pp. 2061–2276. Philadelphia, PA: Saunders Elsevier, 2006.
2. Buchman AL. Etiology and initial management of short bowel syndrome. *Gastroenterology* 2006;130:S5–S15.
3. Goulet O and Ruemmele F. Causes and management of intestinal failure in children. *Gastroenterology* 2006;30:S16–S28.

4. Ross MH, Romrell LJ, and Kaye GI. Digestive system II: Esophagus and gastrointestinal tract. In *Histology, A Text and Atlas*, 3rd Edition, Chapter 16, pp. 440–495. Baltimore, MD: Williams & Wilkins, 1995.

5. Gartner LP and Hiatt JL. Digestive system II. In *Color Atlas of Histology*, 2nd Edition, Chapter 14, pp. 256–278. Baltimore, MD: Williams & Wilkins, 1994.

6. Berne RM and Levy MN. The gastrointestinal system. In *Physiology*, 4th Edition, Section VI, pp. 589–674. St. Louis, Missouri: Mosby, 1998.

7. Cotran R, Kumar V, and Collins T. The gastrointestinal tract. In *Textbook: Robbins Pathologic Basis of Disease*, Section 18, pp. 775–843. Philadelphia, PA: W.B. Saunders Company, 1999.

8. Inui A, Asakawa A, Bowers CY, Mantovani G, Laviano A, Meguid MM, and Fujimiya M. Ghrelin, appetite, and gastric motility: The emerging role of the stomach as an endocrine organ. *FASEB J* 2004;18(3):439–456.

9. Waseem T, Duxbury M, Ito H, Rocha F, Lautz D, Whang E, Ashley S, and Robinson M. Ghrelin ameliorates TNF-a induced anti-proliferative and pro-apoptotic effects and promotes intestinal epithelial restitution. *J Am Coll Surg* 2004;199(3 Suppl):16–17.

10. Cummings D, Weigle D, Frayo R, Breen PA, Ma MK, Dellinger EP, and Purnell JQ. Plasma ghrelin levels after diet-induced weight loss or gastric bypass surgery. *N Engl J Med* 2002;346(21):1623–1630.

11. Appleton GVN, Bristol JB, and Williamson RCN. Proximal enterectomy provides a stronger systemic stimulus to intestinal adaptation than distal enterectomy. *Gut* 1987;28:165–168.

12. Chaves M, Smith MW, and Williamson RCN. Increased activity of digestive enzymes in ileal enterocytes adapting to proximal small bowel resection. *Gut* 1987;28:981–987.

13. Meier JJ, Nauck MA, Pott A, Heinze K, Goetze O, Bulut K, Schmidt WE, Gallwitz B, and Holst JJ. Glucagon-like Peptide 2 stimulates glucagon secretion, enhances lipid absorption, and inhibits gastric acid secretion in humans. *Gastroenterology* 2006;130:44–54.

14. Drucker DJ, Erlich P, Asa SL, and Brubaker PL. Induction of intestinal epithelial proliferation by glucagon-like peptide 2. *Proc Natl Acad Sci USA* 1996;93:7911–7916.

15. Burrin DG, Stoll B, Guan X, Cui L, Chang X, and Holst JJ. Glucagon-like peptide 2 dose-dependently activates intestinal cell survival and proliferation in neonatal piglets. *Endocrinology* 2005;146:22–32.

16. Liu C, Aloia T, Adrian T, Newton TR, Bilchik AJ, Zinner MJ, Ashley SW, and McFadden DW. Peptide YY. A potential proabsorptive hormone for the treatment of malabsorptive disorders. *Am Surg* 1996;62(3):232–236.

17. Mannon PJ. Peptide YY as a growth factor for intestinal epithelium. *Peptides* 2002;23(2):383–388.

18. Iqbal J and Hussain MM. Intestinal lipid absorption. *Am J Physiol Endocrinol Metab* 2009;296(6): E1183–E1194.

19. Abumrad N, Harmon C, and Ibrahimi A. Membrane transport of long-chain fatty acids: Evidence for a facilitated process. *J Lipid Res* 1998;39:2309–2318.

20. Phan CT and Tso P. Intestinal lipid absorption and transport. *Front Biosci* 2001;6:299–319.

21. Andrews N. Disorders of iron metabolism. *N Engl J Med* 1999;341:1986–1995.

22. Gunshin H, Mackenzie B, Berger UV, Gunshin Y, Romero MF, Boron WF, Nussberger S, Gollan JL, and Hediger MA. Cloning and characterization of a mammalian proton-coupled metal-ion transporter. *Nature* 1999;388:482–488.

23. Zhou B and Gitschier J. hCTR1: A human gene for copper uptake identified by complementation in yeast. *Proc Natl Acad Sci USA* 1997;94:7481–7486.

24. Williamson RCN and Chir M. Intestinal adaptation. I. Structural, functional, and cytokinetic changes. *N Engl J Med* 1978;298:1444–1450.

25. Williamson RCN and Chir M. Intestinal adaptation. II. Mechanisms of control. *N Engl J Med* 1978;298:1393–1402.

26. Sham J, Martin G, Meddlings JB, and Sigalet DL. Epidermal growth factor improves nutritional outcomes in a rat model of SBS. *J Pediatric Surg* 2002;37:765–769.

27. Rhoads JM, Argenzio RA, Chen W, Rippe RA, Westwick JK, Cox AD, Berschneider HM, and Brenner DA. L-Glutamine stimulates intestinal cell proliferation and activates mitogen-activated protein kinases. *Am J Physiol* 1997;272:G943–G953.

28. Luk G and Baylin SB. Polyamines and intestinal growth-increased polyamine biosynthesis after jejunectomy. *Am J Physiol* 1983;245:G656–G660.

29. Byrne TA, Wilmore DW, Iyer K, Dibaise J, Clancy K, Robinson MK, Chang P, Gertner JM, and Lautz D. Growth hormone, glutamine, and an optimal diet reduces parenteral nutrition in patients with short bowel syndrome. A prospective, randomized, placebo-controlled, double-blind clinical trial. *Ann Surg* 2005;242:655–661.

30. Jeppesen PB, Hartmann B, Thulesen J, Graff J, Lohmann J, Hansen BS, Tofteng F et al. Glucagon-like peptide 2 improves nutrient absorption and nutritional status in short-bowel patients with no colon. *Gastroenterology* 2001;120:806–815.

31. Jeppesen PB, Sanguinetti EL, Buchman A, Howard L, Scolapio JS, Ziegler TR, Gregory J, Tappenden KA, Holst J, and Mortensen PB. Teduglutide (ALX-0600), a dipeptidyl peptidase IV resistant glucagon-like peptide 2 analogue, improves intestinal function in short bowel syndrome patients. *Gut* 2005;54:1224–1231.

32. O'Keefe SJ, Gilroy R, Jeppesen PB, Messing B, Allard JP, Seidner DL, Pertkiewicz M, Kapikian R, McGraw N, and Caminis J. Teduglutide, a novel GLP-2 analog, in the management of short bowel syndrome (SBS) patients dependent on parenteral nutrition: A multicenter, multinational placebo-controlled clinical trial. *Gastroenterology* 2008;134:A-37.

33. Jeppesen PB, Gilroy R, Pertkiewicz M, Allard JP, Messing B, and O'Keefe SJ. Randomised placebo-controlled trial of teduglutide in reducing parenteral nutrition and/or intravenous fluid requirements in patients with short bowel syndrome. *Gut* 2011;60(7):902–914. Epub 2011 Feb 11.

34. Jeppesen PB, Hartmann B, Hansen BS, Thulesen J, Holst JJ, and Mortensen PB. Impaired meal stimulated glucagon-like peptide 2 response in ileal resected short bowel patients with intestinal failure. *Gut* 1999;45:559–563.

35. Jeppesen PB, Hartmann B, Thulesen J, Hansen BS, Holst JJ, Poulsen SS, and Mortensen PB. Elevated plasma glucagon-like peptide 1 and 2 concentrations in ileum resected short bowel patients with a preserved colon. *Gut* 2000;47:370–376.

36. American Gastroenterological Association Medical Position Statement. Short bowel syndrome and intestinal transplantation. *Gastroenterology* 2003;124:1105–1110.

37. Hofmann AF and Poley JR. Cholestyramine treatment of diarrhea associated with ileal resection. *N Engl J Med* 1969;281(8):397–402.

38. Scolapio JS, Fleming CR, Kelly DG, Wick DM, and Zinsmeister A. Survival of home parenteral nutrition-treated patients: 20 years of experience at Mayo Clinic. *Mayo Clin Proc* 1999;74:217–222.

39. Messing B, Crenn P, Beau P, Boutron-Ruault MC, Rambaud J-C, and Matuchansky C. Long-term survival and parenteral nutrition dependence in adult patients with the SBS. *Gastroenterology* 1999;117:1043–1050.

# 3 Motility Disorders in Intestinal Failure

*Leonel Rodriguez and Samuel Nurko*

## CONTENTS

## 3.1 INTRODUCTION

The main function of the gastrointestinal (GI) tract is to absorb nutrients and energy. The human body has, therefore, evolved multiple mechanisms to ingest food, digest nutrients, transport them through the intestine for their absorption, and eventually eliminate by-products as waste. This transport or motility function is accomplished by sophisticated mechanisms orchestrated by a complex interaction between muscle and the enteric, peripheral, and central nervous systems.

Gastrointestinal motility may be affected in patients with intestinal failure (IF) by a variety of mechanisms, and alternatively diseases that affect intestinal motility may lead to IF. Motility dysfunction can be manifested either as rapid transit as seen in short bowel syndrome (SBS) and congenital causes of intractable diarrhea, or as irregular and/or decreased motility with slow transit as in chronic intestinal pseudo-obstruction (CIPO) and other congenital anomalies such as gastroschisis. Motility can also be affected by medical or surgical interventions used to treat children with IF, or its complications.

In this chapter, we divide the GI motility problems seen in patients with IF as conditions leading either to rapid transit or to hypomotility. Since intestinal transplantation has emerged as a potential cure for IF, we also discuss the effects of transplantation on intestinal motility.

## 3.2 NORMAL PHYSIOLOGY

Ingestion of food starts with voluntary chewing and swallowing. Food is then propelled to the oropharynx by a coordinated centrally mediated mechanism of pharyngeal contractions followed by relaxation of the upper esophageal sphincter. There is an immediate relaxation of the lower esophageal sphincter to allow the bolus to be transferred into the esophagus by the peristaltic contractions of the esophageal body and then into the stomach.

During fasting, the antrum and the small intestine show a motility pattern known as migrating motor complex (MMC), described initially in animals [1] and found later in humans [2]. This MMC is generated at the intracellular level as a "slow wave" of electrical activity. This rhythmic enteric activity is generated by the enteric nervous system (ENS) composed of the interstitial cell of Cajal (ICC), neurons, and glial cells. The ICCs are believed to act as the pacemaker of the GI tract, generating the slow wave. The proto-oncogene C-Kit encodes a transmembrane tyrosine kinase receptor C-Kit that is critical for the development of the ICCs and has become the marker for identifying these cells in tissues. The MMC is composed of three phases, phase 1 is characterized by motor quiescence, phase 2 (the longest) shows irregular and intermittent phasic contractions, and phase 3 shows regular and rhythmic contractions that progress from the antrum to the ileum [3] (Figure 3.1). The MMC is shorter in children and its duration increases with age [3], and occurs approximately once every 3 h during fasting. The presence of an MMC is a marker of neurenteric integrity, and its absence has been associated with feeding intolerance and bacterial overgrowth. After a meal, the MMC is interrupted and the antrum and intestine show irregular contractions of larger duration and amplitude that are known as the fed pattern (Figure 3.2). The fed pattern is a result of extrinsic input, mostly mediated by the vagus nerve.

Small bowel motility is clinically measured with the use of antroduodenal manometry (ADM). This is accomplished with a motility catheter positioned over the antrum and duodenum via fluoroscopy and/or endoscopy. In patients with jejunostomy, the manometry catheter can be placed in the jejunum via the stoma to evaluate jejunal motility. ADM includes a recording during fasting to evaluate the intrinsic motility of the intestine, followed by stimulation with a meal, to analyze the

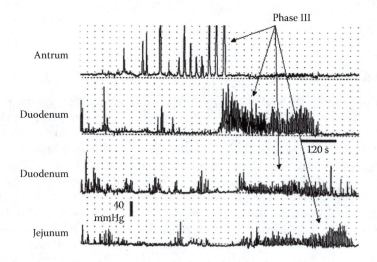

**FIGURE 3.1** Normal fasting ADM. A normal phase-3 front originating in the antrum and migrating aborally along the duodenum into the jejunum can be observed. During phase 3, the antrum contracts at a frequency of 3 min, whereas, the small bowel contracts at a frequency of 11–12 min. Phase 3 is followed by a period of quiescence (phase 1) and is preceded by intermittent irregular contractions (phase 2). (Reprinted from Nurko S. In Kleinman R. et al. (eds) *Pediatric Gastrointestinal Disease*, 5th edn. Philadelphia, PA; B.C. Decker Inc., 2008, pp. 1375–91. With permission.)

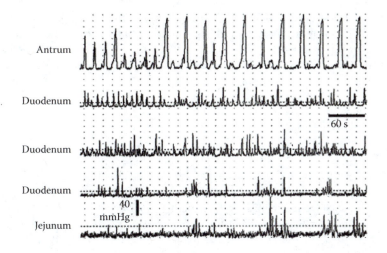

**FIGURE 3.2** Normal postprandial pattern in ADM. There are irregular persistent phasic contractions in the antrum and small bowel. (Reprinted from Nurko S. In Kleinman R. et al. (eds) *Pediatric Gastrointestinal Disease*, 5th edn. Philadelphia, PA; B.C. Decker Inc., 2008, pp. 1375–91. With permission.)

fed response. Provocative medication can be used, mainly erythromycin to elicit antral activity and phase 3 of the MMC via stimulation of motilin receptors, and octreotide that stimulates mainly phase 3 of the MMC by a direct action on the myenteric plexus [4].

The human colon has two primary functions: to absorb water, electrolytes, and some nutrients, and to propel waste aborally and store it in the distal colon until defecation occurs. The propelling function is accomplished by haustrations (segmental contractions) and mass movement (high-amplitude peristaltic contractions [HAPCs]). These activities are believed to be regulated by the colon pacemaker (ICC network) located in the cecum/ascending colon region. The anorectal function has evolved mechanisms that allow for the continence of stool and voluntary defecation.

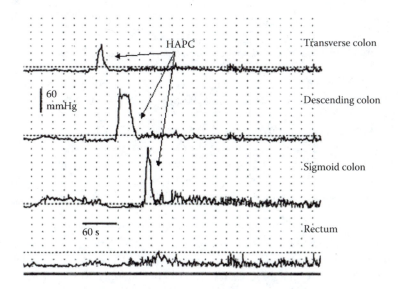

**FIGURE 3.3** Normal colon manometry. The tracing shows the presence of a high-amplitude propagating contraction that is originating in the transverse colon, advancing aborally along the large bowel, and stopping in the sigmoid colon. [Reprinted from Nurko S. In Kleinman R. et al. (eds) *Pediatric Gastrointestinal Disease*, 5th edn. Philadelphia, PA; B.C. Decker Inc., 2008, pp. 1375–91. With permission.]

Colonic motility can be evaluated indirectly by a colon transit study or directly with colonic manometry (CM). CM is performed by inserting a motility catheter in the colon to the cecum via colonoscopy and/or fluoroscopy. The CM test includes recording of fasting followed by a stimulation with a meal and then by provocative medications such as bisacodyl. The presence of HAPCs is a hallmark of normal colonic function (Figure 3.3).

## 3.3   RAPID INTESTINAL TRANSIT

### 3.3.1   SHORT BOWEL SYNDROME

SBS results from insufficient intestinal absorptive capacity due to loss of intestinal mass from congenital malformations such as intestinal atresia or massive resections for necrotizing enterocolitis, gastroschisis, or other congenital malformations. In most patients with SBS, intestinal transit is fast (shortened), given the shortened length of the intestine. As mentioned below, this transit can be modified with bowel-lengthening procedures as well as medications. The following is a description of how motility in different organs may be affected in SBS.

*Esophagus*: Swallowing and esophageal motility do not seem to be affected in SBS, as long as there is no central nervous system or other neurological problems.

*Stomach*: Gastric motility does not seem to be significantly altered in short gut syndrome. Some studies have shown no change in the rate of gastric emptying and postprandial motor activity in patients with SBS compared to controls [5]. In patients with SBS without a colon there is a rapid gastric emptying of liquids [6,7] that has been associated to elevated serum levels of peptide YY, probably because the peptide YY is thought to regulate the colonic brake [6]. Gastric emptying can also be altered after certain surgical procedures. Patients who have undergone fundoplication, pyloroplasty, or distal gastrectomy may develop dumping syndrome. Similar fast gastric emptying can result from the placement of G-tubes too close to the antrum, resulting in the direct dumping of feedings into the antropyloric region.

*Small bowel*: A faster transit occurs because there is a decreased absorptive surface and a shorter bowel length. This faster transit allows less time for the absorption of nutrients, and predisposes to malabsorption and resultant diarrhea. This transit velocity is also faster in patients with ileostomies, and slower in those in which there is still an ileocecal valve and colon. In fact, the duration of parenteral nutrition (PN) seems to decrease (although does not correlate with successful weaning) [8,9] by the presence of an ileocecal valve, probably as a result of decreasing transit, and subsequent better absorption of nutrients [9,10].

Transit in small bowel can be measured by fluoroscopy, breath testing, or by more simple, readily available, and easy-to-interpret methods such as the time for blue food color to appear in ostomy effluent or stools.

Animal studies show that soon after intestinal resection, the frequency of MMCs is unchanged, but there is an increase in cluster contractions [11]. From adult studies, we know that small bowel motility in the SBS is characterized by more frequent interdigestive motor complexes, marked reduction in phase 2 activity and a normal feeding pattern long after intestinal resection; so there is a possibility that adaptation occurs not only by improved absorption but by improved motility as well [5].

The effect of intestinal surgery on intestinal transit varies. The performance of bowel-lengthening/tapering procedures typically cause slowing of the transit. This slowing can be secondary to the increasing length of intestine, but most likely is related to intestinal dysfunction, and probably reduced motility. There exist no studies that have established intestinal motility after Bianchi, but it is known that the procedure increases the intestinal transit time, thereby allowing nutrients more contact time with absorptive surface [12].

Motility effects after the serial transverse enteroplasty (STEP) procedure seem to be more physiologic and better understood compared to the Bianchi procedure. Animal models have shown that the

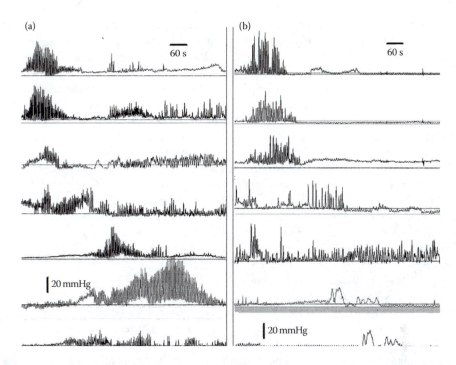

**FIGURE 3.4** Small bowel manometry in STEP (a) and control (b) animals. In these examples, both animals demonstrated the phase 3 activity that started proximally and migrated distally. In the STEP animal, the progression of phase 3 showed some simultaneous activity in the distal channels. In the control animal, the lower segments showed abnormal contractions with a tonic component. [Reprinted from Modi, B.P. et al., *J Pediatr Surg* 2009;44(1):229–35. With permission.]

STEP procedure does not seem to affect the intestinal transit [13], and in a recent STEP model in pigs, we demonstrated that the STEP procedure does not seem to affect the presence and characteristics of spontaneous and octreotide-induced phase 3 of the MMC. In fact, the duration of phase-3 MMC after octreotide was significantly increased compared to non-STEP controls, suggesting a potential benefit of the STEP procedure on small bowel motility by prolonging the MMC and potentially helping absorption [14] (Figure 3.4).

The presence of postoperative adhesions may also change intestinal transit, and produce obstruction, or blind intestinal loops, and a good clinical judgment is needed in the evaluation of children with SBS in which there is evidence of acute slowing of the transit.

*Colon*: Colon motility does not seem to be affected in SBS. In cases with no ileocecal valve, or with malabsorption, colonic transit may be faster. At times dietary changes and/or medications to slow colonic transit are required to decrease water losses. As mentioned above, SBS patients with a residual colon in continuity seem to be able to absorb more nutrients.

### 3.3.1.1 Treatment

Dietary modifications may be useful to manipulate gastric emptying. Higher caloric density and increased dietary fat intake prolong gastric emptying, while the use of human milk versus cow's milk [15,16], decreasing caloric density [17] or increasing viscosity [18] may accelerate it. Although the gastroduodenal motility fed pattern is not different after human milk when compared with cow's milk, the return of phase 3 of the MMC occurs faster and more consistently with human milk, which may explain its overall improved tolerance over cow's milk [19].

Rapid transit and hypermotility in SBS have been treated by dietary changes and medications. Among the medications, loperamide and octreotide have been the most studied.

Treatment with loperamide slows intestinal transit. It decreases intestinal secretions, prolongs the fasting phase 3, delays the postprandial surge of phase 3, and increases the motility index and frequency of contractions [5], potentially assisting in absorption of nutrients by allowing more exposure time to intestinal epithelium. The usual dose is 0.1–0.8 mg/kg, and should be titrated according to the response. Another antidiarrheal that has been used is lomotil. This contains a combination of diphenoxylate and atropine. Given the atropine component, anticholinergic side effects are not uncommon, so patients need close monitoring. The usual dose is 0.3–0.4 mg PO divided QID.

Octreotide, a somatostatin analogue, has been shown to reduce intestinal transit as well as gastric and intestinal secretions [20]. Studies on adults have shown that somatostatin and its analogues may be useful in the short-term management of SBS by reducing fecal mass and improving intestinal net sodium absorption [21] and also has shown significant effects when used for a long term by delaying small bowel transit time [22]. In children, isolated reports suggest a decrease on intestinal transit and improvement on the ostomy output [23]. Although there is controversy in studies on the rat if octreotide inhibits intestinal adaptation [24] or not [25], it is probably wise to use it after some adaptation has occurred. The usual dose is 1 µg/kg, two or three times a day and it needs to be given SC. Given that it has a slowing effect on antral motility, if evidence of delayed gastric emptying appears, it may need to be given with a prokinetic.

*Cisapride* is a prokinetic that improves motility by promoting acetylcholine release at the myenteric plexus. It is available only through a limited access program in the United States since it was removed from the market due to cardiac side effects including fatal arrhythmias. It is useful to improve feeding tolerance and control gastroesophageal reflux. We have recently reported our experience in 11 patients with SBS and feeding intolerance with no mechanical obstruction. They all received 0.1–0.2 mg/kg/dose for 3–4 doses per day. Seven patients had some improvement in enteral tolerance during treatment (two weaned completely from PN). We found a strong positive association between cisapride duration and improved enteral tolerance; the mean percentage of enteral intake increased by 7.3% for every 100 days on cisapride [26].

## 3.4  HYPOMOTILITY

### 3.4.1  Chronic Intestinal Pseudo-Obstruction

CIPO is a severe and disabling disorder characterized by episodes of continuous symptoms and signs of bowel obstruction in the absence of a fixed lumen-occluding lesion [27]. The majority of patients have these symptoms during the first year of life [28–33]. Abdominal distention is the most common sign [31,34], and can be present soon after birth [33] associated with bilious vomiting [30], and beyond the neonatal period with episodic vomiting and constipation [30]. With time, there is an inability to tolerate feedings and IF, requiring the use of PN, and multiple surgeries to decompress the bowel. Bacterial overgrowth is another complication associated to CIPO. Other organs can also be affected in patients with CIPO. Among the associated anomalies, urological involvement is prominent in 36–71% [29–32,35,36].

Potential causes of dysmotility in CIPO include abnormalities in the ICC network [37], delayed maturation of ICCs [38], increase in nitric oxide synthase (NOS) containing ganglionic cells [39], and other causes of inflammation and autoimmune responses. The main resulting problem in children with pseudo-obstruction is that the alterations in the motility lead to abnormal intestinal transit, and inability to tolerate enteral feedings.

Based on which portion of intestinal function is abnormal, there seem to be two main types of pseudo-obstruction, myopathic and neuropathic, although some cases showed mixed pictures. In those patients with myopathic predominant pseudo-obstruction, intestinal motility has the normal characteristics in periodicity and contraction frequency, but there is an inability of the muscle to produce effective contractions. In cases of neuropathic predominant pseudo-obstruction, there are abnormalities in contraction frequency, configuration, speed, or direction.

Diseases of the ENS or the smooth muscle may be familial or sporadic, and may be limited to the colon, or may be part of a more generalized disorder that can affect the whole GI tract. In some cases there may also be extraintestinal involvement (e.g., urological and cardiovascular), or the enteric dysfunction is a result of an abnormal extraintestinal regulation (like in mitochondrial dysfunction).

In children, most cases of pseudo-obstruction are primary, and in many cases congenital. From the primary diseases that affect the smooth muscle, the majority suffer either from hollow visceral myopathy, or megacystis microcolon hypoperistalsis syndrome (MMIHS). MMIHS is the most severe form of pseudo-obstruction, and affects predominantly female infants. It is characterized by marked dilatation of the bladder, a dilated nonperistaltic small bowel, and a malrotated microcolon. Most patients require multiple surgeries and are dependent on PN. The prognosis is poor and most patients die very young from renal insufficiency or sepsis.

There are cases of pseudo-obstruction that occur secondarily to systemic, autoimmune, or mitochondrial diseases and those need to be considered in the differential diagnosis.

The diagnosis of pseudo-obstruction is usually made by manometry (see below). Full-thickness intestinal biopsies should be performed only when a surgical operation is planned, and if possible from both dilated and undilated segments. Changes associated with neuropathies include aganglionosis, neuronal intranuclear inclusions and apoptosis, neural degeneration, intestinal neuronal dysplasia, hypoganglionosis, hypergangliogonosis, neuronal hyperplasia and ganglioneuromas, findings consistent with autoimmune inflammatory neuropathies, and abnormalities on mitochondria, neurotransmitter, and ICC network [40]. Myopathies show the following histological changes: inflammation, fibrosis, and atrophy of the outer longitudinal smooth muscle layer [41], abnormalities in intestinal muscle layering and intrinsic myocyte defects, and/or changes in the extracellular matrix [42]. The neuropathic type carries a better prognosis than myopathic [29,30,33] and is the most common type in children, possibly because myopathic is more likely to be secondary to GI involvement from systemic diseases that are more common in adults (e.g., amyloidosis and myasthenia gravis) and also take long time to develop (e.g., systemic lupus erythematosus, rheumatoid arthritis, and scleroderma).

Specific motor abnormalities seen in pseudo-obstruction include the following:

- *Esophagus*: Esophageal dysmotility is present in most adult patients with CIPO [43]. Children with visceral neuropathies show low amplitude, low duration, and/or simultaneous esophageal waves [44]. These abnormalities are not consistently found in children suggesting that esophageal involvement is a late development. Esophageal manometry may be useful when ADM is not available.
- *Stomach*: Gastric motility is greatly affected in CIPO. Gastric emptying by scintigraphy is delayed in most patients, and antral motility shows hypomotility during ADM (described in detail below) [45,46]. Myoelectrical abnormalities measured by the noninvasive method electrogastrography including an abnormal variation normal frequency, dominant power (voltage) and post-prandial bradygastria [47], and gastric dysrhythmias [48,49] are present in higher number in CIPO patients compared to controls.
- *Small bowel*: Dysmotility of small intestine is the hallmark of CIPO. Motility of the small bowel is evaluated by ADM; ADM is abnormal in CIPO, while a normal ADM in a patient with feeding intolerance excludes CIPO [50]. Typical manometric findings in neuropathic CIPO include absence of MMC during fasting, abnormal configuration of the phase-3 MMC with tonic and retrograde complexes, the presence of the phase-3-like activity during feeding, or the lack of a fed response after a meal [44] (Figure 3.5).

    In the myopathic variety of CIPO, the typical findings include low amplitude or absence of contractions [45,51] (Figure 3.6). The absence of phase 3 of the MMC has been associated with the need for PN [46,52,53] and its presence correlates with feeding tolerance, and a good response to jejunal feedings [54]. The presence of waves that are simultaneous, in clusters, and/or of long duration should raise concern for a missed mechanical obstruction [55,56]. The overall clinical result from these motility abnormalities is an

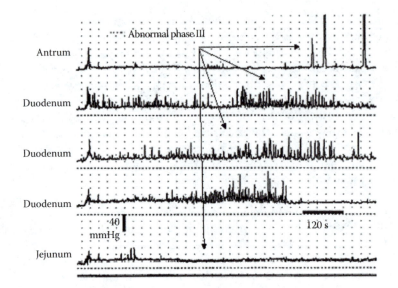

**FIGURE 3.5** ADM in neuropathic pseudo-obstruction. The tracing shows abnormalities in phase 3 of the MMC. Some uncoordinated clusters, as well as isolated irregular phasic contractions can be observed. Throughout the study, there was no organized activity, and irregular phasic contractions were seen. No phase 3 could be observed, even after provocative medications. [Reprinted from Nurko S. In Kleinman R. et al. (eds) *Pediatric Gastrointestinal Disease*, 5th edn. Philadelphia, PA; B.C. Decker Inc., 2008, pp. 1375–91. With permission.]

abnormal intestinal transit, with distention, bacterial overgrowth, and pain. This abnormal transit usually complicates enteral feedings, and in the most severe cases, PN is needed.

ADM is useful not only to confirm abnormal upper GI motility [45,57] but may also help to differentiate between neuropathic and myopathic subtypes [45]. A normal ADM in the suitable clinical setting should raise the concern of pediatric falsification disorder, Munchausen by proxy or pain-associated disability syndrome.

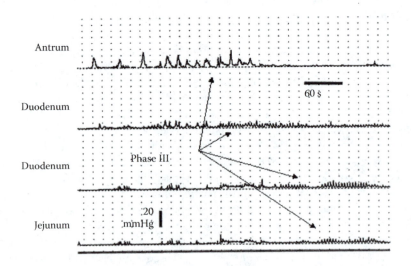

**FIGURE 3.6** ADM in myopathic pseudo-obstruction. The tracing shows the normal propagation of the interdigestive motor complex, although the amplitude is much lower than normal. [Reprinted from Nurko S. In Kleinman R. et al. (eds) *Pediatric Gastrointestinal Disease*, 5th edn. Philadelphia, PA; B.C. Decker Inc., 2008, pp. 1375–91. With permission.]

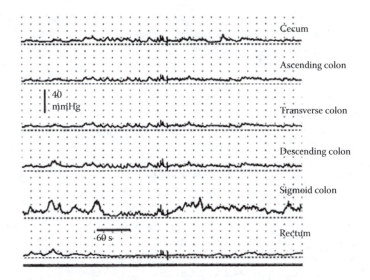

**FIGURE 3.7** Abnormal colon manometry. No high-amplitude propagating contractions or changes in the motility index were seen in this patient with a colonic neuropathy. No HAPCs were seen even after the administration of bisacodyl. [Reprinted from Nurko S. In Kleinman R. et al. (eds) *Pediatric Gastrointestinal Disease*, 5th edn. Philadelphia, PA; B.C. Decker Inc., 2008, pp. 1375–91. With permission.]

Since one of the mechanisms to control bacterial overgrowth in the intestine is motility, particularly the presence of phase-3 activity, it is not surprising that patients with CIPO commonly develop bacterial overgrowth in the small intestine, Common symptoms include diarrhea, abdominal distention, weight loss, and macrocytic anemia. See Chapter 24, Bacterial Overgrowth of the Small Intestine.

- *Colon*: The large bowel is also greatly affected in CIPO. Colonic motility is abnormal in the majority of children with CIPO. In the neuropathic type, abnormal basal activity and absence of HAPCs and gastrocolic response are observed. In the myopathic type, colonic motility shows no contractions [58] (Figure 3.7). Segmental abnormalities can also be noted; the most common one being abnormal sigmoid motility.

- *Anorectum*: Evaluated by anorectal manometry is normal in almost all patients with CIPO [28,44]. It has no significant clinical utility unless indicated to rule out Hirschsprung's disease or defecation disorders such as internal anal sphincter achalasia.

### 3.4.1.1  Treatment

The treatment of patients with CIPO is focused on two main aspects: (a) the optimization of GI motor function and (b) support to maintain an adequate nutrition, while preventing complications (e.g., electrolyte imbalance, malnutrition, and bacterial overgrowth) and controlling symptoms (e.g., abdominal distention and pain).

### 3.4.2  Improving Motility

### 3.4.2.1  Medications

Few prokinetic agents are effective for the treatment of delayed gastric emptying. *Erythromycin* is effective in inducing antral motility and intestinal phase-3 MMC in children with chronic GI functional symptoms. The usual dose is 3 mg/kg three times a day; higher doses are more likely to obtain a clinical response but are also more likely to lead side effects [59]. Although erythromycin seems ineffective for intestinal dysmotility [60], it may be useful in combination with octreotide since octreotide-related antral motility inhibition may be counteracted [61].

*Metoclopramide* has been the most widely used prokinetic in the United States. It is useful for delayed gastric emptying, but has little if any effect in small bowel motility [62]. The usual dose is 0.1–0.2 mg/kg QID. Its use has been associated with multiple side effects, including dystonic reactions, irritability, and the long-term possibility of producing tardive dyskinesia. In February 2009, the US Food and Drug Administration ordered a "black box warning" for metoclopramide-containing products against chronic use of these products to treat GI disorders.

Very few medications can be used to stimulate small intestinal motility. Among those, oral *cisapride* has been associated with increases in the number and amplitude of duodenal contractions after a complex-liquid meal [52] and has resulted in an increase in feeding tolerance and weight gain in children with short gut [26]. As mentioned above, cisapride can only be obtained through the Limited Access Program, and the usual dose is 0.1–0.2 mg/kg per dose, three or four times per day. Subcutaneous *octreotide*, which induces phase 3 of the MMC, has been shown in adult studies to increase feeding tolerance and improve intestinal transit [63,64]. It may, however, decrease antral motility; so its use may need to be associated with a prokinetic, such as erythromycin [65]. The usual dose is 1 µg/kg two or three times per day. We recently reported our experience in the use of octreotide in nine patients with CIPO. All were dependent on PN via central venous access, and their enteral tolerance was less than 1 ounce of formula per day. All had an abnormal ADM (seven with no phase-3 MMC). They all received intravenous octreotide 0.1–0.2 µg/kg/day for a mean of 6 months (range 2–15 months). Seven patients responded satisfactorily, with six tolerating enteral feedings of >4 ounces/day with reduction in PN, and one tolerating full feeds and the complete weaning of PN. One patient had an allergic reaction to octreotide after the second dose, so had to be discontinued, and one patient did not respond [66]. These results indicate that octreotide may also be useful in the chronic management of children with CIPO.

Medications are usually ineffective to stimulate colonic motility in the setting of CIPO. Some have anecdotally responded to daily doses of *bisacodyl* but in general they require surgical procedures to decompress colon. The usual bisacodyl dose is 0.25 mg/kg.

### 3.4.2.2 Surgery

Surgical consultation is helpful in the management of CIPO patients. The main role of the surgeon in cases of pseudo-obstruction is to rule out a mechanical obstruction and to provide central venous access for the delivery of PN. Surgical resections are rarely indicated in the management of CIPO. Gastrostomy is primarily indicated for venting the upper GI tract, usually not useful for feeding purposes. In cases where prokinetics do not work, in the setting of gastroparesis, botulinum toxin injection to the pylorus via endoscopy may be indicated, as it has been reported to be effective improving gastric emptying and symptoms in adults [67] and children [68,69] with gastroparesis. Often bypassing the stomach improves feeding tolerance, or the use of gastrojejunal tubes is common. Jejunostomy may be used for feedings but is not suitable for venting. In cases of severe dysmotility, diverting ostomies, particularly ileostomies have been recommended to decompress the abdomen. Diversion of the intestine may also minimize bacterial overgrowth by eliminating the colon as the source of bacteria, potentially minimizing bacterial translocation as a source of bloodstream infections.

It is important to remember that after any abdominal surgery, adhesions may develop and lead to small bowel obstruction. In patients with pseudo-obstruction who have had surgery and develop an acute episode of pseudo-obstruction, the presence of an anatomic problem always needs to be considered and excluded. Since many patients with CIPO have had at least one exploratory laparotomy, often before the diagnosis of CIPO has been confirmed, this is a common clinical issue.

### 3.4.3 PREVENTION OF COMPLICATIONS

### 3.4.3.1 Nutrition and Electrolytes

Close attention needs to be provided to electrolyte imbalances, as the episodes of obstruction, as well as loss of gastric and bile via gastrostomy, or ileostomy, may lead to fluid and electrolyte imbalances.

Nutritional support is essential in patients with CIPO. Diet can be modified (e.g., lower fat diet) to improve gastric emptying. The enteral route is always preferred, but the abnormal intestinal transit and abdominal pain may limit its administration. The use of trophic feedings in patients dependent on PN may decrease complications, and the presence of phase 3 of the MMC may be a prognostic indicator for the successful achievement of enteral feedings. Enteral feedings may be attempted via a gastrostomy tube, and jejunal feedings may be required when gastric feedings are not tolerated. A gastrostomy can also be used to vent the stomach. Home PN has proven to be safe and has slightly higher survival rates compared to chronic dialysis programs [70]. The age at the start of home PN and the degree of enteral independence are important prognostic factors in the survival rates in irreversible IF [71]. See Chapter 32, Home Parenteral and Enteral Nutrition.

### 3.4.3.2 Other Complications

Medications to treat bacterial overgrowth are also frequently needed, and those include the use of probiotics, and rotating antibiotics.

Pain control is very important, and the use of opiates needs to be avoided. Medications like antidepressants at a low dose (specifically selective serotonin reuptake inhibitors [SSRIs]) and gabapentin can modulate the pain sensation but they may take several weeks to exert their effect.

Finally, medical therapy includes treatment of the underlying cause when possible; replacement of nutritional deficits including vitamins and antibiotics and the role for probiotics is currently being explored.

### 3.4.4 GASTROSCHISIS

Even though different congenital abnormalities may lead to motility disorders, gastroschisis has been shown to have a profound effect on GI motility, so it will be used as a model of congenital malformations associated with dysmotility. Gastroschisis is a condition where a defect on the abdominal wall leads to prenatal exposure of the midgut to the amniotic cavity. Animal studies have shown that early exposure to urine may be deleterious and cause the dysmotility. The mechanism explaining the motility disturbance does not seem to be related to morphological damage to the ganglion cells [72–74] but rather to an effect on the ICC network [75], delayed cytoskeletal organization and reduced synaptic activity in the myenteric neurons [76], or increased NOS activity [77] before surgical correction. After surgery, the mechanism seems to be related to ischemic damage to the bowel wall [78].

*Esophagus*: Feeding difficulties are common in infants with gastroschisis and have been attributed exclusively to intestinal dysmotility, but a recent study in infants with gastroschisis and adequate intestinal length undergoing esophageal manometry showed that during fasting there was a lower frequency and poor propagation of spontaneous swallows, a shorter duration of upper esophageal spincter (UES) relaxation, a faster rate of relaxation and slower esophageal peristaltic propagation velocity. After wet swallows, there was a low frequency of UES contractile reflex and lower esophageal spincter (LES) relaxation. These findings suggest that esophageal motility problems may contribute to feeding problems in these infants [79].

*Stomach*: Gastric myoelectrical abnormalities have been reported in children that persist after surgical correction of the gastroschisis [80], but therapy with prokinetics does not seem to be effective in their treatment. Erythromycin showed no effect helping achieve full enteral autonomy after primary repair in a multicenter double-blind placebo-controlled study [81].

*Small bowel*: Dysmotility of the small intestine is the main limiting factor in establishing enteral tolerance. The mechanism seems to be related to ENS damage due to exposure to amniotic fluid in uterus. Many prokinetics have been attempted with limited success, which is similar to the response to prokinetics seen in CIPO. Studies evaluating prokinetics such as erythromycin, metoclopramide, and octreotide have shown no increase in smooth muscle contractility on the ileum in newborn rabbits with gastroschisis. Cisapride not only improved ileum contractility in that animal model, but also among adult rabbits [82].

*Anorectum*: In our experience, select patients with gastroschisis and internal anal sphincter dysfunction have responded to rectal dilatations and the administration of botulinum toxin.

## 3.5   INTESTINAL TRANSPLANTATION

Since intestinal transplantation has emerged as the potential cure for IF, it is important to understand the effects transplantation has on intestinal motility, particularly because the extrinsic innervation is lacking in the transplanted intestine and the GI motility has to rely on the preservation and function of the ENS. From the studies on dogs, we know that motility function soon after intestinal transplantation may be characterized by gastroduodenal emptying, reduced intestinal flow rates, faster intestinal transit, and similar postprandial phasic contractions compared to short bowel controls [83]. Since these changes are seen immediately after transplantation, they can probably be explained by postoperative and autoimmune responses leading to a temporary impairment of the ICC network associated to a delay in the recovery of spontaneous contractility as seen in rats after transplantation [84]. Interestingly, some have reported that motility changes (abnormalities in frequency and quality of the MMC) in a swine model of transplantation correlate with early rejection by histology and, therefore, might be helpful as a marker for early rejection [85,86]. Some have also reported the utility of octreotide on improving small bowel motility and bacterial overgrowth after intestinal autotransplantation in dogs [87].

The effects of intestinal transplantation on small bowel motility in children have not been well studied. In a study of eight children it was noted that the frequency and amplitude of contractions were normal. During fasting, five patients had spontaneous MMCs with normal manometric characteristics in the allograft small bowel. All phase 3 propagated distally and were dissociated from the native gut MMCs. A normal postprandial increase in motility was seen only in the patient who had multivisceral transplantation. Two patients had giant migrating contractions propagating from the native to the allograft small bowel. They concluded that interdigestive motor activity with normal manometric characteristics was seen in the allograft small bowel in 62% of patients. Discontinuation of the ENS from native to allograft gut disrupts the orderly propagation of MMCs across the anastomosis. Abnormal postprandial motility was present in the majority of patients and could be responsible for an abnormal intestinal transit and mixing, leading to diarrhea and poor absorption [88].

## 3.6   CONCLUSION

The effect of IF on GI motility varies depending on the underlying process. In SBS, esophageal and colonic functions seem unaffected, while gastric motility is affected only if gastric surgery has been performed. Intestinal motility may be increased in SBS and in concert with the decreased absorptive surface and a shorter bowel length, it may lead to faster transit which limits nutrients absorption predisposing to malabsorption and malnutrition. Dietary changes may help to slow the rapid transit, and medications such as loperamide, octreotide, and cisapride have been shown to increase feeding tolerance in SBS patients.

Patients with intestinal pseudo-obstruction have underlying GI motility abnormalities that prevent normal intestinal transit. In these patients, esophageal, gastric, intestinal, and colonic motility may be abnormal, leading to poor enteral tolerance of feeds and resulting in PN dependence in most. The treatment is focused on the optimization of GI motor function to maintain an adequate nutrition, to prevent complications from PN use, or to treat complications like bacterial overgrowth. Prokinetics may have a limited role; erythromycin helps with gastric emptying, cisapride may help gastric emptying and intestinal feeding tolerance, and recently, octreotide has been found useful in helping enteral tolerance.

Intestinal transplantation has emerged as the only potential curative treatment for life-threatening IF. Even though transplantation seems to disrupt the MMC through the anastomosis and to decrease the postprandial activity, it does not seem to alter interdigestive intestinal motility, and most patients achieve full enteral feedings.

## ACKNOWLEDGMENT

This work was supported by NIH grant 1K24DK82792-1 to S.N.

## REFERENCES

1. Szurszewski JH. A migrating electric complex of canine small intestine. *Am J Physiol* 1969;217:1757–63.
2. Vantrappen G, Janssens J, Hellemans J, and Ghoos Y. The interdigestive motor complex of normal subjects and patients with bacterial overgrowth of the small intestine. *J Clin Invest* 1977;59:1158–66.
3. Uc A, Hoon A, Di Lorenzo C, and Hyman PE. Antroduodenal manometry in children with no upper gastrointestinal symptoms. *Scand J Gastroenterol* 1997;32:681–5.
4. Di Lorenzo C, Lucanto C, Flores AF, Idries S, and Hyman PE. Effect of sequential erythromycin and octreotide on antroduodenal manometry. *J Pediatr Gastroenterol Nutr* 1999;29:293–6.
5. Remington M, Malagelada JR, Zinsmeister A, and Fleming CR. Abnormalities in gastrointestinal motor activity in patients with short bowels: Effect of a synthetic opiate. *Gastroenterology* 1983;85:629–36.
6. Nightingale JM, Kamm MA, van der Sijp JR, Ghatei MA, Bloom SR, and Lennard-Jones JE. Gastrointestinal hormones in short bowel syndrome. Peptide YY may be the 'colonic brake' to gastric emptying. *Gut* 1996;39:267–72.
7. Nightingale JM, Kamm MA, van der Sijp JR, Morris GP, Walker ER, Mather SJ, Britton KE, and Lennard-Jones JE. Disturbed gastric emptying in the short bowel syndrome. Evidence for a 'colonic brake' *Gut* 1993;34:1171–6.
8. Georgeson KE and Breaux CW, Jr. Outcome and intestinal adaptation in neonatal short-bowel syndrome. *J Pediatr Surg* 1992;27:344–8; discussion 348–50.
9. Spencer AU, Neaga A, West B, Safran J, Brown P, Btaiche I, Kuzma-O'Reilly B, and Teitelbaum DR. Pediatric short bowel syndrome: Redefining predictors of success. *Ann Surg* 2005;242:403–9; discussion 409–12.
10. Ladd AP, Rescorla FJ, West KW, Scherer LR, 3rd, Engum SA, and Grosfeld JL. Long-term follow-up after bowel resection for necrotizing enterocolitis: Factors affecting outcome. *J Pediatr Surg* 1998;33:967–72.
11. Quigley EM and Thompson JS. The motor response to intestinal resection: Motor activity in the canine small intestine following distal resection. *Gastroenterology* 1993;105:791–8.
12. Weber TR and Powell MA. Early improvement in intestinal function after isoperistaltic bowel lengthening. *J Pediatr Surg* 1996;31:61–3; discussion 63–4.
13. Kaji T, Tanaka H, Wallace LE, Kravarusic D, Holst J, and Sigalet DL. Nutritional effects of the serial transverse enteroplasty procedure in experimental short bowel syndrome. *J Pediatr Surg* 2009;44:1552–9.
14. Modi BP, Ching YA, Langer M, Donovan K, Fauza DO, Kim RB, Jaksic T, and Nurko S. Preservation of intestinal motility after the serial transverse enteroplasty procedure in a large animal model of short bowel syndrome. *J Pediatr Surg* 2009;44:229–35; discussion 235.
15. Cavell B. Gastric emptying in infants fed human milk or infant formula. *Acta Paediatr Scand* 1981;70:639–41.
16. Ewer AK, Durbin GM, Morgan ME, and Booth IW. Gastric emptying in preterm infants. *Arch Dis Child Fetal Neonatal Ed* 1994;71:F24–7.
17. Siegel M, Lebenthal E, and Krantz B. Effect of caloric density on gastric emptying in premature infants. *J Pediatr* 1984;104:118–22.
18. Shimoyama Y, Kusano M, Kawamura O, Zai H, Kuribayashi S, Higuchi T, Nagoshi A, Maeda M, and Mori M. High-viscosity liquid meal accelerates gastric emptying. *Neurogastroenterol Motil* 2007;19:879–86.
19. Tomomasa T, Hyman PE, Itoh K, Hsu JY, Koisumi T, Itoh Z, and Kurome T. Gastroduodenal motility in neonates: Response to human milk compared with cow's milk formula. *Pediatrics* 1987;80:434–8.
20. Farthing MJ. Octreotide in dumping and short bowel syndromes. *Digestion* 1993;54(Suppl 1):47–52.

21. Ladefoged K, Christensen KC, Hegnhoj J, and Jarnum S. Effect of a long acting somatostatin analogue SMS 201–995 on jejunostomy effluents in patients with severe short bowel syndrome. *Gut* 1989;30:943–9.

22. Nehra V, Camilleri M, Burton D, Oenning L, and Kelly DG. An open trial of octreotide long-acting release in the management of short bowel syndrome. *Am J Gastroenterol* 2001;96:1494–8.

23. Ohlbaum P, Galperine RI, Demarquez JL, Vergnes P, and Martin C. Use of a long-acting somatostatin analogue (SMS 201–995) in controlling a significant ileal output in a 5-year-old child. *J Pediatr Gastroenterol Nutr* 1987;6:466–70.

24. Sukhotnik I, Khateeb K, Krausz MM, Sabo E, Siplovich L, Coran AG, and Shiloni E. Sandostatin impairs postresection intestinal adaptation in a rat model of short bowel syndrome. *Dig Dis Sci* 2002;47:2095–102.

25. Vanderhoof JA and Kollman KA. Lack of inhibitory effect of octreotide on intestinal adaptation in short bowel syndrome in the rat. *J Pediatr Gastroenterol Nutr* 1998;26:241–4.

26. Raphael B, Nurko S, Jiang H, Hart K, Jaksic T, and Duggan C. Cisapride for enteral intolerance in pediatric short bowel syndrome. *J Pediatr Gastroenterol Nutr* 2009.

27. Rudolph CD, Hyman PE, Altschuler SM, Christense J, Colletti RB, Cuchiara S, Di Lorenzo C et al. Diagnosis and treatment of chronic intestinal pseudo-obstruction in children: Report of consensus workshop. *J Pediatr Gastroenterol Nutr* 1997;24:102–12.

28. Vargas JH, Sachs P, and Ament ME. Chronic intestinal pseudo-obstruction syndrome in pediatrics. Results of a national survey by members of the North American Society of Pediatric Gastroenterology and Nutrition. *J Pediatr Gastroenterol Nutr* 1988;7:323–32.

29. Mousa H, Hyman PE, Cocjin J, Flores AF, and Di Lorenzo C. Long-term outcome of congenital intestinal pseudoobstruction. *Dig Dis Sci* 2002;47:2298–305.

30. Heneyke S, Smith VV, Spitz L, and Milla PJ. Chronic intestinal pseudo-obstruction: Treatment and long term follow up of 44 patients. *Arch Dis Child* 1999;81:21–7.

31. Martinez Martinez L, Lopez Santamaria M, Prieto Bozano G, Molina Arias M, Jimenez Alvarez C, and Tovar Larrucea JA. Diagnosis and therapeutic options in chronic idiopathic intestinal pseudo-obstruction: Review of 16 cases. *Cir Pediatr* 1999;12:71–4.

32. Goulet O, Jobert-Giraud A, Michel JL, Jaubert F, Lortat-Jacob S, Colomb V, Cuenod-Jabri B et al. Chronic intestinal pseudo-obstruction syndrome in pediatric patients. *Eur J Pediatr Surg* 1999;9:83–9.

33. Faure C, Goulet O, Ategbo S, Breton A, Tounian P, Ginies JL, Roquelaure B et al. Chronic intestinal pseudoobstruction syndrome: Clinical analysis, outcome, and prognosis in 105 children. French-Speaking Group of Pediatric Gastroenterology. *Dig Dis Sci* 1999;44:953–9.

34. Fang X, Ke M, and Liu X. Clinical characteristics and diagnosis of chronic intestinal pseudo-obstruction. *Zhonghua Nei Ke Za Zhi* 2001;40:666–9.

35. Almeida PS and Penna FJ. Chronic intestinal pseudo-obstruction in children—Report of seven cases. *J Pediatr (Rio J)* 2000;76:453–7.

36. Lapointe SP, Rivet C, Goulet O, Fekete CN, and Lortat-Jacob S. Urological manifestations associated with chronic intestinal pseudo-obstructions in children. *J Urol* 2002;168:1768–70.

37. Feldstein AE, Miller SM, El-Youssef M, Rodeberg D, Lindor NM, Burgart U, Szurszewski JH, and Farrugia G. Chronic intestinal pseudoobstruction associated with altered interstitial cells of cajal networks. *J Pediatr Gastroenterol Nutr* 2003;36:492–7.

38. Kenny SE, Vanderwinden JM, Rintala RJ, Connell MG, Lloyd DA, Vanderhaegen JJ, and De Laet MH. Delayed maturation of the interstitial cells of Cajal: A new diagnosis for transient neonatal pseudoobstruction. Report of two cases. *J Pediatr Surg* 1998;33:94–8.

39. Bosman C, Devito R, Fusilli S, and Boldrini R. A new hypothesis on the pathogenesis of intestinal pseudo-obstruction by intestinal neuronal dysplasia (IND). *Pathol Res Pract* 2001;197:789–96.

40. De Giorgio R and Camilleri M. Human enteric neuropathies: Morphology and molecular pathology. *Neurogastroenterol Motil* 2004;16:515–31.

41. Darvishian F and Basham K. Familial visceral myopathy with carcinoma of unknown primary. *Ann Clin Lab Sci* 2002;32:93–7.

42. Smith VV and Milla PJ. Histological phenotypes of enteric smooth muscle disease causing functional intestinal obstruction in childhood. *Histopathology* 1997;31:112–22.

43. Schuffler MD and Pope CE, 2nd. Esophageal motor dysfunction in idiopathic intestinal pseudoobstruction. *Gastroenterology* 1976;70:677–82.

44. Boige N, Faure C, Cargill G, Cordeiro-Ferreira G, Viarme F, Cezard JP, and Nacano J. Manometrical evaluation in visceral neuropathies in children. *J Pediatr Gastroenterol Nutr* 1994;19:71–7.

45. Hyman PE, McDiarmid SV, Napolitano J, Abrams CE, and Tomomasa T. Antroduodenal motility in children with chronic intestinal pseudo-obstruction. *J Pediatr* 1988;112:899–905.
46. Watanabe Y, Ito T, Ando H, Seo T, and Nimura Y. Manometric evaluation of gastrointestinal motility in children with chronic intestinal pseudo-obstruction syndrome. *J Pediatr Surg* 1996;31:233–8.
47. Bracci F, Iacobelli BD, Papadatou B, Ferretti F, Lucchetti MC, Cianchi D, Francalanci P, and Pnticelli A. Role of electrogastrography in detecting motility disorders in children affected by chronic intestinal pseudo-obstruction and Crohn's disease. *Eur J Pediatr Surg* 2003;13:31–4.
48. Devane SP, Ravelli AM, Bisset WM, Smith VV, Lake BD, and Milla PJ. Gastric antral dysrhythmias in children with chronic idiopathic intestinal pseudoobstruction. *Gut* 1992;33:1477–81.
49. Debinski HS, Ahmed S, Milla PJ, and Kamm MA. Electrogastrography in chronic intestinal pseudo-obstruction. *Dig Dis Sci* 1996;41:1292–7.
50. Cucchiara S, Borrelli O, Salvia G, Lula VD, Fecarotta S, Gaudiello G, Boccia G, and Annese V. A normal gastrointestinal motility excludes chronic intestinal pseudoobstruction in children. *Dig Dis Sci* 2000;45:258–64.
51. Tomomasa T, DiLorenzo C, Morikawa A, Uc A, Hyman PE. Analysis of fasting antroduodenal manometry in children. *Dig Dis Sci* 1996;41:2195–203.
52. Hyman PE, Napolitano JA, Diego A, Patel S, Flores AF, Grill BB, Reddy SN, Garvey TQ 3rd, and Tomomasa T. Antroduodenal manometry in the evaluation of chronic functional gastrointestinal symptoms. *Pediatrics* 1990;86:39–44.
53. Fell JM, Smith VV, and Milla PJ. Infantile chronic idiopathic intestinal pseudo-obstruction: The role of small intestinal manometry as a diagnostic tool and prognostic indicator. *Gut* 1996;39:306–11.
54. Di Lorenzo C, Flores AF, Buie T, and Hyman PE. Intestinal motility and jejunal feeding in children with chronic intestinal pseudo-obstruction. *Gastroenterology* 1995;108:1379–85.
55. Frank JW, Sarr MG, and Camilleri M. Use of gastroduodenal manometry to differentiate mechanical and functional intestinal obstruction: An analysis of clinical outcome. *Am J Gastroenterol* 1994;89:339–44.
56. Loftus EV, Jr., Farrugia G, Donohue JH, and Camilleri M. Duodenal obstruction: Diagnosis by gastroduodenal manometry. *Mayo Clin Proc* 1997;72:130–2.
57. Stanghellini V, Camilleri M, and Malagelada JR. Chronic idiopathic intestinal pseudo-obstruction: Clinical and intestinal manometric findings. *Gut* 1987;28:5–12.
58. Di Lorenzo C, Flores AF, Reddy SN, Snape WJ, Jr., Bazzocchi G, and Hyman PE. Colonic manometry in children with chronic intestinal pseudo-obstruction. *Gut* 1993;34:803–7.
59. Di Lorenzo C, Flores AF, Tomomasa T, and Hyman PE. Effect of erythromycin on antroduodenal motility in children with chronic functional gastrointestinal symptoms. *Dig Dis Sci* 1994;39:1399–404.
60. Quigley EM. Chronic Intestinal Pseudo-obstruction. *Curr Treat Options Gastroenterol* 1999;2:239–250.
61. Verne GN, Eaker EY, Hardy E, and Sninsky CA. Effect of octreotide and erythromycin on idiopathic and scleroderma-associated intestinal pseudoobstruction. *Dig Dis Sci* 1995;40:1892–901.
62. Lux G, Katschinski M, Ludwig S, Lederer P, Ellermann A, and Domschke W. The effect of cisapride and metoclopramide on human digestive and interdigestive antroduodenal motility. *Scand J Gastroenterol* 1994;29:1105–10.
63. Sorhaug S, Steinshamn SL, and Waldum HL. Octreotide treatment for paraneoplastic intestinal pseudo-obstruction complicating SCLC. *Lung Cancer* 2005;48:137–40.
64. Lecomte T, Cavicchi M, and Delchier JC. Small bowel pseudo-obstruction revealing an early scleroderma. Long-term efficacy of octreotide and erythromycin. *Gastroenterol Clin Biol* 2000;24:361–3.
65. Di Lorenzo C, Lucanto C, Flores AF, Idries S, and Hyman PE. Effect of octreotide on gastrointestinal motility in children with functional gastrointestinal symptoms. *J Pediatr Gastroenterol Nutr* 1998;27:508–12.
66. Rodriguez LFA. Daily intravenous octreotide promotes enteral feeding tolerance in children with chronic intestinal pseudo-obstruction. *J Pediatr Gastroenterol Nutr* 2009;49(1):E50.
67. Miller LS, Szych GA, Kantor SB, Bromer MQ, Knight LC, Maurer AH, Fisher RS, and Parkman HP. Treatment of idiopathic gastroparesis with injection of botulinum toxin into the pyloric sphincter muscle. *Am J Gastroenterol* 2002;97:1653–60.
68. Woodward MN and Spicer RD. Intrapyloric botulinum toxin injection improves gastric emptying. *J Pediatr Gastroenterol Nutr* 2003;37:201–2.
69. Muniz-Crim A, Rodriguez L, and Flores A. Effect of pyloric injection of botulinum toxin in children with gastroparesis. *J Pediatr Gastroenterol Nutr* 2005;41:521.

70. Llop Talaveron J, Juvany Roig R, Tubau Molas M, Virgili Casas N, Pita Merce A, and Jodar Masanes R. Quality of the home parenteral nutrition program: 14 years of experience at a general university hospital. *Nutr Hosp* 2000;15:64–70.

71. Vantini I, Benini L, Bonfante F, Talamini G, Semenini C, Chiarioni G, Maragnolli O, Benini F, and Capra F. Survival rate and prognostic factors in patients with intestinal failure. *Dig Liver Dis* 2004;36:46–55.

72. Kluck P, Tibboel D, van der Kamp AW, and Molenaar JC. The effect of fetal urine on the development of the bowel in gastroschisis. *J Pediatr Surg* 1983;18:47–50.

73. Langer JC, Longaker MT, Crombleholme TM, Bond SJ, Finkbeiner WE, Rudolph CA, Verrier ED, and Harrison MR. Etiology of intestinal damage in gastroschisis. I: Effects of amniotic fluid exposure and bowel constriction in a fetal lamb model. *J Pediatr Surg* 1989;24:992–7.

74. Oyachi N, Lakshmanan J, Ross MG, and Atkinson JB. Fetal gastrointestinal motility in a rabbit model of gastroschisis. *J Pediatr Surg* 2004;39:366–70.

75. Vargun R, Aktug T, Heper A, and Bingol-Kologlu M. Effects of intrauterine treatment on interstitial cells of Cajal in gastroschisis. *J Pediatr Surg* 2007;42:783–7.

76. Vannucchi MG, Midrio P, Zardo C, and Faussone-Pellegrini MS. Neurofilament formation and synaptic activity are delayed in the myenteric neurons of the rat fetus with gastroschisis. *Neurosci Lett* 2004;364:81–5.

77. Bealer JF, Graf J, Bruch SW, Adzick NS, and Harrison MR. Gastroschisis increases small bowel nitric oxide synthase activity. *J Pediatr Surg* 1996;31:1043–5; discussion 1045–6.

78. Tibboel D, Kluck P, van der Kamp AW, Vermey-Keers C, and Molenaar JC. The development of the characteristic anomalies found in gastroschisis—Experimental and clinical data. *Z Kinderchir* 1985;40:355–60.

79. Jadcherla SR, Gupta A, Stoner E, Fernandez S, Caniano D, and Rudolph CD. Neuromotor markers of esophageal motility in feeding intolerant infants with gastroschisis. *J Pediatr Gastroenterol Nutr* 2008;47:158–64.

80. Cheng G, Langham MR, Jr., Sninsky CA, Talbert JL, and Hocking MP. Gastrointestinal myoelectric activity in a child with gastroschisis and ileal atresia. *J Pediatr Surg* 1997;32:923–7.

81. Curry JI, Lander AD, and Stringer MD. A multicenter, randomized, double-blind, placebo-controlled trial of the prokinetic agent erythromycin in the postoperative recovery of infants with gastroschisis. *J Pediatr Surg* 2004;39:565–9.

82. Langer JC and Bramlett G. Effect of prokinetic agents on ileal contractility in a rabbit model of gastroschisis. *J Pediatr Surg* 1997;32:605–8.

83. Johnson CP, Sarna SK, Zhu YR, Buchrnann E, Bonham L, Telford GL, Roza AM, and Adams MB. Effects of intestinal transplantation on postprandial motility and regulation of intestinal transit. *Surgery* 2001;129:6–14.

84. Matsuura T, Masumoto K, Ieiri S, Nakatsuji T, Akiyoshi J, Nishimoto Y, Takahashi Y, Hayashida M, and Taguchi T. Morphological and physiological changes of interstitial cells of Cajal after small bowel transplantation in rats. *Transpl Int* 2007;20:616–24.

85. Matsuura T, Taguchi T, Hayashida M, Ogita K, Takada N, Nishimoto Y, Taguchi S et al. Relationship between real-time monitoring of the graft motility and mucosal histology in swine intestinal transplantation. *Transpl Proc* 2006;38:1851–2.

86. Matsuura T, Taguchi T, Hayashida M, Ogita K, Takada N, Nishimoto Y, Taguchi S et al. The influence of rejection on graft motility after intestinal transplantation in swine: The possibility of using this method for the real-time monitoring of acute cellular rejection. *J Pediatr Surg* 2007;42:1377–85.

87. Nakada K, Ikoma A, Suzuki T, Reynolds JC, Campbell WL, Todo S, and Starzl E. Amelioration of intestinal dysmotility and stasis by octreotide early after small-bowel autotransplantation in dogs. *Am J Surg* 1995;169:294–9.

88. Mousa H, Bueno J, Griffiths J, Kocoshis S, Todo S, Reyes J, and Di Lorenzo C. Intestinal motility after small bowel transplantation. *Transpl Proc* 1998;30:2535–6.

89. Nurko S. Gastrointestinal manometry, methodology, and indications. In Kleinman RE, Sanderson IR, Goulet O, Sherman P, Miele-Vergani G, Shneider BL (eds) *Pediatric Gastrointestinal Disease*, 5th edn. Philadelphia, PA; B.C. Decker Inc., 2008, pp. 1375–91.

# 4 Clinical Assessment of Intestinal Failure in Children

*Jason S. Soden*

## CONTENTS

Intestinal failure (IF) is a functional diagnosis that encompasses a spectrum of disease states in which the end result is dependence on parenteral nutrition (PN). In the pediatric population, the management of the patient with IF is challenging and requires assessment of an infant's or child's growth, development, bowel adaptation, nutritional status, psychosocial well-being, and any complications of IF and/or PN therapy. The clinical assessment of the pediatric patient with IF must take into account an understanding of the patient's underlying disease, anthropometric and biochemical evaluation of nutritional status, and recognition of the important complications of IF and PN that limit survival and stratify prognosis in the pediatric patient.

## 4.1   IDENTIFICATION OF THE UNDERLYING DISEASE AND ANATOMY

The initial assessment of the infant or child with IF should include identification of the patient's underlying disease and anatomy. Table 4.1 summarizes the etiologies of IF, which include short bowel syndrome (SBS), motility disorders, and congenital enteropathies leading to chronic malabsorption. SBS is the most frequent cause of IF in children [1]. In the more rare setting of an infant with prolonged PN requirement and no clear underlying diagnosis, a thorough evaluation for other etiologies (congenital enteropathy and primary motility disorder) should be completed. For the neonate with intractable diarrhea, evaluation should include endoscopy with careful review of small intestinal and ultrastructural histopathology. The assessment of the infant or child with presumed bowel dysmotility leading to IF requires a complex, coordinated evaluation that may include specialized motility evaluations. See Chapter 1, Etiology and Epidemiology of Intestinal Failure for further details on this topic.

The significance of identifying the underlying diagnosis is relevant in the concept of "irreversible" or "permanent" IF. Certain etiologies of IF, including primary enterocyte disorders, severe dysmotility states, and, potentially, long segment aganglionosis will not, by current and available

**TABLE 4.1**

**Causes of IF in Children**

**Short Bowel Syndrome**

Neonatal/infants
  Intestinal atresia
  Midgut volvulus
  Gastroschisis
  Necrotizing enterocolitis
  Long segment aganglionosis
  Congenital SBS
Older children
  Trauma
  Mesenteric infarction
  Radiation enteritis
  Inflammatory bowel disease (rare)

**Motility Disorders**

Primary (congenital)
  Neuropathic
  Myopathic
Secondary (acquired)
  Neuropathic
  Myopathic

**Mucosal Abnormalities**

Primary enteropathies
  Microvillous inclusion disease
  Primary epithelial dysplasia (tufting enteropathy)
  Congenital disorders of glycosylation
Immune mediated
  Primary immunodeficiency syndromes
  Autoimmune enteropathies

therapies, adapt or improve [2,3]. The pediatric patient with irreversible IF, therefore, has an expected prognosis of permanent PN requirement (via current available standards of treatment), and referral for evaluation by an intestinal transplantation center should be considered at an early stage.

In the setting of a patient with SBS, where the goal in management is to optimize bowel adaptation, the initial evaluation involves establishment of a firm understanding of the infant's postsurgical anatomy. Historically, a large emphasis has been placed on small bowel length, either as length resected or residual length, as the primary prognostic factor. Short residual bowel length (<40 cm), compared to the length of residual small bowel (>100–150 cm), has traditionally been associated with more guarded outcomes. This concept, requisite on absolute bowel length, does not take into account the dynamic changes in infant bowel length through gestational development. As noted by the classic study by Touloukian and Smith [6] (Figure 4.1), where bowel lengths from 30 stillborn fetuses/infants of various gestational ages were measured, small bowel length may double in the developing fetus from 19 to 27 weeks gestation compared to 35 weeks gestation. At term, a mean length of 240 cm increases to 380 cm at 12 months [4–6]. Wide interindividual variations are seen in bowel length, however, More accurate description of bowel length may include percentage of bowel resected (or remaining) compared to gestational age-expected bowel length [7,8]. Thus, the 29-week preterm infant with necrotizing enterocolitis (NEC) and 20 cm resection may lose a much larger percentage bowel than a term infant with similar absolute length of resection.

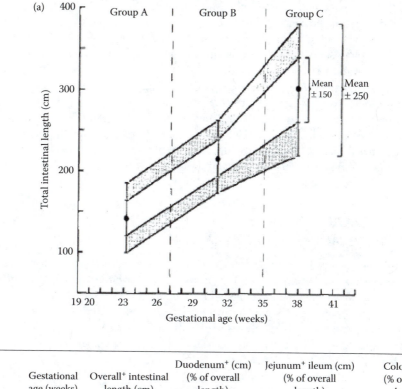

| Group | Gestational age (weeks) | Overall+ intestinal length (cm) | Duodenum+ (cm) (% of overall length) | Jejunum+ ileum (cm) (% of overall length) | Colon+ (cm) (% of overall length) |
|---|---|---|---|---|---|
| A (n = 11) | 19–27 | 142 ± *22 | 3.8 ± 1.0 (2.7) | 114.8 ± *21 (80.8) | 23.4 ± *4 (16.5) |
| B (n = 13) | 27–35 | 217 ± *24 | 5.3 ± 1.9 (2.4) | 172.1 ± *29 (79.3) | 40.9 ± *8 (18.8) |
| C (n = 6) | >35 | 304 ± *44 | 6.5 ± 1.9 (2.1) | 248.0 ± *40 (81.6) | 49.1 ± *6 (16.2) |

$*p < 0.05 \times$ mean ± SD.

**FIGURE 4.1** Measurements of total intestinal length from autopsy data in 30 preterm infants, gestational ages 19–40 weeks. (a) Mean total intestinal lengths ± two standard deviations, comparing groups A (19–27 weeks), B (27–35 weeks), and C (greater than 35 weeks), with data summarized in table (b). (From Touloukian RJ and Smith GJ. *J Pediatr Surg* 1983;18:720–3. With permission.)

The description of the SBS patient should also summarize relevant anatomic details, with consideration of not only bowel length, but equally important postsurgical anatomy. The jejunal resection leads to at least a temporary reduction in nutrient absorption, although adaptation of the ileum may favor long-term outcome. A high jejunostomy implies generally a very limited absorptive potential. Loss of the ileum subsequently leads to fluid and electrolyte losses, in addition to bile acid, fat, fat-soluble vitamin, and vitamin B12 malabsorption. The presence of the ileocecal valve allows an important anatomic barrier against reflux of colonic bacteria into the small bowel, and also helps to regulate the exit of fluids, electrolytes, and nutrients out of the small bowel [9]. The colon itself has important functions in improving water and electrolyte absorption, allowing carbohydrate fermentation and energy absorption via short-chain fatty acid salvage pathways, and may play an important role in promoting adaptation, possibly via its unique microbiota [10]. Thus, residual bowel in continuity (e.g., jejuno-colonic versus jejuno-ileal anastomoses) should be distinguished anatomically, with implied pathophysiology in mind.

Finally, aside from bowel length and anatomy, assessment of residual bowel function is imperative. Bowel dilation and dysmotility may promote stasis, and, secondarily, small bowel bacterial overgrowth (SBBO), potentially contributing to malabsorption, translocation/infection, and liver disease. Furthermore, the presence of SBBO may negatively impact bowel adaptation or ability to wean from PN [11,12]. See Chapter 23, Bacterial Overgrowth of the Small Intestine. Underlying diseases, notably gastroschisis, result in dilated, dysfunctional bowel despite length and anatomy that would otherwise be suitable for adaptation. Phillips et al. reviewed their experience with neonatal gastroschisis from 1993 to 2007, and identified nine patients with gastroschisis/intestinal atresia/dysmotility. These selected patients had adequate postresection small bowel length; however, small bowel dilation and secondary stasis led to significant dysmotility. Survival rate in this group of patients, despite adequate bowel length, was only 43% [13]. In another series, Payne et al. [14] identified bowel dilation on prenatal ultrasound greater than 10 mm as a significant factor in predicting infants with gastroschisis that would develop gastrointestinal complications, including atresia, perforation, or resection.

## 4.2  CONSIDERATION OF PREDICTORS OF ADAPTATION, PN DEPENDENCE, AND SURVIVAL IN INTESTINAL FAILURE

In general, the diagnosis of IF implies a guarded outcome. The survival rates for pediatric patients with SBS varies between 73% and 89%, and survival rates for children on chronic PN has been reported as low as 60% [15,16]. For patients with irreversible IF, the only therapeutic option aside from indefinite PN is bowel transplantation, which still carries significant risks of morbidity and mortality. Transplantation is traditionally reserved for patients with persistent IF despite attempts at bowel rehabilitation, especially those patients with progressive complications of or limitations to parenteral therapy.

In the clinical assessment of the patient with IF, it is therefore important to try and stratify each individual patient within the realm of factors that may predict either favorable or poor outcomes. Because there is a markedly heterogeneous population of pediatric patients with IF as a common end road, the task of predicting outcomes is especially difficult. Published data are largely from single center, retrospective studies that are carried out over a number of years with a diverse population of IF patients, primarily SBS. Definitions of SBS and IF varied in published series; and this has led to variability in key reported outcomes, such as patient mortality [17]. Furthermore, as novel therapies are pioneered and utilized by individual centers (including parenteral lipid modification for liver disease and surgical lengthening procedures), individual patient factors that were, in previous years, more static (e.g., residual small bowel length and presence of persistent cholestasis), may be considered more dynamic variables in the current era.

With these limitations of the available, retrospective data in mind, the clinical assessment of the patient with IF should be performed with consideration of the factors that predict successful or poor outcomes. Table 4.2 highlights some of the key positive and negative prognostic factors in pediatric SBS and IF that have been identified by more recent retrospective studies [7,15,18–22]. Regarding the SBS patient's postsurgical anatomy, the residual length of small intestine, presence of ileocecal

**TABLE 4.2**
**Predictors of Outcomes in Pediatric SBS and IF**

| Positive Factors | Negative Factors |
|---|---|
| Residual bowel length > 35–40 cm | Residual bowel length < 15–20 cm or < 10% age-expected normal |
| Presence of ICV and/or colon | |
| Older infants/children | |
| | Prematurity/neonates |
| | Presence of persistent liver disease |
| | Presence of bacterial overgrowth |
| | Underlying disease: gastroschisis, mucosal inflammation |

valve or colon, and establishment of intestinal continuity have all been demonstrated relatively consistently to help predict the ability to wean PN [3,23,24]. In separate retrospective analyses, residual bowel length of >15–40 cm, or >10% of actual small bowel length at time of resection have been associated with a higher prediction of successful adaptation [19,21,22]. The percentage of daily kilocalories provided enterally at 6, 12, or 24 weeks may provide predictive information as to the ability to wean of PN as well [18,25]. Other patient factors, including the underlying disease (gastroschisis), prematurity, or other systemic complications may impact patient prognosis.

No discussion regarding the clinical assessment of pediatric IF is complete without due mention of the importance of PN-associated liver disease, referred to in this review as intestinal failure-associated liver disease (IFALD). Across the retrospective studies in pediatric IF, the most consistent negative prognostic indicator for overall survival is the presence of IFALD. IFALD is seen in 40–60% of pediatric IF patients, and up to 16.6% may progress to end state liver disease [26,27]. In multiple studies, IFALD is an established predictor of patient mortality or PN dependence [21,22,28,29]. IFALD is a multifactorial disease, likely resulting from several factors unique to the pediatric patient on long-term parenteral nutrition, including the presence of infection/sepsis, bowel stasis, anatomic factors that affect enterohepatic bile acid circulation, susceptibility of the neonatal liver to cholestatic injury, and factors relevant to the PN itself, including macronutrient composition, contamination/toxicity, and/or micronutrient excesses/deficiencies [30]. Because of the multifactorial etiopathogenesis of IFALD, there has been no single patient factor that has been identified to predict occurrence or severity of disease. Age may be an important predicting factor for liver disease, in that neonatal patients are more likely to develop aggressive, cholestatic liver disease in contrast to the histologic steatosis classically seen in adults [30,31]. Sepsis is also an important cofactor for IFALD development, and retrospective studies have illustrated that the timing (early onset) and frequency of catheter associated infections (CAIs) in SBS predict both the occurrence and severity of IFALD [27,32]. Andorsky and colleagues have illustrated that advancement of enteral nutrition (or discontinuation of PN) is an important factor in predicting reversal of biochemical cholestasis [18]. Thus, the clinical assessment of the child with IF requires establishment of risk factors for IFALD development, and, when indicated, defining the presence and severity of liver disease. See Chapter 20, Intestinal Failure–Associated Liver Disease for more details.

## 4.3 FROM RETROSPECTIVE DATA TO CLINICAL ASSESSMENT OF PATIENTS WITH INTESTINAL FAILURE

The management of pediatric patients with IF entails a balance between promotion of growth/bowel adaptation versus recognition and treatment of the complications of IF/SBS and PN therapy. Table 4.3 summarizes the complications seen in IF patients. In general, the most severe complications are those related to the necessity to provide PN. Complications of the underlying disease, especially in SBS, are dependent on the child's anatomy, enteral intake, and other factors. The assessment of IF patients requires a generalized understanding of these complications so that problems can be identified and managed aggressively, if not prevented in the first place.

### 4.3.1 ASSESSMENT OF NUTRITIONAL AND FLUID STATUS

Clinically, the first task in assessment is to ascertain the child's nutritional status. Accurate measurements of weight, height, and head circumference are critical, and these should be compared with standardized, normal values. Plotting along normative growth curves should be corrected for gestational age in the former premature infant. Growth data should be measured, recorded, and compared to each individual patient's own historical data. Fluid shifts, changes in stool and ostomy output, ascites, and bowel wall edema may alter the ability to rely on weight values alone. Reliance

**TABLE 4.3**

**Complications in the Management of IF Patients**

| Complications Related to PN Therapy | Complications Related to SBS or Underlying Disease |
|---|---|
| IF-associated liver disease | Malabsorptive |
| Fluid, electrolyte, micronutrient imbalances | Growth failure |
| Catheter-associated problems | Fluid, electrolyte, micronutrient |
| Infection/sepsis | Deficiency states |
| Thrombosis | Diaper/stoma skin breakdown |
| Mechanical/breakage | Bone demineralization |
| Cholelithiasis | Medication/pharmacologic |
| | Nephrolithiasis |
| | Motility disturbances |
| | Mechanical obstruction |
| | Bacterial overgrowth |
| | D-Lactic acidosis |
| | Gastric acid hypersecretion |
| | GI mucosal |
| | Noninfectious colitis |
| | Anastomotic ulcerations |

on weight or weight/height alone may underestimate the degree of acute malnutrition in children with chronic liver disease, due to inflated patient weight caused by organomegaly [33]. Therefore, assessment of body composition by measuring mid-arm circumference and triceps skinfold thickness is important, especially in the child with fluid shifts and/or IFALD.

In a retrospective series of 87 patients with SBS and IF, nine patients remained on chronic PN and had a mean body weight of $-0.5 \pm 0.64$ standard deviation scores (SDS) and height of $-0.75 \pm 0.99$ SDS. Twelve patients were weaned off PN, but due to a failure to maintain adequate linear growth, PN was restarted. SBS patients who were successfully weaned from all artificial enteral and parenteral nutritional support ($n = 57$) achieved normal long-term growth and pubertal development [19]. Similarly, in a small retrospective series, Wu et al. [34] verified normal anthropometric measurements, weight for age, and height for age in nine patients weaned from PN for more than 2 years. In summary, normal growth may be achieved on PN, and patients successfully weaned from PN may have normal long-term growth. However, anthropometric status should be followed very closely in the period during and after PN weaning.

Assessment of fluid status includes estimation of the patient's hydration status, stoma/stool losses, and serum electrolytes. Gastrointestinal fluid and electrolyte losses vary depending on losses from nasogastric tubes, gastrostomy tubes, or enterostomy output. Fluid and electrolyte management is an integral part of PN management, and serum electrolyte levels should be monitored routinely. Typically, electrolytes should be monitored frequently (at least 2–3 times per week) during more dynamic clinical phases, such as PN advancement, changes in stool/stoma output, or concerns for dehydration or fluid overload. When the patient is more stable, such as in routine, ambulatory settings and electrolytes should be monitored at least monthly. Urine sodium level is traditionally a more accurate estimate of total body sodium content, and a low urine sodium (<10–20 mmol/L) may detect sodium depletion earlier than serum values [4,35].

In a child who has been on long-term PN, or graduated successfully from PN, periodic surveillance of micronutrient status is recommended. Recommendations regarding parenteral supply of minerals and trace elements have been published [36]. For the child on long-term PN, iron deficiency may occur, and laboratory indications of iron status (ferritin, iron level, and iron-binding capacity) should be followed. Dahlstrom et al. [37] demonstrated that patients on long-term PN had decreased levels of serum trace elements compared to age-matched controls; however no clinical signs or symptoms of deficiencies were detected. Fluctuations in serum levels of copper, zinc, manganese, and lead were reported during PN administration in a group of adult patients [4,38]. Other trace elements, including chromium, copper, zinc, and selenium should also be periodically monitored [36]. Zinc deficiency may occur in patients with gastrointestinal fluid losses, and therefore zinc levels should be monitored. Selenium, an important antioxidant, has been shown to be deficient in chronic PN patients. Better biomarkers of micronutrient and trace mineral status, including copper, zinc, selenium, and iodine, need to be developed in order to validate the optimal assays and cutoff values, especially in infants and children [39–43].

Standard PN formulations routinely contain multivitamin components, and guidelines on recommended dosing have been published [36]. There is insufficient evidence to support the routine measurement of serum vitamin levels in all patients with IF that remains on long-term PN. However, certain disease states, especially cholestasis and pancreatic insufficiency, may predispose the patient with IF to greater gastrointestinal fat-soluble vitamin losses, and in these patients, surveillance of fat-soluble vitamin levels is advised. Measurement of water-soluble vitamin levels should be obtained in the child on continued PN therapy if a clinical deficiency syndrome is suspected. In the long-term follow-up of IF and SBS patients that have graduated from PN, micronutrient deficiencies are common and should be surveyed for clinically and via laboratory studies [34,44,45]. The expectation of when to predict micronutrient deficiencies in a patient who has been on long-term PN is not well-established, and more studies are needed to clearly define the timing of laboratory evaluations if clinical deficiency syndromes are not suspected. In general, one should direct the laboratory evaluation toward monitoring for expected micronutrient deficiencies Table 4.4 outlines important minerals and vitamins to follow in the clinical assessment of the pediatric patient with IF, including a summary of clinical deficiency syndromes and recommended laboratory evaluations.

In patients receiving parenteral lipid therapy, serum triglyceride levels should be routinely followed. In patients who are on primarily omega-3 fatty acid-based lipid solutions, or in patients with significant fat malabsorption and who have been weaned off parenteral lipids, surveillance for essential fatty acid deficiency is advised. Essential fatty acid deficiency may present clinically in an infant with sparse hair, poor weight gain, poor wound healing, and thrombocytopenia, and laboratory evaluation confirms an elevated ratio of eicosatrienoic acid:arachidonic acid (triene:tetraene) [46].

## 4.3.2 Assessment of Bowel Length and Function

Along with the nutritional evaluation of the IF patient, the clinical assessment should involve an estimation of the child's residual bowel function. The relevance of postsurgical bowel length and anatomy in the SBS patient has been previously emphasized, and the physical and radiographic examinations may help to assess bowel dilation, motility, and length. In the setting of SBS or primary motility disorders, abdominal radiographs may demonstrate dilated loops of small bowel. Air fluid levels may be demonstrated in areas of mechanical obstruction, or in chronic intestinal pseudoobstruction. Other objective evaluations of bowel motility including manometry and transit studies may provide insight into pathophysiology or bowel function in suspected primary motility disorders with IF [47]. Patients with SBS may have disordered motility due to disruption in normal neuroendocrine patterns in the postsurgical bowel. See Chapter 3, Motility Disorders in Intestinal Failure, for details.

When indicated, contrast radiology may be used as a clinical tool to assess dilation, motility, and length. Nightingale and Woodward [48] reported a high correlation between radiographic and surgical measurements of small bowel length in 18 adult SBS patients. Recently, Rossi et al. [49] reported their experience in the estimation of small bowel length on radiological films with a hand-held opsiometer, and they were able to correlate objective evidence of bowel growth by this method with bowel adaptation and ability to wean off PN in eight pediatric patients.

**TABLE 4.4**

**Micronutrient Deficiency or Overload Syndromes in IF**

| Micronutrient | Pathophysiology | Clinical Deficiency Syndrome | Clinical Overload Syndrome | Laboratory Evaluation |
|---|---|---|---|---|
| **Minerals and Trace Elements** | | | | |
| Calcium | Fat malabsorption | Paresthesias, tetany, bone demineralization | GI, GU, bone complaints[a] | Serum Ca, PTH, DEXA scan |
| Magnesium | Fat malabsorption and high GI fluid losses | Weakness, cardiac arrhythmias, CNS | Weakness, cardiac arrhythmias[a] | Serum Mg |
| Zinc | GI fluid losses | Poor growth, skin, hair, diarrhea | Vomiting, headache, diarrhea, Cu deficiency[a] | Serum Zn, low alkaline phosphatase |
| Copper | Overload more common in cholestasis | Hemolytic anemia, neutropenia[a] | Hepatic overload, neuropsychiatric | Serum Cu |
| Manganese | Overload more common in cholestasis | Poor growth, ataxia, skeletal[a] | Neurotoxicity | Serum Mn |
| Iron | Absorbed proximally; not routinely in PN | Microcytic anemia, irritability | Hepatotoxicity, GI bleeding, vomiting | Ferritin, TIBC, Hgb, Hct, smeared blood cell morphology |
| Selenium | Absorbed throughout small bowel | Myopathy, cardiomyopathy | Thyroid enlargement[a] | Serum selenium |
| **Fat-Soluble Vitamins** | | | | |
| A | Fat malabsorption, cholestasis | Xerophthalmia, night blindness | Increased ICP, hepatitis, vomiting | Vitamin A: retinol binding protein ratio |
| D | Fat malabsorption, cholestasis | Hypocalcemia, hypophosphatemia rickets | Emesis, renal impairment | 25-OH vitamin D |
| E | Fat malabsorption, cholestasis | Myopathy, neuropathy, ataxia, hemolytic anemia | Coagulopathy | Vitamin E: total serum lipid ratio |
| K | Fat malabsorption, cholestasis | Bleeding | Hemolytic anemia | Prothrombin time, PIVKA assay |
| **Water-Soluble Vitamins** | | | | |
| B12 | Gastric or ileal resection | Megaloblastic anemia, CNS including ataxia | None known | Serum B12, methylmalonic acid, homocysteine |
| Folate | Absorbed proximally | Anemia, thrombocytopenia, stomatitis, glossosis | None known | Serum folate |

[a] Rare in pediatric IF.

Aside from estimation of bowel length and motility, estimation of bowel dilation by gastrointestinal (GI) contrast series may play a role in predicting the important pathophysiologic consequences of bacterial overgrowth. Stagnant, dilated loops of bowel, especially in the setting of a patient with an enterocolonic anastomosis, may precipitate small intestinal bacterial overgrowth (SIBO). Figure 4.2 demonstrates pathologic small bowel dilation in a patient with SBS and IF. Objective

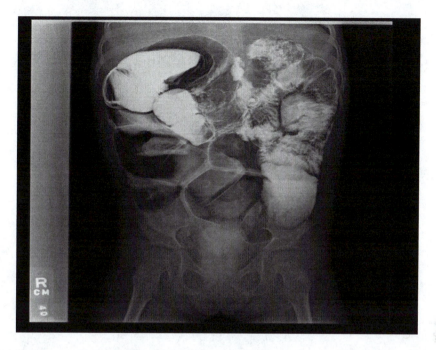

**FIGURE 4.2** Upper GI with small bowel follow through series in a child with short bowel syndrome and an ileo-rectal anastomosis. Note the dilated loops of bowel which contribute to the clinical presentation of abdominal distension, bloating, enteral intolerance, and bacterial overgrowth in the patient.

assessment for SIBO includes hydrogen breath testing or quantitative culture from small intestinal fluid, although the clinical utility of these evaluations in the management of pediatric IF and SBS remains controversial. Furthermore, in the present era, where nontransplant surgical intervention may be considered to relieve intestinal dysmotility and promote intestinal lengthening and adaptation, demonstration of adequate bowel dilation on GI contrast series is important before these procedures are considered.

A direct correlate to bowel function is the assessment of a child's enteral progress. Sondheimer et al. [25] reviewed their experience in 27 infants with SBS and IF and found that the percentage of daily calories provided enterally at 12 weeks adjusted age significantly correlated with the duration of PN dependence (Figure 4.3). Therefore, progress in enteral nutrition serves an indicator of bowel adaptation. Since 100% enteral adaptation is the ultimate goal in IF management, one must carefully assess the patient's enteral access. Frequently, the patient with IF requires continuous feeding, generally via a gastrostomy tube, to optimize both absorption and adaptation. Alternative enteral access routes, including gastrojejunal tubes or direct jejunal feeding tubes are considered in the setting of gastric or proximal bowel dysmotility and/or feeding intolerance. A secondary goal in clinical management is for pediatric IF patients to achieve both oral and enteral autonomy, without dependence on supplemental enteral support. Oral aversion and feeding difficulties are relatively common in the pediatric IF population, namely due to chronic dependence on nutritional support since the neonatal period. Thus, the clinical assessment should include evaluation of enteral caloric intake as an indicator of adaptation and bowel function, and should also be focused on appreciation of enteral access and oral feeding skills and progress.

Recently, serum or plasma citrulline levels have been identified as a potential biomarker of functional enterocyte mass. Citrulline is a nonessential amino acid produced primarily in the enterocyte by the metabolism of glutamine and ornithine. Several studies have correlated circulating citrulline level with functional small bowel enterocyte mass and absorptive capacity [50–59]. Data available from the clinical utility of this assay are promising, and warrants further investigation.

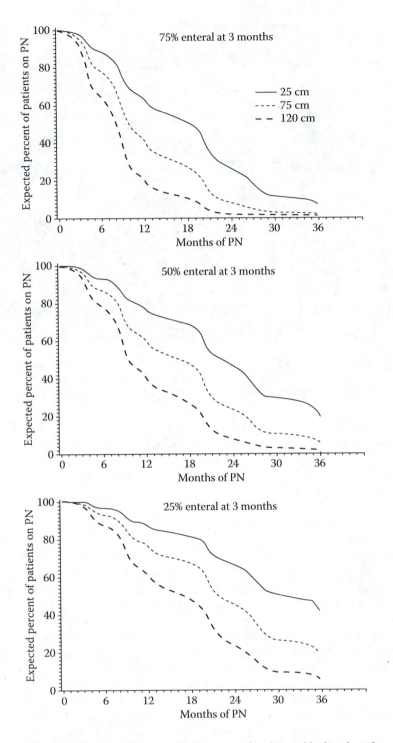

**FIGURE 4.3** Cox Proportional Hazard equation for 3 groups of patients with short bowel syndrome from retrospective series of 44 neonates dependent on PN for >3 months. The three graphs stratify patients by percentage daily calories at 3 months' adjusted age, shown versus residual small intestinal length after surgery. The y-axis contains the percent of patients expected to remain on PN, graphically demonstrated as a survival curve. (From Sondheimer JM et al. *J Pediatr* 1998;132:80–4. With permission.)

### 4.3.3 Assessment of Critical Complications of PN Therapy

Despite meticulous management of nutrition, fluids, and electrolytes, as well as proactive measures to assess and promote bowel adaptation, life-threatening complications of parenteral therapy are unavoidable in the majority of IF patients. In a retrospective cohort of 302 pediatric patients receiving home PN, the mortality rate in children with primary digestive disorders was 9%. Of this subset, 48% died from either liver disease or sepsis [60]. Similarly, Wales et al. [17] identified a mortality rate in 37.5% of a cohort of 40 infants with SBS (defined as bowel length < 25% age-expected normal, or PN > 6 weeks), with the majority of deaths occurring from liver disease or sepsis. Because of the complex causal relationship between infection and liver disease in PN patients, and because of their important impact on patient survival, these complications should be evaluated for vigilantly. Furthermore, in the assessment of the child with IF and either recurrent life-threatening infections or progressive liver disease, referral to a center with experience in aggressive bowel rehabilitation, PN modification strategies, or bowel transplantation should be considered.

## 4.4 CATHETER-ASSOCIATED COMPLICATIONS, INCLUDING INFECTION

Because the provision of PN is dependent on a functioning, central venous catheter (CVC), complications related to the CVC in the IF patient are both relatively common and important to assess and manage. In a retrospective series of 60 pediatric IF patients in Italy, the incidence of CAI was 1.4/1000 CVC days, and thromboses occurred at a rate of 0.2/1000 CVC days [61]. Potential sources for CAI include infection from the skin at the time of placement, catheter lumen infection during connection/disconnection, seeding from a distal site, or contamination [62]. In addition, in IF patients, SBBO, immune dysfunction, compromised bowel permeability, and liver disease may predispose to translocation of enteric bacteria into circulation, creating a setup for catheter colonization or sepsis. In 1992, Kurkchubasche et al. determined a sixfold increase in the incidence of catheter sepsis events in pediatric SBS patients compared to non-SBS patients [63]. SBS patients are also more likely to have Gram-negative infections compared to other patients with indwelling CVC, and patients with a shorter bowel are more likely to develop CAI [64,65]. Thus, infection should be considered with a high index of suspicion in the clinical assessment of the IF patient who presents with either typical presenting signs (fever, lethargy, and shock) or atypical symptoms (irritability, change in baseline stool/stoma output).

The occurrence of CAI may lead to further complications in the patient's parenteral therapy. Despite antimicrobial therapy, catheter salvage only occurs in 42–52% of patients with CAI [63,66] as reported in published data, although in clinical experience, higher rates of catheter salvage are possible. Aside from sepsis, other mechanical and thrombotic complications may occur that require CVC removal. Impaired central venous access is an indication for bowel transplantation; the frequency of infections or mechanical problems should be carefully assessed in each patient, taking into account any pending loss of venous access. Patients who are at risk for loss of central venous access may require sonography or venography for assistance in localization of access sites, or referral to a center with a team skilled at complicated vascular access [67].

## 4.5 INTESTINAL FAILURE–ASSOCIATED LIVER DISEASE

Because of its importance in prognosticating the IF patient's course, the clinical assessment must define the presence and severity of liver disease. Biochemically, elevated transaminases and bilirubin are common in infants on PN, but typically resolve in short-term PN courses. Persistent cholestatic injury is characterized by progressive/persistent elevation in bilirubin, transaminases, and gamma-GT. Histopathologic features include cholestasis, bile duct proliferation, periportal inflammation, and fibrosis [68]. Ultimately, sequelae of chronic liver disease arise in patients with persistent PN requirement and progressive injury. These complications include cirrhosis, portal hypertension, coagulopathy, and ongoing risks of bleeding and death [26,30]. Weber et al. [28]

correlated the severity of liver disease (by Child's classifications) with negative indicators of bowel adaptation (prolonged time to feed, total PN time).

The laboratory assessment of the patient with IFALD should include hepatobiliary enzymes and routine monitoring of synthetic liver function (prothrombin time and albumin) and interval surveillance for fat-soluble vitamin deficiency. The examiner should carefully evaluate the evidence of portal hypertension (splenomegaly, ascites, hypersplensim with thrombocytopenia). When accessible (e.g., during surgery for stoma closure or revision), a liver biopsy should be obtained for evaluation and follow-up of histologic injury. Recently, the $^{13}$C-methionine breath test has been evaluated in a small cohort of patients as a potentially noninvasive and reliable measure of liver function in children with IF [69]. Other noninvasive serum biomarkers and imaging modalities to assess liver fibrosis have not yet been evaluated in the setting of IFALD, but may potentially have important roles in the future [70,71].

## 4.6   OTHER COMPLICATIONS IN THE PEDIATRIC IF PATIENT

Key features of the clinical evaluation of the IF patient have been addressed thus far, including assessment of nutritional status, residual bowel function, enteral tolerance and access, infection rate, catheter access, and liver disease. Long-term follow-up of the patient requires ongoing assessment of these key areas, in addition to awareness of other complications that may occur.

Metabolic bone disease has been reported in pediatric and adult patients with IF [45,72]. The etiology of bone demineralization is likely multifactorial, related to malabsorption of minerals (calcium, phosphorus) and vitamin D. In a series of 18 patients with SBS who had been weaned off parenteral support, subjects were found to have decreased bone mineral content measured by dual-energy x-ray absoptiometry (DEXA) compared to controls. However, these differences were not significant when adjusted for differences in weight and height between the subjects and control group [72]. More studies into this area will optimally help define parameters for surveillance bone densitometry imaging in the IF population.

Luminal bacterial fermentation of malabsorbed carbohydrates in SBS may lead to production and accumulation of D-lactate, which causes the clinical syndrome of D-lactic acidosis [73]. The child with D-lactic acidosis presents with the onset of neurologic symptoms including altered mental status accompanied by an anion gap positive metabolic acidosis. Diagnosis is confirmed by confirming elevated D-lactate levels in plasma or urine.

Fat malabsorption in the setting of a patient with an intact colon (and increased colonic oxalate absorption) may lead to renal stones. Specifically, ongoing fat malabsorption binds luminal calcium, leaving luminal oxalate unbound and free to accumulate in the kidneys. The resultant calcium oxalate precipitation may lead to nephrolithiasis. Although this is an uncommon problem in infants and younger children, adults with SBS and intact colon have up to a 25% chance of developing symptomatic kidney stones [35].

Luminal injury from malabsorption of carbohydrates and bile acids, potentially coupled with SBBO, may lead to a spectrum of mucosal injury in SBS and IF patients. Noninfectious colitis was reported in 81% of infants in Denver with SBS during 1985–1988, and is clinically characterized as bloody, watery, malabsorptive diarrhea [74]. In addition, anastomotic ulcers have been reported in pediatric patients as a long-term complication following enterocolonic resection, and may present with frank gastrointestinal hemorrhage or occult blood loss [44,75].

## 4.7   SUMMARY

The clinical assessment of the pediatric IF patient should include attention to bowel anatomy and function, nutritional status, and the important complications that influence clinical outcomes, including liver disease. Referral to a center with nutritional, medical, and surgical expertise in the multispecialty care of these complex patients is advised. More studies on novel and potentially noninvasive diagnostic tools are warranted, and prospective, multicenter studies are needed to better assess relevant outcomes and therapies.

# REFERENCES

1. De Marco G, Barabino A, Gambarara M, Diamanti A, Martelossi S, and Guarino A. Network approach to the child with primary intestinal failure. *J Pediatr Gastroenterol Nutr* 2006;43(Suppl 1):S61–7.
2. Goulet O, Fusaro F, Lacaille F, and Sauvat F. Permanent intestinal failure. *Indian Pediatr* 2008;45:753–63.
3. Goulet O, Ruemmele F, Lacaille F, and Colomb V. Irreversible intestinal failure. *J Pediatr Gastroenterol Nutr* 2004;38:250–69.
4. Wessel JJ and Kocoshis SA. Nutritional management of infants with short bowel syndrome. *Semin Perinatol* 2007;31:104–11.
5. Weaver LT, Austin S, and Cole TJ. Small intestinal length: A factor essential for gut adaptation. *Gut* 1991;32:1321–3.
6. Touloukian RJ and Smith GJ. Normal intestinal length in preterm infants. *J Pediatr Surg* 1983;18:720–3.
7. Goday PS. Short bowel syndrome: How short is too short? *Clin Perinatol* 2009;36:101–10.
8. Spencer AU, Neaga A, West B, Safran J, Brown P, Btaiche I, Kuzma-O'Reilly B, and Teitelbaum DH. Pediatric short bowel syndrome: Redefining predictors of success. *Ann Surg* 2005;242:403–9; discussion 409–12.
9. Vanderhoof JA and Langnas AN. Short-bowel syndrome in children and adults. *Gastroenterology* 1997;113:1767–78.
10. Goulet O, Colomb-Jung V, and Joly F. Role of the colon in short bowel syndrome and intestinal transplantation. *J Pediatr Gastroenterol Nutr* 2009;48(Suppl 2):S66–71.
11. Kaufman SS, Loseke CA, Lupo JV, Young RJ, Murray ND, Pinch LW, and Vanderhoof JA. Influence of bacterial overgrowth and intestinal inflammation on duration of parenteral nutrition in children with short bowel syndrome. *J Pediatr* 1997;131:356–61.
12. Cole CR and Ziegler TR. Small bowel bacterial overgrowth: A negative factor in gut adaptation in pediatric SBS. *Curr Gastroenterol Rep* 2007;9:456–62.
13. Phillips JD, Raval MV, Redden C, and Weiner TM. Gastroschisis, atresia, dysmotility: Surgical treatment strategies for a distinct clinical entity. *J Pediatr Surg* 2008;43:2208–12.
14. Payne NR, Pfleghaar K, Assel B, Johnson A, and Rich RH. Predicting the outcome of newborns with gastroschisis. *J Pediatr Surg* 2009;44:918–23.
15. Duro D, Kamin D, and Duggan C. Overview of pediatric short bowel syndrome. *J Pediatr Gastroenterol Nutr* 2008;47(Suppl 1):S33–6.
16. Ruiz P, Kato T, and Tzakis A. Current status of transplantation of the small intestine. *Transplantation* 2007;83:1–6.
17. Wales PW, de Silva N, Kim JH, Lecce L, Sandhu A, and Moore AM. Neonatal short bowel syndrome: A cohort study. *J Pediatr Surg* 2005;40:755–62.
18. Andorsky DJ, Lund DP, Lillehei CW, Jaksic T, Dicanzio J, Richardson DS, Collier SB, Lo C, and Duggan C. Nutritional and other postoperative management of neonates with short bowel syndrome correlates with clinical outcomes. *J Pediatr* 2001;139:27–33.
19. Goulet O, Baglin-Gobet S, Talbotec C, Fourcade L, Colomb V, Sauvat F, Jais JP, Michel JL, Jan D, and Ricour C. Outcome and long-term growth after extensive small bowel resection in the neonatal period: A survey of 87 children. *Eur J Pediatr Surg* 2005;15:95–101.
20. Mian SI, Dutta S, Le B, Esquivel CO, Davis K, and Castillo RO. Factors affecting survival to intestinal transplantation in the very young pediatric patient. *Transplantation* 2008;85:1287–9.
21. Quiros-Tejeira RE, Ament ME, Reyen L, Herzog F, Merjanian M, Olivares-Serrano N, and Vargas JH. Long-term parenteral nutritional support and intestinal adaptation in children with short bowel syndrome: A 25-year experience. *J Pediatr* 2004;145:157–63.
22. Spencer AU, Kovacevich D, McKinney-Barnett M, Hair D, Canham J, Maksym C, and Teitelbaum DH. Pediatric short-bowel syndrome: The cost of comprehensive care. *Am J Clin Nutr* 2008;88:1552–9.
23. Mayr JM, Schober PH, Weissensteiner U, and Hollwarth ME. Morbidity and mortality of the short-bowel syndrome. *Eur J Pediatr Surg* 1999;9:231–5.
24. Gupte GL, Beath SV, Kelly DA, Millar AJ, and Booth IW. Current issues in the management of intestinal failure. *Arch Dis Child* 2006;91:259–64.

25. Sondheimer JM, Cadnapaphornchai M, Sontag M, and Zerbe GO. Predicting the duration of dependence on parenteral nutrition after neonatal intestinal resection. *J Pediatr* 1998;132:80–4.

26. Kelly DA. Intestinal failure-associated liver disease: What do we know today? *Gastroenterology* 2006;130:S70–7.

27. Sondheimer JM, Asturias E, and Cadnapaphornchai M. Infection and cholestasis in neonates with intestinal resection and long-term parenteral nutrition. *J Pediatr Gastroenterol Nutr* 1998;27:131–7.

28. Weber TR and Keller MS. Adverse effects of liver dysfunction and portal hypertension on intestinal adaptation in short bowel syndrome in children. *Am J Surg* 2002;184:582–6; discussion 586.

29. Coran AG, Spivak D, and Teitelbaum DH. An analysis of the morbidity and mortality of short-bowel syndrome in the pediatric age group. *Eur J Pediatr Surg* 1999;9:228–30.

30. Carter BA and Shulman RJ. Mechanisms of disease: Update on the molecular etiology and fundamentals of parenteral nutrition associated cholestasis. *Nat Clin Pract Gastroenterol Hepatol* 2007;4:277–87.

31. Kelly DA. Liver complications of pediatric parenteral nutrition—Epidemiology. *Nutrition* 1998;14:153–7.

32. Hermans D, Talbotec C, Lacaille F, Goulet O, Ricour C, and Colomb V. Early central catheter infections may contribute to hepatic fibrosis in children receiving long-term parenteral nutrition. *J Pediatr Gastroenterol Nutr* 2007;44:459–63.

33. Sokol RJ and Stall C. Anthropometric evaluation of children with chronic liver disease. *Am J Clin Nutr* 1990;52:203–8.

34. Wu J, Tang Q, Feng Y, Huang J, Tao Y, Wang Y, Cai W, and Shi C. Nutrition assessment in children with short bowel syndrome weaned off parenteral nutrition: A long-term follow-up study. *J Pediatr Surg* 2007;42:1372–6.

35. Nightingale J and Woodward JM. Guidelines for management of patients with a short bowel. *Gut* 2006;55(Suppl 4):iv1–12.

36. Koletzko B, Goulet O, Hunt J, Krohn K, and Shamir R. 1. Guidelines on Paediatric Parenteral Nutrition of the European Society of Paediatric Gastroenterology, Hepatology and Nutrition (ESPGHAN) and the European Society for Clinical Nutrition and Metabolism (ESPEN), Supported by the European Society of Paediatric Research (ESPR). *J Pediatr Gastroenterol Nutr* 2005;41(Suppl 2):S1–87.

37. Dahlstrom KA, Ament ME, Medhin MG, and Meurling S. Serum trace elements in children receiving long-term parenteral nutrition. *J Pediatr* 1986;109:625–30.

38. Papageorgiou T, Zacharoulis D, Xenos D, and Androulakis G. Determination of trace elements (Cu, Zn, Mn, Pb) and magnesium by atomical absorption in patients receiving total parenteral nutrition. *Nutrition* 2002;18:32–4.

39. Lowe NM, Fekete K, and Decsi T. Methods of assessment of zinc status in humans: A systematic review. *Am J Clin Nutr* 2009;89:2040S–2051S.

40. Hooper L, Ashton K, Harvey LJ, Decsi T, and Fairweather-Tait SJ. Assessing potential biomarkers of micronutrient status by using a systematic review methodology: Methods. *Am J Clin Nutr* 2009;89:1953S–1959S.

41. Harvey LJ, Ashton K, Hooper L, Casgrain A, and Fairweather-Tait SJ. Methods of assessment of copper status in humans: A systematic review. *Am J Clin Nutr* 2009;89:2009S–2024S

42. Ashton K, Hooper L, Harvey LJ, Hurst R, Casgrain A, and Fairweather-Tait SJ. Methods of assessment of selenium status in humans: A systematic review. *Am J Clin Nutr* 2009;89:2025S–2039S.

43. Ristic-Medic D, Piskackova Z, Hooper L, Ruprich J, Casgrain A, Ashton K, Pavlovic M, and Glibetic M. Methods of assessment of iodine status in humans: A systematic review. *Am J Clin Nutr* 2009;89:2052S–2069S.

44. Duro D, Jaksic T, and Duggan C. Multiple micronutrient deficiencies in a child with short bowel syndrome and normal somatic growth. *J Pediatr Gastroenterol Nutr* 2008;46:461–4.

45. Leonberg BL, Chuang E, Eicher P, Tershakovec AM, Leonard L, and Stallings VA. Long-term growth and development in children after home parental nutrition. *J Pediatr* 1998;132:461–6.

46. Friedman Z, Shochat SJ, Maisels MJ, Marks KH, and Lamberth EL, Jr. Correction of essential fatty acid deficiency in newborn infants by cutaneous application of sunflower-seed oil. *Pediatrics* 1976;58:650–4.

47. Connor FL and Di Lorenzo C. Chronic intestinal pseudo-obstruction: Assessment and management. *Gastroenterology* 2006;130:S29–36.

48. Nightingale JM, Bartram CI, and Lennard-Jones JE. Length of residual small bowel after partial resection: Correlation between radiographic and surgical measurements. *Gastrointest Radiol* 1991;16:305–6.

49. Rossi L, Kadamba P, Hugosson C, De Vol EB, Habib Z, and Al-Nassar S. Pediatric short bowel syndrome: Adaptation after massive small bowel resection. *J Pediatr Gastroenterol Nutr* 2007;45:213–21.

50. Santarpia L, Catanzano F, Ruoppolo M, Alfonsi L, Vitale DF, Pecce R, Pasanisi F, Contaldo F, and Salvatore F. Citrulline blood levels as indicators of residual intestinal absorption in patients with short bowel syndrome. *Ann Nutr Metab* 2008;53:137–42.

51. Crenn P, Coudray-Lucas C, Thuillier F, Cynober L, and Messing B. Postabsorptive plasma citrulline concentration is a marker of absorptive enterocyte mass and intestinal failure in humans. *Gastroenterology* 2000;119:1496–505.

52. Crenn P, De Truchis P, Neveux N, Galperine T, Cynober L, and Melchior JC. Plasma citrulline is a bio-marker of enterocyte mass and an indicator of parenteral nutrition in HIV-infected patients. *Am J Clin Nutr* 2009;90:587–94.

53. Crenn P, Messing B, and Cynober L. Citrulline as a biomarker of intestinal failure due to enterocyte mass reduction. *Clin Nutr* 2008;27:328–39.

54. Crenn P, Vahedi K, Lavergne-Slove A, Cynober L, Matuchansky C, and Messing B. Plasma citrulline: A marker of enterocyte mass in villous atrophy-associated small bowel disease. *Gastroenterology* 2003;124:1210–9.

55. Fitzgibbons S, Ching YA, Valim C, Zhou J, Iglesias J, Duggan C, and Jaksic T. Relationship between serum citrulline levels and progression to parenteral nutrition independence in children with short bowel syndrome. *J Pediatr Surg* 2009;44:928–32.

56. Bailly-Botuha C, Colomb V, Thioulouse E, Berthe MC, Garcette K, Dubern B, Goulet O, Couderc R, and Girardet JP. Plasma citrulline concentration reflects enterocyte mass in children with short bowel syndrome. *Pediatr Res* 2009;65:559–63.

57. Celik Y and Celik F. Serum citrulline levels in infants with short bowel syndrome. *J Pediatr* 2006;148:848; author reply 848–9.

58. Rhoads JM, Plunkett E, Galanko J, Lichtman S, Taylor L, Maynor A, Weiner T, Freeman K, Guarisco JL, and Wu GY. Serum citrulline levels correlate with enteral tolerance and bowel length in infants with short bowel syndrome. *J Pediatr* 2005;146:542–7.

59. Jianfeng G, Weiming Z, Ning L, Fangnan L, Li T, Nan L, and Jieshou L. Serum citrulline is a simple quantitative marker for small intestinal enterocytes mass and absorption function in short bowel patients. *J Surg Res* 2005;127:177–82.

60. Colomb V, Dabbas-Tyan M, Taupin P, Talbotec C, Révillon Y, Jan D, De Potter S et al. Long-term outcome of children receiving home parenteral nutrition: A 20-year single-center experience in 302 patients. *J Pediatr Gastroenterol Nutr* 2007;44:347–53.

61. Diamanti A, Basso MS, Castro M, Calce A, Pietrobattista A, and Gambarara M. Prevalence of life-threatening complications in pediatric patients affected by intestinal failure. *Transplant Proc* 2007;39:1632–3.

62. Hodge D and Puntis JW. Diagnosis, prevention, and management of catheter related bloodstream infection during long term parenteral nutrition. *Arch Dis Child Fetal Neonatal Ed* 2002;87:F21–4.

63. Kurkchubasche AG, Smith SD, and Rowe MI. Catheter sepsis in short-bowel syndrome. *Arch Surg* 1992;127:21–4; discussion 24–5.

64. Terra RM, Plopper C, Waitzberg DL, Cukier C, Santoro S, Martins JR, Song RJ, and Gama-Rodrigues J. Remaining small bowel length: Association with catheter sepsis in patients receiving home total parenteral nutrition: Evidence of bacterial translocation. *World J Surg* 2000;24:1537–41.

65. Piedra PA, Dryja DM, and LaScolea LJ, Jr. Incidence of catheter-associated gram-negative bacteremia in children with short bowel syndrome. *J Clin Microbiol* 1989;27:1317–9.

66. Moukarzel AA, Haddad I, Ament ME, Buchman AL, Reyen L, Maggioni A, Baron HI, and Vargas J. 230 patient years of experience with home long-term parenteral nutrition in childhood: Natural history and life of central venous catheters. *J Pediatr Surg* 1994;29:1323–7.

67. Rodrigues AF, van Mourik ID, Sharif K, Barron DJ, de Giovanni JV, Bennett J, Bromley P et al. Management of end-stage central venous access in children referred for possible small bowel transplantation. *J Pediatr Gastroenterol Nutr* 2006;42:427–33.

68. Zambrano E, El-Hennawy M, Ehrenkranz RA, Zelterman D, and Reyes-Mugica M. Total parenteral nutrition induced liver pathology: An autopsy series of 24 newborn cases. *Pediatr Dev Pathol* 2004;7:425–32.

69. Duro D, Duggan C, Valim C, Bechard L, Fitzgibbons S, Jaksic T, and Yu YM. Novel intravenous (13) C-methionine breath test as a measure of liver function in children with short bowel syndrome. *J Pediatr Surg* 2009;44:236–40; discussion 240.

70. Guha IN and Rosenberg WM. Noninvasive assessment of liver fibrosis: Serum markers, imaging, and other modalities. *Clin Liver Dis* 2008;12:883–900.

71. Manning DS and Afdhal NH. Diagnosis and quantitation of fibrosis. *Gastroenterology* 2008;134:1670–81.
72. Dellert SF, Farrell MK, Specker BL, and Heubi JE. Bone mineral content in children with short bowel syndrome after discontinuation of parental nutrition. *J Pediatr* 1998;132:516–9.
73. Petersen C. D-Lactic acidosis. *Nutr Clin Pract* 2005;20:634–45.
74. Taylor SF, Sondheimer JM, Sokol RJ, Silverman A, and Wilson HL. Noninfectious colitis associated with short gut syndrome in infants. *J Pediatr* 1991;119:24–8.
75. Sondheimer JM, Sokol RJ, Narkewicz MR, and Tyson RW. Anastomotic ulceration: A late complication of ileocolonic anastomosis. *J Pediatr* 1995;127:225–30.

# 5 Clinical Assessment of Intestinal Failure in Adults

*Kuang Horng (Jamie) Kang and George Blackburn*

## CONTENTS

## 5.1 ADULT INTESTINAL FAILURE OVERVIEW

Intestinal failure (IF) is defined as the inability of the alimentary tract to digest or absorb nutrients to sustain normal growth and health in life [1]. Similar to children, in which necrotizing enterocolitis requiring multiple bowel resections is the leading cause for IF, 75% of cases of short bowel syndrome in adults occur from massive intestinal resection [2]. In adults, IF is most commonly associated with recurrent Crohn's disease and accounts for ~25% of patients. Other causes include: mesenteric occlusion or injuries, radiation enteritis, midgut volvulus, and traumatic injury of the bowel [3]. In addition, motility disorders and intestinal neoplasms can also cause functional IF in adults [4] (see Table 5.1).

## 5.2 REVERSIBLE VERSUS IRREVERSIBLE IF

When assessing an adult patient with IF, it is important to determine whether the failure is likely to be permanent. Ultimately this may affect the timing of referral for intestinal transplant. Factors associated with reversibility of IF include the length of bowel resected, the area of bowel resected, the amount of functional bowel length remaining, age at initiation of PN and enteral dependence (Table 5.2) [5,6].

It is difficult to predict the reversibility of IF based solely upon the measure of residual bowel length. The small intestine achieves its maximum length of 600–800 cm in adulthood. Unlike the bowel in children, especially neonates, which continues to grow in length with time until at least 4 years of age, the adult small intestine adapts mostly by dilatation [7]. Surgeons generally classify intestinal resection into one of three categories after measuring the residual length of the small intestine along the antimesenteric border. As noted in Table 5.3, a short resection leaves more than 100–150 cm of small intestine; a large resection leaves between 40 and 100 cm; and a massive resection leaves <40 cm [5]. A 1999 study conducted by Messing et al. [8] showed that a residual

### TABLE 5.1
### Common Causes of IF in Adults

Massive bowel resection
Crohn's disease
Radiation enteritis
Superior mesenteric artery thrombosis
Trauma
Motility disorders
Neoplasms

### TABLE 5.2
### Factors Associated with Reversibility of IF

Bowel length resected
Bowel part resected
Functional bowel length remaining
Age at the initiation of PN
Enteral dependence

### TABLE 5.3
### Impact of Resection Size on Residual Bowel Length

| Category | Remaining Small Bowel Length after Resection |
|---|---|
| Short resection | 100–150 cm |
| Large resection | 40–100 cm |
| Massive resection | <40 cm |

small bowel length of <100 cm is highly predictive of permanent IF in adult patients with short bowel syndrome. In other words, patients with a large and massive resection are at greatest risk for irreversible IF.

Several etiologies of IF are known to cause permanent PN dependence regardless of bowel length. Neuromuscular diseases involving the gastrointestinal tract such as total aganglionosis or chronic intestinal pseudo-obstruction can render patients with normal length of small bowel on long-term PN [5]. According to a study conducted by Vantini et al., of the 68 subjects studied with intestinal insufficiency, excluding those with ultrashort bowel (<50 cm), it was reported that long-term PN use was more frequently required in patients with chronic intestinal pseudo-obstruction [6].

Outcome of bowel adaptation may vary depending on the part of bowel resected or remaining. Presence of ileum, colon, and ileocecal valve (ICV) have been shown to bring favorable outcomes after massive bowel resection [9]. Generally, absorption takes place along the length of the small intestine. According to work conducted by Borgstron and colleagues and by Johansson, about 90% of digestion and absorption of significant macro- and micronutrients occur in the proximal 100–150 cm of jejunum [10,11]. This may be secondary to the taller villi, deeper crypts, and greater enzyme activity found in jejunum as compared to ileum [12]. However, absorption of proteins, carbohydrates, and most vitamins and minerals can be unaffected because of ileal adaptation that occurs even after extensive jejunal resection [13]. On the other hand, ileal resection can have deleterious effects to water and electrolyte absorption. As the ileum serves as an important site for bile salt and vitamin B12 absorption, ileal resection often leads to diarrahea requiring aggressive fluid supplementation, fat malabsorption, steatorrhea, and loss of fat-soluble vitamins. Preservation of colon may have positive attributes in adult patients. As shown by Philips and Giller, water absorption in colon can increase to 5 times its normal capacity after small bowel resection [14]. The residual bacteria in the colon has the inherent capacity to metabolize undigested carbohydrates into short fatty acids, the preferred fuel source for the colon. Interestingly, it was found that colon can absorb up to 500 kcal of these metabolites daily [15]. Retention of the ICV is believed to slow down transit time, allowing more time for absorption. Moreover, the presence of an ICV may decrease the possibility of bacterial colonization of small bowel from colon. However, a large clinical trial has not been done to validate this claim.

Interestingly, patients whose PN is initated before 45 years of age have been shown to have a longer life expectancy [6]. In that study, survival rates were significantly higher in those who started PN before 45 years of age. The 4-year actuarial survival rate for those below and those above 45 years of age was 100% and 44%, respectively [6]. Longer survival allows more time for bowel adaptation and achievement of enteral autonomy.

Last but not least, tolerance to enteral feedings is a favorable predictor in the reversibility of IF and is correlated with better survival rate and time [6]. Oral and enteral feeding stimulate the secretion of enterotrophic hormones, including gastrin, cholecystokinin and neurotensin, which may potentially promote bowel adaptation. Additionally, enteral feedings enhance absoption by permiting total saturation of the transporters within the bowel [16,17].

## 5.3 CONSIDERATIONS IN ASSESSING ADULTS WITH IF

Not all IF is permanent. Studies in France found that 75% of adults with nonmalignant IF eventually achieved intestinal autonomy, a majority of them within their first 2 years of diagnosis [18]. Another study conducted in 2004 showed that enteral independence can be achieved in time by about 40% of patients with IF [6]. This is because bowel adaptation takes place after resection, hence making IF reversible [9]. Thus, careful assessment and management of patients with reversible IF are crucial in sustaining their lives, thereby allowing bowel adaptation and full intestinal autonomy to be achieved (see Table 5.4).

### 5.3.1 ASSESSMENT OF NUTRITION

Nutritional status of adult patients should be assessed by accurate measurement of weight and height on a regular basis. For patients on PN, these measurements, together with urine dipstick for glucose,

**TABLE 5.4**
**Considerations in Assessing Adults with IF**

Nutrition
Hydration
Bowel adaptation
PN-associated complications
PNALD
CRBSI
Other IF-related factors
SIBO
Metabolic bone disease
Calcium oxalate nephrolithiasis
D-Lactic acidosis

should be obtained and recorded by patients on a daily basis [19]. In addition, mid-arm circumference and triceps skin-fold thickness should be measured periodically during follow-up in addition to other growth benchmarks, especially in patients with chronic liver disease. This is because these patients can have normal or even increased weight secondary to organomegaly and/or ascites [20]. Routine laboratory work should include serum complete blood count, electrolytes, albumin, liver/biliary function markers (hepatic enzymes, bilirubin, and prothrombin time), phosphorus, magnesium, and calcium. In PN-dependent patients, these studies are usually performed weekly and then monthly as the patient stabilizes [21]. With long-term PN therapy, iron deficiency may occur and require supplementation; serum iron, ferritin, and iron-binding capacity should be followed. Moreover, data by Dahlstrom et al. [22] demonstrated decreased serum levels of trace elements in asymptomatic patients on prolonged PN as compared to age-matched controls. Therefore, periodic laboratory surveillance should include serum level of copper, zinc, manganese, chromium, and selenium [23–25]. Serum trace elements should be checked initially and then every 6 months. If deficiency is detected, however, laboratory monitoring should be more frequent, especially after supplementation has been initiated to assess responsiveness to the therapy. Moreover, while weaning patients off PN, periodic monitoring of micronutrient status is still warranted.

Although standard PN formulations routinely contain vitamins, but there are certain disease states (e.g., cholestasis or pancreatic insufficiency) or postsurgical anatomy that can predispose patients to lose additional fat-soluble and water-soluble vitamins. Despite supplementation, serum levels of fat-soluble vitamins (A, D, E, and K) should be monitored regularly. For patients on continuous PN, water-soluble vitamins levels should be obtained if deficiency is suspected during clinical assessment. In patients who underwent ileal resection, vitamin B12 levels should be closely monitored [26–28].

Most patients on PN will also receive fat-emulsion infusion. Serum triglyceride and cholesterol levels should be followed in these patients. Additionally, monitoring essential fatty acid profiles is recommended for patients who are receiving an omega-3 fatty acid-based lipid as monotherapy or those patients with significant fat malabsorption who have been weaned off parenteral lipids [29].

## 5.3.2 Assessment of Hydration

The gastrointestinal tract processes about 8–9 L of fluid per day, with most of this derived from endogenous secretions. A healthy gastrointestinal tract is capable of reabsorbing the majority of this fluid (98%) and only 100–200 mL is lost in fecal matter each day. Of note, 80% of this reabsorption takes place in the small intestine [30]. Therefore, assessment of hydration status for patients with short bowel syndrome should consider fluid loss from stool, stoma, or nasogastric tube. Serum electrolyte levels should be followed closely. However, a urine sodium level is actually a more accurate estimate of total body sodium content than serum values [31].

## 5.3.3 Assessment of Bowel Adaptation

Intestinal physiology changes take place immediately after resection and is generally divided by three phases, namely an acute phase, an adaptation phase, and a maintenance phase [32]. Progress of adaptation should be monitored during follow-up. Contrast radiography may be used as a tool to assess length, dilatation, and motility of the bowel. By using barium follow-through, Nightingale et al. [33] demonstrated a correlation between radiographic and surgical measurement of small bowel length in 18 adult patients with short bowel syndrome. Since stagnant and dilated loops of bowel may precipitate small intestinal bacterial overgrowth (SIBO), bowel dilatation estimation by contrast radiography may play a role in predicting such overgrowth. Furthermore, imaging from contrast studies can also provide a road map for a tapering and lengthening procedure.

Progress in enteral tolerance is a reliable indicator of bowel adaptation. To enhance enteral nutrition, enteral access including gastrostomy tube, gastro-jejunal tube, or jejunal feeding tube should be considered in patients unable to tolerate adequate oral intake. Furthermore, patients with oral aversion should be referred to an appropriate therapist for prompt rehabilitation [34].

A novel means of assessing the absorptive capacity of the small intestine is the use of serum citrulline levels. Citrulline is a nonessential amino acid synthesized almost exclusively in entero-cytes and its serum level has been shown to correlate with functional small bowel enterocyte mass and absorptive capacity [35–38]. Hence, serum citrulline levels may serve as a biomarker for intes-tinal function in patients with IF [39]. Chapter 31, Assessment of Mucosal Mass and Hormonal Therapy, discusses this topic in greater detail.

### 5.3.4 Assessment of PN-Associated Complications

Similar to pediatric patients, one of the most common causes of death in adults with short bowel syndrome is parenteral-nutrition–associated liver disease (PNALD) [40]. Chemical and histological changes have been described in about 1.4–15% of patients with chronic IF who require PN [41–44]. Besides routine physical examination to evaluate for hepatomegaly or splenomegaly, regular labora-tory assessment should include liver function tests (alanine aminotransferase, aspartate aminotrans-ferase [AST], total bilirubin) and other liver function markers such as albumin levels and prothrombin time. Persistent elevation of hepatobiliary enzymes should prompt investigations including abdomi-nal sonogram to examine biliary anatomy, a review of all medications, and assessment of the com-position of PN and fat emulsion. A liver biopsy should be obtained when other investigations are inconclusive or when the patient undergoes a surgical procedure. A study published in 2003 demon-strated that AST-to-platelet ratio index could predict significant fibrosis and cirrhosis in 51% and 81% of patients with chronic hepatitis C, respectively [45]. However, this index is not widely used in patients with PNALD as fibrosis and cirrhosis are both late findings of this complication. Detection should be made at an early stage so that prompt intervention can take place to prevent disease pro-gression or even to reverse the damage.

The need for PN in patients with IF has led to an increased use of indwelling central venous catheters (CVCs). Catheter-related blood stream infection (CRBSI) and thrombotic events are the common complications associated with these devices. According to one Italian study, the incidence of CRBSI among home parenteral nutrition (HPN) patients was 0.30/year with an incidence of venous thrombosis of 0.05/year in patients with chronic IF [46]. Recent evidence suggests that patients with IF may be predisposed to this common complication. Data have shown that IF patients receiving long-term PN have decreased splenic function and tufsin deficiency, thereby weakening their immunological defenses [47–49]. Tufsin is a physiologic tetrapeptide which has been shown to possess immunoadjuvant properties including the stimulation of macrophage and granulocyte phagocytosis, migration, bactericidal, and tumoricidal activities [50]. Therefore, function of the CVC and its placement site should be examined thoroughly during assessment. Common signs and symptoms of CRBSI include fever, lethargy, redness, or tenderness around insertion site or along the catheter tract and purulent discharge from the catheter insertion site. If CRBSI is suspected, blood cultures should be obtained from both a peripheral venous site and through the catheter. If catheter preservation is not possible, the tip of the CVC should be cultured upon removal. If resis-tance is encountered when infusing fluid into the CVC or there is difficulty in withdrawing blood from the catheter, thrombosis or catheter misplacement should be suspected. A chest x-ray and a vascular sonogram can help with the diagnosis (see Chapters 19, Central Venous Catheter Infections: Prevention and Treatment, and 26, Central Venous Catheter Care).

### 5.3.5 Other IF-Related Complications

Malabsorption of calcium, phosphorus, and vitamin D can lead to metabolic bone disease in patients with IF [51]. In 1980, Klein described an unusual metabolic bone disease characterized by insidious onset of severe bone pain in 11 adults with chronic IF receiving PN for more than 3 months. All 11 patients had normal serum levels of calcium, phosphorus, 25-hydroxy-vitamin D, and parathyroid hormone at that time. However, low bone turnover and patchy osteomalacia were seen on histomorphometric analysis of bone biopsy specimens [52]. Based on these observations, in addition to serological tests, bone mineral content should be monitored periodically by dual-energy x-ray absorptiometry (see Chapter 22, Osteopenia and Bone Health in Patients with Intestinal Failure).

Preservation of the colon after small bowel resection in adults increases the incidence of urinary calcium oxalate stone formation. Oxalate usually binds to calcium in the small intestine, making it insoluble in the colon. After small bowel resection, most of this calcium binds to free intraluminal fats, leaving free oxalate to be absorbed in the colon. Saturation of urine with calcium oxalate can eventually lead to nephrolithiasis [31]. A urinalysis and a KUB should therefore be obtained in patients presenting with hematuria and persistent back pain.

Bowel dilatation and dysmotility in patients with IF predispose them to the colonization bacteria in the small intestine [53]. Studies have shown that SIBO is a negative factor for bowel adaptation, and can lead to prolonged PN dependence [54]. Patients usually present with diarrhea or vomiting, oral or enteral intolerance, excessive ostomy output, and failure to thrive despite maximal nutritional support. These symptoms, however, can also be attributed to other complications of IF. Work-up should include a stool culture and detection of *Clostridium difficile* toxin, contrast study to evaluate for obstruction and careful clinical examination to look for CRBSI. There are a variety of noninvasive breath tests available for the diagnosis of SIBO, including $C_{14}$-glycocholic acid, glucose hydrogen, lactulose, lactose, $C_{14}$-xylose, and $C_{13}$-xylose [55]. However, endoscopy with culture of jejunal aspirate remains the gold standard diagnostic test for SIBO (see Chapter 24, Bacterial Overgrowth of the Small Intestine). The presence of microorganism of more than $10^4$ CFU/mL of jejunal aspirate is diagnostic [56,57].

Altered mental status, ataxia, nystagmus, and muscle weakness are some of the neurological symptoms that should alert a clinician of D-lactic acidosis in patients with IF [58]. After bowel resection, poorly absorbed carbohydrates serve as substrate for D-lactate-producing bacteria and lead to high level of colonic D-lactic acid. This excessive amount of lactic acid is then absorbed into circulation, causing D-lactic acidosis [59,60]. A serum level of D-lactate >3 mmol/L is diagnostic [61]. A urinary D-lactate assay may be used when serum assay is not available [62,63].

## 5.4   QUALITY OF LIFE ON HPN

HPN has made it possible for patients with IF who need PN to be discharged from the hospital. An individual on HPN is a "technology-dependent person," federally defined as someone who needs both a medical device to compensate for the loss of a vital body function and substantial, ongoing nursing care to avoid death or disability [64]. Administration of HPN requires time and skills, which can in turn affect daily lifestyle of a patient and his or her family [65]. Thus, quality of life (QOL) on HPN becomes one of the key components in assessing adults with IF. According to a study conducted on adult patients with IF receiving HPN, most perceived HPN as a "lifeline" and "nutritional safety net." Many were frustrated by the need to be on HPN, but at the same time, they also understood how necessary PN is to sustain their lives [66]. The World Health Organization clarifies that QOL is not merely the absence of disease or infirmity but that health is a resource for everyday life, influenced by social and personal resources, as well as physical capabilities. Many adults on HPN secondary to IF defined QOL as "enjoying life," "being happy, satisfied, or content with life," and "being able to do what you want to do when you want to do it" [66]. In contrast to literature reporting poor QOL for individuals on HPN compared to normal population or to others who have chronic health conditions [67,68], individuals with IF described their QOL as "good" and "wonderful" [66]. In addition, Persoon et al. demonstrated that HPN-dependent individuals were able to attribute physical symptoms to their underlying diseases and psychosocial problems to PN dependency [69]. There are a number of factors affecting QOL of an adult patient receiving HPN, which include problems from underlying diseases, PN dependence, inability to eat, family coping skills, and financial instability [66,70]. Chapters 32,

---

**TABLE 5.5**

**Factors Affecting QOL of Adult Patients Receiving Home PN**

Symptoms or physical problems from underlying diseases

Presence of an ostomy

Unpredictable diarrhea

Abdominal pain

PN dependence

Long duration on PN

Infusion schedule

Inability to eat

Social restrictions

Family coping skills

Financial instability

---

Home Parenteral and Enteral Nutrition in Adults and Children, and 33, Health Related Quality of Life, discuss these matters in greater detail. Table 5.5 summarizes the factors impacting the QOL in adult HPN patients.

The Oley Foundation (Chapter 38, Support Groups) is a national, independent, nonprofit organization founded by Dr. Lyn Howard and her patient, Clarence "Oley" Oldenburg in 1983. This foundation provides information and psychosocial support to patients on HPN and home enteral nutrition (HEN) (home enteral nutrition) and also serves as a resource for patients' families to meet others (http://www.oley.org/programs.html). Participants in one study reported receiving better information from other people receiving HPN than from their doctors [66].

In summary, healthcare professionals should prepare their patients physically, psychologically and socially to live with HPN. An individual's personal definition of QOL and factors influencing his or her QOL should be discussed at the initiation of HPN and throughout its course. In addition, connecting individuals to others with a similar experience or to the Oley Foundation should also be considered.

## 5.5 REFERRAL TO TRANSPLANT

Early referral to transplant should be made if permanent IF is highly suspected. Liver and small bowel transplantation is recommended for individuals with irreversible liver injury and IF (Chapter 17). Improvements in intestinal transplant outcomes have been made by advances in surgical technique, refinements in recipient selection criteria and organ allocation, identification and management of previously unrecognized complications, standardized grading of rejection and better understanding of transplant immunology [71]. The 1-year survival rate for patients undergoing intestinal transplantation after 1995 was ~65%, and the 1-year graft survival rate was 60%. Data analysis from the International Transplant Registry revealed that the factors significant for determining outcome included center size and type of allograft. Transplantation centers where more than 10 intestinal transplantations were performed had better survival. A patient survival advantage was also noted for those patients receiving either an isolated small bowel transplantation or liver-small bowel transplantation compared with those receiving a multivisceral transplant. However, there is no apparent survival advantage conferred by the use of living-related donors [72]. The International Transplant Registry and several large centers have shown that 77–93% of surviving recipients remain independent of PN beyond 6–12 months after transplant [72–74].

Indications to refer an adult patient for transplant are similar to that of a pediatric patient, with PNALD being the most common condition [75]. Other indications are irreversible IF with exhaustion of vascular access, life-threatening sepsis associated with CRBSI and cases of IF that usually lead to early death such as ultra-short bowel, refractory diarrhea, and PN incompliance [76]. Table 5.6 lists

**TABLE 5.6**

**Indications for Intestinal and Multivisceral Transplantation**

Impending or overt liver disease

Thrombosis of major central venous channels (two thromboses in subclavian, jugular, or femoral veins)

Frequent CRBSI related sepsis (two episodes of systemic sepsis secondary to line infection per year,
  one episode of line related fungemia, septic shock, or acute respiratory distress syndrome)

Frequent severe dehydration

*Source:* Adapted from Mailloux RJ, DeLegge MH, and Kirby DF. *JPEN J Parenter Enteral Nutr*
1993;17:578–82; Farmer DG. et al., *Transplant Proc* 2002;34:896–7.

the indications in which Medicare has approved payment for intestinal transplant in patients who fail PN therapy.

## 5.6  SUMMARY

The majority of adult patients with IF will eventually achieve enteral autonomy. Intestinal rehabilitation therefore plays a significant role in reaching that goal. More research should be done to improve assessment of reversibility, prevention, and treatment of PN-associated complications and other IF related complications. With the advancement in surgical techniques and immunosuppression therapy, intestinal transplant may become a practical alternative to treat IF in near future.

## REFERENCES

1. Beath S, Pironi L, Gabe S. et al., Collaborative strategies to reduce mortality and morbidity in patients with chronic intestinal failure including those who are referred for small bowel transplantation. *Transplantation* 2008;85:1378–84.
2. Casey L, Lee KH, Rosychuk R, Turner J, and Huynh HQ. 10-year review of pediatric intestinal failure: Clinical factors associated with outcome. *Nutr Clin Pract* 2008;23:436–42.
3. Scolapio JS and Fleming CR. Short bowel syndrome. *Gastroenterol Clin North Am* 1998;27:467–79, viii.
4. Moreno JM, Planas M, Lecha M. et al., The year 2002 national register on home-based parenteral nutrition. *Nutr Hosp* 2005;20:249–53.
5. Goulet O, Ruemmele F, Lacaille F, and Colomb V. Irreversible intestinal failure. *J Pediatr Gastroenterol Nutr* 2004;38:250–69.
6. Vantini I, Benini L, Bonfante F. et al., Survival rate and prognostic factors in patients with intestinal failure. *Dig Liver Dis* 2004;36:46–55.
7. Ulshen MTW, editor. *Small Intestine.* New York City: Lippincott Williams and Wilkins; 2004.
8. Messing B, Crenn P, Beau P, Boutron-Ruault MC, Rambaud JC, and Matuchansky C. Long-term survival and parenteral nutrition dependence in adult patients with the short bowel syndrome. *Gastroenterology* 1999;117:1043–50.
9. Weale AR, Edwards AG, Bailey M, and Lear PA. Intestinal adaptation after massive intestinal resection. *Postgrad Med J* 2005;81:178–84.
10. Borgstrom B, Dahlqvist A, Lundh G, and Sjovall J. Studies of intestinal digestion and absorption in the human. *J Clin Invest* 1957;36:1521–36.
11. Johansson C. Studies of gastrointestinal interactions. VII. Characteristics of the absorption pattern of sugar, fat and protein from composite meals in man. A quantitative study. *Scand J Gastroenterol* 1975;10:33–42.
12. Clarke RM. Mucosal architecture and epithelial cell production rate in the small intestine of the albino rat. *J Anat* 1970;107:519–29.
13. Vanderhoof JA and Langnas AN. Short-bowel syndrome in children and adults. *Gastroenterology* 1997;113:1767–78.
14. Phillips SF and Giller J. The contribution of the colon to electrolyte and water conservation in man. *J Lab Clin Med* 1973;81:733–46.

15. Pomare EW, Branch WJ, and Cummings JH. Carbohydrate fermentation in the human colon and its relation to acetate concentrations in venous blood. *J Clin Invest* 1985;75:1448–54.
16. Jeppesen PB and Mortensen PB. Enhancing bowel adaptation in short bowel syndrome. *Curr Gastroenterol Rep* 2002;4:338–47.
17. Sham J, Martin G, Meddings JB, and Sigalet DL. Epidermal growth factor improves nutritional outcome in a rat model of short bowel syndrome. *J Pediatr Surg* 2002;37:765–9.
18. Carbonnel F, Cosnes J, Chevret S. et al., The role of anatomic factors in nutritional autonomy after extensive small bowel resection. *JPEN J Parenter Enteral Nutr* 1996;20:275–80.
19. Shatnawei A, Parekh NR, Rhoda KM. et al., Intestinal failure management at the Cleveland Clinic. *Arch Surg* 2010;145:521–7.
20. Sokol RJ and Stall C. Anthropometric evaluation of children with chronic liver disease. *Am J Clin Nutr* 1990;52:203–8.
21. Sacks G, editor. *Parenteral Nutrition Implementation and Management*. 2nd ed. Silver Spring: American Society For Parenteral and Enteral Nutrition; 2005.
22. Dahlstrom KA, Ament ME, Medhin MG, and Meurling S. Serum trace elements in children receiving long-term parenteral nutrition. *J Pediatr* 1986;109:625–30.
23. Koletzko B, Goulet O, Hunt J, Krohn K, and Shamir R.1. Guidelines on paediatric parenteral nutrition of the European Society of Paediatric Gastroenterology, Hepatology and Nutrition (ESPGHAN) and the European Society for Clinical Nutrition and Metabolism (ESPEN), supported by the European Society of Paediatric Research (ESPR). *J Pediatr Gastroenterol Nutr* 2005;41(Suppl 2):S1–87.
24. Papageorgiou T, Zacharoulis D, Xenos D, and Androulakis G. Determination of trace elements (Cu, Zn, Mn, Pb) and magnesium by atomical absorption in patients receiving total parenteral nutrition. *Nutrition* 2002;18:32–4.
25. Lowe NM, Fekete K, and Decsi T. Methods of assessment of zinc status in humans: A systematic review. *Am J Clin Nutr* 2009;89:2040S–51S.
26. Wu J, Tang Q, Feng Y. et al., Nutrition assessment in children with short bowel syndrome weaned off parenteral nutrition: A long-term follow-up study. *J Pediatr Surg* 2007;42:1372–6.
27. Duro D, Jaksic T, and Duggan C. Multiple micronutrient deficiencies in a child with short bowel syndrome and normal somatic growth. *J Pediatr Gastroenterol Nutr* 2008;46:461–4.
28. Leonberg BL, Chuang E, Eicher P, Tershakovec AM, Leonard L, and Stallings VA. Long-term growth and development in children after home parental nutrition. *J Pediatr* 1998;132:461–6.
29. Friedman Z, Danon A, Stahlman MT, and Oates JA. Rapid onset of essential fatty acid deficiency in the newborn. *Pediatrics* 1976;58:640–9.
30. Sellin J, editor. *Intestinal Electrolyte Absoption and Secretion*, 6th ed. Philadelphia: W.B. Saunders Co; 1998.
31. Nightingale J and Woodward JM. Guidelines for management of patients with a short bowel. *Gut* 2006;55(Suppl 4):iv1–12.
32. Sundaram A, Koutkia P, and Apovian CM. Nutritional management of short bowel syndrome in adults. *J Clin Gastroenterol* 2002;34:207–20.
33. Nightingale JM, Bartram CI, and Lennard-Jones JE. Length of residual small bowel after partial resection: Correlation between radiographic and surgical measurements. *Gastrointest Radiol* 1991;16:305–6.
34. Soden JS. Clinical assessment of the child with intestinal failure. *Semin Pediatr Surg* 2010;19:10–9.
35. Santarpia L, Catanzano F, Ruoppolo M. et al., Citrulline blood levels as indicators of residual intestinal absorption in patients with short bowel syndrome. *Ann Nutr Metab* 2008;53:137–42.
36. Crenn P, Coudray-Lucas C, Thuillier F, Cynober L, and Messing B. Postabsorptive plasma citrulline concentration is a marker of absorptive enterocyte mass and intestinal failure in humans. *Gastroenterology* 2000;119:1496–505.
37. Celik Y and Celik F. Serum citrulline levels in infants with short bowel syndrome. *J Pediatr* 2006;148:848; author reply-9.
38. Bailly-Botuha C, Colomb V, Thioulouse E. et al., Plasma citrulline concentration reflects enterocyte mass in children with short bowel syndrome. *Pediatr Res* 2009;65:559–63.
39. Jianfeng G, Weiming Z, Ning L. et al., Serum citrulline is a simple quantitative marker for small intestinal enterocytes mass and absorption function in short bowel patients. *J Surg Res* 2005;127:177–82.
40. Raman M and Allard JP. Parenteral nutrition related hepato-biliary disease in adults. *Appl Physiol Nutr Metab* 2007;32:646–54.
41. Messing B, Lemann M, Landais P. et al., Prognosis of patients with nonmalignant chronic intestinal failure receiving long-term home parenteral nutrition. *Gastroenterology* 1995;108:1005–10.
42. Pironi L, Miglioli M, Ruggeri E. et al., Home parenteral nutrition for the management of chronic intestinal failure: A 34 patient-year experience. *Ital J Gastroenterol* 1993;25:411–8.

43. Chan S, McCowen KC, Bistrian BR. et al., Incidence, prognosis, and etiology of end-stage liver disease in patients receiving home total parenteral nutrition. *Surgery* 1999;126:28–34.

44. Bowyer BA, Fleming CR, Ludwig J, Petz J, and McGill DB. Does long-term home parenteral nutrition in adult patients cause chronic liver disease? *JPEN J Parenter Enteral Nutr* 1985;9:11–7.

45. Wai CT, Greenson JK, Fontana RJ. et al., A simple noninvasive index can predict both significant fibrosis and cirrhosis in patients with chronic hepatitis C. *Hepatology* 2003;38:518–26.

46. Pironi L, Paganelli F, Labate AM. et al. Safety and efficacy of home parenteral nutrition for chronic intestinal failure: A 16-year experience at a single centre. *Dig Liver Dis* 2003;35:314–24.

47. Howard L, Heaphey L, Fleming CR, Lininger L, and Steiger E. Four years of North American registry home parenteral nutrition outcome data and their implications for patient management. *JPEN J Parenter Enteral Nutr* 1991;15:384–93.

48. Howard L, Ament M, Fleming CR, Shike M, and Steiger E. Current use and clinical outcome of home parenteral and enteral nutrition therapies in the United States. *Gastroenterology* 1995;109:355–65.

49. Zoli G, Corazza GR, Wood S, Bartoli R, Gasbarrini G, and Farthing MJG. Impaired splenic function and tuftsin deficiency in patients with intestinal failure on long term intravenous nutrition. *Gut* 1998;43:759–62.

50. Phillips JH, Babcock GF, and Nishioka K. Tuftsin: A naturally occurring immunopotentiating factor. I. *In vitro* enhancement of murine natural cell-mediated cytotoxicity. *J Immunol* 1981;126:915–21.

51. Dellert SF, Farrell MK, Specker BL, and Heubi JE. Bone mineral content in children with short bowel syndrome after discontinuation of parental nutrition. *J Pediatr* 1998;132:516–9.

52. Klein GL, Targoff CM, Ament ME. et al., Bone disease associated with total parenteral nutrition. *Lancet* 1980;2:1041–4.

53. Ziegler TR and Cole CR. Small bowel bacterial overgrowth in adults: A potential contributor to intestinal failure. *Curr Gastroenterol Rep* 2007;9:463–7.

54. Cole CR and Ziegler TR. Small bowel bacterial overgrowth: A negative factor in gut adaptation in pediatric SBS. *Curr Gastroenterol Rep* 2007;9:456–62.

55. Rana SV and Bhardwaj SB. Small intestinal bacterial overgrowth. *Scand J Gastroenterol* 2008;43:1030–7.

56. Justesen T, Nielsen OH, Jacobsen IE, Lave J, and Rasmussen SN. The normal cultivable microflora in upper jejunal fluid in healthy adults. *Scand J Gastroenterol* 1984;19:279–82.

57. Donaldson RM, Jr. Normal bacterial populations of the intestine and their relation to intestinal function. *N Engl J Med* 1964;270:1050–6; CONCL.

58. James PD, Black D, Kuper A, and Saibil F. D-Lactic acidosis and ataxia in a man with Crohn disease. *CMAJ* 2010;182:276–9.

59. Bakhru MR, Kumar A, and Aneja A. A 58-year-old woman with mental status changes. *Cleve Clin J Med* 2007;74:457–62.

60. Halperin ML and Kamel KS. D-Lactic acidosis: Turning sugar into acids in the gastrointestinal tract. *Kidney Int* 1996;49:1–8.

61. Uchida H, Yamamoto H, Kisaki Y, Fujino J, Ishimaru Y, and Ikeda H. D-Lactic acidosis in short-bowel syndrome managed with antibiotics and probiotics. *J Pediatr Surg* 2004;39:634–6.

62. Haschke-Becher E, Baumgartner M, and Bachmann C. Assay of D-lactate in urine of infants and children with reference values taking into account data below detection limit. *Clin Chim Acta* 2000;298:99–109.

63. Inoue Y, Shinka T, Ohse M. et al., Changes in urinary level and configuration ratio of D-lactic acid in patients with short bowel syndrome. *J Chromatogr B Analyt Technol Biomed Life Sci* 2007;855:109–14.

64. Smith CE. Quality of life and caregiving in technological home care. *Annu Rev Nurs Res* 1996;14:95–118.

65. Huisman-de Waal G, Schoonhoven L, Jansen J, Wanten G, and van Achterberg T. The impact of home parenteral nutrition on daily life-a review. *Clin Nutr* 2007;26:275–88.

66. Winkler MF, Hagan E, Wetle T, Smith C, Maillet JO, and Touger-Decker R. An exploration of quality of life and the experience of living with home parenteral nutrition. *JPEN J Parenter Enteral Nutr* 2010;34:395–407.

67. Richards DM and Irving MH. Assessing the quality of life of patients with intestinal failure on home parenteral nutrition. *Gut* 1997;40:218–22.

68. O'Keefe SJ, Emerling M, Koritsky D. et al., Nutrition and quality of life following small intestinal transplantation. *Am J Gastroenterol* 2007;102:1093–100.

69. Persoon A, Huisman-de Waal G, Naber TA. et al., Impact of long-term HPN on daily life in adults. *Clin Nutr* 2005;24:304–13.

70. Smith CE. Quality of life in long-term total parenteral nutrition patients and their family caregivers. *JPEN J Parenter Enteral Nutr* 1993;17:501–6.

71. Fishbein TM, Kaufman SS, Florman SS. et al. Isolated intestinal transplantation: Proof of clinical efficacy. *Transplantation* 2003;76:636–40.

72. Grant D. Intestinal transplantation: 1997 Report of the international registry. Intestinal Transplant Registry. *Transplantation* 1999;67:1061–4.

73. Abu-Elmagd K, Reyes J, Todo S. et al., Clinical intestinal transplantation: New perspectives and immunologic considerations. *J Am Coll Surg* 1998;186:512–25; discussion 25–7.

74. Sudan DL, Kaufman SS, Shaw BW, Jr. et al., Isolated intestinal transplantation for intestinal failure. *Am J Gastroenterol* 2000;95:1506–15.

75. Messing B, Corcos O, Amiot A, and Joly F. Intestinal failure: From adaptation to transplantation. *Gastroenterol Clin Biol* 2009;33:648–59.

76. Lopez Santamaria M and Hernandez Oliveros F. Indications, techniques, and outcomes of small bowel transplant. *Nutr Hosp* 2007;22(Suppl 2):113–23.

77. Mailloux RJ, DeLegge MH, and Kirby DF. Pulmonary embolism as a complication of long-term total parenteral nutrition. *JPEN J Parenter Enteral Nutr* 1993;17:578–82.

78. Farmer DG, McDiarmid SV, Yersiz H. et al., Outcomes after intestinal transplantation: A single-center experience over a decade. *Transplant Proc* 2002;34:896–7.

# 6 Gastrointestinal Endoscopy and Pathologic Findings

*Debora Duro*

## CONTENTS

## 6.1 INTRODUCTION

Patients with intestinal failure (IF) suffer from a variety of gastrointestinal pathologies that are best assessed by endoscopic examination and mucosal biopsy. When parenteral feedings are weaned and enteral feedings are advanced, it is common for patients to suffer from occasional setbacks due to feeding intolerance and/or infections. Persistent or recurrent feeding difficulties should prompt consideration for endoscopic evaluation. Although limited prospective data exist to estimate the role of endoscopic exam, a recent retrospective study suggested that there is a high diagnostic yield of endoscopy. Ching et al.[1] performed 61 endoscopies in 27 patients with IF and found gross endoscopic, histologic, or microbiologic abnormalities in 89% (24) of these.

Gastrointestinal endoscopy can be diagnostic as well as therapeutic in IF. One case report of intraoperative enteroscopy diagnosed a partial intestinal obstruction in an infant on prolonged parenteral nutrition (PN), a lesion that had eluded detection via previous contrast studies and laparotomy.[2] Auvin et al.[3] reported a case of an infant with short bowel syndrome and chronic intestinal obstruction syndrome secondary to gastroschisis who developed extensive necrotic bowel with obstruction. This patient needed continuous nasogastric decompression, so a percutaneous jejunostomy was successfully placed endoscopically in order to avoid recurrent bowel obstruction. Liu et al.[4] reported a case of endoscopic balloon dilatation under fluoroscopic guidance of an ileocolonic stricture secondary to an intestinal anastomosis in an infant with short bowel syndrome. Gama-Rodrigues et al.[5] described the role of a combined intraoperative enteroscopy and a small resection through a minimal enterostomy in an adolescent who developed intestinal intussusception and obstruction due to small bowel polyps. Moreover, this endoscopic method was used with the objective of avoiding intestinal resection in this patient with Peutz–Jeghers syndrome.[5]

This chapter focuses on the role of gastrointestinal endoscopy in the evaluation of patients with IF, emphasizing common endoscopic and pathological findings.

## 6.2   ANASTOMOTIC ULCER

Anastomotic ulcers are usually a late complication of intestinal resection in children who have undergone surgical ileo-colonic anastomosis. Signs and symptoms include refractory iron-deficiency anemia, overt rectal bleeding, and/or occult blood in stool. Patients can also present with hematochezia, tarry stools, and severe signs of anemia which require recurrent blood transfusions.[6] The precise etiology of anastomotic ulcers remains speculative, although a combination of possible factors include reduced intestinal blood flow, the presence of a foreign body (e.g., suture material), poor motility, and bacterial overgrowth could all be at play.

The endoscopic appearance of anastomotic ulcers is similar to other ulcerations of the gastrointestinal tract: a defect in the mucosal lining that is often superficial and can be marked by an exudative covering with or without active bleeding (Figure 6.1a). An important clue to their etiology is physical proximity to a bowel anastomosis, as identified by surgical history, radiographic finding, or the presence of suture material.

The pathologic appearance of the anastomotic ulcer is variable. Both multiple, small, and superficial ulcers and single large, deep ulcers have been described, either at the anastomosis itself or just proximally in the ileal segment. Perianastomotic ileo-colic ulceration is likely to reflect a process of chronic inflammation and repair. The histopathological appearance consist of inflammatory infiltrate composed predominantly of neutrophils and vessels that have plump endothelial cells characteristic of the newly formed vessels in granulation tissue (Figure 6.1b).

A common characteristic of the anastomotic ulcer is recurrence and resistance to medical treatment. These ulcers are often unresponsive to common anti-inflammatory therapy, antibiotics, and immunosuppressive medication. One case series described that the surgical revision of the anastomosis and ulcer resection in five patients was followed by rapid recurrence in four.[7]

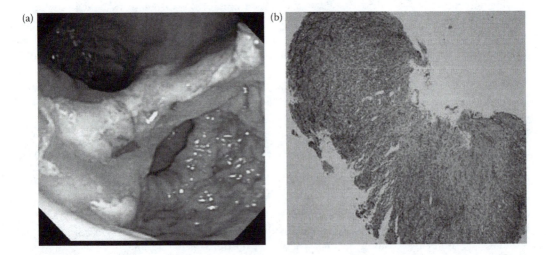

**FIGURE 6.1**   (a) Anastomotic ulcer at the level of ileo-colonic anastomosis in a patient with refractory iron anemia. (b) H&E 10× anastomosis site showing granulation tissue with dense inflammation and prominent vascular channels.

## 6.3  ALLERGY/HYPERSENSITIVITY

Food allergy is a common condition affecting 2–8% of children younger than two years of age.[8] In patients with IF, food allergy can manifest as diarrhea, malabsorption, and difficulty in advancing enteral feedings or by the presence of overt or occult rectal bleeding. In addition to reducing mucosal surface area for nutrient absorption, massive resection can reduce gut barrier function, thereby predisposing the patient with IF to protein hypersensitivity.[9] Rectal bleeding is a common symptom of allergy in these patients and endoscopic evaluation can help differentiate among infection (e.g., *Clostridium difficile*), anastomotic ulcer, and allergies.

Figure 6.2a shows an endoscopic photograph from a colonoscopy in a patient with IF who presented with persistent rectal bleeding and negative stool cultures. The colonoscopy revealed erythema, mucosal friability, and focal erosions (Figure 6.2b). Histology revealed an increased number of eosinophils throughout the lamina propria of the colon (Figure 6.2c). Usually the number of eosinophils varies ranging from >6 to more than 20 per high-power field, and is frequently a focal finding.[10] Another less specific finding of hypersensitivity is mucosal nodularity, suggestive of lymphoid nodular hyperplasia.

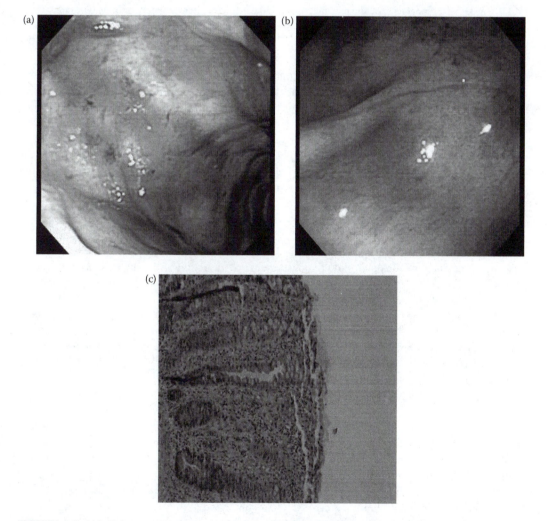

**FIGURE 6.2**  (a) Colonoscopy revealed erythema, mucosa friability, and focal erosions. (b) This patient presented with rectal bleeding. Biopsies confirmed high eosinophil count throughout his colon. (c) H&E 40× colonic mucosa with a markedly increased number of eosinophils in the lamina propria.

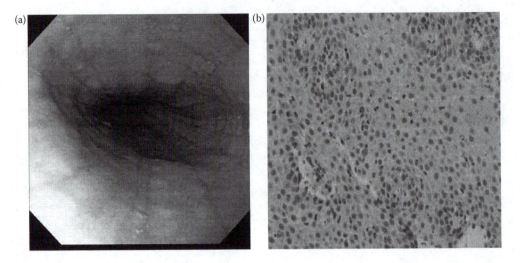

**FIGURE 6.3**   (a) Esophagus showing pale mucosa and linear furrows in a patient with IF who presented with occasional vomiting. (b) H&E 40× histologic findings confirmed the presence of eosinophilic esophagitis >15 eosinophils per high-power field.

Eosinophilic esophagitis (EoE) is another condition in the spectrum of allergic disorders and can be difficult to distinguish from gastroesophageal reflux-induced esophagitis. The symptoms are similar (e.g., vomiting and difficulty advancing enteral feeds) and EoE should be considered when patients fail conventional antireflux therapy. Endoscopic findings of EoE include pale mucosa, absence of vascular pattern, and vertical furrows (Figure 6.3a). The histopathologic criteria of increased eosinophils, that is, more than 15 per high-power field, presence of eosinophils in the intramuscular layers (Figure 6.3b), and presence of clusters of eosinophils in the esophageal mucosa are required to classify allergic esophagitis[11] in patients with IF.

## 6.4   BACTERIAL OVERGROWTH

Bacterial overgrowth of the small intestine is a very common entity in patients with IF. Predisposing factors include anatomical changes in the bowel including resection of the ileocecal valve, dilation of small bowel during intestinal adaptation, impaired motility, and the use of acid suppression therapy. The standard method for diagnosis of small intestinal bacterial overgrowth is a duodenal aspirate and the diagnosis confirmation rests on the abnormally high bacterial population level in the small bowel, exceeding $10^5$ organisms/mL and a positive clinical response to antibiotic therapy.[12] Because endoscopy is an invasive procedure, the lactulose or glucose breath hydrogen tests are considered noninvasive alternatives. This topic is discussed in detail in Chapter 24, Bacterial Overgrowth of the Small Intestine.

Clinical symptoms suggestive of bacterial overgrowth can be quite broad and may include abdominal pain, bloating, diarrhea, feeding intolerance, and signs of malabsorption.[6] Because bacterial overgrowth can mimic many conditions in IF, diagnostic endoscopy and quantitative cultures of small intestinal fluid may be helpful to assess this diagnosis.

Intestinal biopsies can be difficult to differentiate from mild cases of gluten-sensitivity and other forms of enteropathy, reinforcing the need for clinical correlation. Upper endoscopy performed in a child with IF who presented with upper gastrointestinal bleeding showed a duodenum bulb (Figure 6.4a) with a nodular and granular pattern. An ulcer was found at the second portion of the duodenum along the gastro-jejunal feeding tube (Figure 6.4b). Bulb biopsies revealed mild villous atrophy, crypt hyperplasia, and intraepithelial lymphocytes, conveys the potential of celiac disease.

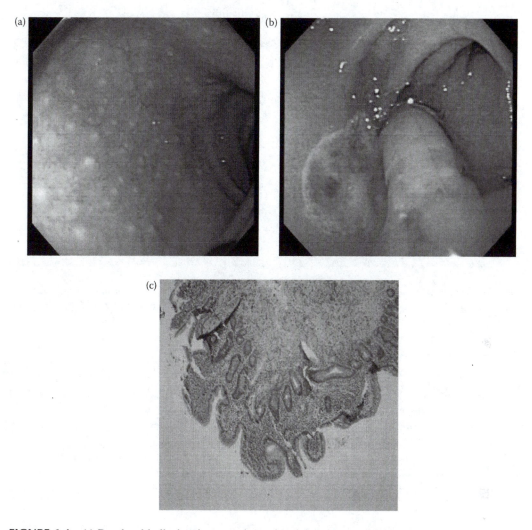

**FIGURE 6.4** (a) Duodenal bulb showing granular and nodular pattern with biopsies in this area demonstrating villous atrophy, increased intraepithelial lymphocytes, and mild villous blunting. (b) A small ulcer along the gastro-jejunal side was found at the second portion of the duodenum; biopsies demonstrated focal duodenitis. (c) H&E 40× duodenal mucosa with villous atrophy, crypt hyperplasia, and intraepithelial lymphocytosis.

Tissue transglutaminase and antiendomysial antibodies were negative. In addition, quantitative cultures of small bowel fluid grew *Escherichia coli*, *Enterobacter cloacae*, and *Enterococcus* species. These findings were, therefore, thought more consistent with enteropathy due to bacterial overgrowth as opposed to celiac disease.

Histological changes of bacterial overgrowth can be normal, or can include villous atrophy, crypt hyperplasia, and mild inflammation (Figure 6.4c). Other features consistent with bacterial overgrowth are signs of chronic inflammatory changes which can be seen in a setting of small ulcerations (Figure 6.5a) found in this ileoscopy. This patient presented with persistent stomal bleeding. An ileoscopy was performed and several small ulcerations were found within 15–20 cm of his ileum. Biopsies were consistent with inflammatory ulcers and inflammatory changes in the mucosa representing bacterial overgrowth (Figure 6.5b). The duodenal aspirate revealed *Klebsiella pneumoniae*, *E. coli*, and *E. cloacae*.

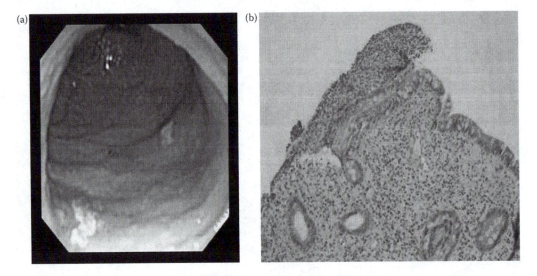

**FIGURE 6.5**    (a) Ileoscopy demonstrating multiple small ulcers in a patient with recurrent ostomy bleeding. Biopsy demonstrating chronic inflammatory changes compatible with bacterial overgrowth. (b) H&E 20× small intestinal mucosa with ulceration and superficial neutrophilic exudates.

## 6.5    PEPTIC DISEASE

Patients with IF are at risk of peptic disease due to increased gastric secretions and hypergastrinemia which follow massive small bowel resection.[13,14] Endoscopy with biopsy is the gold standard of peptic disease diagnosis when signs of esophagitis or gastritis are present. Ching et al.[1] found peptic disease (gastritis or esophagitis) in nine of 34 upper gastrointestinal endoscopies (26%) in pediatric IF patients. Peptic disease can present as vomiting or epigastric or chest pain in IF patients. Of note, an increase in stool output may also occur due to high acid production in patients with proximal small bowel resection stimulating intestinal motility. Figure 6.6a demonstrates erythematous mucosa in a patient with IF who had chest pain and heartburn; Figure 6.6b shows the histopathologic results of mild esophagitis.

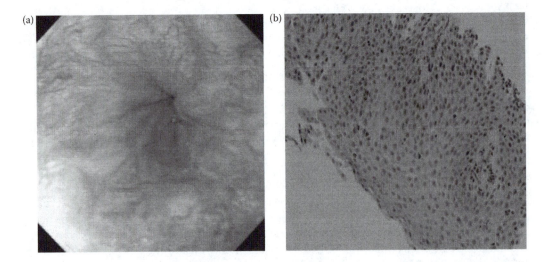

**FIGURE 6.6**    (a) Esophagitis in a child with IF whose chief complaint was chest pain. (b) H&E 40× squamous epithelium with scattered intraepithelial eosinophils.

## 6.6 ANATOMICAL ABNORMALITIES AND OTHER PATHOLOGICAL FINDINGS

### 6.6.1 DUODENAL WEBS

Duodenal webs are a rare finding in children, with a reported incidence ranging from one in 10,000 to one in 40,000.[15] Common presentations include vomiting and failure to advance enteral feeds. Figure 6.7 shows a duodenal web in a child with IF who had recurrent vomiting and poor enteral tolerance. An upper endoscopy found a blind loop (Figure 6.7) that had no opening after the duodenal bulb. A prior upper gastrointestinal series had failed to demonstrate the web, although a second one after the endoscopic finding confirmed the presence of a duodenal web. After surgical correction of the web, feedings were advanced.

### 6.6.2 INTESTINAL STRICTURE

Intestinal stricture is a common finding in patients who have undergone intestinal resection due to necrotizing enterocolitis (NEC). The etiology of intestinal strictures after NEC is ischemic in nature. The clinical presentation varies from indolent process to signs of obstruction and significant decreased stool output in patients with IF. Figure 6.8 shows a colonic stricture in a patient who had been born with gastroschisis and had undergone a serial transverse enteroplasty procedure and who presented with feeding intolerance. Figure 6.9 demonstrates an ileal stricture in a patient with IF who showed signs of decreased ostomy output and abdominal discomfort.

### 6.6.3 ESOPHAGEAL VARICES

Esophageal varices can be the sole and first manifestation of severe liver disease in patients with IF who develop portal hypertension due to PN-associated liver disease. The age of manifestation can be as early as the first year of life, but usually ranges from 5 to 13 years. Patients with IF who have established cirrhosis should undergo close endoscopic monitoring if portal hypertension is suspected in order to assess the development of esophageal varices. Figure 6.10 shows esophageal varices that

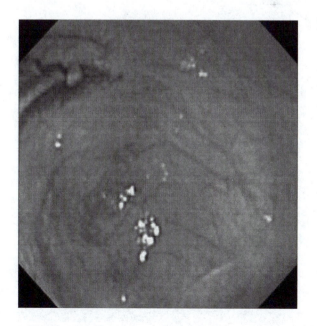

**FIGURE 6.7** Endoscopy finding associated with a duodenal pouch confirmed by upper gastrointestinal series which demonstrated a duodenal web.

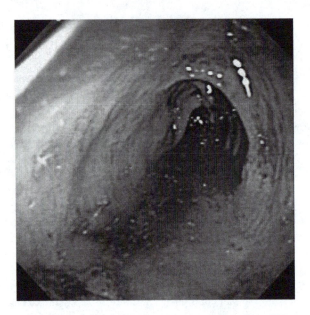

**FIGURE 6.8**   Colonic stricture.

developed in a girl with IF due to NEC who presented with upper GI bleeding requiring ICU observation.

### 6.6.4   FOREIGN BODY

Foreign bodies should always be considered in children. A young child with IF due to NEC presented with hematochezia and underwent colonoscopy; Figure 6.11 shows the presence of a small square foreign body in his descending colon. After removal of the foreign body, bleeding did not recur.

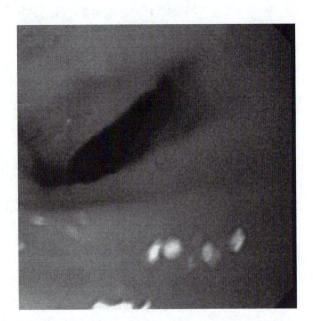

**FIGURE 6.9**   Ileal stricture.

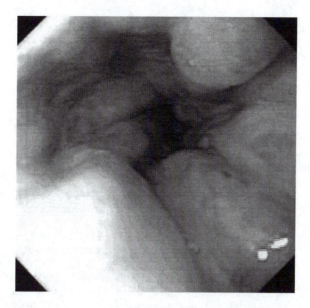

**FIGURE 6.10**   Esophageal varices in the lower esophagus of the child presented with upper GI bleeding. This child developed cirrhosis after several years of PN.

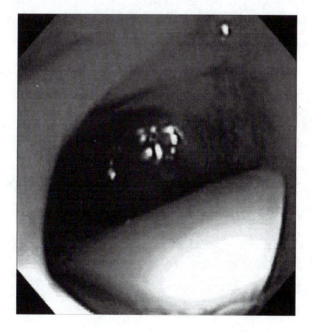

**FIGURE 6.11**   A foreign body (a piece of plastic) was found in the descending colon of the child with IF who presented with rectal bleeding.

## 6.7   SUMMARY

Patients with IF are prone to develop a variety of symptoms related to their remnant bowel function and anatomy. Gastrointestinal endoscopy with biopsy is an important diagnostic tool in the management of these patients, and a growing literature supports therapeutic endoscopy as well. As with all endoscopic procedures, careful patient selection and collaboration with a gastrointestinal pathologist are critical in optimizing diagnostic efforts and patient care.

## ACKNOWLEDGMENT

Debora Duro was supported by the Junior Faculty Career Development Award from Children's Hospital, Boston.

## REFERENCES

1. Ching YA, Modi BP, Jaksic T, and Duggan C. High diagnostic yield of gastrointestinal endoscopy in children with intestinal failure. *J Pediatr Surg* 2008;43:906–10.
2. Duggan C, Shamberger RC, Antonioli D, and Leichtner AM. Intraoperative enteroscopy in the diagnosis of partial intestinal obstruction in infancy. *Dig Dis Sci* 1995;40:2236–8.
3. Auvin S, Michaud L, Guimber D, Sfeir R, Gottrand F, and Turck D. Percutaneous endoscopic jejunostomy for decompression in an infant with short-bowel syndrome. *Endoscopy* 2002;34:240.
4. Liu E, Hoffenberg EJ, Kaye RD, and Sokol RJ. Endoscopic dilation of an ileocolonic stricture in an infant with short gut syndrome. *Gastrointest Endosc* 2001;54:533–5.
5. Gama-Rodrigues JJ, Silva JH, Aisaka AA, Jureidini R, Falci R, Jr., Maluf Filho F, Chong AK, Tsai AW, and Bresciani C. Intestinal intussusception and occlusion caused by small bowel polyps in the Peutz–Jeghers syndrome. Management by combined intraoperative enteroscopy and resection through minimal enterostomy: Case report. *Rev Hosp Clin Fac Med Sao Paulo* 2000;55:219–24.
6. Duro D, Jaksic T, and Duggan C. Multiple micronutrient deficiencies in a child with short bowel syndrome and normal somatic growth. *J Pediatr Gastroenterol Nutr* 2008;46:461–4.
7. Sondheimer JM, Sokol RJ, Narkewicz MR, and Tyson RW. Anastomotic ulceration: A late complication of ileocolonic anastomosis. *J Pediatr* 1995;127:225–30.
8. Sicherer SH. Food protein-induced enterocolitis syndrome: Clinical perspectives. *J Pediatr Gastroenterol Nutr* 2000;30(Suppl):S45–9.
9. Mazon A, Solera E, Alentado N, Oliver F, Pamies R, Caballero L, Nieto A, and Dalmau J. Frequent IgE sensitization to latex, cow's milk, and egg in children with short bowel syndrome. *Pediatr Allergy Immunol* 2008;19:180–3.
10. Odze RD, Bines J, Leichtner AM, Goldman H, and Antonioli DA. Allergic proctocolitis in infants: A prospective clinicopathologic biopsy study. *Hum Pathol* 1993;24:668–74.
11. Antonioli DA and Furuta GT. Allergic eosinophilic esophagitis: A primer for pathologists. *Semin Diagn Pathol* 2005;22:266–72.
12. Singh VV and Toskes PP. Small bowel bacterial overgrowth: Presentation, diagnosis, and treatment. *Curr Treat Options Gastroenterol* 2004;7:19–28.
13. Frederick PL, Sizer JS, and Osborne MP. Relation of massive bowel resection to gastric secretion. *N Engl J Med* 1965;272:509–14.
14. Straus E, Gerson CD, and Yalow RS. Hypersecretion of gastrin associated with the short bowel syndrome. *Gastroenterology* 1974;66:175–80.
15. Rehbein F and Boix-Ochoa J. Duodenal stenosis—Duodenal atresia. Problems of diagnosis and treatment. *Dtsch Med Wochenschr* 1963;88:1240–5.

# 7 Radiographic Evaluation

*Stephanie DiPerna and Carlo Buonomo*

## CONTENTS

The role of imaging in the child with short bowel syndrome (SBS) is, first and foremost, to demonstrate and define, as completely and accurately as possible, the anatomy of the gastrointestinal tract. That this seemingly simple task is often difficult to realize in practice is a fact with which all radiologists who work with children with SBS are only too aware. The gastrointestinal anatomy of the child with SBS is, of course, never normal and the abnormality is rarely limited to the length of the intestine. The complexity of the pathologic anatomy is a consequence, in most instances, of both the underlying disorder that led to the SBS and the subsequent, often multiple, surgical procedures. A complete and accurate map of the intestine is essential for effective management of SBS, but will rarely be drawn without persistence and expertise on the part of the radiologist.

An additional secondary goal of imaging in SBS is to estimate the function and viability of the intestine. In practical terms, the task usually amounts to gauging intestinal motility. This assessment of physiology is, of course, notoriously subjective and even more dependent upon the experience of the radiologist than that of the anatomy. Still, this assessment, however tentative, may provide indispensable information to those caring for these patients. Very little has been written about the radiology of SBS in children (Ching et al. 2007; Duro et al. 2008). What follows in this chapter is an outline of our approach to the imaging of children with SBS.

## 7.1 GENERAL PRINCIPLES

Most children with SBS have complicated medical and surgical histories and a thorough review of available medical records, especially operative notes, is essential. Obviously, the more detailed the knowledge of the (expected) postoperative anatomy the easier it will be to organize and tailor the imaging workup and to avoid serious errors in interpretation such as labeling a stricture as a normal anastomosis, or completely ignoring long sections of defunctionalized bowel. In addition, an understanding of the condition which led to the SBS may alert the radiologist to potential pertinent and common findings. For example, in a child with a history of necrotizing enterocolitis we might expect segmental and patchy bowel involvement and a high incidence of colonic strictures. Children with a history of gastroschisis will frequently have multiple areas of stenoses and very poor motility. In a child with a single or multiple atresias anastomotic strictures as well as dilated segments of nonfunctioning or poorly functioning bowel are common.

Review of prior radiographic studies may make additional studies unnecessary or redundant and spare the child trauma and radiation exposure. Repeat or serial studies may provide useful information on the functional significance of specific findings.

All this being said, many children with SBS are referred from other institutions and frequently arrive with few, if any, records. Furthermore, in some patients, such as those with severe diffuse necrotizing enterocolitis, even the attending surgeon may be unsure of the postoperative anatomy. Ultimately, our approach to the imaging of SBS is similar in all patients: review available records and studies; talk with the child's parents and/or caregivers who often provide invaluable information; examine the child, looking for evidence of fistulae, and stomas, if present; and, finally, and most importantly, opacify with contrast *all* bowel which is accessible, not only by mouth and by rectum, but also via stomas and fistulae, if present, and if necessary. All the "dots" should be connected: failure to do so may lead to critical diagnostic errors (Figure 7.1).

## 7.2   RADIOGRAPHIC EVALUATION: GENERAL APPROACH

The plain abdominal radiograph is the fundamental first step in the imaging evaluation of the child with SBS. The radiographs, usually in two projections (supine and tangential beam, either upright, left-side down decubitus or cross-table lateral) allow an initial assessment of the amount, distribution, and caliber of both small and large bowel.

Many children with SBS have chronically, diffusely dilated bowel. This dilatation may be "adaptive" and if not normal is at least expected (Figure 7.2). This diffuse dilatation may be difficult to distinguish from an obstructive pattern. A prone (PA) film of the abdomen may be useful in making this distinction. In prone position air will rise into the nondependent segments of the intestine, including the rectum. If air does fill the rectum an obstruction is much less likely. Even more helpful than additional views, however, is comparison with prior radiographs, if available. An unchanging pattern of dilatation over time is usually comforting.

The most important imaging modality in the evaluation of the child with SBS is fluoroscopy with enteral contrast. Commonly performed studies are the upper gastrointestinal series (UGI), UGI with small bowel follow through (UGI/SBFT), contrast enema, stomagram, and fistulagram. Again, as noted above, our goal is to opacify all accessible bowel, including if possible, diverted loops, and estimate its length, caliber, and function. The choice of contrast medium will be determined by a number of factors, including the potential for perforation or leak, the age and size of the patient, the route of administration, the possibility of obstruction, the length of bowel to be opacified and the functional status of the bowel (i.e., diverted or not).

Some general principles of contrast selection are worth noting. We never use Gastrografin (diatrizoate meglumine and diatrizoate sodium) in children. Its high osmolality makes it extremely dangerous if aspirated (our patients not infrequently aspirate when given contrast by mouth, and frequently reflux and aspirate the refluxed contrast); Gastrografin used for enemas may cause significant fluid shifts. We use barium only for UGI/SBFT in older children in whom water-soluble contrast will usually not provide dense enough opacification. We of course always use water-soluble contrast if there is any possibility of perforation or in recently postoperative patients in whom there may be an anastomotic leak.

For UGI /SBFT in infants and young children we use nonionic, iso-osmolar water soluble contrast, such as Omnipaque 180 (Nycomed Inc., New York) which is 411 mOsm. The advantage of this type of contrast is that since it is water soluble it does not flocculate (like barium) and since it is nearly iso-osmolar it does not draw in water. This allows for longer imaging in these patients who frequently have prolonged intestinal transit.

For enemas, stomagrams, and fistulagrams we usually use Cysto-Conray II (Mallincrodt, Inc., St. Louis, Missouri) which is ~400 mOsm. This contrast is much less expensive than the nonionic products, and will nearly always provide adequate opacification. It cannot be stressed enough that only water-soluble contrast should be employed in diverted, defunctionalized bowel, for example, in

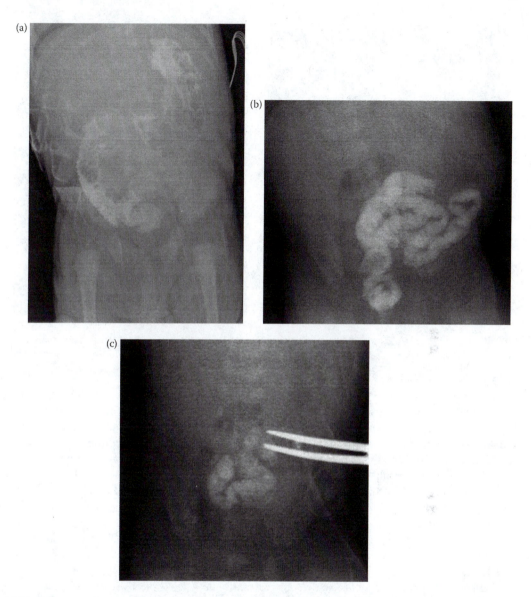

**FIGURE 7.1**   One-month-old boy with SBS due to complicated intestinal atresia. Surgery performed at out-side institution. (a) UGI demonstrates proximal jejunostomy. (b) Contrast enema demonstrates small caliber (unused) rectum, sigmoid, and descending colon. More proximal bowel could not be opacified. (c) Injection of mucus fistula fills bowel distal to jejunostomy and proximal to colon.

the colon of a child with a diverting upstream ostomy. Barium administered in this situation may be impossible to remove from the defunctionalized loop.

## 7.3   RADIOGRAPHIC EVALUATION: SPECIFIC EXAMINATIONS

### 7.3.1   GASTROINTESTINAL/SMALL BOWEL FOLLOW-THROUGH

The most frequently performed study in the child with SBS will be the UGI/SBFT. In children with complete intestinal continuity it will demonstrate anatomy and allow an estimate of intestinal function and length.

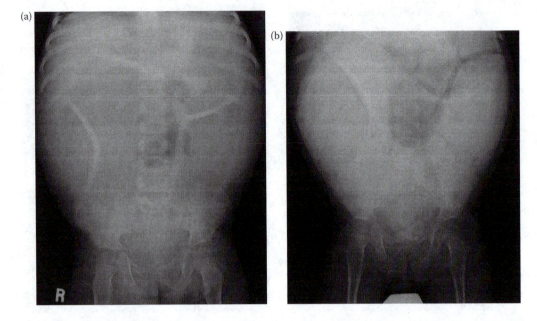

**FIGURE 7.2**   Five-year-old boy with SBS secondary to necrotizing enterocolitis. (a) Plain abdominal radiograph demonstrates massive diffuse distention. (b) UGI/SBFT delayed radiograph demonstrates distention but no obstruction.

There has been very little work done on the reliability of measurements of small bowel length from the SBFT, and none that we are aware of in children with SBS. In adults, accuracy seems to be better when the entire bowel can be visualized on a single radiograph, without overlapping bowel (Nightingale et al. 1991; Shatari et al. 2004). In our experience, only relatively imprecise measurements are possible, since the frequently dilated bowel loops nearly always overlap and multiple procedures and radiographs are often required in order to visualize the bowel in its entirety. In addition, the transit time from stomach to rectum (or ostomy) can rarely be used to help in the estimation of length since, in children with markedly dilated bowel of any length, transit time is often extremely long.

As noted earlier, radiographic estimates of function are even less reliable than those of length. The single most useful finding which suggests poor function is a prolonged transit time through a dilated segment. Patients will often benefit from resection of such segments.

The UGI/SBFT will of course also demonstrate anastomotic leaks or obstruction (Figure 7.3).

Performance of the UGI/SBFT is generally straightforward. Contrast selection depends on the indication. Older infants and children with intestinal continuity and/or end ostomies who are not in the immediate post-operative state should generally be given barium. Newborns, especially those with underlying motility disorder such as gastroschisis, and all patients with risk of leak or perforation, are better served with Omnipaque 180 for reasons noted above. Contrast for the UGI/SBFT may be given by mouth, nasogastric tube, or gastrostomy tube. (It must be remembered that while the flavored barium used in most pediatric institutions is quite palatable, water-soluble contrast is not, and more often than not, will be refused.) The only difference in our protocol for the UGI/SBFT in patients with SBS is that we usually follow the contrast into the rectum (or ostomy bag). That is sometimes the only way to assure that the entirety of the intestine has been imaged (Figure 7.4).

## 7.3.2   Contrast Enema

There are several indications for contrast enemas in children with SBS. In our institution, the enema is most frequently requested for evaluation of the defunctionalized colon in children with proximal

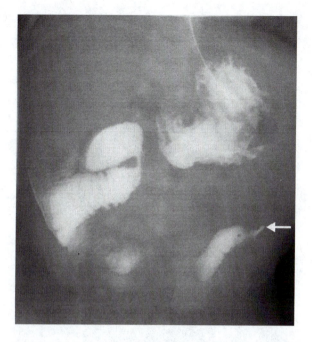

**FIGURE 7.3**   Five-week-old boy with repaired gastroschisis and bilious vomiting. SBFT demonstrates high-grade jejunal stricture (arrow).

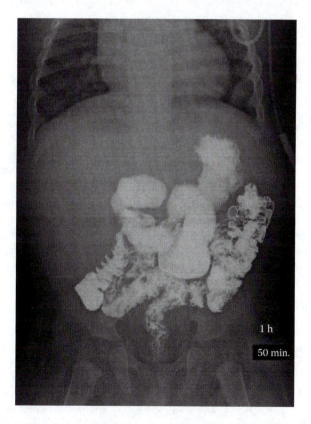

**FIGURE 7.4**   Sixteen-month-old boy with SBS due to necrotizing enterocolitis. Overhead film from UGI/SBFT demonstrates very short small bowel with contrast reaching rectum in 1 h 50 min.

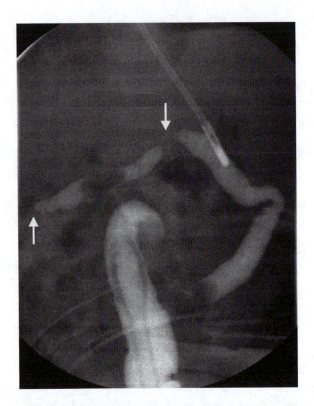

**FIGURE 7.5**　Six-month-old boy with a history of necrotizing enterocolitis with end ileostomy. Contrast enema demonstrates two focal strictures (arrows).

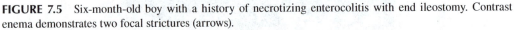

diverting ostomies. This examination is particularly critical in children with SBS due to necrotizing enterocolitis in whom there is a 20% incidence of stricture, usually in the left colon (Figure 7.5) (Buonomo 1999).

Enemas are also performed in order to evaluate colonic anastomoses. These anastomoses are always better evaluated with retrograde studies.

For all enemas we use Cysto-Conray II. It bears repeating that barium should *never* be used in defunctionalized colon. We use the largest catheter possible. Most children with SBS will be large enough for an enema tip but infants may require something smaller. In these cases we use a balloon tip catheter with the balloon inflated outside the patient, to obturate the anus. We very rarely tape the catheter as most children have good natural tone and will retain the contrast. Even in cases in which the contrast leaks taping is usually not helpful. We *never* inflate the balloon within the rectum in a child and *never* inject contrast with a syringe. Contrast should always be instilled via gravity. Forceful injection with a syringe may result in perforation.

### 7.3.3　STOMAGRAMS AND FISTULAGRAMS

Stomagrams are most often performed in a retrograde fashion, either to evaluate for stomal obstruction or to evaluate segments of bowel that cannot be reached antegrade by UGI/SBFT, either because of proximal obstruction or poor motility. Antegrade studies are occasionally requested to opacify bowel that cannot be reached by enema either because of diversion or obstruction.

Stomagrams are always performed with water-soluble contrast (Cysto-Conray II or equivalent). We generally perform the study by using a balloon catheter with the balloon inflated outside of the stoma, using the balloon to obturate the lumen. Rarely, in older children, we carefully inflate the balloon within the lumen to create a tight seal. The critical point of technique is to position the

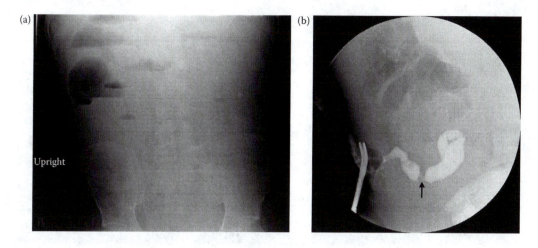

**FIGURE 7.6** Twenty-five-year-old man with pseudoobstruction and ileostomy. (a) Upright abdominal radiograph demonstrates dilated small bowel with air fluid levels. (b) Stomagram demonstrates stricture ~2 cm from stoma (arrow).

catheter as close to the skin surface as is possible. Most stomal obstructions occur just beneath the skin and are caused by "kinks" rather than true strictures; a catheter positioned even a few centimeters into the lumen may bypass the point of obstruction (Figure 7.6).

Fistulae may be spontaneous or surgically created. A spontaneous fistula is usually the result of chronic infection or inflammation. We inject the fistula with water-soluble contrast in order to demonstrate any connection with bowel, if present. Occasionally, the fistula may be demonstrated in antegrade study (Figure 7.7).

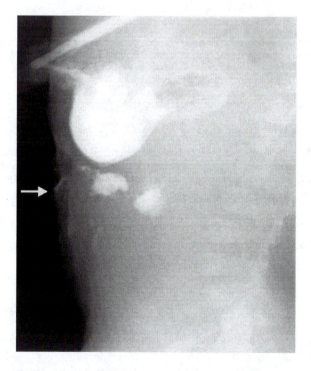

**FIGURE 7.7** Five-month-old girl with SBS due to necrotizing enterocolitis and multiple surgeries. Spot radiograph from UGI/SBFT demonstrates enterocutaneous fistula (arrow).

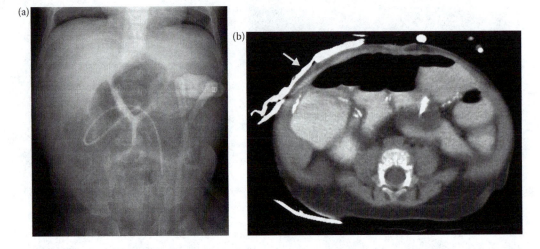

**FIGURE 7.8**  Ten-month-old boy with SBS due to gastroschisis with bilious emesis. (a) Abdominal radiograph demonstrates diffuse bowel dilation. (b) Image from CT scan demonstrates bowel dilatation with no obstruction. Contrast is present is ostomy bag (arrow).

Surgically created fistulae, like stomas, are studied in order to identify bowel which is not demonstrable by other antegrade or retrograde studies (Figure 7.1c).

### 7.3.4  COMPUTERIZED TOMOGRAPHY

Computerized tomography (CT) scanning is frequently helpful in children with SBS and very dilated bowel, which occurs frequently in SBS, in whom there is a question of obstruction. Fluoroscopic studies are very difficult to perform and interpret in the setting of extreme dilatation because the contrast usually becomes too dilute (Figure 7.8).

Administration of oral contrast is usually not necessary in the evaluation of obstruction since the intraluminal fluid, invariably present, serves as an excellent contrast medium.

## 7.4  EVALUATION OF SURGICAL TREATMENTS OF SBS

There are two major surgical approaches to SBS: bowel lengthening and intestinal (or multi visceral) transplantation. There are two common approaches to bowel lengthening, the Bianchi procedure and the STEP procedure. The Bianchi procedure is a method of longitudinal intestinal lengthening and tailoring (Bianchi 1980) in which dilated bowel is divided in half, longitudinally, preserving the blood supply of each leaf of the mesentery. This effectively doubles the bowel length while halving its caliber.

In the newer STEP (serial transverse enteroplasty) procedure the bowel is divided in a serial fashion at right angles with a stapler, thereby creating a zig-zag pattern of longer, narrower bowel (Kim et al. 2003). The STEP procedure is a simpler approach to bowel lengthening, and can be performed on asymmetrically dilated bowel eliminating the need for enterotomies.

Little, if anything, has been written about the radiographic appearance of surgically lengthened bowel. In our experience, the bowel lengthened by either the Bianchi or STEP does not have atypical or unusual appearance (Figure 7.9).

Small bowel transplantation either isolated or as part of multi visceral transplantation, is another option for treatment of SBS and intestinal failure. As is the case with bowel lengthening, little has been written about the radiology of intestinal transplantation in children and, as is also the case with bowel lengthening, it is remarkable how normal the intestine appears (Figure 7.10) (Bach et al. 1991, 1992).

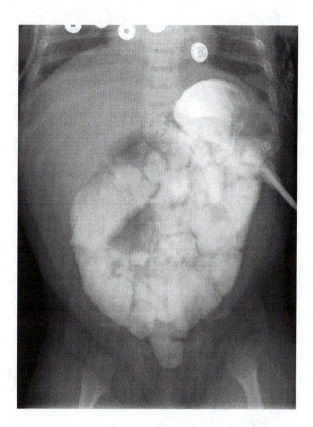

**FIGURE 7.9** Four-month-old boy with SBS due to jejunal atresia status post STEP procedure. Overhead radiograph from UGI/SBFT demonstrates diffuse moderate bowel dilatation without obstruction.

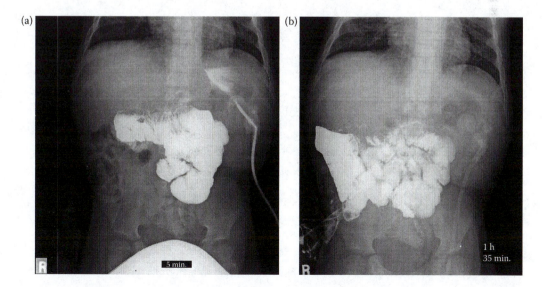

**FIGURE 7.10** (a, b) Six-year-old boy with SBS due to multiple intestinal atresias status postmulti visceral transplant, including small bowel. Overhead radiographs demonstrate relatively normal appearance of small bowel with satisfactory progression of contrast into ostomy bag.

## REFERENCES

Bach, D. B., D. J. Hurlbut, W. M. Romano, F. R Sutherland, B. M. Garcia, W. J. Wall, C. N. Ghent, and D. R. Grant. 1991. Human orthotopic small intestine transplantation: Radiologic assessment. *Radiology* 180(1):37–41.

Bach, D. B., M. F. Levin, A. D. Vellet, D. B. Downey, P. L. Munk, D. R. Grant, W. J. Wall et al. 1992. CT findings in patients with small-bowel transplants. *AJR Am J Roentgenol* 159(2):311–5.

Bianchi, A. 1980. Intestinal loop lengthening—A technique for increasing small intestinal length. *J Pediatr Surg* 15(2):145–51.

Buonomo, C. 1999. The radiology of necrotizing enterocolitis. *Radiol Clin North Am* 37(6):1187–98, vii.

Ching, Y. A., K. Gura, B. Modi, and T. Jaksic. 2007. Pediatric intestinal failure: Nutrition, pharmacologic, and surgical approaches. *Nutr Clin Pract* 22 (6):653–63.

Duro, D., D. Kamin, and C. Duggan. 2008. Overview of pediatric short bowel syndrome. *J Pediatr Gastroenterol Nutr* 47(Suppl 1):S33–6.

Kim, H. B., D. Fauza, J. Garza, J. T. Oh, S. Nurko, and T. Jaksic. 2003. Serial transverse enteroplasty (STEP): A novel bowel lengthening procedure. *J Pediatr Surg* 38(3):425–9.

Nightingale, J. M., C. I. Bartram, and J. E. Lennard-Jones. 1991. Length of residual small bowel after partial resection: Correlation between radiographic and surgical measurements. *Gastrointest Radiol* 16(4):305–6.

Shatari, T., M. A. Clark, J. R. Lee, and M. R. Keighley. 2004. Reliability of radiographic measurement of small intestinal length. *Colorectal Dis* 6(5):327–9.

# Part II

Medical and Surgical Management

# 8 Principles of Bowel-Preserving Surgery

*Milissa A. McKee*

## CONTENTS

## 8.1 GENERAL PRINCIPLES

The primary cause of intestinal failure (IF) in children is catastrophic loss of intestinal length due to congenital or acquired conditions. Depending on the length of bowel remaining, the patient may suffer from short bowel syndrome (SBS). SBS is generally defined as loss of intestinal length resulting in a malabsorptive state and inability to maintain adequate hydration and nutrition.[1] Most of these conditions are surgical in nature and pediatric patients requiring emergency surgical intervention for abdominal problems tend to be young infants, frequently premature, with associated small size and delicate conditions. They are often unstable or even moribund. The decisions that are made at the time of the initial procedure will, in many cases, have long-term consequences. Once bowel has been resected it cannot be replaced short of intestinal transplantation. The medical and surgical management of SBS will be discussed at length in other chapters of this text. The goal of this chapter is to discuss general principles of management during abdominal surgery with the intent to preserve as much bowel as possible. In some cases, SBS can be avoided entirely and in others, the severity of their condition may be improved.

A primary goal of management in infants undergoing abdominal exploration should be preservation of as much functional intestinal length as possible. This important principle must be balanced with the risks to the patients life of ongoing metabolic derangement due to ischemia and intraabdominal sepsis. In the majority of cases, there will be adequate lengths of viable bowel such that consideration of SBS would be unlikely and the appropriate corrective procedure can be carried out without undue concern. Unfortunately, emergent surgical conditions, not infrequently, are associated with inadequate intestinal length that results in SBS and resultant significant morbidity and mortality.

The most common conditions resulting in severe SBS and IF with possible eventual need for small bowel transplantation are necrotizing enterocolitis (NEC), gastroschisis, intestinal atresia, and midgut volvulus (Table 8.1).[2–4] There are other less common entities such as visceral loss (anatomical or functional) due to long segment Hirschsrung's disease, trauma, dysmotility syndromes,

**TABLE 8.1**

**Most Common Diagnoses in Patients with Short Bowel Syndrome**

| Diagnosis | Spencer et al.[2] (N = 102) | Nayyar et al.[3] (N = 210) |
|---|---|---|
| Necrotizing enterocolitis | 36 | 24 |
| Gastroschisis | 19 | 52 |
| Intestinal atresia | 14 | 21 |
| Midgut volvulus | 14 | 48 |
| Miscellaneous | 10 | 65 |

and inflammatory bowel disease. While reports differ as to which is most common, the combination of NEC and complicated gastroschisis account for half or more of all pediatric patients undergoing small bowel transplantation.[3,4] By making a conscious effort to preserve bowel length, SBS may be avoided in borderline cases. In more severe cases, retention of as much bowel as possible increases the possibility of success from future adaptation of the bowel or the application of gut-lengthening techniques.

## 8.2  BOWEL LENGTH AND VIABILITY

Under ideal circumstances, the bowel is of normal length and completely viable. This is unfortunately often not the case. Normal bowel length varies by age and size of the patient. There are significant reserves in terms of function and large lengths can be resected with minimal long-term consequences. Classic descriptions of normal intestinal length in neonates were based on postmortem measurements.[5] This resulted in the general belief that a normal intestinal length at term was around 300 cm. More recent reports question the validity of these estimates as postmortem measurements in adults have been shown to be significantly longer than in live patients due to loss of contractility and tensile strength of the wall. More recent published norms based on live infants estimate the normal small bowel length at term to be closer to 200 cm.[6] What is clear is that the small bowel length varies widely, increases markedly in the latter weeks of pregnancy and continues to increase through the first years of life. Absolute bowel length is associated with the development of SBS but because normal bowel length is variable by age and size it cannot be generalized between patients. A more appropriate indicator of likelihood of SBS is percentage of normal bowel remaining for the patient's size. Infants with less than 10% of normal bowel have an increased risk of mortality and significantly lower likelihood of achieving independence from parenteral nutrition.[2] Obviously there is a continuum of probability of developing SBS between nearly normal bowel length to no bowel at all. In addition to actual bowel length, the functional status of the bowel must also be considered. This is even more difficult to predict or measure. Certain conditions such as gastroschisis are often associated with dysmotility and malabsorption even in the setting of what would usually be considered adequate lengths of small bowel.[7] Ischemic insults, such as in cases of NEC or midgut volvulus, may also impair the function of the bowel.[8] Even if the bowel ultimately survives, normal bowel function including motility and absorption may not normalize for an extended period of time, if at all.

Whether or not SBS develops is a function of both length and function of the intestine. Historic estimates of absolute length necessary for survival have been challenged and there are increasing case reports of patients with very short lengths of small bowel that eventually achieve full enteral nutrition. There remains a significant ethical issue for the operating surgeon when confronted with catastrophic intraabdominal bowel loss. Classically, this occurs in midgut volvulus or NEC. Virtually all of the small bowel from ligament of Treitz to ileocecal valve may be nonviable. When this is obviously the case, the surgeon must decide whether potentially lifesaving intestinal resection should be performed in an unstable infant knowing that without it they will most likely succumb.

With resection, the patient will be an intestinal cripple with their only hope for long-term survival based on small bowel transplantation. As the success and survival of small bowel transplant patients continue to improve, more patients are being offered that chance but not without significant morbidity, mortality, and issues of quality of life.[3–4] This remains a controversial area that will continue to evolve as medical care progresses.

Assessment of viability at the time of surgery is another complicated issue in infants and children. Techniques that are useful in adults such as using a Doppler to assess the mesenteric vessels are of little practical value in smaller patients. The appearance of the bowel and wall integrity by inspection and palpation are more useful. At the two extremes of normal appearing bowel and completely necrotic bowel it is relatively easy to decide what should be resected. It is more difficult to make this decision when evaluating bowel that is impaired but not clearly dead. As a general rule, significant lengths of bowel of marginal viability should not be removed. As an alternative, the abdomen can be packed open with the intention of reassessing the bowel in 24–48 hours, a so-called "second look" operation.[9–11] This allows for an additional period of time for resuscitation and hopefully, improvement in the overall hemodynamic condition of the patient. It also gives additional time for the questionable bowel to demarcate into a more obvious level of viability or necrosis. This approach is appropriate for any patient with severe illness and bowel of questionable appearance that would result in extensive resection. For short resections, it is probably more expedient to simply complete the procedure without planning one or more additional procedures. In those patients where bowel length is obviously going to be an issue, preserving as much bowel as possible by smaller sequential resections is worthwhile. Leaving the abdomen open has the additional benefit of avoiding compartment syndrome and the deleterious effects of increased intra-abdominal pressure on already compromised bowel. A temporary closure of the abdomen is accomplished in infants by gently covering the bowel with a nonadherent dressing followed by a drain and adhesive dressings. Patients in this condition are usually markedly edematous with ongoing third spacing of fluid. This type of dressing allows for the controlled egress of fluid and prevents increasing intra-abdominal pressure in this critical phase.

## 8.3  CREATION OF STOMAS

An issue that is frequently encountered during emergent abdominal exploration and intestinal resection is whether to restore intestinal continuity during the primary procedure or create an enterostomy. Historically, creation of a stoma has generally been considered to be the "safest" choice, but there are certainly advantages and disadvantages to this option. Advantages include in most cases more rapid visible return of bowel function and protection by diverting the fecal stream of any distal areas of abnormality. It tends to be relatively quick and is most appropriate for the bowel that is of questionable ability to heal an anastamosis especially in patients who are critically ill or unstable. There are, however, significant disadvantages. There is a significant rate of associated morbidity with stomas.[12,13] Stomal prolapse, ischemia with retraction and potential obstruction, herniation at the site, local skin breakdown, and high volume loss of fluid and electrolytes are all well described. Enteral feeding tolerance may be limited by stoma output and in cases where intestinal length is already short the creation of a stoma and subsequent takedown procedure will result in the loss of additional precious centimeters of bowel length.

The decision to create a stoma or not must be individualized to the patients underlying pathology and overall condition. A more aggressive approach with primary anastamosis is becoming more common but must be weighed against the risk of anastomotic failure with resultant intra-abdominal sepsis.[11,14,15] This is where the individual surgeon's judgement must be exercised. In general, extremely sick and small infants with bowel of marginal viability would be most likely to benefit from ostomy creation. In infants who do have a stoma, most surgeons now favor early takedown to restore intestinal continuity. This is typically done 4–6 weeks after the initial surgical resection provided that the infant is medically stable and of sufficient size (generally >2 kg) to undergo an additional abdominal procedure. Again, these rules are relative with regards to what is medically stable and what is an appropriate size, but the general trend over the past 20 years is to be more aggressive about stoma closure to optimize the patient's overall recovery and allow achievement of as much enteral nutrition as possible. The percentage of enteral nutrition achieved with the stoma in place may be limited depending on the relative position in the gastrointestinal tract and will in most cases improve after stoma closure.

## 8.4   NECROTIZING ENTEROCOLITIS

NEC is the most common surgical condition requiring laparotomy in the neonate.[8] It is a disease almost exclusively associated with prematurity and as smaller and sicker babies survive the overall incidence rises. The current incidence of NEC is estimated at one in 3000 live births. NEC has become one of the most common, if not the most common, underlying diagnoses in patients referred for intestinal transplantation.[3,4]

Around one-third to one-half of patients diagnosed with NEC will require surgical intervention. The most common indication for surgical intervention is perforation, usually evidenced by free air. In many cases there will be an isolated perforation in the ileum or evidence of ischemia or necrosis in relatively limited areas of the bowel. This situation is relatively straightforward and should be treated by resection of the involved bowel and usually creation of a stoma. In select cases, primary anastamosis can also be considered under ideal conditions.[14–16]

When perforation is not present or extensive amounts of the bowel are involved the decision to explore the abdomen and intraoperative judgements become more difficult. Approximately 10–15% of infants with NEC will have involvement of the entire small bowel, the so-called NEC totalis (Figure 8.1).[17,18] Resecting all of the involved bowel would result in complete absence of the midgut. There are some reports in these cases of simply draining the abdominal cavity while leaving the bowel in place. The likelihood of survival is low. If the patient survives, it is possible that the bowel would also recover. This is still an area fraught with difficulty and most patients do not survive. Given that the likelihood of survival is minimal with such extensive disease, many surgeons would opt to close and recommend comfort care.

When NEC involves large portions of the small bowel resection will be required. Clearly necrotic portions of bowel should be resected and in most cases diverted with an ostomy proximal to the diseased area. Bowel of marginal viability may not require resection. A planned second look procedure may be useful to reassess the bowel in 24–36 h. Diversion of the fecal stream may also allow

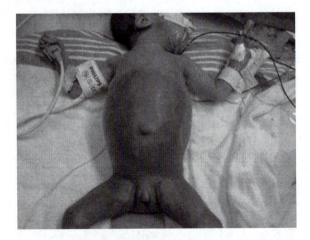

**FIGURE 8.1**   This premature infant was not perforated but spontaneously developed compartment syndrome as a result of NEC totalis.

for the survival of bowel of marginal viability that can be replaced in continuity at a later date. More aggressive approaches including anastamosis with a "patch, drain, and wait" philosophy have been reported with some success.[19,20] This involves preserving bowel of questionable quality, placing drains throughout the abdominal cavity, and allowing for the development of frequently multiple enterocutaneous fistulas. If the patient recovers, these fistulas may heal spontaneously or additional procedures may be required to resect strictures and close fistulas.

Surgical treatment of NEC is common and it is useful to have a knowledge of a number of options for more complex cases.[16] The pathway chosen will be impacted by the patient's overall condition, the extent of involvement, and the family's wishes. With thoughtful consideration of these factors the surgeon must then ultimately decide what surgical intervention will result in the best outcome for the patient under potentially dire circumstances.

## 8.5   GASTROSCHISIS

The incidence of gastroschisis is estimated at one in 5000 live births. Worldwide there has been an increasing number of cases with the treatment of gastroschisis becoming commonplace in tertiary care centers.[21] Gastroschisis is also one of the most common diagnoses in pediatric patients undergoing intestinal transplantation for IF.

The vast majority of these infants have an excellent prognosis with overall survival rates now exceeding 95%.[22] The excellent survival rate reflects advances in medical care and the predominance of "uncomplicated" cases. Uncomplicated cases include those where the bowel is intact and viable without visible atresia or perforation. The goal of surgical care is to replace the viscera in the abdominal cavity and close the abdominal wall. This can be done by way of silo placement and bedside closure or primary operative closure. Silo placement has become increasingly common as it has many benefits in simplifying the patient's care.[23] It can be performed rapidly at the bedside, does not require anesthesia, and results in immediate protection of the bowel from fluid and heat losses. If primary closure is pursued one must be cognizant of the risk of compartment syndrome which may result in ischemia and should be carefully avoided. The development of compartment syndrome may be life threatening or could result in the loss of the entire gut, which is an unacceptable outcome in a survivable condition. The average length of hospital stay for straightforward cases is around 3–4 weeks.

The only congenital anomaly associated with gastroschisis is intestinal atresia which occurs in 10–15% of patients.[7,24,25] These more "complicated" cases of gastroschisis are frequently associated with prolonged hospitalization, multiple surgeries, prolonged parenteral nutrition dependence, and complications of care which may eventually increase the risk of mortality. In addition to the anatomic defect there is often associated dysfunction of the remaining bowel with both dysmotility and/or malabsorption.[7] Atresia may be associated with vascular accidents *in utero*, which is also a postulated mechanism for development of the abdominal wall defect. Alternatively, *in utero* midgut volvulus may occur or in a rare variant termed vanishing gastroschisis, the defect may close around the root of the exposed viscera effectively strangulating the blood supply and resulting in catastrophic intestinal loss[26] (Figure 8.2).

When an atresia is identified in association with gastroschisis the bowel should be carefully examined and measured for remaining length. There is the caveat that dilated bowel will measure longer than it probably is in reality and also interpreted with respect to gestational age as these infants are frequently if modestly premature. The classical teaching in pediatric surgery is to defer the treatment of atresia in gastroschisis to a second operation 4–6 weeks after abdominal closure. This may still be the most appropriate treatment in cases where the bowel is compromised with ischemia or severe inflammation. The disadvantage to this plan is the mandatory period of parenteral nutritional support that will be required even before they begin to recover from their exploration to restore intestinal continuity.

With a more aggressive approach many surgeons would now choose to preserve bowel that is perhaps compromised but not overtly gangrenous. In addition, primary anastamosis should be

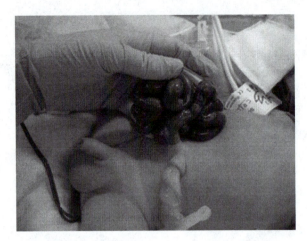

**FIGURE 8.2**   A case of vanishing gastroschisis. Despite the appearance of the bowel, almost all of it was salvaged and eventually the infant achieved full enteral nutrition after resection of an ileal stricture 6 weeks after visceral reduction.

considered relative to the patients overall condition and the appearance of the bowel. In almost every case, there will be a significant size mismatch between the two limbs of bowel. Frequently, limited tapering of the proximal limb will be helpful in creating an anastamosis between the proximal and distal bowel and theoretically may be helpful in promoting function of the anastamosis (Figure 8.3). Extensive tapering should be avoided particularly in patients who are likely to have short gut as them may benefit from gut-lengthening procedures in the future. From the beginning forethought must be given to what future treatment might be required. Depending on the assessment of likelihood of short gut, consideration should also be given to placing a gastrostomy for long-term continuous tube feeding to optimize their care and avoid unnecessary additional operations. Intravenous access should also be established. Initially a peripherally inserted central catheter is likely ideal, but failing success a long-term tunneled line should be placed. Ultimately, the vast majority of patients with gastroschisis will recover with adequate bowel function. Even in complicated cases many patients will eventually have a good outcome.

## 8.6   INTESTINAL ATRESIA

Jejunoileal atresia (JIA) is the most common intestinal atresia (Figure 8.4). There are several subtypes of JIA ranging from a simple web obstructing the lumen to numerous atresias. Surgical treatment in most cases consists of resection of the atretic ends with primary anastomosis.[27] The bowel length is typically normal or near normal. There is often some degree of dysmotility associated with the transition of proximal dilated to distal small caliber bowel. This may result in prolonged return of bowel function, but within several weeks most patients will be able to spontaneously stool and be initiated on enteral feeds.[28,29]

More complex cases may have congenitally short bowel with loss of significant portions of the mesenteric blood supply. Bowel viability may be dubious with retrograde flow through collateral arcades. In these cases care must be taken to avoid losing any further bowel length and appropriately orienting the bowel to avoid any volvulus or ischemia based on bowel position. Intestinal atresia as an isolated congenital anomaly would, in general, be managed similarly to those associated with gastroschisis. One significant difference is that the bowel is likely to be more normal in appearance because of its intra-abdominal location. This allows for primary anastomosis in almost all cases. The main technical difficulty is related to the size mismatch between the proximal and distal limbs. Limited tapering may be useful to allow for anastamosis of limbs of more similar caliber. The distal

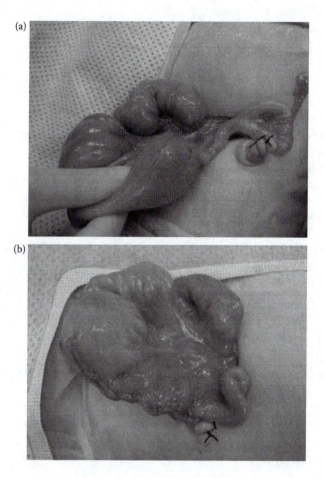

FIGURE 8.3 (a) A proximal atresia related to vanishing gastroschisis. The blind ending loops of jejunum and colon have been amputated at the level of the abdominal wall. (b) A tapered anastamosis was created between the two limbs.

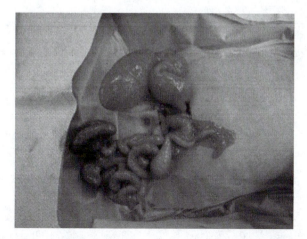

FIGURE 8.4 Proximal jejunal atresia with dilated proximal and small caliber bowel distal to the atresia.

limb may also be spatulated to increase the overall size of the anastamosis. Rarely, when the proximal limb is extremely dilated, diversion with an ostomy may allow it to approach a more reasonable size for anastamosis.

## 8.7  MIDGUT VOLVULUS

Malrotation is a classic pediatric surgical condition. The congenital lack of normal fixation of the bowel results in a narrow-based mesentery prone to twisting. Midgut volvulus occurs when the bowel torses at the base of the mesentery around the superior mesenteric artery. The result is ischemia which left untreated would result in loss of the entire small bowel in a matter of hours. Presentation can occur at any age but is most likely in the newborn period. The hallmark symptom is bilious emesis which should be considered a surgical emergency until proven otherwise. Immediate upper gastrointestinal series should be obtained. The optimal treatment when the diagnosis is established is immediate exploration to reduce the volvulus. When the ischemia has been prolonged variable amounts of the gut may be nonviable up to and including the entire midgut. There is often some sparing of the proximal jejunum near the ligament of Treitz due to collateral flow. In addition, there if frequently sparing of the very distal ileum with flow through the ileocolic vascular arcades. The bowel may improve with observation after reduction of the volvulus. This is a classic example where strong consideration should be given to restoring vascular inflow and performing a second-look laparotomy in 24–48 h to reevaluate. At reexploration, the bowel may have improved significantly or at minimum the areas that are nonviable will be more obviously demarcated. The length of salvaged bowel will be critical to the survival and quality of life of this type of patient. Ultimately, nonviable areas will likely require resection but maximizing the retained bowel will allow for adaptation and the possibility of survival off parenteral nutrition and without transplantation. There are patients in whom no bowel is salvageable and these patients require prolonged nutritional support and transplant evaluation.

## 8.8  MISCELLANEOUS

There are multiple other conditions which occur less commonly but result in SBS. Inflammatory bowel disease with repeated resections, long-segment Hirschsprung's disease, and congenital dysmotility disorders as well as other sporadic entities may result in SBS. Each condition has its own features which must be considered when surgical intervention is required.

## 8.9  CONCLUSIONS

SBS in the pediatric population is almost always the result of a surgical emergency and associated required treatment. While extensive bowel loss is oftentimes unavoidable, every effort should be made to maximize the bowel salvaged even under difficult circumstances. What has been historically considered the most conservative treatment frequently involved aggressive resection and diversion. Modern surgical practice requires consideration of options and an effort to balance the short- and long-term risks and benefits to the individual patient with the intention to minimize morbidity and mortality.

## REFERENCES

1. Duro, D., Kamin D., and Duggan, C. Overview of pediatric short bowel syndrome. *J Pediatr Gastroenterol Nutr* 2008;47(Suppl 1):33–36.
2. Spencer, A., Neaga, A., West, B. et al. Pediatric short bowel syndrome, redefining predictors of success. *Ann Surg* 2005;242(3):403–412.
3. Nayyar, N., Mazariegos, G., Ranganathan, S. et al. Pediatric small bowel transplantation. *Semin Pediatr Surg* 2010;19:68–77.

4. Nathan, J., Rudolph, J., Kocoshis, S. et al. Isolated liver and multivisceral transplantation for total paren-teral nutrition-related end-stage liver disease. *J Pediatr Surg* 2007;42:143–147.
5. Touloukian, R. and Walker Smith, G. Normal intestinal length in preterm infants. *J Pediatr Surg* 1983;18:720–723.
6. Strujis, M., Diamond, I., Silva, N. et al. Establishing norms for intestinal length in children. *J Pediatr Surg* 2009;44:933–938.
7. Phillips, J., Raval, M., Redden, C. et al. Gastroschisis, atresia, dysmotility: Surgical treatment strategies for a distinct clinical entity. *J Pediatr Surg* 2008;43:2208–2212.
8. Duro, D., Kalish, L., Johnston, P. et al. Risk factors for intestinal failure in infants with necrotizing enterocolitis: A Glaser Pediatric Research Network study. *J Pediatr* 2010;157(2):203–208.
9. Hoffman, M., Johnson, C., Moore, T. et al. Management of catastrophic neonatal midgut volvulus with a silo and second-look laparotomy. *J Pediatr Surg* 1992;27(10):1336–1339.
10. Weber, T. and Lewis, J. The role of second-look laparotomy in necrotizing enterocolitis. *J Pediatr Surg* 1986;21(4):323–325.
11. Hunter, C., Chokshi, N., and Ford, H. Evidence vs experience in the surgical management of necrotizing enterocolitis and focal intestinal perforation. *J Perinatol* 2008;28(Suppl 1):S14–S17.
12. Aguayo, P., Fraser, J., St Peter, S. et al. Stomal complications in the newborn with necrotizing entero-colitis. *J Surg Res* 2009;157(2):257–258.
13. Nour, S., Beck, J., and Stringer, M. Colostomy complications in infants and children. *Ann R Coll Surg Engl* 1996;78(6):526–530.
14. Singh, M., Owen, A., Gull, S. et al. Surgery for intestinal perforation in preterm neonates: Anastamosis vs stoma. *J Pediatr Surg* 2006;41(4):725–729.
15. Hall, N., Curry, J., Drake, D. et al. Resection and primary anastamosis is a valid surgical option for infants with necrotizing enterocolitis who weigh less than 1000 g. *Arch Surg* 2005;140(12):1149–1151.
16. Petty, J. and Ziegler, M. Operative strategies for necrotizing enterocolitis: The prevention and treatment of short-bowel syndrome. *Semin Pediatr Surg* 2005;14:191–198.
17. Ricketts, R. and Jerles, M. Neonatal necrotizing enterocolitis: Experience with 100 consecutive surgical patients. *World J Surg* 1990;14(5):600–605.
18. Rees, C., Eaton, S., and Pierro, A. National prospective surveillance study of necrotizing enterocolitis in neonatal intensive care units. *J Pediatr Surg* 2010;45(7):1391–1397.
19. Moore, T.C. The management of necrotizing enterocolitis by "patch, drain, and wait." *Pediatr Surg Int* 1989;4:110–113.
20. Moore, T.C. Successful use of the "patch, drain, and wait" laparotomy approach to perforated necrotizing enterocolitis: *Is* hypoxia-triggered "good angiogenesis" involved? *Pediatr Surg Int* 2001;16:356–363.
21. Clark, R., Walker, M., and Gauderer, M. Prevalence of gastroschisis and associated hospital time con-tinue to rise in neonates who are admitted for intensive care. *J Pediatr Surg* 2009;44(6):1108–1112.
22. Skarsgard, E., Claydon, J., Bouchard, S. et al. Canadian pediatric surgical network: A population-based pediatric surgery network and database for analyzing surgical birth defects. The first 100 cases of gastros-chisis. *J Pediatr Surg* 2008;43(1):30–34.
23. Pastor, A., Phillips, J., Fenton, S. et al. Routine use of a SILASTIC spring-loaded silo for infants with gastroschisis: A multicenter randomized controlled trial. *J Pediatr Surg* 2008;43(10):1807–1812.
24. Kronfli, R., Bradnock, T., and Sabharwal, A. Intestinal atresia in association with gastroschisis: A 26-year review. *Pediatr Surg Int* 2010;26:891–894.
25. Snyder, C., Miller, K., Sharp, R. et al. Management of intestinal atresia in patients with gastroschisis. *J Pediatr Surg* 2001;36(10):1542–1545.
26. Vogler, S., Fenton, S., Scaife, E. et al. Closed gastroschisis: Total parenteral nutrition-free survival with aggressive attempts at bowel preservation and intestinal adaptation. *J Pediatr Surg* 2008;43:1006–1010.
27. Stolman, T., de Blaauw, I., Wijnen, M. et al. Decreased mortality but increased morbidity in neonates with jejunoileal atresia: A study of 114 cases over a 34-year period. *J Pediatr Surg* 2009;44(1):217–221.
28. Burjonrappa, S., Crete, E., and Bouchard, S. Prognostic factors in jejuno-ileal atresia. *Pediatr Surg Int* 2009;25(9):795–798.
29. Piper, H., Alesbury, J., Waterford, S. et al. Intestinal atresias: Factors affecting clinical outcomes. *J Pediatr Surg* 2008;43(7):1244–1248.

# 9 Medical and Nutritional Management

*Clarivet Torres*

## CONTENTS

## 9.1 INTRODUCTION

The main goal of therapy for intestinal failure (IF) is to facilitate bowel adaptation and enteral autonomy. To accomplish this goal, a comprehensive, multidisciplinary management program is required to provide frequent monitoring, early identification and treatment of complications and efforts to help establish normal growth and development. Continual parent/patient education and support is also an important part of the treatment. Patients with IF encounter multiple acute and chronic problems including nutrient loss, diarrhea, and fluid and electrolyte abnormalities. Ideally, the multidisciplinary management team should include a gastroenterologist, a surgeon, a nurse practitioner/coordinator, a dietitian, a pharmacist as well as social and psychological support. To determine the most appropriate therapy, a comprehensive evaluation is necessary. This chapter will review the medical and enteral nutritional management of patients who have acquired IF as a result of short bowel syndrome (SBS).

## 9.2 CLINICAL MANAGEMENT

The management of SBS is a multistage process [1,2]. It begins with the use of parenteral nutrition (PN) (see Chapters 10 and 11, Parenteral Nutrition in Children and Adults, respectively) followed by gradual introduction of enteral feedings combined with PN. As enteral tolerance improves, the nutritional support advances to oral and continuous enteral feeding alone and then to weaning to bolus feeding and solid foods, with the ultimate goal of attaining regular intake of a solid and liquid diet.

## 9.3 INITIAL PHASE

The immediate postoperative state following bowel resection is usually characterized by a period of intestinal ileus (2–5 days) with high gastric output, followed by profuse diarrhea and massive electrolyte loss. PN is the only nutritional support possible during the perioperative period and it provides the maintenance fluids and the nutrients required to replenish the energy stores depleted during the stress of the presurgery and transient postoperative ileus phases [1]. PN requires continuous nutritional monitoring, both clinically and via laboratory evaluations, to ensure adequate nutritional rehabilitation.

During this initial phase, it is crucial to strictly monitor fluid and electrolyte losses and give the patient the appropriate replacement solutions. If the patient is on ventilator support, has cardiac dysfunction or renal impairment postoperatively, the maintenance fluids should be reduced by 10–20% based on the patient's specific condition. Gastric and ostomy losses need to be replaced milliliter for milliliter with a saline solution, with careful monitoring of serum electrolytes and/or the electrolytes of the gastric or ostomy losses. Gastric secretions and serum gastrin levels are often significantly elevated in patients with SBS and treatment with IV H2 blockers or proton pump inhibitors may be given in the immediate postoperative period [3,4]. Gastric hypersecretion tends to be transient, and this therapy could be discontinued later. However, the treatment needs to be continued in patients who develop gastroesophageal reflux disease or peptic ulcers [1].

Once the ileus disappears, and the fluid and electrolyte losses have diminished, enteral feedings should be instituted. Controversy exists about the optimal enteral feeding regimen to use in the patient with SBS. Many intestinal rehabilitation programs use continuous enteral feedings to gradually advance the enteral formula tolerated by the infants with SBS [5,6]. In our experience, the use of continuous enteral feedings, even in patients with a history of severe enteral intolerance and advance liver disease, can lead to successful outcomes [7]. The theory of continuing enteral feedings to improve absorption is based on a study by Parker et al., which showed better nutrient absorption in infants with damaged intestine [8]. Supporting the data are the results of a recent randomized crossover study in SBS adult patients, which compared absorption between isocaloric tube feedings (CEF) and oral feedings (OF) in 15 SBS patients. An oral feeding period combined with enriched tube feeding (OCEF) was also tested in nine patients [9]. This study demonstrated that CEF exclusively or in conjunction with oral feedings significantly increased net absorption of lipids, proteins, and energy compared with oral feedings alone (see Figure 9.1) [9]. The net gain per day was clinically relevant with a total energy gain of 700 kcal/day with the group of CEF, corresponding to 33% of the total energy expenditure. The energy gain for the combined group OCEF was 1036 kcal/day corresponding to 57% of the total energy expenditure for SBS patients. The total energy expenditure estimated for SBS patient is calculated as basal energy expenditure multiplied by 1.5, a figure necessary to obtain energy balance equilibrium in SBS patients [10].

Continuous enteral feedings have numerous advantages over bolus feedings. CEF allows a gradual infusion of a liquid diet, permitting a greater percentage of total nutritional requirements to be delivered by the enteral route and reducing the tendency for emesis [2]. Use of CEF also stimulates the increase in carrier protein saturation, which helps maximize the overall functional capacity of the intestine [1,2]. Normal patients fed continuously compared with patients fed with boluses showed a reduction in thermal energy losses [11]. There are many ways to advance feedings but slow, gradual advancement of continuous tube feedings is usually the most successful and it aids the close monitoring of hydration status and electrolyte balance. A marked increase in stool losses by more than 50% or stool output greater than 40–50 mL/kg/day is an indication to slow the advancement of tube feedings. In patients with an intact large bowel, a decrease in stool pH below 5.5 is indicative of carbohydrate malabsorption and osmotic diarrhea. It is important to maintain good hydration during the process of advancing enteral fluids, as mild dehydration makes the pediatric patient more prone to emesis and decreased absorption [1,7].

Patients with SBS need between 1.5 and 2 times maintenance fluids between enteral feedings and IV fluids to compensate for intestinal losses. Accurate measurements of stool output with adequate replacement of fluid loss is difficult in SBS patients unless they have an ostomy. Patients with renal dysfunction, respiratory problems or CNS involvement require some fluid restriction and should be evaluated individually.

The route of enteral nutrition is selected according to the needs of the patient. Nasogastric tube feedings are usually an initial good temporary option. Nasoduodenal (ND) or nasojejunal (NJ) feeding

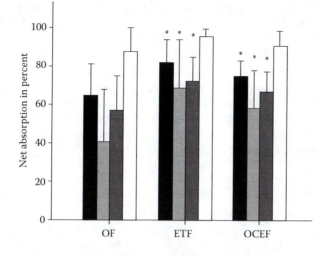

**FIGURE 9.1** Net absorption (in percent) of total calories, lipids, proteins, and carbohydrates during the three study periods. The histogram represents the percent net absorption of total calories, lipids, proteins, and carbohydrates, respectively, in black, light gray, dark gray, and white. The coefficient of net intestinal absorption, expressed as a percentage of total calories ingested and of the main energy sources (lipids, proteins, and carbohydrates), represents the proportion of ingested calories and of the main energy sources not recovered in stool output. *Macronutrient absorption in percent was significantly increased in ETF and OCEF versus OF, for total calories ($P < .001$), lipids ($P < .001$), and proteins ($P < .001$). Mean ± SD. ETF, exclusive tube feeding; OCEF, oral combined with tube feeding; OF, oral feeding. [Reproduced from Joly F and Dray X. *Gastroenterology* 2009;136(3):824–831. Epub 2008 Nov. With permission.]

is an alternative option when delayed gastric emptying or gastroesophageal reflux disease limits gastric feeding. The frequent dislodgement of the NJ tube and the difficulty in replacing it makes transpyloric feeding less attractive [12]. Patients with SBS often need long-term continuous enteral feedings, and they may benefit from the placement of a gastrostomy tube (GT). A GT may be converted to a gastro-jejunal tube later, if necessary.

The ideal formula for feeding children with SBS has not yet been determined. Breast milk, if available and tolerated by the patient, is the best formula to start with. Human milk, particularly colostrum, contains a unique combination of specific immunoglobulins, nutrients, hormones, and growth factors for the infant. It plays an important role in the development of the intestinal, immunologic, and neurologic systems. Epidermal growth factor, glucagon-like peptide (GLP) 2, insulin-like growth factor-1, growth hormone, and interleukin-11, have been identified in colostrum and these factors may have a trophic effect on bowel mucosa and intestinal adaptation. Polymeric infant formula supplemented with colostrum protein concentrate was associated with improved intestinal adaptation in juvenile pigs with SBS compared with animals fed an unmodified polymeric infant formula diet [13,14].

Breast milk may not always be available and some patients with protein or lactose intolerance may not tolerate breast milk. For these patients, hydrolysate formulas or elemental (amino acid) formulas are nutritionally well balanced and are formulated to deliver all necessary macro- and micronutrients for infants and older children. Protein hydrolysate formulas may be more easily tolerated, since most proteins are absorbed in the form of di- and tripeptides. Elemental formulas are beneficial in reducing the risk of secondary protein intolerance [1], which may occur more frequently in children with SBS due to conditions that predispose them to enhanced intestinal permeability. Carbohydrates in elemental and hydrolyzed formulas are usually glucose polymers in the form of corn syrup, maltodextrins, hydrolyzed starch; sometimes disaccharidases such as sucrose are used.

Although intestinal feeding is one of the major trophic factors that stimulates intestinal adaptation after small bowel resection, not all nutrients have equal stimulatory trophic effects. For example, long-chain fatty acids are slightly less well absorbed than medium-chain fatty acids; however, they offer a very strong stimulus for adaptation and are more efficient and calorically dense than protein and carbohydrates [15,16]. They should constitute a significant percentage of the total enteral caloric intake for children with SBS. Support for this approach comes from animal studies. The early use of a high-fat diet in rats with SBS resulted in increased absorptive capacity of the intestinal remnant as measured by increased food and fat absorption [17].

In the initial phase of nutritional therapy, very small volume of oral bolus feedings of the specialized formula or oral electrolyte solution are beneficial in stimulating normal development of oral feeding. Pacifier use in infants is not sufficient to meet these needs. As little as 10–15 mL of formula, two to three times a day may help to prevent feeding aversion in infants [1,6,18] (see Chapter 35).

## 9.4   LATER PHASES

As enteral feedings are tolerated, PN is weaned proportionally. The calculation of the caloric requirements for patients with short bowel syndrome (SBS) is made by multiplying the recommended dietary allowance (RDA) for age by a factor of 1.2–1.5 to account for malabsorption [1,10]. Precise energy needs for IF patients are unknown, however, and anecdotally enteral energy intakes as high as 150–180 kcal/kg/day are sometimes needed to achieve adequate growth. PN infusion time is progressively weaned during the day as the child gets older, to allow for activities unencumbered by catheter infusion. Careful monitoring of glucose and hydration status throughout this time is important. When the total volume and caloric content provided by PN or the number of hours of infusion are reduced, PN, or hydration fluids, can be eliminated one or two nights per week Progressive advancement of days without PN is the goal for patients who continue to tolerate enteral nutrition. This entire process is very gradual and may take weeks, months, or even years to complete [7].

A small number of patients tolerate the necessary enteral feedings to maintain nutritional balance, but still require extra fluids for the maintenance of good hydration and electrolyte status. In these patients, extra IV fluids at night may be used to replace the fluids and electrolytes they need. This fluid/electrolyte deficit may also be replaced using the enteral route. Oral rehydration solution (ORS), boluses of normal saline or half-normal saline may be added to the patient's feeding regimen or mixed with the 24-h formula to meet the patient's fluid needs [7].

Once adequate growth is achieved in children, the normal stimulation of eating should be introduced (including both chewing and swallowing) at the appropriate developmental times. While solid food feedings traditionally start with high carbohydrate foods, children with SBS do better with high fat, high protein foods. Meats are an example of a potentially well-designed food group for SBS patients, as they provide less osmotic load to the small bowel and the fat provides an additional stimulus for intestinal adaptation [2,7]. Red meat is also rich in iron and zinc, critical minerals for which the SBS patient may be shortchanged (see Chapter 35).

In adult patients with SBS, the diet needs to be individualized, depending on the underlying disease, the bowel anatomy, the presence or absence of the colon and individual taste and tolerance [19,20]. Patients with jejunocolic anastomosis should receive 30–35 kcal/day of complex carbohydrates with soluble fiber, with 20–30% of caloric intake as fat in the form of medium-chain (MCT) and long-chain triglycerides (LCT) and 1.0–1.5 g/kg/day of intact protein. In patients without a colon there is no need for fiber supplementation and LCT alone is recommended [19]. The types of carbohydrate chosen should be those that help to reduce abdominal cramping, flatulence, and stool output [20]. It is important to avoid concentrated simple sugars (candies, fruit juices) as they produce a high osmotic load and tend to exacerbate the underlying osmotic diarrhea. Complex carbohydrates such as bread, pasta, potatoes, and rice are usually well tolerated and should provide about 50% of energy intake [20]. Oxalate restriction is important in patients with a colon, as 25% of patients with less than 200 cm of small bowel and a colon develop nephropathy [21]. In these patients, the use of a low oxalate diet and administration of citrate may help to prevent stone formation. Low oxalate diets exclude cocoa, peanut products, tea, coffee,

**Table 9.1**

**Composition of Selected Oral Electrolyte Solutions**

| | | Reduced-Osmolality | |
| --- | --- | --- | --- |
| | C-ORS | WHO-ORS | Standard WHO-ORS |
| Sodium, mmol/L | 45 | 75 | 90 |
| Potassium, mmol/L | 20 | 20 | 20 |
| Chloride, mmol/L | 35 | 65 | 80 |
| Base, mmol/L | 10 | 10 | 10 |
| Glucose, mmol/L | 139 | 75 | 111 |
| Osmolality, mmol/kg $H_2O$ | 250 | 245 | 311 |

*Source:* Adapted from King CK et al. *MMWR* 2003; 52 (No. RR-16):1–16.

*Note:* C-ORS indicates commercially prepared oral rehydration solution; WHO-ORS, World Health Organization-oral rehydration solution.

wheat germ, rhubarb, beets, collards, spinach, tofu and soybeans, tomatoes, fruit, and the use of citrus drinks should be restricted.

The best-tolerated meal pattern usually involves 5–6 smaller meals spread over the course of the day. Other general strategies are to avoid drinking water without food, spreading fluid intake out over the course of the day, avoidance of hypotonic fluids, and drinking oral rehydration solutions that contain salt and carbohydrates [22,23]. Currently, tube feedings in adults are recommended only in the early postoperative state. However, Joly and Dray. [9] have demonstrated a significant improvement in the net percent macronutrient absorption using tube feeding during the postoperative adaptive and postadaptive periods. These results were independent of the type of intestinal remnant.

In the later phases of the advancement of feeding of patients with SBS, dehydration can occur more readily with viral gastroenteritis or environmental exposure to extreme heat. This is because these patients usually have a small margin for adaptation when their intestinal function is adversely affected by infection or other stresses. Constant intake of small volumes of fluid, such as ORS, as well as avoidance of excessive heat, is necessary to avoid hospitalization. ORS is important in the maintenance of adequate fluid balance and helps to decrease the need for parenteral fluids. This is especially significant in patients with proximal jejunostomies who are net fluid and sodium excretors. The jejunum is permeable to sodium and chloride; therefore, solutions with a high NaCl content are readily and passively absorbed [23]. Several commercially available ORS products are available; however probably the best are the ones with high sodium content (90 mmol/L) and low osmolality (less than 300 mmol/L) (Table 9.1). Watery diarrhea is one of the most common complications of SBS, mostly due to the osmotic effect of the enteral intake of formula and/or the effect of bacterial overgrowth. Careful review and control of the oral dietary intake is an essential part of the management of the diarrhea. A change from bolus to continuous enteral feedings as well as dilution of the formula may be helpful in lessening the diarrhea. Decreasing the carbohydrate content and adding long-chain fatty acids to the formula may be also useful. For patients who have intravenous access, consideration should be given to keep an extra supply of intravenous solutions on hand for emergencies, as this may prevent rehospitalization [1,2].

## 9.5   VITAMIN AND MINERAL SUPPLEMENTATION

At any stage, careful monitoring of weight gain and growth is the most beneficial tool to evaluate nutritional status and nutrient absorption. Efforts to identify malabsorbed nutrients in the stool are not helpful [1,2]. The careful monitoring of weight is also important to ensure that the patient's weight gain is appropriate for his or her height. Serial measures of body mass index are important in this regard as well (see Chapters 4 and 5). Patients are screened more frequently for micronutrient deficiencies, as the enteral feeding becomes the primary nutritional source. Macronutrients such as fat, proteins, and carbohydrates are usually absorbed in adequate amounts. In contrast, micronutrients such as zinc, magnesium, fat-soluble vitamins, and iron are frequently deficient in SBS patients. Serum zinc concentration is neither a sensitive nor specific indicator of zinc deficiency. Reduced concentrations of serum zinc in association with low serum alkaline phosphatase level and/or normal serum albumin suggest deficiency. Patients with SBS have difficulty absorbing fat-soluble vitamins because they often lack bile salts and have insufficient absorptive surface. They frequently require large doses of vitamins A, D, and E to avoid deficits. Liquid preparations may be necessary, because tablets or capsules are often excreted intact. Patients with significant resection of the ileum will require routine vitamin B12 supplementation. Some patients may absorb high doses of oral vitamin B12 while others will require parenteral or intranasal preparations. Enteral feeding can also be supplemented with the specific deficient micronutrient, although magnesium supplements often result in osmotic diarrhea. Supplementation with magnesium lactate or gluconate is preferred because these preparations do not increase output as much as other forms such as magnesium oxide [1,19,20].

## 9.6   DIETARY SUPPLEMENTS AND TROPHIC FACTORS

During later therapy, many other additional dietary supplements are used to enhance enteral tolerance. Insoluble fiber such as wheat bran can cause bulking of the stool and increase intestinal transit time. Soluble fiber, such as pectin, guar gum, slows gastric emptying and overall transit time. In addition, aerobic bacteria of the colon metabolize unabsorbed fiber (pectins) to short-chain fatty (SCFA) acids. These SCFA are rapidly absorbed by the colonic mucosa and used for energy [24].

Numerous other additives, such as glutamine and growth hormone, have been attempted with varying degrees of success. The use of high-dose recombinant human growth hormone in uncontrolled [25] and controlled studies [26,27,28] has led to variable results. The benefits of this therapy must be weighed against the potential side effects, which include fluid retention, edema, arthralgias, and carpal tunnel syndrome [29]. Clearly, the dose, the optimal timing of administration and the safety and efficacy of long-term treatment with growth hormone has not yet been determined.

Glucagon-like peptide 2 (GLP-2) is an enteroendocrine peptide produced in the L-cells localized in the distal small bowel and colon. Evidence from both animal studies and clinical trials demonstrate that GLP-2 is a trophic hormone that plays an important role in the regulation of intestinal adaptation and in nutrient absorption [30,31]. Although GLP-2 is not commercially available, investigational studies of a longer acting, genetically engineered analog of GLP-2 are underway. In an open-label cross-over study, Jeppessen et al. described the effects of administration of 400 μg of GLP-2, by subcutaneous injection TID, to 11 SBS patients for two consecutive years [32]. The study showed that GLP-2 treatment reduced fecal weight by approximately 1000 g/day and enabled SBS patients to maintain their intestinal fluid and electrolyte absorption at lower oral intakes. This was accompanied by a 28% improvement in creatinine clearance. No significant changes were demonstrated in energy intake or absorption, and GLP-2 did not significantly affect mucosal morphology, body composition, bone mineral density or muscle function. See Chapter 31 for a detailed discussion of this topic.

## 9.7   OTHER MEDICATIONS USED IN THE MANAGEMENT OF SBS

Antiperistaltic agents such as loperamide have been used safely in the pediatric age group. They can prolong transit time, reduce daily fecal volume, and diminish loss of fluids and electrolytes. Loperamide has been effective in reducing the volume of discharge from ileostomies [33,34]. However, these medications have been associated with increased small bowel bacterial overgrowth and must be used carefully [2,35]. Transdermal administration of clonidine has resulted in improvement in diarrhea and sodium loss in patients with proximal jejunostomies, decreasing daily fecal volume and weight [36].

Somatostatin, and its analog octreotide, may improve diarrhea by increasing the transit time, reducing salt and water excretion and reducing gastric hypersecretion. Although these therapeutic agents can be beneficial in the short term, they have not resulted in long-term benefits, and they may have some important potential deleterious effects. These effects include the inhibition of intestinal regeneration, which may delay or inhibit intestinal adaptation, the development of cholelithiasis due to delayed gallbladder emptying, decreased hepatico-biliary secretion, and sphincter of Oddi dysfunction [37–39]. They may also exacerbate steatorrhea because of impaired pancreatic exocrine function. Therefore, octreotide should not be used routinely for the management of chronic diarrhea in these patients.

Ursodeoxycholic acid, an effective choleretic, is frequently used in patients with SBS; however, it may be poorly absorbed in patients with no ileum causing more diarrhea. Gallbladder stasis from lack of enteral feedings and a reduction of bile salts may lead to the formation of cholesterol stones. Ursodeoxycholic acid therapy and early cholecystectomy are recommended treatments for cholelithiasis [40,41].

The main fraction of bile acid is absorbed in the distal third of the terminal ileum by an active sodium couple transport (enterohepatic circulation) [42,43]. Patients with an ileal resection of 30 cm or more may develop malabsorption of the bile acid, resulting in an increased passage of bile acids into the colon, where dihydroxy bile acid induces the secretion of salt and water causing diarrhea [42]. However, with major ileal resections (>100 cm), fecal bile salt loss exceeds the rate of hepatic synthesis of bile acids. Lack of bile salt absorption inhibits fat absorption, and consequently causes fat-soluble vitamins (A,D,E,K) and divalent cations (calcium, magnesium, and zinc) deficiencies, requiring large doses of vitamins to compensate deficits [44].

The use of cholestyramine in powder, which releases the active substance into the small bowel, has been used with some success to sequester bile in SBS patients who have bile salt-induced watery diarrhea. Nevertheless, such treatment has two physiological disadvantages [45]. First, the jejunal concentration of nonsequestered bile acids is suboptimal for sufficient solubilization of the lipolytic products after meals resulting in the malabsorption of fat, steatorrhea, and diarrhea induced by fatty acids. Second, malabsorption of bile acid is increased because sequestered bile acids are not available for small intestinal reabsorption. In the adult population, Jacobsen et al. [45] have observed reduction of diarrhea, without noticeably interfering with the metabolism of fat or bile acid, with the use of cholestyramine entercoated with cellulose acetate phthalate (tablets), which mostly releases the active substance in the distal ileum/colon. In children with SBS the use of cholestyramine entercoated has not been studied. The use of cholestyramine in children is limited because the diagnosis of bile acid-induced diarrhea is not easily made as the measurement of either fecal bile acid excretion or postprandial plasma levels of bile acids is not performed in most clinical laboratories [46] and because of the inability to determine the ileal length. Its use may cause more secondary complications (steatorrhea, fat-soluble vitamin deficiency, and osteoporosis) than benefits.

## 9.8  CONCLUSION

The successful management of patients with SBS is complex and requires a multidisciplinary approach. The basic goals of medical treatment are to promote bowel adaptation and enteral autonomy, to maintain fluid electrolyte and nutrient balance and prompt and effective treatment of complications. The length and function of the remaining bowel are major factors that determine the successful advancement of enteral feedings and the concomitant weaning of parenteral nutrition. The use of aggressive enteral feeding programs, support of good nutrition, and hydration status by intestinal rehabilitation programs with experienced medical and other staff are also important factors in the long-term survival of patients with SBS. Many controversial issues still exist in the management of these patients, including the type and route of optimal enteral feeding, the timing of the initiation and advancement of enteral and oral feedings, and the use of parenteral nutritional additives and dietary supplements. However, it is clear from clinical practice that thoughtful and carefully managed nutritional intervention, combined with appropriate patient education and monitoring can facilitate successful weaning from PN. The current assessment of the efficacy and outcome of the different medical treatment options are limited by the small number of SBS patients in any one center. There is a great need to join efforts between centers to comprehensively study the care of these patients in order to develop and standardize optimal treatment protocols.

## REFERENCES

1. Torres C and Vanderhoof JA. Short bowel syndrome. In: Rolandelli RH, Bankhead R, Boullata JI, and Compher CW, eds. *Short Bowel Syndrome in Clinical Nutrition, Enteral and Tube Feedings*. 4th ed. Philadelphia, PA: Elsevier-Saunders, 2004. pp. 451–463.
2. Vanderhoof JA and Young RJ. Short bowel syndrome. In: Lifschitz,CH, editor. *Pediatric Gastroenterology and Nutrition in Clinical Practice*. New York: Marcel Dekker; 2002. pp. 701–723.
3. Hyman PE and Garvey TQ. Effect of ranitidine on gastric acid hypersecretion in an infant with short bowel syndrome. *J Pediatr Gastroenterol Nutr* 1985;4:316–319.
4. Hyman PE and Everett SL. Gastric acid hypersecretion in short bowel syndrome in infants. Association with extent of resection and enteral feeding. *J Pediatr Gastroenterol Nutr* 1987;5:191–197.
5. Quiros–Tejeira RE, Ament ME, Reyen L, Herzog F, Merjanian M, Olivares-Serrano N, and Vargas JH. Long term parenteral nutritional support and intestinal adaptation in children with short bowel syndrome: A 25-year experience. *J Pediatr* 2004;145:157–163.
6. Wessel JJ and Kocoshis SA. Nutritional management of infants with short bowel syndrome. *Semin Perinatol* 2007;31(2):104–111.
7. Torres C and Sudan D. Role of an intestinal rehabilitation program in the treatment of advanced intestinal failure. *J Pediatr Gastroenterol Nutr* 2007;45(2):204–212.
8. Parker P and Stroop S. A controlled comparison of continuous versus intermittent feeding in the treatment of infants with intestinal disease. *J Pediatr* 1987;99:360.
9. Joly F and Dray X. Tube feeding improves intestinal absorption in short bowel syndrome patients. *Gastroenterology* 2009;136(3):824–831. Epub 2008 Nov.
10. Messing B, Pigot F, Morin MC, Ndeïndoum U, and Rambaud JC. Intestinal absorption of free oral hyperalimentation in the very short bowel syndrome. *Gastroenterology* 1991;100(6):1502–1508.
11. Heymsfield SB, Casper K, and Grossman GD. Bioenergetic and metabolic response to continuous vs intermittent nasoenteric feeding. *Metabolism* 1987;36:570.
12. Marchand V, Baker SS, and Baker RD. Enteral nutrition in the pediatric population. *Gastro Endosc Clin North Am* 1998;8(3):669–703.
13. Torres C. Intestinal failure: Is it permanent? *Curr Opin Organ Transplant* 2005;10:132–136.
14. Nagy ES, Paris MC, and Taylor RG. Colostrum protein concentrate enhances intestinal adaptation after massive small bowel resection in juvenile pigs. *J Pediatr Gastroenterol Nutr* 2004;39(5):487–492.
15. Morin CL, Grey VI, and Garafalo C. Influence of lipids on intestinal adaptation after resection. In: Robinson JW, Dowling RH, Riecken EO, editors. *Mechanisms of Intestinal Adapation*. Lancaster: MTP Press; 1982. pp. 175–185.
16. Vanderhoof AJ, Park JH, Herrington MK, and Adrian TE. Effects of dietary menhaden oil on mucosal adaptation after small bowel resection in rats. *Gastroenterology* 1994;106:94–99.
17. Sukhotnik I, Mor-Vaknin N, Drongowski RA, Coran AG, and Harmon CM. Effect of dietary fat on fat absorption and concomitant plasma and tissue fat composition in a rat model of short bowel syndrome. *Pediatr Surg Int* 2004;20(3):185–191.
18. Goulet O, Ruemmele F, Drongowski RA, Coran AG, and Harmon CM. Irreversible intestinal failure. *J Pediatr Gastroenterol Nutr* 2004;38(3):250–269.
19. Buchman AL and Scolapio J. AGA technical review on short bowel syndrome and intestinal transplantation. *Gastroenterology* 2003;124(4):1111–1134.
20. Matarese LE, O'Keefe SJ, Kandil HM, Bond G, Costa G, and Abu-Elmagd K. Short bowel syndrome: Clinical guidelines for nutrition management. *Nutr Clin Pract* 2005;20(5):493–502.
21. Nightingale JM, Lennard-Jones JE, Gertner DJ, Wood SR, and Bartram CI. Colonic preservation reduces need for parenteral therapy, increases incidence of renal stones, but does not change high prevalence of gall stones in patients with a short bowel. *Gut* 1992;33(11):1493–1497.

22. Jeejeebhoy KN. Short bowel syndrome: A nutritional and medical approach. *CMAJ* 2002;166(10): 1297–1302.

23. Buchman AL. The medical and surgical management of short bowel syndrome. *MedGenMed* 2004;6(2):12.

24. Rombeau JL and Kripke SA. Metabolic and intestinal effects of short-chain fatty acids. *J Parenter Enteral Nutr* 1990;14(Suppl):181–185.

25. Byrne TA and Persinger RL. A new treatment for patients with short-bowel syndrome. Growth hormone, glutamine, and a modified diet. *Ann Surg* 1995;222(3):243–54; discussion 254–255.

26. Szkudlarek J, Jeppesen PB, and Mortensen PB. Effect of high-dose growth hormone with glutamine and no change in diet on intestinal absorption in short bowel patients: A randomized, double blind, crossover, placebo-controlled study. *Gut* 2000;47(2):199–205.

27. Scolapio JS, Camilleri M, Fleming CR, Oenning LV, Burton DD, Sebo TJ, Batts KP, and Kelly DG. Effect of growth hormone, glutamine, and diet on adaptation in short-bowel syndrome: A randomized, controlled study. *Gastroenterology* 1997;113(4):1074–1081.

28. Byrne TA, Wilmore DW, Iyer K, Dibaise J, Clancy K, Robinson MK, Chang P, Gertner JM, and Lautz D. Growth hormone, glutamine, and an optimal diet reduces parenteral nutrition in patients with short bowel syndrome: A prospective, randomized, placebo-controlled, double-blind clinical trial. *Ann Surg.* 2005;242(5):655–661.

29. Jackson C and Buchman AL. Advances in the management of short bowel syndrome. *Curr Gastroenterol Rep* 2005;7(5):373–378.

30. Lovshin J and Drucker DJ. New frontiers in the biology of GLP-2. *Regul Pept* 2000;90:27–32.

31. Martin GR, Beck PL, and Sigalet DL. Gut hormones, and short bowel syndrome: The enigmatic role of glucagon-like peptide-2 in the regulation of intestinal adaptation. *World J Gastroenterol* 2006;12(26):4117–4129.

32. Jeppesen PB, Lund P, Gottschalck IB, Nielsen HB, Holst JJ, Mortensen J, Poulsen SS, Quistorff B, and Mortensen PB. Short bowel patients treated for two years with glucagon-like peptide 2: Effects on intestinal morphology and absorption, renal function, bone and body composition, and muscle function. *Gastroenterol Res Pract* 2009;2009:616054. Epub 2009 Aug 20.

33. Tytgat GN, Huibregtse K, Dagevos J, and van den Ende A. Effect of loperamide on fecal output and composition in well-established ileostomy and ileorectal anastomosis. *Am J Dig Dis* 1977;22(8):669–676.

34. King RF, North RT, and Hill GL. A double-blind crossover study of the effect of loperamide hydrochloride and codeine phosphate on ileostomy output. *Aust N Z J Surg* 1982;52(2):121–124.

35. Duval-Iflah Y, Berard H, Baumer P, Guillaume P, Raibaud P, Joulin Y, and Lecomte JM. Effects of racecadotril and loperamide on bacterial proliferation and on the central nervous system of the newborn gnotobiotic piglet. *Aliment Pharmacol Ther* 1999;13(Suppl 6):9–14.

36. Buchman AL, Fryer J, Wallin A, Ahn CW, Polensky S, and Zaremba K. Clonidine reduces diarrhea and sodium loss in patients with proximal jejunostomy a controlled study. *JPEN* 2006;30:487–491.

37. Bass BL, Fischer BA, Richardson C, and Harmon JW. Somatostatin analogue treatment inhibits postresectional adaptation of the small bowel in rats. *Am J Surg* 1991;161:107–112.

38. Redfern JS and Fortuner WJ 2nd. Octreotide-associated biliary tract dysfunction and gallstone formation: Pathophysiology and management. *Am J Gastroenterol* 1995;90:1042–1052.

39. Thompson JS, Nguyen BLT, and Harty RF. Somatostatin analogue inhibits intestinal regeneration. *Arch Surg* 1993;128:385–389.

40. Balistreri WF, A-Kader HH et al. Biochemical and clinical response to UDCA administration in pediatric patients with chronic cholestasis. In: Paumgartner G, Stiehl A, Gerok W, editors. *Bile Acids as Therapeutic Agents*. Lancaster, UK: Kluwer; 1991. pp. 323–333.

41. Roslyn JJ, Pitt HA, Mann L, Fonkalsrud EW, and DenBensten L. Parenteral nutrition-induced gall bladder disease: A reason for early cholecystectomy. *Am J Surg* 1984;148(1):58–63.

42. Hofmann AF. Bile acid malabsorption caused by ileal resection. *Arch Intern Med* 1972;130:597–596.

43. Hofmann AF. Chemistry and enterohepatic circulation of bile acids. *Hepatology* 1984;4:4S–14S.

44. Torres C and Vanderhoof JA. Chronic complications of short bowel syndrome. *Current Paediatrics* 2006;16:291–297.

45. Jacobsen O, Højgaard L, Møller EH, Wielandt TO, Thale M, Jarnum S, and Krag E. Effect of enterocoated cholestyramine on bowel habit after ileal resection: A double blind crossover study. *Br Med J (Clin Res Ed)* 1985;290(6478):1315–1318.

46. Hofmann AF. Chronic diarrhea caused by idiopathic bile acid malabsorption: An explanation at last. *Expert Rev Gastroenterol Hepatol* 2009;3(50):461–464.

47. King CK, Glass RI, Bresee JS, Duggan C. Managing acute gastroenteritis among children: Oral rehydration, maintenance and nutritional therapy. *MMWR* 2003;52 (No. RR-16):1–16.

# 10 Parenteral Nutrition in Children

*Sharon Collier, Kathleen M. Gura, and Christopher P. Duggan*

## CONTENTS

## 10.1 INTRODUCTION

Parenteral nutrition (PN) for the pediatric population has now been available for about 40 years [1]. It is often a life-saving means of nutrition support and serves as a bridge until enteral feedings can be initiated and advanced. Over the years there have been many modifications in the components and method of delivery in the quest to meet the needs of the patients and provide a safe and efficacious product. Pediatric patients with intestinal failure are particularly dependent on PN and in fact this dependence is incorporated into common case definitions of intestinal failure. (Although some authors refer to parenteral nutrition as "total parenteral nutrition" or TPN, we prefer "PN" to avoid the implication that PN is a complete source of human nutrition and/or that it meets all nutrient requirements in humans.)

## 10.2 INDICATIONS

For the pediatric population there are many conditions for which PN is indicated. In general, it is used for patients who cannot be enterally fed. The clinical conditions leading to this situation can often be divided into medical and surgical conditions (Table 10.1). The medical indications include: chronic diarrhea, acute flare in inflammatory bowel disease, gastrointestinal motility disorders, and prematurity. Typical surgical conditions include congenital anomalies of the gastrointestinal tract that require surgical repair such as gastroschisis and intestinal atresias. All of these conditions, whether medical or surgical based, require a period where enteral feeding could pose a greater risk and/or would not be tolerated.

**TABLE 10.1**

**Possible Indications for PN Support**

| Medical | Surgical |
|---|---|
| Prematurity | Gastroschisis |
| Chronic diarrhea | Midgut volvulus/malrotation |
| Inflammatory bowel disease | Congenital diaphragmatic hernia |
| Necrotizing enterocolitis | Intestinal atresias |
| Pseudo-obstruction | Perforated necrotizing enterocolitis |
| Microvillous inclusion disease | Omphalocele |
| Pancreatitis | |
| Burns | |

## 10.3   ACCESS

Venous catheter placement and efforts to reduce technical and infectious complications of their use are important aspects of care in the safe delivery of the PN solution. The location of the catheter tip in the central venous circulation is crucial for the infusion of hypertonic PN solutions [2]. Central locations reduce the risk of thrombus formation due to the presence of a foreign object as well as the likelihood of vascular intimal damage. A central catheter tip also allows for instantaneous dilution of hypertonic PN solution (>900 mOsm/L). In children, the superior vena cava (SVC), the junction of the SVC and the right atrium and the inferior vena cava above the bifurcation of the iliac veins, can offer the largest caliber lumen and very high blood flow; all are considered central, locations for the catheter tip placement [2]. Peripheral locations, namely all others not included as central, preclude hyperosmolar solutions and therefore PN solutions should be limited to 900 mOsm/L or less to help reduce the risks of phlebitis infiltration and infection [3]. Chapters 12 and 26 discuss issues associated with vascular access devices in more detail.

## 10.4   COMPONENTS OF PN

Fluid requirements for the patient should be assessed based on weight and/or clinical condition. Typically the maintenance fluid is provided with the PN solutions. Maintenance fluid requirements can be assessed using the Holliday–Segar method [4]. In certain clinical situations, such as liver or kidney dysfunction, the fluids may need to be restricted.

In pediatric PN solutions the dextrose, amino acids, electrolytes, and micronutrients are typically provided in a single solution. Due to stability limitations, the lipid emulsions are usually infused separately from the dextrose–protein solution although in most adult and a limited number of pediatric facilities, total nutrient admixtures (TNAs), in which the lipid emulsions mixed directly with the PN solution are used. In circumstances where severe fluid restriction is necessary, the fluid from the fat emulsion is considered in the total fluid allotment. In most cases however, it is calculated in addition to the PN volume.

Of the macronutrients, dextrose provides the primary source of energy of the PN solution. In the intravenous form it is dextrose monohydrate with a caloric density of 3.4 kcal/g. This is slightly less than the 4 kcal/g caloric density attributed to all other carbohydrate (CHO) sources. In PN, dextrose infusions are typically initiated at a glucose infusion rate (GIR) of 5 mg CHO/kg/min which approximates endogenous glucose production of premature infants and neonates [5]. Incremental increases of the GIR (either by infusion rate or by dextrose concentration) are performed on a daily basis with careful blood glucose monitoring. The increase in GIR will vary depending on the age, size, and tolerance to the dextrose infusion although in most cases, dextrose advancement is done in increments of 2–5 mg/kg/min. The recommended maximum GIR for infants is 12–14 mg/kg/min [6].

There may be clinical situations where the rate needs to be slightly greater; however there is a potential risk of overfeeding and a high dextrose intake may contribute toward the development of cholestasis [7]. Excess CHO intake is metabolized to fat and stored in the liver leading to hepatic steatosis. Monitoring tolerance to the dextrose infusion is performed by blood glucose checks as well as urine dipsticks to assess for glucosuria as the GIR is increased. Urine glucose checks are advantageous as they are noninvasive and can be checked regularly. Routine monitoring of urine for glucose can be helpful as a positive result may be the first sign of sepsis in a situation of stable GIR. If hyperglycemia and positive urine glucose occurs, the GIR may need to be reduced even if temporarily. If hyperglycemia persists with inadequate total energy intake, insulin therapy may need to be considered. Insulin therapy can be initiated at doses as low as 0.01 U/kg/h in a separate infusion from the PN solution and titrated up as needed to maintain normoglycemia [8]. Although studies in adults admitted to the surgical ICU suggest a benefit to tight glycemic control [9], well-controlled prospective data in pediatric patients are lacking but are needed.

Crystalline amino acids provide the protein source in PN solutions. Most commonly used in the United States in the pediatric population is Trophamine (B. Braun Medical), Premasol (Baxter), or Aminosyn PF (Hospira). The neonatal amino acid solutions have greater amounts of aspartic and glutamic acid and taurine with lower quantities of methionine, glycine, and phenylalanine. See Table 10.2 for composition differences between the different amino acid solutions. In premature infants, the conditionally essential amino acid cysteine hydrochloride is routinely added due to the premature infants' reduced ability to metabolize methionine to cysteine and taurine. Taurine plays an important role in solubilizing bile salts and is necessary for adequate biliary secretion and reabsorption from the ileum [10]. It supports the formation of a more water-soluble conjugated bile acid which protects against lithocholate toxicity.

In most infants, the amino acids provision is initiated at 1–2 g protein/kg/day and advanced by 1 g/kg/day increments to 3–4 g/kg/day. A higher dose is typical for the premature infant <1000 g supported by data that suggest prompt initiation of parenteral protein (e.g., 2 g/kg in the first 24–48 h of life) is associated with optimal metabolic profiles [11]. For older children (i.e., <12 years of age), up to 2 g/kg/day is usually adequate [3]. Monitoring the safety for protein intake include blood urea nitrogen, and in the rare instance of liver failure, serum ammonia levels. If the patient is not in a catabolic state prealbumin, along with C-reactive protein levels, are monitored for adequacy of protein and energy intake. Reduced protein intake usually occurs in the situation of renal failure before dialysis is initiated or in severe liver failure; otherwise provision of protein according to standard Dietary Reference Intakes (DRI) is a typical practice.

Intravenous fat emulsions (IFE) provide a rich source of energy, essential fatty acids and a balance of macronutrients. IFEs available in the United States are soybean oil based (and are therefore contraindicated in patients with severe and documented soy allergy). Chapters 21 and 28 discuss the various lipid emulsion products in greater detail. Current practice is to initiate lipid infusions at 1 g fat/kg/day and advance to 3 g fat/kg/day for neonates and 1–2 g/kg/day for older children and adults [3]. Among infants who are likely to remain PN dependent for one or more months, we commonly limit the use of IFE to 1 g/kg/day. IFEs should not exceed 50% of the total calories since a higher percentage may cause ketosis. Tolerance to intravenous fats is performed by monitoring serum triglyceride (TG) concentrations, which ideally should remain <150 mg/dL. Since data linking adverse metabolic effects of hypertriglyceridemia are usually noted at far higher concentrations, higher TG levels are often tolerated. Although some cases of hypertriglyceridemia are attributable solely to excessive amounts of IFE, many patients receiving PN will have other reasons to have high serum TG levels, including acute phase stress response, sepsis, or hepatic and/or renal dysfunction [12]. Multiple medications are also associated with hypertriglyceridemia (Table 10.3). If persistent hypertriglyceridemia is noted, options include reducing the infusion time to 20 or fewer hours (and monitoring TG concentrations after this 4 h "fast") [13], or infusing lipids on alternating days of the week [14].

Recent research has linked excessive IFE intake with a higher incidence of PN-associated liver disease [15–17], and the practice of limiting IFE to 1 g fat/kg/day is emerging in some centers. Among

**TABLE 10.2**

**Brand-Specific Composition of Common Pediatric Parenteral Amino Acid Solutions**

| Product (Manufacturer) | Solutions Designed for Infants | | Standard Solutions Suitable for Ages 1 Year and Above | | | | | |
|---|---|---|---|---|---|---|---|---|
| | Aminosyn PF (Hospira) | Trophamine (B. Braun) Premasol (Baxter) | Aminosyn (Hospira) | Aminosyn II (Hospira) | Freamine III (B. Braun) | Novamine (Hospira) | Travasol (Baxter) | Prosol (Baxter) |
| Nitrogen mg/100 mL of 1% soln | 152 | 155 | 157 | 153 | 153 | 158 | 165 | 161 |
| **Amino Acids (Essential) mg/100 mL of a 1% Solution** | | | | | | | | |
| Isoleucine | 76 | 82 | 72 | 66 | 69 | 50 | 60 | 54 |
| Leucine | 120 | 140 | 94 | 100 | 91 | 69 | 73 | 54 |
| Lysine | 68 | 82 | 72 | 105 | 73 | 79 | 58 | 68 |
| Methionine | 18 | 34 | 40 | 17 | 53 | 50 | 40 | 38 |
| Phenylalanine | 43 | 48 | 44 | 30 | 56 | 69 | 56 | 50 |
| Threonine | 51 | 42 | 52 | 40 | 40 | 50 | 42 | 49 |
| Tryptophan | 18 | 20 | 16 | 20 | 15 | 17 | 18 | 16 |
| Valine | 67 | 78 | 80 | 50 | 66 | 64 | 58 | 72 |
| **Amino Acids (Nonessential) mg/100 mL of a 1% Solution** | | | | | | | | |
| Alanine | 70 | 54 | 128 | 99 | 71 | 145 | 207 | 138 |
| Arginine | 123 | 120 | 98 | 102 | 95 | 98 | 115 | 98 |
| Histidine | 31 | 48 | 30 | 30 | 28 | 60 | 48 | 59 |
| Proline | 81 | 68 | 86 | 72 | 112 | 60 | 68 | 67 |
| Serine | 50 | 38 | 42 | 53 | 59 | 39 | 50 | 51 |
| Taurine | 7 | 2.5 | | | | | | |
| Tyrosine | 4 | 4.4 | 4.4 | 27 | | 2.6 | 4 | 2.5 |
| Glycine | 39 | 36 | 128 | 50 | 140 | 69 | 103 | 103 |
| Glutamic acid | 62 | 50 | | 74 | | 50 | | 51 |
| Aspartic acid | 53 | 32 | | 70 | | 29 | | 30 |
| Cysteine | <1.6 | | | | <2.4 | | | |
| N-ac-L-tyrosine | 0 | 24 | 0 | | 0 | 0 | 0 | |

---

**TABLE 10.3**

**Medications Associated with Hypertriglyceridemia**

| | | |
|---|---|---|
| Abacavir | Dexrazoxane | Mirtazapine |
| Acitretin | Didanosine | Mitotane |
| Adalimumab | Efavirenz | Nafarelin |
| Amiodarone | Eplerenone | Olanzapine |
| Amprenavir | Eprosartan | Olmesartan |
| Aripiprazole | Estrogen | Paclitaxel |
| Atevirdine | Estropipate | Propofol |
| Bazedoxifene | Febuxostat | Raloxifene |
| Beta-blockers | Fluconazole | Retinoids/vitamin A |
| Calcitriol | Fluoxetine | Risperidone |
| Candesartan | Fomepizole | Ritonavir |
| Capecitabine | Glucocorticoids | Sertraline |
| Cholestyramine | Indinavir | Sirolimus |
| Carevedilol | Interferons | Somatropin |
| Clomiphene | Isotretinoin | Tacrolimus |
| Clozapine | Itraconazole | Tamoxifen |
| Cyclosporine | Ketoconazole | Thiazide diuretics |
| Darunavir | L-Asparaginase | Thyrotropin |
| Delavirdine | Leflunomide | Tipranavir |
| | | Vitamin E |

*Source:* Adapted from Henkin J, Como JA, and Oberman A. *JAMA* 1992;267:961–968, and the *Online Formulary,* Children's Hospital Boston.

---

infants who are likely to remain PN dependent for one or more months, we commonly limit the use of IFE to 1 gram/kg/day. Fat restriction however potentially increases the risks of essential fatty acid deficiency (EFAD), in adequate energy intake for growth and/or excessive carbohydrate intake. Three to five percent of total calories as fat are recommended to prevent EFAD, and in infants this can be met with as little as 0.5 g/kg/day of standard soy-based IFE. In cases of limited fat intake, monitoring for EFAD with a total fatty acid profile is prudent. The biochemical hallmark of EFAD is an elevated ratio of triene to tetraene fats (>0.2). Conversely a "fat overload" syndrome has been described with excessive administration of lipids characterized by focal seizures, fever, hepatosplenomegaly, and thrombocytopenia [18]. This typically occurs when infusion rates exceed 0.17 g/kg/h.

More recently, the use of an alternate fish oil based (IFE) has been found to be efficacious in reducing serum bilirubin levels commonly seen in patients who have been on long-term PN support. The mechanism for its effectiveness remains unclear but could be due to the high amount of the ω-3 fatty acid docosohexanoic acid (DHA) along with reduced amounts of the ω-6 fatty acid, arachidonic acid (AA), resulting in less production of inflammatory thromboxanes, prostaglandins, and leukotrienes [19]. It could also be related to the absence of phytosterols as compared to the high phytosterol content present in soybean oil-based IFE [20]. See Chapter 21 for further details.

## 10.5 PERIPHERAL PARENTERAL NUTRITION

Peripheral parenteral nutrition (PPN) is often used in situations where central venous access is not possible. In some cases of central venous catheter sepsis, PPN is often used until the blood stream infection has resolved and/or a new catheter can be placed. PPN is not suitable for all intestinal failure patients due to provision of inadequate energy. Because PPN solutions have low caloric concentrations,

**TABLE 10.4**
**Osmolarity and Energy Density of Select PN Solutions**

| Solution | Osmolarity (mOsm/L) | Energy Density (kcal/mL) |
|---|---|---|
| 5% Dextrose | 300 | 0.17 |
| 10% Dextrose | 600 | 0.34 |
| 20% Dextrose | 1200 | 0.68 |
| 10% Dextrose + 2% amino acids | 900 | 0.42 |
| 20% + 2% | 1500 | 0.75 |
| 25% + 3% | 1800 | 0.95 |
| 30% + 3% | 2200 | 1.12 |
| 10% IFE | 276 | 1.1 |
| 20% IFE | 258 | 2.0 |

large volumes of fluid are necessary in order to deliver adequate calories. Thus, children with significant fluid restrictions would probably not benefit from the few calories provided from such solutions. Moreover, due to risks of phlebitis and sclerosis, the maximum osmolarity of PN for peripheral vein administration is 900 mOsm/L [3]. This corresponds to a solution of 10% dextrose and 2% amino acid with standard amounts of electrolytes and minerals. Table 10.4 lists the osmolarity and estimated caloric density of several common PN solutions. It should be noted that IFE both 10% and 20%, provide an isotonic source of calories and be infused through either a peripheral or central vein.

## 10.6   MICRONUTRIENTS IN PN

The importance of vitamins in patients receiving PN has been underscored in the United States by several widespread shortages of parenteral multivitamins and reports of symptomatic thiamine deficiency [21]. Fatal vitamin deficiencies have been reported in patients receiving PN without vitamins in as short a time as a few weeks. Table 10.5 lists the current parenteral vitamin products available in the United States. The pediatric versions of multivitamins are notable for the inclusion of vitamin K, higher amounts of vitamin D, and lower amounts of B vitamins, as compared to formulations designed for adults. Certain patient conditions may require adjustments to their parenteral vitamin intake. For example, patients with large gastrointestinal fistula output may require a double dose of multivitamins due to increased losses [22]. Patients with prolonged prothrombin times may benefit from short courses of supplemental phytonidione.

In the event of another parenteral multivitamin shortage, it is imperative that practitioners provide adequate thiamine so as to avoid metabolic lactic acidosis. Adult parenteral multivitamins should never be used in the neonate because the propylene glycol and polysorbates contained in many of these products could be toxic [23]. Moreover, adult products contain less vitamin D and may increase the risk of metabolic bone disease in pediatric patients receiving them for extended periods of time. Neonates who must receive PN without conventional pediatric parenteral multivitamins should always receive parenteral thiamine in the PN at a dose of 0.03 mg/kg/day [24]. In patients with intestinal failure with malabsorption if an *oral* multivitamin is given, it should be done so in conjunction with parenteral thiamine.

Monitoring vitamin levels depends on the clinical situation. If serum vitamin A is monitored, the level should be drawn with a retinol binding protein level if liver failure is present since it is the carrier protein for transport of vitamin A from the liver. It is often helpful to include a parathyroid hormone level when checking 25 OH D levels. Chapter 23 provides a detailed discussion on the more commonly micronutrients and vitamins used in patients with intestinal failure.

Currently there is no parenteral vitamin preparation designed especially for premature infants and there is some controversy concerning vitamin requirements for these patients [25]. Recommendations for pediatric parenteral vitamin doses for full-term and preterm infants are shown in Table 10.6.

**TABLE 10.5**
**Comparison of Parenteral Multivitamin Preparations**

| Product | Supplier | A (IU) | B$_1$ (mg) | B$_2$ (mg) | B$_6$ (mg) | B$_{12}$ (µg) | Biotin (µg) | C (mg) | Folic Acid (µg) | D (IU) | E (IU) | K (µg) | Niacinamide (mg) | Dexpanthenol (mg) |
|---|---|---|---|---|---|---|---|---|---|---|---|---|---|---|
| | | | | | | Pediatric (<11 Years of Age) | | | | | | | | |
| Infuvite pediatric (per 5 mL) | Baxter | 2300 | 1.2 | 1.4 | 1 | 1 | 20 | 80 | 140 | 400 | 7 | 200 | 17 | 5 |
| M.V.I. pediatric (per 5 mL) | Hospira | 2300 | 1.2 | 1.4 | 1 | 1 | 20 | 80 | 140 | 400 | 7 | 200 | 17 | 5 |
| | | | | | | Adolescents and Adults (≥11 Years of Age) | | | | | | | | |
| Infuvite adult (per 10 mL) | Baxter | 3300 | 6 | 3.6 | 6 | 5 | 60 | 200 | 600 | 200 | 10 | 150 | 40 | 15 |
| M.V.I.-12 (per 10 mL) | Hospira | 3300 | 3 | 3.6 | 4 | 12.5 | 60 | 100 | 400 | 200 | 10 | — | 40 | 15 |
| M.V.I. adult (per 10 mL) | Hospira | 3300 | 6 | 3.6 | 6 | 5 | 60 | 200 | 600 | 200 | 10 | 150 | 40 | 15 |

**TABLE 10.6**

**Recommended Levels of Intake for Intravenous Multivitamins for Term and Preterm Infants**

| Vitamin | Term Infants (Dose per Day)[b] | Preterm Infants (Dose per kg)[a] | |
| | | Current Suggestion[c] | Best New Estimate[d] |
|---|---|---|---|
| A (IU) | 2300 | 920 | 1643 |
| D (IU) | 400 | 160 | 160 |
| E (mg) | 7 | 2.8 | 2.8 |
| K (µg) | 200 | 80 | 80 |
| Ascorbic acid (mg) | 80 | 32 | 25 |
| Thiamine (mg) | 1.2 | 0.48 | 0.35 |
| Riboflavin (mg) | 1.4 | 0.56 | 0.15 |
| Niacin (mg) | 17 | 6.8 | 6.8 |
| Pantothenate (mg) | 5 | 2.0 | 2.0 |
| Pyridoxine (mg) | 1.0 | 0.4 | 0.18 |
| Vitamin B12 (µg) | 1.0 | 0.4 | 0.3 |
| Biotin (µg) | 20 | 8.0 | 6.0 |
| Folate (µg) | 140 | 56 | 56 |

[a] Maximum dose not to exceed term infant dose.
[b] These are all met by currently available pediatric parenteral multivitamins.
[c] These are met by 40% of the single dose (0.4 × 5 mL = 2 mL) of a pediatric multivitamin per kg per day.
[d] Based on data suggesting a reduced need for water-soluble vitamins and increased need for vitamin A in preterm infants.

Trace elements commonly added to PN solutions include zinc, copper, manganese, and chromium. Table 10.7 lists recommendations for trace elements in PN. Due to biliary excretion of copper and manganese, these should be reduced in patients with cholestasis. Copper however should not be eliminated totally without careful monitoring. Individuals on long-term PN with cholestatic jaundice can develop hypocupremia. This can result in significant hematologic complications including severe anemia, thrombocytopenia, and neutropenia [26]. Routine monitoring of serum copper and ceruloplasmin levels is necessary to help guide Cu dosing. Monitoring manganese status is not commonly performed as serum levels are difficult to interpret. There are reports [27,28] of abnormal cranial MRI findings consistent with manganese deposition, a concern for pediatric patients on long-term PN who may be at risk of neurocognitive dysfunction due to prematurity and other medical problems already.

Parenteral intake of selenium, chromium, zinc, and molybdenum should be reduced or held in cases of renal dysfunction. Addition of selenium and carnitine may be necessary after 30 days of PN and no or minimal enteral intake. For patients with intestinal failure there may be greater zinc losses due to their higher diarrhea/ostomy losses. It is common practice to add additional zinc to help replace those losses [29]. If a multi-ingredient trace element cocktail is used, practitioners should take the amount provided by the product into consideration when determining the additional amount to supplement.

The use of parenteral iron to treat iron deficiency anemia has been controversial due to the risk of anaphylaxis and the possible effect of encouraging microbial growth and sepsis. Nonetheless, a judicious use of iron dextran is recommended in those patients with iron deficiency (as noted by biochemical assessment of iron status) and for whom the enteral route is contraindicated. Patients

**TABLE 10.7**
**Suggested Intake of Trace Nutrients (Concentration per 1000 mL PN)**

| Element | Weight <2 kg | Weight >2 kg | Comments |
|---|---|---|---|
| Zinc | 3 mg | 1 mg | Increase dose with increased intestinal losses |
| Manganese | 50 µg | 60 µg | Decrease dose with cholestatic liver disease |
| Copper | 200 µg | 200 µg | Decrease dose with cholestatic liver disease |
| Chromium | 1.7 µg | 2 µg | Increase dose with intestinal losses and decrease with renal dysfunction |
| Iron | 1 mg/day (see text) | | Monitor for anaphylaxis with initial infusion |
| Selenium[a] | 1–3 µg/kg/day max dose 30–40 µg/day | | Reduce dose with renal disease; may have increased requirements with increased intestinal losses |
| Carnitine[a] | 8–16 mg/kg/day | | Patients with primary carnitine deficiency will require higher doses |

*Source:* From Collier SB et al. *Manual of Pediatric Nutrition.* 4th ed. Hamilton Ontario: BC Decker; 2005. With Permission.
[a] May be added after 30 days of NPO status and/or minimal enteral intake.

who receive blood transfusions however typically will not require supplemental iron as a single blood transfusion provides approximately 3 months' worth of iron [30].

The total amount of parenteral iron (as iron dextran) needed to normalize hemoglobin level can be estimated according to the following formula:

$$\text{mg Fe} = \text{weight (kg)} \times 4.5 \times (13.5\text{—patient's Hgb [g/dL]})$$

An initial test dose of 0.5 mL (25 mg Fe) (0.25 mL/12.5 mg Fe in infants) should be given on the first day at a rate of <1 mL/h to monitor for an anaphylactic response. Epinephrine and diphenhydramine should be readily available. If well tolerated, daily doses of 25–100 mg may be given IV for a few days needed to replenish stores. Long-term maintenance dose at 1 mg/day may be indicated in some patients and may be added directly to lipid-free PN solutions.

Iodine is a required trace element for the synthesis of thyroid hormones and until recently was not routinely added to PN solutions. PN-dependent infants and children are likely to be at risk of iodine deficiency but limited data do not support this as an important occurrence [31]. Although lower circulating levels of thyroid hormones in preterm infants have been associated with increased rates of mortality and morbidity, at least one randomized trial of higher iodine intake was not associated with reduced morbidity [32]. Given that topical absorption has been postulated as one potential reason why parenterally fed patients have been able to maintain normal iodine status, reduced use of iodine containing topical sterilization solutions (e.g., povidone iodine) suggests that patients who prolonged courses of PN may be at risk for developing iodine deficiency. Although there exist limited data in this regard, both the European Society for Parenteral and Enteral Nutrition (ESPGHAN) guidelines and the American Society for Clinical Nutrition (ASCN) recommendations suggest that parenteral iodine supplementation of 1 µg/kg/d occur in infants and children receiving PN for >30 days [18,25].

## 10.7 CALCIUM, PHOSPHORUS, MAGNESIUM, SODIUM, POTASSIUM, CHLORIDE, AND ACETATE

Calcium, phosphorus, and magnesium balance are interrelated. Inadequate intakes of each may result in rickets, fractures, failure of appropriate bone mineralization, and reduced linear growth. In the PN-dependent child, relatively high amounts of calcium and phosphorus are needed. The provision of these nutrients in PN is particularly challenging due to the physicochemical limitations of current PN additives. When compounding a solution with high amounts of calcium and phosphorus it is imperative that the pH is low enough to optimize solubility and that the additions of calcium and phosphorus salts are done in the correct order. According to the FDA Safety Alert, calcium should always be the last ingredient added to the PN solution [33]. Phosphorus salts should be one of the first additives so that it is well diluted prior to the addition of the calcium. Currently, calcium gluconate is the preferred salt for use in PN solutions since it dissociates less than chloride salts and thereby remains in solution more readily. Other factors favoring the formation of calcium–phosphorus precipitates include low amino acid content, low dextrose content, high temperature, and high pH. Since pH is primarily determined by amino acid concentration increasing amino acid intake, the use of more acidic brands of amino acid solutions and/or the addition of cysteine hydrochloride are common strategies used to prevent precipitation. It is also recommended that if a PN solution contains <1% amino acids either calcium or phosphorus (not both) should be added [34]. Published nomograms are useful for specific compatibility information. A conservative estimate may be obtained by adding the sum of calcium and phosphorus concentrations (mmol/L); if the sum of these numbers exceeds 40, the risk of precipitation is high [34]. It should be noted that these recommendations do not apply to TNAs since calcium and phosphorus solubility is lower in these solutions [35].

Like calcium, approximately 60% of magnesium is found in bone with the remainder being intracellular [36]. Serum magnesium levels do not accurately reflect total body magnesium stores because of the slow rate of magnesium exchange. It is imperative that baseline magnesium levels are obtained prior to initiation of PN in infants born to mothers treated for hypertension or preeclampsia as these infants tend to have elevated serum magnesium levels due to poor renal elimination of magnesium. Although not as well described as calcium–phosphorus incompatibility PN solutions high in magnesium and phosphorus are also prone to precipitation. Patients receiving drugs that increase magnesium wasting (i.e., amphotericin) may require additional supplementation.

Sodium and potassium are typically included to provide standard electrolyte requirements. Oftentimes in patients with intestinal failure sodium requirements are greater due to intestinal losses

**TABLE 10.8**
**Gastrointestinal Electrolyte Losses and Suggested Replacement Regimen**

| Source of Body Fluid Loss | Sodium (mEq/L) | Potassium (mEq/L) | Chloride (mEq/L) | Typical Replacement Fluid |
|---|---|---|---|---|
| Gastric (nasogastric gastrostomy drainage) | 20–80 | 5–20 | 100–150 | 1/2 NS with 10 K+ per liter[a]: mL replacement for mL losses unless total fluid concerns |
| Ileostomy | 45–135 | 3–15 | 20–115 | 1/2–3/4 NS: mL replacement for mL losses unless total fluid concerns; if $CO_2$ is low, could use Lactated Ringer's solution or may need 50% of sodium to be provided as NaCl and 50% of sodium from Na acetate salts |
| Colostomy | 50–120 | 30–40 | 90–95 | 1/2–3/4 NS with 20 K+ per liter[a]: mL replacement for mL losses unless total fluid concerns |

*Source:* From Walker WA et al. *Pediatric Gastrointestinal Disease.* 4th ed. vol. 2. Ontario: BC Decker; 2004. With permission.

[a] Any replacement solution with potassium needs to be infused over a few to several hours depending on the total amount of potassium and total volume of replacement fluid required.

via nasogastric or gastrostomy tube drainage and/or high ostomy output (Table 10.8). Potassium requirements could also be greater in these situations of higher losses. Chloride and acetate are also important electrolytes that are included in PN solutions. The total amount varies depending on the amino acid concentration and the total sodium and potassium content. Acetate salt concentrations may need to be higher in cases where there are high ostomy losses.

## 10.8   MEDICATION AND PN

Patients requiring PN are often on multiple medications and questions frequently arise concerning whether these medications can be coadministrated with PN. Because of the risks of precipitation and/or infection coadministration of medications and PN should be avoided whenever possible. Moreover medications should not be added directly to the PN bag except by pharmacy staff. Medications not directly added to PN should be coinfused via a "y" connection with the intravenous setup proximal to a filter. Whenever the PN formula changes coadministered medications and potential compatibility problems should be reviewed. This also includes whenever there are changes in the brands of amino acids or lipid emulsions.

---

**TABLE 10.9**
**Medications Compatible with PN Solutions**

| | | |
|---|---|---|
| Albumin[a] | Enalaprilat | Mezlocillin |
| Aldesleukin | Epinephrine[d] | Miconazole |
| Amikacin[b] | Erythromycin | Morphine |
| Aminophylline[c] | Famotidine | Nafcillin |
| Atracurium | Fentanyl | Norepinephrine |
| Atropine | Fluconazole | Ondansetron |
| Aztreonam | Gentamicin[b] | Oxacillin |
| Bumetanide | Glycopyrrolate | Pancuronium |
| Cefepime | Granisetron | Penicillin G+ (aqueous) |
| Cefotaxime | Heparin | Phenobarbital |
| Cefoxitin | Hydralazine | Phytonidione |
| Ceftazidime | Hydrocortisone | Piperacillin |
| Ceftriaxone | Hydromorphone | Piperacillin/tazobactam |
| Cefuroxime | Insulin (U-100 regular) | Promethazine |
| Chloramphenicol | Iron dextran | Pyridoxine |
| Chlorpromazine | Isoproterenol | Ranitidine |
| Cimetidine | Leucovorin | Tacrolimus |
| Clindamycin | Levocarnitine | Ticarcillin |
| Dexamethasone | Lorazepam | Ticarcillin/clavulanic acid |
| Digoxin | Magnesium sulfate | Tobramycin[b] |
| Diphenhydramine | Meperidine | Tolazoline |
| Dobutamine[b] | Mesna | Vancomycin[b] |
| Doxycycline | Methylprednisolone[e] | Vecuronium |
| | | Zidovudine |

*Source:*   Adapted from the *2011 Online Formulary*, Children's Hospital Boston.

[a]   Will clog filter if albumin concentration >25 g/L.
[b]   Incompatible with heparin-containing PN solutions.
[c]   Do not exceed 3 mg/mL for piggyback administration.
[d]   Incompatible with iron-containing PN solutions.
[e]   Contains phosphate buffers which may precipitate in solutions high in calcium or phosphorous.

---

**TABLE 10.10**
**Medications Compatible with IFE**

| | |
|---|---|
| Aldesleukin | Erythromycin |
| Aztreonam | Famotidine |
| Bumetanide | Gentamicin |
| Cefotaxime | Hydrocortisone |
| Cefoxitin | Hydromorphone |
| Ceftazidime | Insulin regular |
| Ceftriaxone | Interlukin-2 |
| Chloramphenicol | Isoproterenol |
| Cimetidine | Lidocaine |
| Clindamycin | Norepinephrine |
| Cyclosporine | Oxacillin |
| Digoxin | Penicillin |
| Diphenhydramine | Ranitidine |
| Dobutamine | Ticarcillin |
| Dopamine | Tobramycin |
| | Vancomycin |

*Source:*   Adapted from the *2011 Online Formulary* Children's Hospital Boston.

Tables 10.9 and 10.10 list medications generally considered safe for coadministration with PN and lipids respectively. Tables 10.11 and 10.12 list medications that are considered incompatible with PN and lipids. In all cases, consultation with the pharmacy is recommended. In the event for which no information is available, the medication should be considerably incompatible with both PN and fat emulsion.

**TABLE 10.11**
**Medications Incompatible with PN Solutions**

| | |
|---|---|
| Acetazolamide | Furosemide |
| Acyclovir | Ganciclovir |
| Amphotericin | Imipenem |
| Amphotericin b lipid complex | Indomethacin |
| Ampicillin | Mannitol |
| Ampicillin/sulbactam | Methotrexate |
| Calcium salts | Metoclopramide |
| Cefazolin | Metronidazole |
| Ciprofloxacin | Midazolam |
| *cis*-platinum | Nitroglycerin |
| Cyclosporine | Nitroprusside |
| Cytarabine | Octreotide |
| Diazepam | Phenytoin |
| Doxorubicin | Piperacillin |
| Filgrastim | Promethazine |
| Foscarnet | Trimethoprim/sulfamethoxazole |
| Flurouracil | Tromethamine |

*Source:*   Adapted from the *2011 Online Formulary,* Children's Hospital Boston.

**TABLE 10.12**

**Medications Incompatible with IFE**

| | |
|---|---|
| Acetazolamide | Furosemide |
| Acyclovir | Ganciclovir |
| Amikacin | Gentamcin |
| Aminophylline | Heparin |
| Amphotericin | Imipenem |
| Amphotericin b lipid complex | Indomethacin |
| Ampicillin | Iron dextran |
| Ampicillin/sulbactam | Magnesium salts |
| Calcium salts | Metronidazole |
| Ciprofloxacin | Midazolam |
| Cyclosporine | Morphine |
| Diazepam | Nitroglycerin |
| Doxorubicin | Nitroprusside |
| Filgrastim | Penicillin |
| Flurouracil | Phenytoin |
| Foscarnet | Trimethoprim/sulfamethoxazole |
| | Tromethamine |

*Source:* Adapted from the *2011 Online Formulary,* Children's Hospital Boston.

In PN patients with limited venous access, it may be a challenge to administer parenteral medications if the medication is incompatible with PN. If possible, a compatible medication should be considered. If that is not an option, the PN infusion needs to be interrupted so that the incompatible medication may be infused. Prior to infusing the medication, the PN infusion must be stopped, the line should be flushed with a neutral fluid compatible with the medication (i.e., saline or dextrose), then the medication is infused followed by another flush with a compatible fluid before the PN infusion is resumed. Children receiving PN with high dextrose concentrations may need to have the PN rate gradually reduced prior to the start of the drug infusion. In cases where the child cannot have their PN infusion interrupted because of an inability to maintain adequate blood glucose levels, the medication should be infused in a carrier fluid with a similar dextrose concentration and infusion rate as the PN. If a lipid infusion needs to be interrupted for the administration of an incompatible medication, no rate reduction before lipid discontinuation is necessary.

## 10.9 OTHER COMPOUNDING CONSIDERATIONS

In addition to the calcium–phosphorus compatibility, other factors have received attention regarding the prevention of PN-related complications: minimizing aluminum exposure, protecting the solutions from light, and avoidance of di(2-ethylhexyl)phthalate DEHP materials. Premature infants and children with intestinal failure have immature or diminished antioxidant defenses which renders them more susceptible to oxidant stress. Moreover, as children with intestinal failure receive prolonged courses of PN, they are especially prone to these complications.

### 10.9.1 ALUMINUM

Aluminum exposure is a risk in patients receiving prolonged courses on PN. This metal is found in raw materials incorporated into products during the manufacturing process and leached from glass containers during autoclaving for sterilization [37]. When aluminum is administered parenterally, it bypasses the protective barrier of the gastrointestinal tract. Specific findings of this toxicity include encephalopathy, impaired neurodevelopment, bone pain with development of osteopenia or osteo-malacia, microcytic anemia, and cholestasis. In July 2004, the U.S. Food and Drug Administration (FDA) issued a mandate that required manufacturers to include the aluminum content on the label of additives commonly used in the compounding of PN solutions [38]. The amount of aluminum provided by PN should be less than 5 μg/kg/day the threshold deemed "safe" by the FDA.

Calcium gluconate salts are a major source of aluminum contamination in PN patients. Since calcium gluconate salts are a large source of contamination, infants and children are at risk for developing toxicity due to their high calcium requirements coupled with renal immaturity. In response to the findings of potential adverse neurodevelopment associated with aluminum exposure [39], the use of calcium chloride in PN solutions has been reevaluated. Calcium chloride salts are inherently less contaminated and in theory could be used as an alternative to calcium gluconate salts. This could predispose patients especially children however to a potentially greater risk of developing metabolic acidosis due to the increased chloride load. Koo et al. [40] suggest that using a 50% calcium gluconate/50% calcium chloride mix in conjunction with the use of potassium and sodium acetate salts in place of sodium and potassium chloride could minimize this risk. Calcium–phosphorus solubility would still be a concern as calcium chloride salts have a higher degree of dissociation and thus less than optimal calcium and phosphate intake would still be problematic [41]. This risk can be minimized if calcium chloride salts are used with an *organic* phosphate salt; however these organic phosphate salts are expensive and not available in many countries.

Since the implementation of the FDA mandate, it has been difficult to incorporate them into clinical practice due to limitations in current product formulations. Currently there are few options available to reduce the aluminum load in PN solutions. One is to replace potassium phosphate with sodium phosphate salts that have considerably less aluminum. Furthermore, not all ingredients (i.e., heparin, albumin, insulin) that are often added to PN solutions are required to list their aluminum on their label which makes it even more difficult to accurately calculate potential aluminum exposure secondary to PN use [42].

### 10.9.2  AMBIENT LIGHT

When PN is exposed to ambient light, lipid peroxides and hydrogen peroxide are generated [43]. Approximately 50% reduction is found in the amount of hydrogen peroxide infused with PN when the entire solution and delivery system is protected from ambient light (i.e., amino acid dextrose bag, lipid syringe, and tubing) [44]. This phenomenon was first reported in the early 1980s when it was observed that light exposure might cause vitamin instability but most practitioners still choose not to cover solutions, especially if the multivitamins are added immediately prior to infusing. Multivitamins, however, are not the only component of PN that may be affected by light. The amino acids tryptophan and tyrosine undergo photooxidation to form free radicals with hepatotoxic properties [45]. Other amino acids such as methionine, histidine, and cysteine are also susceptible to photo-xidation. Riboflavin appears to facilitate the photooxidation process by serving as a photosensitizing agent [46].

In addition to its impact on vitamins and amino acids, phototherapy might cause significant peroxidation in IFEs resulting in the formation of cytotoxic triglyceride hydroperoxides [47]. Lipid hydroperoxides could theoretically cause pulmonary vasoconstriction via an interference with endogenous prostaglandin synthesis [48]. It has been recommended by some that fat emulsion containers be covered with aluminum foil or that fat emulsion be supplemented with sodium ascorbate prior to light exposure [49]. However, results from a study on a large cohort of premature infants demonstrated no beneficial effect of partial light protection of PN on clinically relevant outcomes [43]. This study did not provide complete protection against ambient light; therefore further investigation is warranted.

### 10.9.3  DEHP TOXICITY

Di-(2-ethylhexyl)phthalate (DEHP) is an industrial additive plasticizer found in polyvinylchloride (PVC). PN infusion systems have been shown to be the most important source of DEHP load.

Although DEHP has a rapid turnover (half-life less than 24 h), this phthalate and its metabolites are consistently detected in human body fluids such as plasma, urine, amniotic fluid or breast milk [50]. In preterm neonates and infants who receive intensive care, DEHP has shown to increase oxidative stress and toxicity [51]. PN infusion sets and containers containing DEHP have been implicated as contributing to this risk. Retrospective data showed that by changing to PVC-free infusion systems, a reduction in the incidence of cholestatic liver disease was noted [52]. Moreover, the use of poly-vinylchloride infusion sets correlated strongly with the development of PN-associated liver disease ($p = 0.0004$). DEHP-free containers and infusion sets should be used whenever possible so as to minimize this risk.

## 10.10   CONCLUSION

Since its introduction in 1968, PN has been the mainstay in the management of children with intestinal failure. Although numerous advancements have been made over the years to provide more balanced and less toxic solutions, PN continues to be an artificial and inherently risky procedure. Clinicians providing long-term PN need to be aware of the many possible complications of this therapy, as well as work toward continued innovations to improve this approach.

## REFERENCES

1. Dudrick SJ, Wilmore DW, Vars HM, and Rhoads JE. Long term total parenteral nutrition with growth development and positive nitrogen balance. *Surgery* 1968;64:134–142.
2. Rocadio JM, Doellman DA, Johnson ND, Bean JA, and Jacobs BR. Pediatric peripherally inserted central cathethers: Complication rates related to catheter tip location. *Pediatrics* 2001;107:e28.
3. American Society for Parenteral and Enteral Nutrition (ASPEN) Board of Directors. Clinical guidelines for the use of parenteral and enteral nutrition in adult and pediatric patients 2009. *JPEN* 2009;33:255–259.
4. Holliday MA and Segar WE. The maintenance need for water in parenteral fluid therapy. *Pediatrics* 1957;19:823–832.
5. Chawla D, Thukral A, Agarwal R, Deorari AK, and Paul VK. Parenteral nutrition. *Indian J Pediatr* 2008;75:377–383.
6. Yu VY. Principles and practice of parenteral nutrition in the neonatal period. *Acta Med Port* 1997;10:185–196.
7. Collier S, Crouch J, Hendricks K, and Caballero B. Use of cyclic parenteral nutrition in infants less than six months of age. *Nutr Clin Pract* 1994;9:65–68.
8. Preissig CM and Rigby MR. Pediatric critical illness hyperglycemia: Risk factors associated with development and severity of hyperglycemia in critically ill children. *J Pediatr* 2009;155:734–739.
9. Van den Berghe G, Wouter P, Weekers F, Verwaest C, Bruyninckx F, Schetz M, Vlasselaers D, Ferdinande P, Lauwers P, and Bouillon R. Intensive insulin therapy in critically ill patients. *N Engl J Med* 2001;345:1359–1367.
10. Spencer AU, Sunkyung Y, Tracy TF et al. Parenteral nutrition-associated cholestasis in neonates: Multivariate analysis of the potential protective effect of taurine. *JPEN* 2005;29:337–344.
11. Embleton ND. Optimal protein and energy intakes in preterm infants. *Early Hum Dev* 2007;83:831–837.
12. Colomb V, Jobert-Giraud A, Lacaille F et al. Role of lipid emulsions in cholestasis associated with long-term parenteral nutrition in children. *JPEN* 2000;24:345–350.
13. Cavicchi M, Beau P, Crenn P et al. Prevalence of liver disease and contributing factors in patients receiving home parenteral nutrition for permanent intestinal failure. *Ann Intern Med* 2000;132:525–532.
14. Shin JI, Namgung R, Park MS et al. Could lipid infusion be a risk for parenteral nutrition-associated cholestasis in low birth weight neonates? *Eur J Pediatr* 2008;167:197–202.
15. Goulet O, Girot R, Maier-Redelsperger M, Bougle D, Virelizier J, and Ricour C. Hematologic disorders following prolonged use of intravenous fat emulsions in children. *JPEN* 198610:284–288.
16. Brans YW, Dutton EB, Andrew DS, Menchaca EM, and West DL. Fat emulsion tolerance in very low birth weight neonates: Effect on diffusion of oxygen in the lungs and on blood pH *Pediatrics* 1986;78:79–84.
17. Heyman MB, Storch S, and Ament ME. The fat overload syndrome. *Am J Dis Child* 1981;135(7):628–630.

18. Koletzko B, Goulet O, Hunt J, Krohn K, and Shamir R. Parenteral Nutrition Guidelines Working Group; European Society for Clinical Nutrition and Metabolism; European Society of Paediatric Gastroenterology Hepatology and Nutrition (ESPGHAN); European Society of Paediatric Research (ESPR). Guidelines on Paediatric Parenteral Nutrition of the European Society of Paediatric Gastroenterology Hepatology and Nutrition (ESPGHAN) and the European Society for Clinical Nutrition and Metabolism (ESPEN), Supported by the European Society of Paediatric Research (ESPR). *J Pediatr Gastroenterol Nutr* 2005;41(Suppl 2):S1–87.

19. Gura KM, Lee S, Valim C et al. Safety and efficacy of a fish-oil-based fat emulsion in the treatment of parenteral nutrition-associated liver disease. *Pediatrics* 2008;121:e678–e686.

20. Clayton PT, Whitfiewl P, and Iyer K. The role of phytosterols in the pathogenesis of liver complications of pediatric parenteral nutrition. *Nutrition* 1998;14:158–164.

21. Hahn JS, Berquist W, Alcorn DM, Chamberlain L, and Bass D. Wernicke encephalopathy and beriberi during total parenteral nutrition attributable to multivitamin infusion shortage. *Pediatrics* 1998;101:E10.

22. Dudrick SJ, Maharaj AR, and McKelvey AA. Artificial nutritional support in patients with gastrointestinal fistulas. *World J Surg* 1999;23:570–576.

23. Reinshagen K, Zahn K, Buch C, Zoeller M, Hagl CI, Ali M, and Waag KL. The impact of longitudinal intestinal lengthening and tailoring on liver function in short bowel syndrome. *Eur J Pediatr Surg* 2008;18:249–253.

24. MacDonald MG, Fletcher AB, Johnson EL, Boeckx RL, Getson PR, and Miller MK. The potential toxicity to neonates of multivitamin preparations used in parenteral nutrition. *JPEN* 1987;11:169–171.

25. Green Hl, Hambridge KM, Schanler R et al. Guidelines for the use of vitamins trace elements calcium magnesium and phosphorus in infants and children receiving total parenteral nutrition. Report of the subcommittee on Clinical Practice Issues of the American Society for Clinical Nutrition. *Am J Clin Nutr* 1988;48:1324–1342.

26. Hurwitz M, Garcia MG, Poole RL, and Kerner JA. Copper deficiency during parenteral nutrition: A report of four pediatric cases. *Nutr Clin Pract* 2004;19:305–308.

27. Fell JM and Reynolds AP. Manganese toxicity in children receiving long-term parenteral nutrition. *Lancet* 1996;347:1218–1221.

28. Takagi Y, Okada A, Sando K et al. Evaluation of indexes of *in vivo* manganese status and the optimal intravenous dose for adult patients undergoing home parenteral nutrition. *Am J Clin Nutr* 2002;75:112–118.

29. Chen W, Wong WK, and Chen TC. A case of zinc deficiency during long-term total parenteral nutrition. *J Formos Med Assoc* 1990;89:388–391.

30. Muñoz M, Breymann C, García-Erce JA, Gómez-Ramírez S, Comin J, and Bisbe E. Efficacy and safety of intravenous iron therapy as an alternative/adjunct to allogeneic blood transfusion. *Vox Sang* 2008;94:172–183.

31. Zimmermann MB and Crill CM. Iodine in enteral and parenteral nutrition. *Best Pract Res Clin Endocrinol Metab* 2010;24:143–158.

32. Biswas S, Buffery J, Enoch H, Bland JM, Walters D, and Markiewicz M. A longitudinal assessment of thyroid hormone concentrations in preterm infants younger than 30 weeks' gestation during the first 2 weeks of life and their relationship to outcome. *Pediatrics* 2002;109:222–227.

33. McKinnon BT. FDA safety alert: Hazards of precipitation associated with parenteral nutrition. *Nutr Clin Pract* 1996;11(2):59–65. Erratum in: *Nutr Clin Pract* 1996;11(3):120.

34. Collier SB, Gura KM, Richardson DS, and Duggan D. Parenteral nutrition In: Hendricks KM and Duggan C, editors. *Manual of Pediatric Nutrition*. 4th ed. Hamilton Ontario: BC Decker; 2005.

35. Driscoll DF, Silvestri AP, Nehne J, Klütsch K, Bistrian BR, and Niemann W. Physicochemical stability of highly concentrated total nutrient admixtures for fluid-restricted patients. *Am J Health Syst Pharm* 2006;63(1):79–85.

36. Rude RK, Singer FR, and Gruber HE. Skeletal and hormonal effects of magnesium deficiency. *J Am Coll Nutr* 2009;28(2):131–141.

37. Bohrer D, Cicero do Nascimento P, Binotto R et al. Contribution of the raw material to the aluminum contamination in parenterals. *JPEN* 2002;26:382–388.

38. Federal Register—*Proposed Rules*. 2002;67(228):70691–70692.

39. Bishop NJ, Morley R, Day JP, and Lucas A. Aluminum neurotoxicity in preterm infants receiving intravenous-feeding solutions. *N Engl J Med* 1997;29:3361557–3361561.

40. Newton DW and Driscoll DF. Calcium and phosphate compatibility: Revisited again. *Am J Health Syst Pharm* 2008;65:73–80.

41. Koo WW, Kaplan LA, Horn J, Tsang RC, and Steichen JJ. Aluminum in parenteral nutrition solution–sources and possible alternatives. *JPEN* 1986;10:591–595.

42. Gura KM and Puder M. Recent developments in aluminum contamination of products used in parenteral nutrition. *Curr Opin Clin Nutr Metab Care* 2006; 9:239–246.

43. Sherlock R and Chessex P. Shielding parenteral nutrition from light: Does the available evidence support a randomized controlled trial? *Pediatrics* 2009;123:1529–1533.

44. Lavoie JC, Belanger S, Spalinger M et al. Admixture of a multivitamin preparation to parenteral nutrition: The major contributor to *in vitro* generation of peroxides. *Pediatrics* 1997;99:3: e6.

45. Shattuck KE, Bhatia J, Grinnell C, and Rassin DK. The effects of light exposure on the *in vitro* hepatic response to an amino acid–vitamin solution. *JPEN* 1995;19:398–402.

46. Laborie S, Lavoie JC, and Chessex P. Paradoxical role of ascorbic acid and riboflavin in solutions of total parenteral nutrition: Implication in photoinduced peroxide generation. *Pediatr Res* 1998;43:601–606.

47. Bhatia J, Moslen MT, Kaphalia L, and Rassin DK. Glutathione and tissue amino acid responses to light-exposed parenteral nutrients. *Toxicol Lett* 1992;63:79–89.

48. Neuzil J, Darlow BA, Inder TE et al. Oxidation of parenteral lipid emulsion by ambient and phototherapy lights: Potential toxicity of routine parenteral feeding. *J Pediatr* 1995;126:785–790.

49. Laborie S, Lavoie JL, Pineault M, and Chessex P. Protecting emulsions of parenteral nutrition from peroxidation. *JPEN* 1999;23:104–108.

50. Silva MJ, Barr DB, Reidy JA et al. Urinary levels of seven phthalate metabolites in the U.S. population from the National Health and Nutrition Examination Survey (NHANES) 1999–2000. *Environ Health Perspect* 2004;112:331–333.

51. Calafat AM, Needham LL, Silva MJ et al. Exposure to di-(2-ethylhexyl) phthalate among premature neonates in a neonatal intensive care unit. *Pediatrics* 2004;113:e429–e434.

52. Von Rettberg H, Hannman T, Subotic U et al. Use of di(2-ethylhexyl)phthalate containing infusion systems increases the risk for cholestasis. *Pediatrics*. 2009;124:710–716.

53. Henkin J, Como JA, and Oberman A. Secondary dyslipidemia: Inadvertent effects of drugs in clinical practice. *JAMA* 1992;267:961–8.

54. Walker WA, Goulet O, Kleinman R, Sherman P, Shneider B, and Sanderson I. Chapter 75, Part 4A, Parental nutrition. *Pediatric Gastrointestinal Disease*, Vol 2, 4th ed. Ontario: BC Decker; 2004.

# 11 Parenteral Nutrition in Adults

*M. Molly McMahon, Erin Nystrom, and John M. Miles*

## CONTENTS

The recognition in 1968 that patients could receive all of their nutritional requirements intravenously was a landmark in the field of nutrition and clinical medicine. Although parenteral nutrition (PN) can be essential or even lifesaving, its substantial cost and potential for complications necessitate judicious initiation and use.

## 11.1 INDICATIONS FOR NUTRITIONAL SUPPORT

Protein catabolism (with eventual depletion of body protein leading to protein-calorie malnutrition) can result from starvation, severe illness, or a combination of the two. Malnutrition is difficult to define and thus inevitably arbitrary. The need for nutritional support in patients with malnutrition is a reflection of the timing and extent of recent (previous 3- to 6-month interval) weight loss, adequacy of fat and protein stores on clinical exam, body mass index, the presence or absence of clinical markers of stress, and the anticipated time that the patient will be unable to meet nutritional requirements orally. Studies that have demonstrated a beneficial influence of nutritional support on clinical outcome have provided nutrition for a minimum of one week. Currently, no evidence suggests that nutritional support of briefer duration is beneficial. Additional research is needed to develop clinical markers for malnutrition and to identify patients who will benefit from nutritional support.

## 11.2 INDICATIONS FOR PN

PN should be selected whenever nutritional support is indicated in a malnourished patient with a nonfunctioning or inaccessible gastrointestinal tract. In intestinal failure, PN is indicated in the patient following massive intestinal resection without sufficient intestinal adaptation to receive adequate enteral nutrition once hemodynamic stability has been achieved. In addition, PN should be considered in malnourished patients with persistent distal bowel obstruction, gastrointestinal fistula in whom enteral intake is contraindicated, severe gastrointestinal bleeding, severe mucositis, chylous effusion, and severe gastrointestinal motility disorders resulting in enteral tube feeding intolerance [1].

## 11.3  PN COMPONENTS

Nutrients are substances that must be provided by the diet because they are not synthesized in the body in required amounts. PN contains protein (amino acids providing nitrogen), carbohydrate (dextrose), fat, electrolytes, trace elements, vitamins, and water delivered either by a central vein (central PN) or via a peripheral vein (peripheral PN).

## 11.4  PROTEIN

Nitrogen is required for protein synthesis and is thus an essential component of PN. All currently manufactured PN solutions use crystalline amino acids as the source of nitrogen. Each gram of protein provides 4.0 kcal. For a well-nourished healthy adult without stress, the recommended dietary allowance of protein is 0.8 g/kg body weight, provided that total caloric intake is adequate. Although protein is a metabolic fuel, its structural functions are as important as its fuel functions. Protein oxidation, which provides energy by generating ATP, equals protein intake at steady state. Therefore, caloric requirements should be estimated as total calories rather than as nonprotein calories; the latter method includes carbohydrate and fat but excludes protein as a caloric source. Protein breakdown and synthesis are dynamic processes. During severe illness, protein catabolism exceeds protein synthesis, and net loss of body protein results. Net protein loss results in a loss of tissue function. The increase in proteolysis is primarily caused by the actions of hormones and cytokines, with additional protein losses occurring in specific disease states. Diminished protein synthesis results from bed rest and decreased food intake. Administering nutrition support to critically ill, immobilized patients can decrease but not prevent the loss of body protein.

In general, hospitalized patients with normal renal and hepatic function should receive 1.0–1.5 g of protein per kilogram of body weight per day. Increasing the amount of protein administered will improve nitrogen balance to some extent [2], but there is a limit to this effect. Maximal rates of repletion occur with 1.5 g/kg in malnourished patients. For the majority of patients, providing greater amounts of protein is not of benefit, and the excess protein results in increased ureagenesis [3]. For obese patients (body mass index ≥30), it may be appropriate to provide 1.5 g of protein per kilogram of estimated ideal weight or to express protein requirements as a fraction of estimated basal energy requirements [4]. Data about how to feed stressed obese patients are limited.

Modified amino acid solutions have been formulated for use in specific disease states. For example, the use of branched-chain enriched, low aromatic amino acid solutions has been suggested for patients with acute hepatic encephalopathy. These patients have decreased plasma levels of branched-chain amino acids and increased levels of aromatic amino acids. Branched-chain amino acids, often depleted in this group, are uniquely oxidized in skeletal muscle and adipose tissue rather than in the liver. Aromatic acids undergo deamination by the liver and this process may be impaired in the setting of hepatic encephalopathy. For patient with refractory hepatic encephalopathy, a specialized branched chain enriched PN formula may be considered, although clinical trials do not demonstrate consistent clinical benefit [5]. Once the encephalopathy has resolved or if the patient does not receive benefit from this solution, the less costly standard amino acid solution should be substituted. Patients with liver disease but no encephalopathy can tolerate the less costly standard amino acid solutions. There is insufficient evidence to support the use of other specialized branched-chain amino acid solutions for patients with renal failure or severe stress.

Currently, glutamine is not present in commercially available PN solutions in the United States because of its limited solubility and stability. Glutamine is considered a nonessential amino acid, however, during critical illness glutamine appears to be a conditionally essential amino acid for the intestinal tract. At this time, limited evidence suggests a possible benefit in reducing mortality in critically ill patients [6]. Data does not support the use of parenteral glutamine to improve bowel adaptation. Additional prospective randomized trials of these modified formulas are needed.

## 11.5  CARBOHYDRATE

Parenteral carbohydrate provided in the form of dextrose is a vital source of fuel and has important nitrogen-sparing effects. Each gram of hydrated dextrose monohydrate provides 3.4 kcal. The minimum daily glucose requirement is the amount necessary to meet brain glucose needs of 100–150 g because body carbohydrate stores are limited. Providing calories as glucose stimulates insulin secretion, reduces muscle protein breakdown, and decreases hepatic glucose release, thus reducing the need for skeletal muscle to provide amino acid precursors for gluconeogenesis. Glucose oxidation also is stimulated which spares oxidation of amino acids.

## 11.6  INTRAVENOUS FAT

Fat emulsion provides a concentrated intravenous source of fat calories and the essential fatty acids, linoleic, and linolenic acid. Currently, intravenous fat emulsion is available as 10% (1.1 kcal/mL), 20% (2 kcal/mL), and 30% (3.0 kcal/mL). The emulsions contain long-chain fatty acids (derived from safflower and/or soybean oil), egg yolk phospholipids as emulsifying agents, and glycerin to make the solution isotonic with plasma. Intravenous fat is calorically dense (9 kcal/g), isotonic, protein sparing, and its use prevents essential fatty acid deficiency. In addition, provision of a portion of calories as fat allows lower rates of dextrose infusion, which results in less hyperglycemia and hyperinsulinemia and a lower incidence of abnormalities in liver function tests. Although the optimal percentage of calories that should be infused as fat is unclear, provision of 20% to 30% of total calories as fat is recommended for most stressed patients receiving PN.

The role of fat extends beyond that of energy substrate alone. Substitution of different fat sources has been reported to beneficially modify the patient's response to illness by influencing prostaglandin and leukotriene synthetic pathways. Active investigation is underway to determine the optimal type and quantity of fat to be provided in PN solutions.

## 11.7  MICRONUTRIENT CONTENT: ELECTROLYTES, VITAMINS, AND TRACE ELEMENTS

The electrolytes required for health are sodium, potassium, chloride, calcium, phosphorus, and magnesium. These minerals are supplied as salts; sodium and potassium as chloride, acetate, or phosphate, calcium as gluconate, and magnesium as sulfate. Sodium and potassium cations are added to the PN solution as chloride or acetate salts after the phosphate requirement is met. Acetate is further metabolized by the liver, kidney, and skeletal muscle to bicarbonate to provide an alkaline buffer.

Electrolyte modification is needed for patients with significant losses due to illness or the use of certain medications. Patients with intestinal failure often require additional fluid and higher amounts of sodium and divalent cations (Table 11.1) due to gastrointestinal losses or impaired absorption. Adjustments in potassium, magnesium, phosphorus, and acetate and chloride are often needed in patients with renal failure, although modifications vary depending on whether the patient is receiving dialysis and the type and frequency of dialysis.

While specific requirements for intravenous trace elements and vitamins have not been well-defined for hospitalized patients, typically standardized intravenous preparation components of combined vitamins and minerals are used [7]. Multiple trace element preparations contain four or five elements (zinc, copper, manganese, and chromium, with or without selenium) formulated for medically stable adult patients. Trace elements are also available as single-item injections, allowing adjustment of components as needed for individual patients. If a four-component trace element package is used, selenium injection must also be added. Iodine and molybdenum are no longer

**TABLE 11.1**

**Mineral and Micronutrient Deficiencies in Intestinal Failure**

| Nutrient | Loss and Mechanism for Deficiency | Dosing |
|---|---|---|
| Sodium | Stomach: 60–100 mEq/L<br>Small bowel: 80–140 mEq/L<br>Colon: 60 mEq/L<br>Colectomy; significant sodium and water reabsorption occurs in the colon | Consider GI losses; provision of sodium above usual parenteral requirement of 1–2 mEq/kg/day may be necessary<br>Monitor sodium and fluid balance closely |
| Potassium | Colon: 10–30 mEq/L<br>Secondary hyperaldosteronism due to depletion of sodium increases urinary losses<br>Magnesium deficiency reduces potassium transport into cells | Usual parenteral requirement 1–2 mEq/kg/day; consider also stool losses<br>Treat magnesium deficiency<br>Ensure adequate sodium and water balance to correct hyperaldosteronism |
| Magnesium | Impaired absorption; primary sites of absorption are the distal jejunum and ileum<br>GI losses<br>Reduced absorption from increased intraluminal binding of magnesium by unabsorbed fatty acids<br>Hyperaldosteronism secondary to sodium loss increases loss in urine | Provision of magnesium above the usual parenteral requirement of 8–24 mEq/day may be necessary<br>Serum levels may not reflect total body stores |
| Bicarbonate | GI losses may lead to metabolic acidosis | Increase sodium and potassium acetate salts and minimize chloride salts in PN |
| Calcium | Impaired absorption<br>Hypomagnesemia-induced reduction in PTH secretion results in increased urinary loss and reduced absorption<br>Vitamin D deficiency | Usual parenteral requirement: 10–15 mEq/day<br>Serum levels may not reflect total body stores |
| Zinc | Impaired absorption<br>15 mg/L of small bowel and colon | Maintenance parenteral dose of 2.5–5 mg/day may be met with standard multiple trace element product<br>Increase PN zinc up to 10–20 mg/day with persistent, high GI losses<br>Serum levels may not reflect total body stores |
| B12 | Impaired absorption with loss of ileum<br>Bacterial overgrowth resulting in increased B12 metabolism | Standard parenteral multivitamin meets needs<br>Additional supplementation outside of PN may be required to treat deficiency |
| Fat-soluble vitamins: A,D,E,K | Fat malabsorption<br>Bacterial overgrowth increases deconjugation of bile acids, reducing fat absorption<br>Colonic bacteria synthesize vitamin K, therefore, deficiency is unlikely without colectomy | Standard parenteral multivitamin meets maintenance needs<br>Additional monitoring of levels and supplementation outside of PN may be required to treat deficiency |

included in combination trace element injections, as they are likely present as contaminants in PN solution. Iron is also not routinely included, so iron levels should be monitored and replaced as needed in patients are on long-term PN.

The composition of intravenous multivitamin products has been established in accordance with the guidelines of the American Medical Association Nutrition Advisory Group and the Food and Drug Administration. The most commonly used commercial multivitamin formulation provides the daily maintenance for four fat-soluble (A, D, E, and K) and nine water-soluble vitamins (C, folic acid, B1, B2, B6, niacin, B12, pantothenic acid, and biotin). A formulation that does not contain vitamin K is also available. Some patients require additional vitamin replacement beyond that provided in these preparations. Serious consequences can result from providing less than the standard replacement amounts of vitamins. Body stores of vitamins vary significantly. For example, folate and thiamine can become depleted within weeks when eating a poor diet, while others, such as B12, take years for deficiency to manifest. Deaths associated with thiamine deficiency due to exclusion of multivitamins from PN during periods of multivitamin shortage have been reported [8].

## 11.8   ESTIMATION OF DAILY CALORIC REQUIREMENTS

Daily caloric requirement of patients can be estimated by use of a predictive formula such as the Harris–Benedict equation or measured by indirect calorimetry. Steady-state conditions must be achieved during the indirect calorimetric measurement. The premise that sick hospitalized patients have elevated caloric requirements, especially when stressed by surgery, trauma, or sepsis, is no longer supported. Substantial variability in energy expenditure among studies in patients with comparable severity of illness has been reported, and may be due to errors in indirect calorimetry measurement. A careful review of the literature has shown that the majority of hospitalized adults have surprisingly normal energy expenditure, in the range of 100% and 120% of estimated basal energy expenditure (Harris–Benedict equation) [9]. Data about how to feed obese patients are limited. Some groups advocate the use of hypocaloric feeding (e.g., 75% of actual basal energy requirements or an amount based on a lower "adjusted" weight).

## 11.9   FLUID REQUIREMENT

The normal daily requirement for water in adults without abnormal renal or gastric losses is 30 mL of volume per kg body weight. Patients with increased total body water and peripheral edema generally should receive fluid-restricted PN formulas. Patients with negative fluid balance and hyponatremia generally require additional volume and sodium. For example, patients with intestinal failure and increased gastrointestinal losses should receive additional fluid as crystalloid because volume of losses may change daily. PN volume may be increased appropriately once it is clear that the gastrointestinal volume loss is relatively stable. Nondextrose-containing crystalloid is recommended, as patients receive adequate dextrose with PN.

## 11.10   SELECTION OF PERIPHERAL VERSUS CENTRAL PN

PN can be administered by peripheral or central vein. The severity of illness, length of anticipated duration of use, caloric need, and fluid requirement aid in choosing central or peripheral PN for a patient. Peripheral PN avoids the use of central vein catheterization for nutrition, as the nutrition is administered by peripheral vein. Peripheral PN may be considered in medically stable patients with good cardiac function who can tolerate higher fluid volumes and who require short-term (e.g., 7–10 days) PN. In general, critically ill patients or patients with renal, hepatic, or cardiac issues will not tolerate the high volume rates required to meet nutritional needs and will require central PN. It is not possible to peripherally administer the high osmolarity solutions used for central PN because of phlebitis. For this reason, the osmolarity of peripheral PN solutions should not exceed 1000 mOsm/L. The addition of isotonic lipid to dextrose and amino acids may enhance vein tolerance to peripheral PN solutions.

## 11.11   MONITORING GUIDELINES

Height, body weight, and body mass index should be recorded at baseline. Before initiation of PN, patients should have glucose, sodium, potassium, phosphorus, magnesium, calcium, creatinine, urea, triglyceride, and aspartate aminotransferase levels measured. The extent and frequency of biochemical monitoring following initiation of PN should be individualized; at a minimum, plasma glucose, electrolytes, and phosphorus levels should be checked daily until stable. A triglyceride level should be checked two to three days postinitiation of intravenous fat emulsion [10]. If triglyceride values are >300–350 mg/dL, the fat emulsion dose should be reduced or stopped and strong consideration should be given to a hypocaloric regimen, since isocaloric fat-free feeding can lead to worsening of hypertriglyceridemia [11].

Although the extent of the daily examination should be individualized, the catheter site, heart, and lungs should always be examined and the possible development of peripheral edema assessed. The source of fever should always be investigated in a patient with a central venous catheter. Hemodynamic data, fluid balance, urine output, and creatinine, urea, and sodium levels should be reviewed to help determine the appropriate PN volume. Daily weights are best interpreted in light of the fluid balance; weight increases exceeding 0.25 kg over a 24-h period usually reflect fluid gain.

While PN should not be used to treat acute abnormalities in volume or electrolyte levels, it is an effective vehicle to replace chronic losses. Knowledge of the magnitude of gastrointestinal and renal losses allows an estimation of electrolyte and mineral losses and appropriate PN supplementation. PN sodium content may need to be increased in patients with significant gastrointestinal tract losses, and magnesium content may need to be increased in the setting of renal losses. The acetate and chloride content (as potassium or sodium salts) of the PN admixture should be adjusted for acid–base disturbances. For example, the PN acetate content may be increased and the chloride content decreased in cases of metabolic acidosis (e.g., diarrhea or small bowel losses); the converse is true for metabolic alkalosis (e.g., gastric losses).

The interpretation of plasma trace elements is challenging. Trace element changes during illness often include a decrease in the plasma concentration of iron and zinc. Low levels of iron and zinc may reflect visceral sequestration [12], however, and not true deficiency. Familiarity with the route of excretion for plasma trace elements is helpful to determine frequency of monitoring and need for replacement. Plasma zinc levels should be measured in patients with impaired absorption or increased gastrointestinal output. More aggressive replacement generally is indicated for patients with a low level and a potential cause for the low level.

Plasma levels of several metal ions are influenced by the plasma albumin concentration. Because circulating calcium, magnesium, and zinc are all bound in part to serum albumin, hypoalbuminemia may be the sole cause of a low plasma level of these cations. Thus, supplementation of the mineral or trace element may not be necessary or appropriate. The threshold for the development of symptoms due to hypocalcemia and hypomagnesemia has not been well-defined, and there is no evidence that administration of parenteral calcium or magnesium improves clinical outcomes. Algorithms developed to correct the plasma calcium value for varying degrees of hypoalbuminemia have been shown to be inaccurate in stressed patients [13]. Moreover, direct measurement of the ionized calcium level, although in theory a desirable practice, may yield spuriously low values in the presence of hypoalbuminemia. Because of the limitations on interpretation of plasma divalent cations concentrations, it is important to rely heavily on data from the history and physical examination. The absence of physical findings of neuromuscular irritability (i.e., no Chvostek sign, Trousseau sign, or clonus) and no electrocardiographic evidence of hypocalcemia (i.e., QT prolongation) in patients with no clinical reason to have an abnormality would suggest that reduced plasma concentrations of these are ions are probably so mild as to be clinically insignificant or due to alterations in binding proteins.

Patients with extensive small bowel disease or post resection are at greater risk for nutrient, mineral, and vitamin deficiencies because of the loss of absorptive surface (Table 11.1). Levels of calcium, magnesium, zinc, and fat-soluble vitamins should be monitored. When measuring vitamin D levels, the 25-hydroxyvitamin D level should be assessed. In addition, the ileum is the site for absorption of vitamin $B_{12}$ and bile salts. Because resection of more than 60 cm of ileum is associated with malabsorption of intrinsic factor-bound vitamin, measurement and supplementation of vitamin $B_{12}$ is important. Resection of more than 100 cm of ileum is associated with insufficient bile salt concentrations in the duodenum that may lead to fat and fat-soluble vitamin malabsorption.

Glucose control is critical in patients receiving PN. Hyperglycemia and hypertriglyceridemia are associated with adverse outcomes and PN can contribute to both, especially when the patient is overfed. We favor "permissive underfeeding" of patients who are overweight and obese. Other causes of hyperglycemia include infection, dehydration, or medications, such as glucocorticoids. During short-term hospitalization, national guidelines suggest aiming for a glucose goal of 140–180 mg/dL in critically ill patients. Available evidence does not permit confident proposal of one overall guideline [14–18]. The proposed glucose goal range should minimize adverse consequences related to hyper and hypoglycemia. Hypoglycemia is defined as a glucose level <70 mg/dL.

In patients with hyperglycemia or at risk for hyperglycemia, initially we recommend limiting PN dextrose to 150–200 g/day. Insulin is the mainstay of management of hyperglycemia in patients receiving PN. In most cases, PN dextrose may be safely "covered" by the addition of 0.1 U of Regular insulin per gram of dextrose (e.g., 10 U/100 g dextrose or 10 U/L for 10% dextrose) for diabetic patients or patients who are hyperglycemic prior to PN initiation [4,19]. This is an effective starting dose of insulin with minimal risk of hypoglycemia in patients with normal renal function. It is often necessary to increase the amount of insulin by 0.05 U/g of dextrose to 0.15 or 0.2 U/g of dextrose infused for dextrose coverage. Some groups place higher amounts in the admixture. If the PN dextrose is reduced or increased, insulin dose should be adjusted proportionately to maintain similar insulin to glucose ratio. The advantage of this approach is that the infusion of dextrose and insulin are linked; if the infusion is interrupted for any reason, the administration of insulin is also stopped. Initiation of subcutaneous regular insulin or long acting insulin or a standardized intravenous insulin infusion program also may be necessary.

Medication profiles should be reviewed daily to identify metabolic parameters that require monitoring. Examples of medications that may affect metabolic tests include amphotericin (hypokalemia, hypomagnesemia, renal tubular acidosis), corticosteroids (hyperglycemia, hypokalemia), insulin (hypokalemia, hypophosphatemia, and hypomagnesemia), and diuretics (hypokalemia, hypomagnesemia, metabolic alkalosis). Intravenous medications may be compounded with dextrose-containing solution. Finally, propofol is an anesthetic agent that is formulated in a 10% fat emulsion, and its administration may necessitate a decrease or complete elimination of intravenous fat. Dextrose content and calories from all sources should be considered when developing PN programs.

The daily goal is to determine whether the PN program (volume or composition) needs modification in light of the patient's current condition. Once the gastrointestinal tract regains function, the enteral route should be used for nutrition.

## 11.12 COMPLICATIONS

PN-associated complications can be categorized into catheter-related (mechanical, infectious, and thrombotic), metabolic, and gastrointestinal. Catheter-related complications are discussed in Chapter 19.

Serious metabolic disturbances can result from PN [20], and the risk can be lessened with awareness of pathophysiology [21]. Complications may result from providing excess calories or too much or too little volume, among other causes. Overfeeding can increase oxygen consumption, carbon dioxide production, minute ventilation, and the work of breathing, which can fatigue patients with impaired lung function. Overfeeding also can cause hyperglycemia, hypertriglyceridemia, and abnormal liver test results.

Serious and life-threatening complications of sudden refeeding, coined the refeeding syndrome, have been recognized since the advent of PN therapy. The refeeding risk increases when chronically malnourished patients are rapidly refed. The risks are related to fluid and electrolyte abnormalities, malnutrition-related organ dysfunction, and vitamin deficiencies. The depleted muscle stores of minerals and acute increase in plasma insulin concentration caused by PN can lead to severe hypokalemia, hypomagnesemia, and hypophosphatemia if electrolyte and mineral replacement is inadequate. If severe baseline deficiencies are present, initiation of PN should be delayed until values are

in the normal reference range. Levels of these electrolytes and minerals should be carefully monitored until results are in the normal reference range. Overfeeding should be avoided. Acute hyperinsulinemia due to refeeding also promotes renal tubular sodium resorption, which can expand the
extracellular fluid and lead to cardiac decompensation in extremely malnourished patients with
decreased left ventricular mass. Thus, excess fluid and excess sodium should be avoided. Thiamine
supplementation should be provided.

Hepatic abnormalities, the most common gastrointestinal complication associated with PN, may be
caused by the therapy itself or by the patient's underlying disease or medications. In adults, PN-related
hepatic abnormalities from short-term use are common and are generally benign and temporary.
Complications may be biochemical (elevation of serum aminotransferase, alkaline phosphatase, or
bilirubin) or histologic (steatosis, portal triaditis). Transaminase elevations generally occur early in
therapy (1–2 weeks after initiation of PN) and often resolve without change in the nutrition program.
Bilirubin and alkaline phosphatase elevations usually appear slightly later (2–3 weeks into therapy).
Biliary complications associated with PN include acalculous cholecystitis, gall bladder sludge, and
cholelithiasis. Sludge, the most common of these complications, occurs when the gastrointestinal tract
is not used. Abnormal liver function test results should not automatically lead to stopping or altering
the PN solution inasmuch as abnormal liver function results may not represent true liver dysfunction.
Other causes of abnormal hepatic function, such as extrahepatic obstruction, medications, or infection,
should be excluded. The nutrition program should be reviewed to be certain that the caloric intake is
not excessive and that a mixed-fuel system (i.e., dextrose, protein, and fat) is being administered.
Further information is provided in Chapter 20, Intestinal Failure-Associated Liver Disease.

Early studies demonstrated that nutrition support teams reduced complications. The importance
of standardized PN order sets and protocols and integration of nutrition education into medical cur-
ricula was found to be important [22].

Systems reliant on information technology show merit in improving patient safety. Information
technology can prevent errors and adverse events, facilitate a more rapid response after an adverse
event has occurred, and provide feedback about adverse events [23]. Systems using this technology
applied to patients receiving PN have shown promise [24]. In our experience, when a nutrition support service consultation was required prior to initiation of PN, significantly fewer patients received
PN for less than 7 days compared with patients who did not receive a mandatory consult (Nystrom
et al. 2009, unpublished data). Hospitals should be encouraged to monitor the use of PN, including
the frequency of short duration (<7 days) use.

## REFERENCES

1. A.S.P.E.N. Board of Directors CGTF. Guidelines for the use of parenteral and enteral nutrition in adult
   and pediatric patients. *JPEN J Parenter Enteral Nutr* 2002;26:1SA–138SA.
2. Elwyn DH, Gump FE, Munro HN, Iles M, and Kinney JM. Changes in nitrogen balance of depleted
   patients with increasing infusions of glucose. *Am J Clin Nutr* 1979;32:1597–611.
3. Shaw JH, Wildbore M, and Wolfe RR. Whole body protein kinetics in severely septic patients: The
   response to glucose infusion and total parenteral nutrition. *Ann Surg* 1987;205:288–94.
4. McMahon MM, Farnell MB, and Murray MJ. Nutritional support of critically ill patients. *Mayo Clin
   Proc* 1993;68:911–20.
5. Als-Nielsen B, Koretz RL, Kjaergard LL, and Gluud C. Branched-chain amino acids for hepatic encephalopathy. *Cochrane Database Syst Rev* 2003;(2):CD001939.
6. McClave SA, Martindale RG, Vanek VW et al. Guidelines for the provision and assessment of nutrition
   support therapy in the adult critically ill patient: Society of Critical Care Medicine (SCCM) and American
   Society for Parenteral and Enteral Nutrition (A.S.P.E.N.). *JPEN J Parenter Enteral Nutr*
   2009;33:277–316.
7. Mirtallo J, Canada T, Johnson D et al. Safe practices for parenteral nutrition. *JPEN J Parenter Enteral
   Nutr* 2004;28:S39–70.
8. Centers for Disease Control. Deaths associated with thiamine-deficient total parenteral nutrition. *MMWR
   Morb Mortal Wkly Rep* 1989;38:43–6.

9. Miles JM. Energy expenditure in hospitalized patients: Implications for nutritional support. *Mayo Clin Proc* 2006;81:809–16.

10. Jurgens DJ, Litzow MR, Baker MR, Clifford LR, McMahon MM, and Miles JM. Serum triglyceride levels during parenteral nutrition in blood and marrow transplant patients. *Annual Meeting of the American Society for Parenteral and Enteral Nutrition*. Phoenix, AZ, 2007.

11. Paluzzi M and Meguid MM. A prospective randomized study of the optimal source of nonprotein calories in total parenteral nutrition. *Surgery* 1987;102:711–7.

12. Goldblum SE, Cohen DA, Jay M, and McClain CJ. Interleukin 1-induced depression of iron and zinc: Role of granulocytes and lactoferrin. *Am J Physiol* 1987;252:E27–32.

13. Ladenson JH, Lewis JW, and Boyd JC. Failure of total calcium corrected for protein, albumin, and pH to correctly assess free calcium status. *J Clin Endocrinol Metab* 1978;46:986–93.

14. Moghissi ES, Korytkowski MT, DiNardo M et al. American Association of Clinical Endocrinologists and American Diabetes Association consensus statement on inpatient glycemic control. *Diabetes Care* 2009;32:1119–31.

15. Van den Berghe G, Wouters P, Weekers F et al. Intensive insulin therapy in the critically ill patients. *N Engl J Med* 2001;345:1359–67.

16. Van den Berghe G, Wilmer A, Hermans G et al. Intensive insulin therapy in the medical ICU. *N Engl J Med* 2006;354:449–61.

17. The NICE-SUGAR Study Investigators. Intensive versus conventional glucose control in critically ill patients. *N Engl J Med* 2009;360:1283–97.

18. Miles JM, McMahon MM, and Isley WL. No, the glycaemic target in the critically ill should not be < or = 6.1 mmol/l. *Diabetologia* 2008;51:916–20.

19. McMahon MM. Diabetes mellitus. In: Merritt R, editor. *The A.S.P.E.N. Nutrition Support Practice Manual. Silver Springs*. MD: American Society for Parenteral and Enteral Nutrition; 2005. pp. 317–31.

20. Weinsier RL and Krumdieck CL. Death resulting from overzealous total parenteral nutrition: The refeeding syndrome revisited. *Am J Clin Nutr* 1981;34:393–99.

21. Mehanna HM, Moledina J, and Travis J. Refeeding syndrome: What it is, and how to prevent and treat it. *BMJ* 2008;336:1495–8.

22. Chrisanderson D, Heimburger DC, Morgan SL et al. Metabolic complications of total parenteral nutrition: Effects of a nutrition support service. *JPEN J Parenter Enteral Nutr* 1996;20:206–10.

23. Bates DW and Gawande AA. Improving safety with information technology. *N Engl J Med* 2003;348:2526–34.

24. Wilson JW, Oyen LJ, Ou NN et al. Hospital rules-based system: The next generation of medical informatics for patient safety. *Am J Health Syst Pharm* 2005;62:499–505.

# 12 Vascular Access Devices

*Ivan M. Gutierrez, Horacio Padua, and Tom Jaksic*

## CONTENTS

## 12.1 INTRODUCTION

The use of vascular access devices (VADs) has become ubiquitous in all branches of medicine. Adequate venous access plays an essential role in many patient populations for the treatment of various disease entities and their use has shifted from the acute care setting to long-term care. In the setting of intestinal failure, VADs are essential for administration of intravenous fluids, medications, intermittent blood draws, and total parenteral nutrition. It is essential to gain an understanding of the various access devices available and placement techniques to properly address each patient's needs. Also, by recognizing the importance of appropriate care it is possible to minimize the risk of morbidity and mortality associated with the use of VADs.

## 12.2 PERIPHERAL VERSUS CENTRAL VENOUS ACCESS

The decision regarding which catheter is most appropriate for a given patient should be based on the following factors: diagnosis, patient preference, length and type of therapy, and history of previous access. Central venous access is mandatory for specific infusion solutions such as vesicant drugs and total parenteral nutrition. Another indication for central venous access is the need for long-term access with the presence of inaccessible peripheral veins. In general, central venous lines are preferred in intestinal failure patients.

## 12.3 CLASSIFICATION OF VADs

VADs can be classified as either venous or arterial. In this review, we will focus on venous VADs as they are the primary access used specifically in patients with intestinal failure. Venous VADs can be classified according to the time intended for their use; short-term, intermediate-term, and long-term use or according to their position in the venous system, peripheral versus central as discussed previously.

### 12.3.1 SHORT-TERM VENOUS ACCESS

Peripheral access venous catheters are the most commonly used in clinical practice and are usually placed in superficial veins of the arms. These catheters range in length from 35 to 52 mm and they are usually made of Teflon. Short-term central venous lines are designed for continuous short-term infusion (1–3 weeks). Temporary central venous catheters (CVCs) are usually placed in the critical care setting. These CVCs are made from polyurethane and range in length from 8 to 30 cm with either single or multiple lumens. They are commonly placed into a central vein (subclavian, internal jugular, innominate, axillary, or femoral). Usually these catheters are not tunneled through the skin; rather they are secured to the skin with interrupted sutures. These lines are recommended for hospitalized patients rather than for outpatient therapy due primarily to their propensity for infection outside a skilled nursing environment.[1]

### 12.3.2 INTERMEDIATE VENOUS ACCESS

Intermediate venous access devices are specifically designed for prolonged intermittent use and are usually nontunneled. The most commonly known device in this category is the peripherally inserted central catheter (PICC). Advantages of a PICC include: (1) its utility as an inpatient or outpatient access device; (2) potential for placement within the central venous system hence allowing for the infusion of total parenteral nutrition; and (3) the likely low risk of pneumothorax and hemothorax associated with their use. Specially trained nursing teams are capable of placing PICCs. Common access sites include peripheral veins such as the basilic, brachial, or cephalic. The Food and Drug Administration has approved the use of PICC lines for up to 12 months, but their longevity depends upon several factors. The most important of these are patient compliance with proper care and frequency of device utilization.[2]

### 12.3.3 LONG-TERM VENOUS ACCESS

For prolonged venous access a tunneled line or an implanted reservoir (port) may be inserted. Tunneled catheters are usually made of silicone and they can have anchoring cuffs. The cuff is thought to induce an inflammatory reaction in the subcutaneous tissue, which leads to fibrosis and fixation of the catheter. Thus, tunneled catheters have lower infection rates when compared to nontunneled catheters.[3] Implanted ports are made up of a subcutaneous reservoir, which is connected to a silicone catheter. Ports are often implanted in a surgically created pocket on the anterior or lateral chest. The advantages of the implantable port system are improved appearance and less interference with activities of daily living (i.e., swimming). Implantable ports also tend to have a reduced risk of infection when compared to tunneled and nontunneled catheters.[3] The major disadvantages are the need to use a needle through the skin to access the port and the higher cost for placement and maintenance. The Centers for Disease Control and Prevention guidelines recommend the use of a tunneled catheter for patients that require continuous access such as patient with intestinal failure. On the other hand, ports are preferred for patients that require venous access intermittently.[4]

### 12.3.4 CATHETER DESIGN AND COMPOSITION CONSIDERATIONS

CVCs have the option of single or multiple lumens. The major advantage of having multiple lumens is the ability to infuse different solutions simultaneously. However, studies have demonstrated that multiple lumens are associated with increased rate of infections.[5] For this reason, it is recommended to maintain the number of lumens to a minimum.[6] If a CVC or a multilumen PICC is used for parenteral nutrition, a dedicated port should be used exclusively for its infusion.[7]

Most central catheters are made of either silicone or polyurethane. One major advantage of silicone catheters is malleability, which in turn makes them less traumatic to the vascular endothelium. However, a downside is a comparatively smaller diameter and thicker catheter wall required to maintain their strength. The polyurethane catheters have improved flow rates due to their larger diameter but often cause more trauma to the vessel increasing the risk of thrombosis.[2] On balance silicone catheters are usually preferred in patients with intestinal failure requiring PN.

## 12.4 INSERTION OF CVCs

Most short- and long-term catheters are introduced using a percutaneous approach and then guided into the central circulation. Placement is performed either in the operating room or the interventional radiology suite. Percutaneous venous approaches are based upon the Seldinger technique where a guide wire is placed into a vein and a catheter is then advanced over it. The advantages of this technique when compared to a cut down procedure (where the vein is actually exposed surgically) include more rapid venous access, less cost, and avoidance of a larger incision.[8] The clinician may deem that a cut down is safer in certain patients where percutaneous access is difficult (i.e., patients who are obese, have skeletal abnormalities, or have had multiple cannulations). Similarly a cut down may be preferred if the target vein is extremely small (i.e., premature neonate).

### 12.4.1 UPPER EXTREMITY APPROACH

The basilic or cephalic veins in the upper arm are the preferred approach for PICC placements. Without image guidance, the antecubital fossa is the usual access site as the veins are easy to visualize. With ultrasound guidance, the access sites tend to be higher in the arm where the vein target has a larger diameter.

### 12.4.2 INTERNAL JUGULAR VEIN APPROACH

The internal jugular veins run laterally within the right and left carotid sheath of the neck. On the right side the internal jugular vein courses more directly into the superior vena cava (SVC) and is thus often the initially preferred route of access. Internal jugular vein catheters should be placed in a sterile environment, and long-term catheters are commonly tunneled to the anterior chest wall. Ultrasound guidance may be useful for the percutaneous access of the jugular veins.[9]

### 12.4.3 SUBCLAVIAN VEIN APPROACH

The subclavian vein has been described as one of the preferred sites for central venous access in the hospital setting because of its defined anatomical landmarks. In the acute care setting, an experienced clinician can access the subclavian vein rapidly without the aid of any imaging modalities. The subclavian vein arches behind the clavicle anterior to the scalene muscle and over the first rib, where it joins the internal jugular vein to form the brachiocephalic vein. There are conditions that predispose patients to a higher risk of complications with a subclavian approach. These include; prior axillary dissection, use of high-pressure ventilation, and the presence of chronic obstructive pulmonary disease.[8]

### 12.4.4 FEMORAL VEIN APPROACH

This approach is usually reserved for patients whose upper arm and neck veins are no longer available. It is very important to perform femoral vein cannulation in a sterile environment as these lines carry an increased risk of infection due their proximity to the inguinal region. The femoral anatomy can be recalled by using the pneumonic NAVEL. The pneumonic describes the location of critical structures from lateral to medial below the inguinal ligament; nerve, artery, vein, empty space, and lymphatics. In the femoral vein approach, the Seldinger technique is usually used to cannulate the vein. If the line is intended for long-term use it may be tunneled. Ultrasound guidance is used as needed.

### 12.4.5 OTHER ALTERNATIVE SITES

It is our experience that patients with intestinal failure are prone to multiple line infections and occasional thromboses. In patients where the upper and lower extremity veins have been exhausted, careful consideration must be given to alternative sites. Alternative sites frequently require the expertise of interventional radiologists with various imaging modalities to place catheters via a translumbar, transhepatic, or internal thoracic approach. These have been reported in the literature often as single case reports.[10] Intestinal failure patients with difficult access should be discussed in a multidisciplinary fashion with a team encompassing surgeons, nursing IV team, and interventional radiologists to determine access options tailored for the specific clinical scenario.

## 12.5 COMPLICATIONS OF CVCs

The frequent use and placement of CVCs expose patients to an array of complications that have been well documented in the literature. The use of CVC for long-term parenteral nutrition has been reported as a primary cause of morbidity in patients dependant on this form of nutrition in the United States and abroad. Prevention of complications and preservation of venous access is critical in intestinal failure patients.

### 12.5.1 EARLY COMPLICATIONS

Early complications refer to problems that occur within the perioperative period. They involve technical aspects of insertion as well as mechanical malfunction of the catheters immediately after placement. Some of the most common early complications include pneumothorax, hemothorax, arrythmias, arterial puncture, and primary malposition or malfunction of the catheter. Early complication rates vary depending upon patient age, access approach, and the location of CVC tip. Pneumothorax is consistently reported to be the most common major complication.

### 12.5.2 PNEUMOTHORAX

Pneumothorax usually results from a percutanous approach for CVC placement with or without ultrasonography guidance. Both subclavian vein and internal jugular vein approaches can result in this complication, but the former has a higher incidence. Operator technical experience is a key component in avoiding this complication. It is estimated that more than 50 implantations are required in order to attain a significant reduction in pneumothorax complication rate.[11] Although the use of ultrasonography has been shown to have some benefit in the process of cannulation in adults and older children, it has not been evaluated in infants, as most of these tend to have their lines placed in the operating room or interventional radiology suite where fluoroscopy is available. Controversy exists regarding the use of ultrasonography as this modality is operator dependant.

When pneumothorax results from CVC insertion the presentation varies according to the size of lung collapse. A pneumothorax estimated to be 30% or less is usually asymptomatic. Patients usually have a confirmatory chest x-ray after line placement; however, some experts suggest that this may be unnecessary if fluoroscopy was used. In the presence of hemodynamic and/or respiratory instability in patients after CVC placement a prompt chest x-ray is highly recommended.

Treatment for an iatrogenic pneumothorax depends upon whether the patient develops symptoms. Asymptomatic patients can be managed with observation alone although serial x-rays are warranted and some have suggested the use of supplemental oxygen. Patients who develop symptoms should be managed with a chest tube placement or with simple aspiration of the pneumothorax with a small-bore catheter. In small pediatric patients sedation or anesthesia is usually required prior to invasive procedures hence primary chest tube placement is the option of choice. In all cases, chest tube placement is the more sure remedy for symptomatic pneumothorax.

### 12.5.3   LATE COMPLICATIONS

Late complications include: catheter dislodgement and migration, catheter-related bloodstream infections (CRBSI), as well as line and vein thrombosis. Other less likely complications include pulmonary embolism and SVC syndrome. Late complications have a great impact upon ultimate morbidity and mortality.

### 12.5.4   INFECTIONS

Infectious complications related to intravascular catheters range widely and include local site infections, CRBSI, septic thrombophlebitis, and endocarditis. The mortality for CRBSI has been reported to be as high as 35% in some prospective studies. CRBSI also have a significant impact with respect to cost. It has been estimated that the cost per infection ranges from $34,508 to $56,000, with an annual cost from $296 million to $2.3 billion.[12] Details of central catether care and methods to reduce the risk of infectious complications are provided in Chapter 26: Central Venous Catheter Care.

The most common organisms isolated from blood stream infection include coagulase-negative staphylococci, *Staphylococcus aureus*, and Gram-negative rods. Understanding the pathogenesis of catheter-related infections is crucial in designing strategies for prevention.

There are three main mechanisms by which CRBSI may arise: external infection at the catheter entry site with subsequent migration of pathogens along the external aspect of the catheter, contamination of the catheter hub with intraluminal microbes and from pathogens that enter the blood stream and seed the catheter hematogenously (Figure 12.1). The inevitable formation of a biofilm on the catheter as well as the presence of translocated bacteria from the intestine of short bowel syndrome patients has been suggested as a further synergistic cause of CRBSI.

The material from which the device is made as well as the intrinsic virulence of the organism causing the infection is the primary determinant of pathogenesis. Catheters made from polyvinyl chloride or polyethylene are more susceptible to adherence by bacteria when compared to those made of silicone or polyurethane.[4] Some organisms such as coagulase-negative bacteria have been found to adhere to polymer surfaces more easily than other pathogens.[4]

More recently, the study of biofilms has added to our understanding of CRBSI. The biofilms can form in patches or as a contiguous layer that completely covers the surface of the catheter. The continuous supply of oxygen and nutrients found in the bloodstream allows for a catheter placed in the vein to become an ideal location for the formation of biofilms. Further the production of adhesion molecules and accumulation of proteins derived from microorganisms allows for the development of an environment suitable for proliferation.[13] The bacterial density in the biofilms can be as large

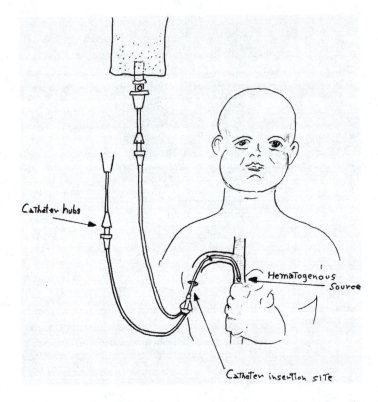

**FIGURE 12.1**    Potential sources for CRBSI in patients receiving parenteral nutrition. (Drawing courtesy of Dr. Neil Feins.)

as $10^7$ cells/cm$^2$ on the surface of a catheter.[14] The dissemination of organisms within biofilms typically occurs from the hydrostatic force from the circulation or by the production of lytic enzymes from the biofilm itself. This results in dislodgement of individual cells or a cluster of cells from the biofilm. Dislodgement of a single cell is resolved quickly by the host's immune system; however, when dissemination is substantial or dislodgment occurs in the setting of immunosuppression infection is manifested clinically. The American College of Surgeons has developed guidelines to aid in the diagnosis and management of CRBSI.[15] A summary of these criteria follows.

Catheters should not be removed on the basis of fever alone and a thorough clinical workup of CRBSI is necessary. Ideally blood cultures (one drawn through the central line and another peripherally) should be sent if CRBSI is suspected. Indications for the removal of venous VADs in the setting of CRBSI are summarized in Table 12.1.

Therapy with antibiotics for CRBSI should be empiric with careful consideration of the likelihood of resistant strains such as methicillin-resistant *S. aureus*. Coverage should include

**TABLE 12.1**

**Indications for Catheter Removal in CRBSI**

Signs of infection at entry site (purulence and erythema)

Bacteremia or sepsis lasting >48 h

Resistant microorganisms

Relapse of infection after antibiotic course completion

Positive quantitative blood cultures

Presence of other complications (infective endocarditis, pulmonary embolus)

Gram-negative bacteria and in neutropenic patients empiric coverage against pseudomonas is recommended.[16] It is very important to institute rapid and appropriate antibiotic therapy as a failure to do so is correlated with higher mortality. Once speciation of organism is determined therapy should be tailored accordingly. Although there is no compelling data to support specific length of antibiotic therapy it is widely accepted that a treatment course of 10–14 days is usual in patients who are not immunocompromised and do not have any underlying valvular heart disease. Recommendations for treatment length of *S. aureus*, CRBSI varies from 4 to 6 weeks. Other specific pathogen treatment protocols are beyond the scope of this review, however, they can be found in the latest set of guidelines from the Infectious Diseases Society of America.[17]

Although there have been some promising reports in using antibiotic lock solutions for prevention of CRBSI, there still remains a concern about development of resistance. Because ethanol has been shown to be an effective microbicidal agent and it also has the ability to penetrate the biofilms it has been used it as a catheter lock solution in pediatric patients with intestinal failure. A regimen of 70% ethanol lock solutions administered three times a week has been noted to decrease the rate CRBSI over fourfold in a cohort of pediatric intestinal failure patients.[18]

## 12.5.5 THROMBOSIS

Thrombosis can occur from fibrin accumulation around the catheter or from clotted blood within the lumen. When thrombosis occurs there are two options for treatment, removal of the catheter or declotting with medical treatment. Surgical and endovascular recanalization is possible, but usually with high risk of bleeding. The absolute indications for catheter removal are an irreversible occlusion or an infected thrombus. It has been shown that bacteria preferentially adhere to platelet-rich thrombus, thus making it a potential nidus for persistent infection.[19]

Prevention of thrombus is paramount in avoiding catheter removal. The use of saline versus heparinized flush solutions has been studied and found to have equal efficacy in maintaining the patency of CVCs.[20] Another promising agent studied has been tetrasodium EDTA, a chelator with both anticoagulant and antimicrobial properties but it has not been used extensively.[21] Episodes of thrombosis detected at an early stage might be amenable to the use of thrombolytic drugs such as urokinase, or recombinant tissue plasminogen activator.

Catheter-related thrombosis can either be asymptomatic or can result in complications such as major venous occlusion, pulmonary embolism, deep-vein thrombosis, SVC syndrome, and intracardiac thrombosis. Management of these severe complications with systemic anticoagulation or thrombolytic therapy is often necessary and specific therapy must be tailored to the individual.

## 12.5.6 MECHANICAL COMPLICATIONS

These complications usually occur after inappropriate handling or inadequate placement. The external part of the catheter can be damaged in the process of changing dressings or inadvertent exposure to chemicals that damage the integrity of the catheters. PICCs and tunneled catheters can often be repaired using commercially available kits at the bedside.

Catheter dislodgement is usually a direct result in failure to secure the CVC to the skin. Many CVCs come with stabilization devices in order to avoid this problem. When considering stabilization devices, stitches should be avoided for intermediate and long-term catheters as stitches have been shown to increase the risk of local and blood stream infections.[6] Dislocation of tunneled catheters is avoided by inserting the cuff at least 2.5 cm beyond the skin entry site.[2]

## 12.6 CONCLUSION

CVCs are a major component in the management of patients with intestinal failure. Understanding their appropriate usage and minimizing associated risks can significantly improve the quality of life for these patients.

## REFERENCES

1. Cheung E, Baerlocher MO, Asch M, and Myers A. Venous access: A practical review for 2009. *Can Fam Phys* 2009;55(5):494–496.

2. Gallieni M, Pittiruti M, and Biffi R. Vascular access in oncology patients. *CA Cancer J Clin* 2008;58(6):323–346.

3. Maki DG, Kluger DM, and Crnich CJ. The risk of bloodstream infection in adults with different intravascular devices: A systematic review of 200 published prospective studies. *Mayo Clin Proc* 2006;81(9):1159–1171.

4. O'Grady NP, Alexander M, Dellinger EP et al., Guidelines for the prevention of intravascular catheter-related infections. The Hospital Infection Control Practices Advisory Committee, Center for Disease Control and Prevention, U.S. *Pediatrics* 2002;110(5):e51.

5. Dezfulian C, Lavelle J, Nallamothu BK, Kaufman SR, and Saint S. Rates of infection for single-lumen versus multilumen central venous catheters: A meta-analysis. *Crit Care Med* 2003;31(9):2385–2390.

6. Bishop L, Dougherty L, Bodenham A et al., Guidelines on the insertion and management of central venous access devices in adults. *Int J Lab Hematol* 2007;29(4):261–278.

7. Waitzberg DL, Plopper C, and Terra RM. Access routes for nutritional therapy. *World J Surg* 2000;24(12):1468–1476.

8. Grant JP. Anatomy and physiology of venous system vascular access: Implications. *JPEN J Parenter Enteral Nutr* 2006;30(Suppl 1):S7–S12.

9. Theodoro D, Krauss M, Kollef M, and Evanoff B. Risk factors for acute adverse events during ultrasound-guided central venous cannulation in the emergency department. *Acad Emerg Med* 2010;17(10):1055–1061.

10. Alomari AI. The use of the internal thoracic vein for percutaneous central venous access in an infant. *J Vasc Interv Radiol* 2010;21(3):400–402.

11. Sznajder JI, Zveibil FR, Bitterman H, Weiner P, and Bursztein S. Central vein catheterization. Failure and complication rates by three percutaneous approaches. *Arch Intern Med* 1986;146(2):259–261.

12. Mermel LA. Prevention of intravascular catheter-related infections. *Ann Intern Med* 2000;132(5):391–402.

13. Costerton W, Veeh R, Shirtliff M, Pasmore M, Post C, and Ehrlich G. The application of biofilm science to the study and control of chronic bacterial infections. *J Clin Invest* 2003;112(10):1466–1477.

14. Ryder M. Evidence-based practice in the management of vascular access devices for home parenteral nutrition therapy. *JPEN J Parenter Enteral Nutr* 2006;30(Suppl 1):S82–S93, S98–S89.

15. Freel AC, Shiloach M, Weigelt JA et al., American college of surgeons guidelines program: A process for using existing guidelines to generate best practice recommendations for central venous access. *J Am Coll Surg* 2008;207(5):676–682.

16. Bouza E, Burillo A, and Munoz P. Catheter-related infections: Diagnosis and intravascular treatment. *Clin Microbiol Infect* 2002;8(5):265–274.

17. Mermel LA, Allon M, Bouza E et al., Clinical practice guidelines for the diagnosis and management of intravascular catheter-related infection: 2009 Update by the Infectious Diseases Society of America. *Clin Infect Dis* 2009;49(1):1–45.

18. Jones BA, Hull MA, Richardson DS et al. Efficacy of ethanol locks in reducing central venous catheter infections in pediatric patients with intestinal failure. *J Pediatr Surg* 2010;45(6):1287–1293.

19. Mohammad SF. Enhanced risk of infection with device-associated thrombi. *ASAIO J* 2000;46(6):S63–S68.

20. Smith S, Dawson S, Hennessey R, and Andrew M. Maintenance of the patency of indwelling central venous catheters: Is heparin necessary? *Am J Pediatr Hematol Oncol* 1991;13(2):141–143.

21. Kite P, Eastwood K, Sugden S, and Percival SL. Use of *in vivo*-generated biofilms from hemodialysis catheters to test the efficacy of a novel antimicrobial catheter lock for biofilm eradication *in vitro*. *J Clin Microbiol* 2004;42(7):3073–3076.

# 13 Enteral Access

*Sara N. Horst and Douglas L. Seidner*

## CONTENTS

## 13.1  INTRODUCTION

Patients with intestinal failure require specialized nutritional support to maintain normal nutritional status and hydration. Interventions may include diet modification, oral supplementation of vitamins and minerals, enteral tube feeding, and parenteral nutrition. Enteral access device placement should be considered when the promotion of intestinal adaptation can be expected to assist in the transition from parenteral nutrition to nutritional autonomy by enteral nutrition, or when oral nutrition fails in patients who are not on parenteral nutrition. Enteral access device placement can also benefit patients with intestinal failure who suffer from intestinal obstruction and required decompression of the gastrointestinal tract. This chapter discusses the rationale for placement of an enteral access device, provide details on appropriate patient selection, and discuss technical aspects of various devices. Although the literature concerning the use of enteral feeding tubes and techniques among patients with intestinal failure is sparse, the physiologic principles concerning access to the gastrointestinal tract is generally similar for patients with and without intestinal failure.

## 13.2  RATIONALE FOR ENTERAL ACCESS DEVICE PLACEMENT

Enteral tube feeding can provide great benefit to patients with intestinal failure, especially those with short bowel syndrome. Enteral nutrition plays a primary role in the maintenance of gut integrity and the promotion of intestinal adaptation after massive intestinal resection [1]. Physiologic changes that have been noted during this adaptive process include mucosal hyperplasia with an increase in villous height and crypt depth, an increase in mucosal blood flow, improvement in segmental absorption of macro- and micronutrients, and an increase in pancreaticobiliary secretions.

These changes are also believed to be responsible for an increase in intestinal transit time. Successful adaptation can take years after surgery.

Human data describing the physiology that occurs in the early phase of intestinal adaptation in short bowel syndrome is relatively rare. One study evaluated enteral feeding through gastrostomy, jejunostomy, or nasoenteric tubes in the early postoperative period (14 days) and found that a specially prepared formula using polysaccharides, medium-chain triglycerides, protein hydrolysates, and fiber supplementation was well tolerated and resulted in decreased fecal volume despite increases in infusion volume [2]. This formula, however, was not compared with oral intake. The only comparative study of tube feeding versus an oral diet was performed in a series of five patients who received a polymeric formula following an extensive ileal resection 5–12 weeks after surgery [3]. These authors found a 35% reduction in steatorrhea during the trial of tube feeding. Studies in pediatric patients also support the use of enteral tube feeding in children with short bowel syndrome [4]. Benefits include improved intestinal absorption and discontinuation of parenteral nutrition.

Patients with short bowel syndrome may need to consume two to four times their resting energy expenditure to achieve autonomy from parenteral nutrition [5]. Supplemental enteral tube feeding can be used when oral intake cannot achieve these goals. The benefit of enteral feedings was demonstrated in a randomized, crossover study comparing isocaloric tube feedings versus oral feedings in 15 patients with short bowel syndrome more than 3 months after small bowel constitution [6]. Orally fed patients ingested their usual dietary intake for 7 days, while tube-fed patients had exclusive enteral feeding via nasogastric tube for 7 days using a 24-h constant infusion of a polymeric formula containing 21% proteins, 18% long-chain triglycerides, 13% medium-chain triglycerides, and 48% carbohydrates. Results were also reported for a subgroup of patients who volunteered to receive oral and enteral tube feeding simultaneously after the controlled portion of the study. The authors found a statistically significant increase in the absorption of proteins, lipids, and energy with the use of continuous enteral feedings. They also found an increase in energy absorption, 600–700 kcal, when tube feeding was combined with oral feeding, compared to oral feeding alone. The pediatric literature also suggests that continuous enteral tube feeding leads to better absorption when compared to intermittent feeding [7].

## 13.3  INDICATIONS FOR ENTERAL ACCESS

As described in Chapter 1, many diagnoses can lead to this condition [8]. Patients with this syndrome have a wide variety of presentation but generally have an inability to maintain protein, energy, fluid, electrolyte, or micronutrient balance without some form of specialized nutrition support.

A list of indications for placement of an enteral access device is shown in Table 13.1. In part because of the heterogeneous nature of the underlying diagnoses, it is difficult to develop an algorithm or set of formal guidelines to choose patients who will benefit from an enteral access device. Anatomic factors are certainly important when deciding whether to place a device or not; however, consideration must also be given to the psychological profile of the patient and the social support systems and economic resources available to the patient as well. When assessing the integrity of the remnant bowel, one must assess the length of residual small intestine, whether there is residual underlying mucosal disease, and the presence or absence of colon and ileocecal valve. The importance of the colon cannot be overstated as it can absorb a significant amount of fluid and energy in addition to increasing intestinal transit time to improve absorption in the small bowel. Patients who are unlikely to benefit from enteral tube feeding are those with extremely short bowel who have been shown to be permanently dependent on parenteral nutrition [9]. This group includes adult patients with a jejunocolostomy with <30 cm residual small intestine anastomosed to the entire colon, jejunocolic or ileocolic anastomosis with <65 cm residual small intestine anastomosed to half of the colon, and an end jejunostomy with <100 residual small intestine. Patients with a greater length of small intestinal length may be candidates for enteral feeding. This approach has in fact

**TABLE 13.1**

**Indications for Enteral Access in Intestinal Failure**

Promote intestinal adaptation

Improve nutrient absorption

Children with oral aversion

Decompression of obstructed bowel

been used in clinical practice for many years [10]. In pediatrics, it is common to place a feeding tube in almost all patients regardless of residual small bowel length, since many infants with intestinal failure also suffer from oral aversion.

## 13.4   CONTRAINDICATIONS TO ENTERAL ACCESS

Absolute contraindications to percutaneous gastrostomy and jejunostomy tube placement include an inability to bring the anterior wall of the stomach or small bowel into apposition with the abdominal wall; pharyngeal or esophageal obstruction; or uncorrectable coagulopathy. The presence of liver disease with portal hypertension or a moderate-to-large amount of ascites is generally considered to be an absolute contraindication though case reports described safe tube placement with aggressive control of ascites [11]. It is especially important to consider these complications of liver disease as patients with intestinal failure who have been maintained on long-term parenteral nutrition are at moderately high risk for developing liver disease. These procedures may be difficult or unsuccessful in patients with prior gastric resection, hepatomegaly, and obesity as these conditions impede abdominal transillumination. Percutaneously placed tubes should not be used for nutritional support when gastrointestinal tract obstruction is present. Relative contraindications to percutaneously placed tubes include neoplastic, inflammatory, and infiltrative diseases of the gastric and abdominal walls [12]. These concerns should not preclude placement of tubes in patients with Crohn's disease, since these devices do not appear to lead to a fistula formation, and healing of the stoma tract occurs when tubes need to be removed [13]. A summary of these contraindications are listed in Table 13.2.

**TABLE 13.2**

**Contraindications for Enteral Access in Intestinal Failure**

**All Devices**

Extreme short bowel syndrome

**Percutaneous Devices**

Portal hypertension

Ascites

Pharyngeal or esophageal obstruction

Neoplastic or inflammatory disease of the gastric or abdominal wall[a]

Previous gastric surgery or multiple laparotomies[a]

Hepatomegaly[a]

Obesity[a]

**Nasoenteric Devices**

Pharyngeal or esophageal obstruction

[a]   Relative contraindication.

## 13.5   TUBE SELECTION

Once the clinician has selected a patient who may be appropriate for enteral nutrition, the next step is to determine the optimal enteral feeding strategy. Important factors to consider include the antici-pated duration of nutritional support, aspiration risk, gastrointestinal tract function, placement tech-nique, and the patient's overall clinical condition. A nasoenteric tube should be used if short-term nutrition is planned. A clinical situation where this might be considered would be in a patient whose tolerance to tube feeding is being tested prior to the placement of a more permanent and higher risk percutaneous feeding tube. Nasoenteric tubes are typically used for less than 4–6 weeks, though long-term use has been described in patients who perform self-cannulation for nocturnal feeding [10]. If longer term feeding is planned, percutaneous, radiologically, or surgically placed enteral feeding tubes should be considered.

The next question to consider is whether feeding should be delivered to the stomach or jejunum. There exist limited data to help decide which approach is best, and much of it is not in patients with intestinal failure/short bowel syndrome. Some experts have suggested that gastric feeding is more physiological, but that small bowel feeding is more reliable in delivering the total daily energy pre-scription [12]. A randomized trial in critically ill patients found a lower incidence of gastro esopha-geal reflux with small bowel feeding and a trend to a decrease in micro aspiration when compared to gastric feeding [14]. This result is in contrast to a systematic review of eight studies on gastric versus postpyloric feeding that showed similar rates of pneumonia and mortality, percentage of caloric goal achieved, and length of intensive care unit stays [15]. Patients with anatomic abnormali-ties of the stomach caused by previous gastric surgery, such as hemigastrectomy for peptic ulcer disease or gastric bypass for morbid obesity, may not be suitable candidates for placement of a gas-tric feeding tube. Percutaneous placement of a gastrostomy tube in a pediatric patient with intestinal failure who has undergone multiple laparotomies can be difficult, since peritoneal adhesions may make isolation of the stomach for safe placement difficult. Delayed gastric emptying may make it undesirable to place a feeding tube in the stomach as well. Other contraindications to gastric feed-ings include severe intractable nausea and vomiting, and abdominal pain with tube feeding, or repeated regurgitation of tube feeding when delivered through a temporary nasogastric tube. Relative contraindications are mild-to-moderate gastroesophageal reflux disease, delayed gastric emptying, pulmonary aspiration of feeding solution, and partial duodenal obstruction [16]. Having said this, one should keep in mind that feeding beyond the ligament of Treitz will result in a diminu-tion in nutrient delivery in patients with short bowel syndrome by virtue of the fact that the duode-num is being bypassed. Therefore, the delivery of enteral tube feeding should be into the stomach unless there is a good reason that this cannot be done.

If enteral feedings are indicated but gastric feedings are contraindicated, then small bowel feeds should be attempted. A decision must then be made on which approach is best; percutaneous gas-trojejunostomy (PEG-J) versus a direct percutaneous jejunostomy (D-PEJ). A few studies suggest that D-PEJ is more likely to maintain placement in the small bowel and decrease the need for endo-scopic replacement. Fan et al. [17] retrospectively reviewed their endoscopic database from two large tertiary care center institutions. They identified 56 patients with D-PEJ and 49 with a PEG-J over a 5-year period and reviewed their medical records for a period of 6 months following tube placement. Tube patency was significantly higher in the patients with D-PEJ placement and proxi-mal migration of the jejunal extension tube was the most common indication for PEG-J reinterven-tion. Over the 6 months following tube placement, five D-PEJ and 19 PEG-J required replacement. Similarly, Wolfsen et al. [18] found that the frequency of PEG-J malfunction as high as 53% and Shike et al. [19] found that the frequency of long-term tube malfunction with D-PEJ to be low at 3%. The data would therefore suggest that D-PEJ is preferred over PEG-J in patients who require long-term jejunal access.

There are a few circumstances where it might be preferable to place a PEG-J. One is where a patient may benefit from gastric decompression with jejunal feeding. Another is when direct jejunal tube placement is not possible because of the presence of dense adhesions. If a PEG-J is placed and the patient gains benefit from these dual function tubes, then a decision needs to be made on what to do when the tube requires replacement. If the PEG-J is maintained for 4–6 months then replacement with the same tube is likely to be the best option. If the durability of the tube is not so long, consideration should be given to placement of both a dedicated gastrostomy and a jejunostomy tube if this is technically feasible.

## 13.6  TECHNIQUES FOR ENTERAL ACCESS DEVICE PLACEMENT

### 13.6.1  SHORT-TERM PREPYLORIC: NASOENTERIC GASTRIC TUBES

Historically, the placement of a nasoenteric feeding tube has been considered to be technically straightforward requiring minimal training to become proficient, especially when the desired location of the tube tip is the stomach. The procedure itself takes only a few minutes and is often well tolerated by the patient. The tube is most often placed blindly at the patient's bedside. Tubes may also be placed blindly following an operative procedure if it is anticipated that a patient will need this device. In both of these instances, radiographic confirmation is required to assure that the tip of the tube is in the stomach and not in the airway. This is necessary since airway placement can occur even in patients who are completely alert with a normal swallowing mechanism [20]. Fluoroscopic assistance is sometimes necessary for patients with dysphagia or anatomic abnormalities of the esophagus, in which case a confirmatory radiograph is not necessary. A tracking device that senses an electromagnetic pulse emitted from the end of the tube has been developed that can also be used to assist in the placement of a nasogastric tube, though its use has not become widespread. This device is more fully discussed below [21]. The final option for nasoenteric tube placement is by endoscopy; however, this is the least frequently used approach and it also does not require a confirmatory radiograph.

### 13.6.2  SHORT-TERM POSTPYLORIC: NASOENTERIC JEJUNAL TUBES

A similar approach is applied to the placement of postpyloric feeding tube. It is most desirable to position these tubes into the jejunum. Large case series have shown a similar rate of postpyloric placement ranging from 80% to 90% whether blind bedside placement, fluoroscopy, or endoscopy is used for tube placement [22–24]. The reason for placement failure is not known but is likely related to the anatomic configuration of the stomach and relative location of the pyloric region. Similarly, only approximately half of tubes placed beyond the pylorus make it to the jejunum, and again the shape of the stomach probably plays a role in these less than optimally placed tubes. Intraoperative tube placement is the only method that assures jejunal positioning, with manual advancement performed prior to closure of the abdominal cavity [25]. The technique which is used depends on operator preferences and institutional resources.

One of the first descriptions of blind placement of a postpyloric nasoenteric feeding tube was described by Thurlow [26]. In his report he describes bending the tip of the stylet to take on an obtuse angle and then pushing the tube from the stomach into the small bowel while simultaneously turning the tube on its long axis in a clockwise direction. Zaloga [22] refined this technique and showed that a core of trained nurses could successfully place tubes into the jejunum for a moderately large percentage of the time. Prokinetic agents, such as metoclopramide, may also be helpful in the placement of a feeding tube, especially in the critical care setting [27]. Devices to assist placement beyond the pylorus have been developed. This included a large magnet that is held above the abdomen and is used to draw the tube into the small bowel using a metal-tipped tube that is designed specifically for this technique [28]. Another device has been designed which allows the operator to monitor the tip of the feeding tube as it passes into and through the gastrointestinal track [21]. This device works by placing a receiver over the upper abdomen that receives an electromechanical signal that is transmitted to the tip of the tube using a specially designed stylet. A major advantage of this device is that the tip of the tube can be monitored as it passes through the oropharynx and can avoid tube placement into the airway [20]. In addition, it has been shown that the location of the tube tip is reliably shown on the device monitor, and that radiographic confirmation adds little to the technique when used by an experienced clinician [29,30].

The technique for endoscopic nasoenteric postpyloric tube placement depends on available resources, as well as provider and institutional experience. One of the first described techniques is the drag and pull technique which involves attaching suture to the end of the feeding tube, grasping it with forceps, and dragging it into position endoscopically [31]. It can be difficult, however, to release the suture, resulting in displacement of the tube into the stomach. Another technique involves the initial placement of guide wire into the small intestine endoscopically. If performed via transnasal endoscopy using an ultrathin endoscope, this technique can avoid an oral-to-nasal tube transfer once it is in the proper position [32]. A prospective randomized trial evaluated this technique in 100 consecutive ICU patients compared to fluoroscopic placement and found that the overall success rate was high (90%) and there was no significant difference in success rates between the two methods [33]. The advantage of this approach is that it can be done at the bedside. The disadvantage is that it is more costly than the other bedside procedures described previously.

Wiggins and DeLegge [34] described a "push" technique by which a 12-French jejunal feeding tube is "stiffened" by placing a 0.035 in. Savary wire guide wire adjacent to the stylet included in the feeding tube kit prior to insertion [34]. A standard diagnostic upper endoscope is normally passed into the stomach followed by blind insertion of the stiffened feeding tube into the stomach. The endoscope allows direct visualization of the feeding tube as it is passed through the pylorus. Following this step, the endoscope and the feeding tube are simultaneously advanced into the jejunum keeping the tube 3–4 cm in front of the tip of the endoscope. The stiffness of the wire prevents the tube from being drawn back into the stomach while the endoscope is withdrawn. In a retrospective review of 42 patients, an average procedure time was reported as 11.6 min (range 5–50 min) with a 97.6% success rate.

### 13.6.3   LONG-TERM PREPYLORIC: PERCUTANEOUS GASTROSTOMY

As with the nasojejunal feeding tube, the percutaneous gastrostomy placement technique depends on the operator and institutional resources. The success rate for percutaneous gastrostomy placement should be expected to be >95% when the procedure is performed by an experienced operator [35].

A variety of approaches are there for gastrostomy tube placement with the percutaneous approach being the most preferred because of the lower costs and risks associated with the procedure when compared to surgical placement. The technique for percutaneous endoscopic gastrostomy (PEG), which was first described in 1980 by Gauderer, revolutionized the placement of permanent feeding tubes [36]. Three techniques are used for PEG placement. These are the Ponsky "pull," the Sachs-Vine "push," and the Russel "poke" techniques [37,38]. This chapter will not discuss in detail these three approaches as most gastroenterologists are familiar and comfortable with at least one of these methods. Subsequently, a radiographic technique that uses fluoroscopy was developed which has a slight advantage over PEG placement in that the location of the transverse colon can be observed during the procedure, and contamination of the tube track is unlikely because the tube does not traverse the oropharynx during placement [39]. Since colon injury and tube track infection or tumor seeding is very unusual with PEG, it is hard to strongly support one approach over the other. There is, however, one situation where radiographic gastrostomy must be used. In patients with intestinal failure and malnutrition after gastric bypass, computer tomography-guided tube placement is the only means to gain access into the digestive tract to provide supplemental feeding [40]. This approach can be used to gain access into the body of the stomach and allow feeding to be delivered to the pancreaticobiliary limb.

## 13.6.4  LONG-TERM POSTPYLORIC: PEG-J

PEG with a jejunostomy (PEG-J) was first described by Ponsky in 1985 [41]. Placement of these devices was often unsuccessful prior to the development of commercially prepared tube kits. These kits contain a PEG that is placed by either the pull or the push technique. A jejunal extension tube is than placed through the PEG and advanced into the small bowel by either passing it over a wire or by grasping the end of the tube and pulling it into the small bowel [42]. The wire can be placed by a variety of methods including pulling it into place by using a forceps passed into the upper endoscope [43], passing the wire through an ultrathin scope that is inserted through the PEG [44], or fluoroscopic observation. A modification of this technique involves using a glide wire that is partially inserted into the proximal duodenum followed by placement of a biliary catheter over the glide wire which serves as a stiffener to avoid kinking of the glide wire [45]. The glide wire is then advanced forward with a steering device for a modest distance followed by further advancement of the stiffening catheter. This is repeated until the tip of the glide wire is beyond the ligament of Treitz. This approach pushes the wire forward which was technically preferred by these investigators. Another option that has been described involves passage of an ultrathin scope through a PEG tract that has been allowed to mature four or more weeks, delivery of a guide wire beyond the ligament of Treitz, and the placement of a single piece gastrojejunostomy (GJ) tube using fluoroscopic control [46]. A modification of this technique that allows initial placement of a single-piece GJ tube involves anchoring the gastric wall to the abdominal wall with T-fasteners, placement of a percutaneous guide wire into the stomach, dilating a stoma tract, and insertion of the GJ tube into position [39]. It is unclear whether a two-piece or one-piece system has a major advantage regarding longevity of the tube, but single-piece tubes with a series of fenestrations in the side of the gastric portion of the tube may allow for better gastric decompression.

## 13.6.5  LONG-TERM POSTPYLORIC: D-PEJ

D-PEJ placement is considerably more difficult to perform and is often most efficiently performed by two physicians. Patients who are thin or have had previous abdominal surgery so that the bowel may be more adherent to the abdominal wall may be more likely to have successful placement, but it is appropriate to try placement with all suitable candidates [47,48]. D-PEJ allows placement of a jejunal tube directly into the small bowel using an endoscope and requires the use of an enteroscope or pediatric colonoscope to reach a position beyond the ligament of Treitz if the stomach is intact. The procedure can be performed on patients who have undergone previous gastric surgery (where the duodenal C-loop is bypassed) with a standard upper endoscope. Transillumination of the abdominal wall during endoscopy is an important step to ensure that there is not an intervening loop of bowel between the abdominal wall and the lumen of the jejunum. Close approximation of the small bowel to the abdominal wall should be confirmed by purposeful indentation with the fingertip which can be confirmed by endoscopic evaluation of bowel wall indentation. In addition, the safe-track technique should also be used to make sure that there is no intervening loop of bowel prior to tube placement [49]. Intravenous glucagon may be used to minimize peristalsis so that a limb of the jejunum can be identified and accessed. Finally, a standard pull-type gastrostomy tube should be pulled into position since a push-type tube may not readily pass through angulated loops of bowel.

One of the original difficulties with D-PEJ was movement of the small bowel after initial localization. Varadarajula and DeLegge [50] described a two-needle stick technique to avoid this problem. A 19 or 21 gauge needle (often the same needle being used to administer local anesthesia and initial jejunal localization) is passed into the small intestine and grasped by the endoscopist using a snare, thus anchoring the small intestine to the abdominal wall. An incision is then made with a scalpel blade on either side of the needle and the larger introducer catheter is passed next to the smaller needle. The snare is then used to anchor the introducer catheter. Endoscopic confirmation of the position of the inner bumper is advised with D-PEJ to minimize the track length [19]. This is in contrast to leaving the external bumper approximately 1 cm off of the abdominal wall of a PEG tube to avoid pressure injury to the tissues of the abdominal wall [51].

## 13.7   COMPLICATIONS OF ENTERAL ACCESS DEVICES

### 13.7.1   Nasoenteric Tubes

Many of the complications that occur with nasoenteric tubes are listed in Table 13.3. Procedure-related complications associated with nasoenteric tubes have been reported to be approximately 10% and include epistaxis, aspiration, and rarely esophageal perforation and circulatory or respiratory compromise [52]. Airway placement of these tubes is a great concern. Technical issues to monitor or avoid this problem have been previously discussed. There are a host of complications that can occur following placement of these tubes. The most common mechanical complication is dysphagia, which can occur in up to 20% of the subjects who are managed with these tubes [53]. Aspiration pneumonia is the most common infectious complication of nasoenteric feeding tube use. This risk of this complication may be as high as 25–40%, though this high rate is most often reported in the critical care setting [54]. There is also difficulty in discerning whether aspiration occurs as a result of tube feeding or from the presence of oropharyngeal secretions. The risk of this complication can be limited by maintaining the head of the bed above 30° and monitoring gastric residual volumes during feeding. Though jejunal feeding is used to avoid or limit the risk of aspiration, one should keep in mind that delivery of feeding at this level limits the amount of nutrients that can be absorbed in these patients who already have compromised gastrointestinal function. Sinusitis appears to be another common infectious complication, though the diagnosis is probably overestimated by radiographic study [53]. The use of a small bore tube may limit the development of this problem. Intestinal ischemia is a rare complication of nasojejunal feeding that is most often described in critically ill patients [52]. This problem occurs when the oxygen demand of the intestinal mucosa exceeds that which is required for absorption and metabolism of nutrients as a result of inadequate mesenteric blood flow from hypotension or the use of systemic vasopressors. It would therefore be highly unusual in patients who are hemodynamically stable.

### 13.7.2   Percutaneous Tubes

Feeding tubes that are placed by the percutaneous approach can result in a number of major and minor complications that are listed in Table 13.4. The frequency of these complications is approximately 4%,

**TABLE 13.3**
**Complications of Nasoenteric Devices**

**During Tube Insertion**

Epistaxis
Aspiration
Perforation
Airway placement
Cardiopulmonary compromise

**During Tube Feeding**

Dysphagia
Aspiration pneumonia
Sinusitis
Tube migration
Tube occlusion
Mucosal ulceration with bleeding

### TABLE 13.4
### Complications of Percutaneous Devices

#### Major

Gastrointestinal or intra-abdominal hemorrhage
Peritonitis or intra-abdominal abscess
Visceral laceration (small and large bowel, liver)
Buried bumper
Gastrocolocutaneous fistula
Necrotizing fasciitis
Neoplastic seeding of the stoma
Aspiration pneumonia

#### Minor

Cellulitis
Peristomal drainage
Cutaneous ulceration
Persistent gastrocutaneous fistula after device removal
Jejunal extention tube migration (PEG-J)

with one half being the major type and the other half being the minor. Of the serious complications, bleeding and peritonitis are the most common and often need operative intervention to manage. Uncommon problems that require surgical intervention includes laceration of the stomach, small bowel, or colon [55,56]. Mortality is very unusual following one of these procedures with a reported frequency of <1% [56].

Of the minor complications, tube site infection is the most common complication following percutaneous tube placement. The true incidence is difficult to estimate because most reports have involved small number of patients; however, it has been estimated to range from 5% to 30% [57–59]. Administration of a broad spectrum antibiotic, usually a first-generation cephalosporin intravenously just prior to tube placement, has been shown to decrease the risk of infection in three separate randomized trials [58,60,61]. Patients who are allergic to penicillin can be given intravenous clindamycin. In addition to peritonitis, another life threatening, and fortunately rare, infectious complications is necrotizing fasciitis [52].

Several complications are believed to be related to the placement of the external bolster too tightly against the skin, thus resulting in excessive pressure on the skin and subcutaneous tissues by the external bolster and gastrointestinal mucosa and tissue by the internal bolster [62]. These complications include local infections, skin ulceration, leaking or drainage of gastrointestinal secretions through the stoma tract, and the buried bumper syndrome. The buried bumper syndrome occurs when chronic pressure is placed at the level of the inner bolster and the bolster gradually erodes through the wall of the bowel [52]. Symptoms from the buried bumper occur when the stoma tract begins to close on the luminal side, leading to difficulty with infusion of feeds, drainage of feeds out onto the skin, and occasionally local exit site infection. To avoid these problems, it is advised that the external bumper be placed 1 cm off of the skin at the time of gastrostomy tube placement and that the bumper be backed off several days after jejunostomy tube placement [19,51]. Similarly, patients should be instructed to avoid excessive traction on the tube to avoid these problems since this traction can lead to excessive pressure on the tube tract and on the luminal side of the tube.

An unusual complication of percutaneous tube placement is the development of a gastrocolocutaneous fistula [52]. Though this problem occurs when the transverse colon comes between the abdominal wall and the stomach during the time of tube placement, it is often not manifest for weeks to months after the procedure. After the initial tube placement, fibrous tissue surrounds the tract of the tube within the peritoneal cavity. This fibrous tissue is also formed when the tube is inadvertently pulled through both sides of the transverse colon. Feeding is initiated and tolerated until the inner bolster migrates from the stomach into the colon at which time the patient will classically begin to complain of diarrhea. Alternatively, symptoms of a buried bumper can occur. The treatment is tube removal that should lead to closure of the tract and resolution of the fistula. Though antibiotics are often administered, it is unclear if they are necessary to treat this problem. The difficult decision is to decide whether a new tube can be placed percutaneously near the old one and avoid placement through the colon or whether an open (laparoscopic) approach should be taken.

A potential complication that is often not discussed is the development of a persistent gastrocutaneous fistula after tube removal [52]. This occurs when the stoma tract becomes epithelialized with intestinal mucosa and thus is more likely to occur with tubes that are maintained for a prolonged duration of time and when the stoma tract is short in length.

Complications from D-PEJ and PEG-J tubes are almost entirely identical to complications from PEG tubes. The most unique and common complication of PEG-J tubes is migration of the jejunal portion of the tube back into the proximal small bowel or stomach [18,63]. Multiple procedures are often necessary to replace the jejunal end of the tube back into position in patients who have prolonged or permanent severe gastroparesis. Occasionally, a patient with poor gastric emptying will have marked improvement or resolution of their gastroparesis and the jejunal extension tube can be entirely removed and gastric feedings can be successfully administered with the usual precautions to prevent regurgitation and aspiration. As discussed earlier, placement of a D-PEJ or PEG and D-PEJ may be the best option for patients with severe persistent gastroparesis.

## 13.8  CONCLUSION

Enteral feeding in patients with intestinal failure is often critical to maintain nutritional balance. The therapy involves careful evaluation of the appropriate patient, as well as thoughtful assessment of length of therapy, the type of tube to be placed, and the placement technique. A collaborative approach with gastroenterology, radiology, surgery, and nutrition staff is advised.

## REFERENCES

1. Buchman AL. Use of percutaneous endoscopic gastrostomy or percutaneous endoscopic jejunostomy in short bowel syndrome. *Gastrointest Endosc Clin N Am* 2007;17(4):787–94.
2. Levy E, Frileux P, Sandrucci S et al. Continuous enteral nutrition during the early adaptive stage of the short bowel syndrome. *Br J Surg* 1988;75(6):549–53.
3. Cosnes J, Parquet M, Gendre JP et al. Continuous enteral feeding to reduce diarrhea and steatorrhea following ileal resection (author's transl). *Gastroenterol Clin Biol* 1980;4(10):695–9.
4. Weizman Z, Schmueli A, and Deckelbaum RJ. Continuous nasogastric drip elemental feeding. Alternative for prolonged parenteral nutrition in severe prolonged diarrhea. *Am J Dis Child* 1983;137(3):253–5.
5. Jeppesen PB and Mortensen PB. Intestinal failure defined by measurements of intestinal energy and wet weight absorption. *Gut* 2000;46(5):701–6.
6. Joly F, Dray X, Corcos O, Barbot L, Kapel N, and Messing B. Tube feeding improves intestinal absorption in short bowel syndrome patients. *Gastroenterology* 2009;136(3):824–31.
7. Parker P, Stroop S, and Greene H. A controlled comparison of continuous versus intermittent feeding in the treatment of infants with intestinal disease. *J Pediatr* 1981;99(3):360–4.
8. Nightingale J and Woodward JM. Guidelines for management of patients with a short bowel. *Gut* 2006;55(Suppl 4):iv1–12.
9. Messing B, Crenn P, Beau P, Boutron-Ruault MC, Rambaud JC, and Matuchansky C. Long-term survival and parenteral nutrition dependence in adult patients with the short bowel syndrome. *Gastroenterology* 1999;117(5):1043–50.
10. McIntyre PB, Wood SR, Powell-Tuck J, and Lennard-Jones JE. Nocturnal nasogastric tube feeding at home. *Postgrad Med J* 1983;59(698):767–9.
11. Wejda BU, Deppe H, Huchzermeyer H, and Dormann AJ. PEG placement in patients with ascites: A new approach. *Gastrointest Endosc* 2005;61(1):178–80.

12. Gopalan S and Khanna S. Enteral nutrition delivery technique. *Curr Opin Clin Nutr Metab Care* 2003;6(3):313–7.

13. Mahajan L, Oliva L, Wyllie R, Fazio V, Steffen R, and Kay M. The safety of gastrostomy in patients with Crohn's disease. *Am J Gastroenterol* 1997;92(6):985–8.

14. Heyland DK, Drover JW, MacDonald S, Novak F, and Lam M. Effect of postpyloric feeding on gastroesophageal regurgitation and pulmonary microaspiration: Results of a randomized controlled trial. *Crit Care Med* 2001;29(8):1495–501.

15. Marik PE and Zaloga GP. Gastric versus post-pyloric feeding: A systematic review. *Crit Care* 2003;7(3):R46–51.

16. DiSario JA. Endoscopic approaches to enteral nutritional support. *Best Pract Res Clin Gastroenterol* 2006;20(3):605–30.

17. Fan AC, Baron TH, Rumalla A, and Harewood GC. Comparison of direct percutaneous endoscopic jejunostomy and PEG with jejunal extension. *Gastrointest Endosc* 2002;56(6):890–4.

18. Wolfsen HC, Kozarek RA, Ball TJ, Patterson D.J, and Botoman VA. Tube dysfunction following percutaneous endoscopic gastrostomy and jejunostomy. *Gastrointest Endosc* 1990;36(3):261–3.

19. Shike M, Latkany L, Gerdes H, and Bloch AS. Direct percutaneous endoscopic jejunostomies for enteral feeding. *Gastrointest Endosc* 1996;44(5):536–40.

20. Koopmann MC, Kudsk KA, Szotkowski MJ, and Rees SM. A Team-based protocol and electromagnetic technology eliminate feeding tube placement complications. *Ann Surg* 2011;253(2):287–302.

21. Rao MM, Kallam R, Flindall I, Gatt M, and Macfie J. Use of Cortrak—An electromagnetic sensing device in placement of enteral feeding tubes. *Proc Nutr Soc* 2008;67(OCE):E109.

22. Zaloga GP. Bedside method for placing small bowel feeding tubes in critically ill patients. A prospective study. *Chest* 1991;100(6):1643–6.

23. Gutierrez ED and Balfe DM. Fluoroscopically guided nasoenteric feeding tube placement: Results of a 1-year study. *Radiology* 1991;178(3):759–62.

24. Stark SP, Sharpe JN, and Larson GM. Endoscopically placed nasoenteral feeding tubes. Indications and techniques. *Am Surg* 1991;57(4):203–5.

25. Jensen GL, Sporay G, Whitmire S, Taraszewski R, and Reed MJ. Intraoperative placement of the nasoenteric feeding tube: A practical alternative? *JPEN* 1995;19(3):244–7.

26. Thurlow PM. Bedside enteral feeding tube placement into duodenum and jejunum. *JPEN* 1986;10(1):104–5.

27. Cresci G and Martindale R. Bedside placement of small bowel feeding tubes in hospitalized patients: A new role for the dietitian. *Nutrition* 2003;19(10):843–6.

28. Gabriel SA and Ackermann RJ. Placement of nasoenteral feeding tubes using external magnetic guidance. *JPEN* 2004;28(2):119–22.

29. Rivera R, Campana J, Seidner D, and Hamilton C. Small bowel feeding tube placement using an electromagnetic tube placement device: Accuracy of tip placement. *JPEN* 2009;33(2):203–4.

30. Hemington-Gorse SJ, Sheppard NN, Martin R, Shelley O, Philp B, and Dziewulski P. The use of the Cortrak enteral access system for post-pyloric (PP) feeding tube placement in a Burns Intensive Care Unit. *Burns* 2011;37(2):277–80.

31. Byrne KR and Fang JC. Endoscopic placement of enteral feeding catheters. *Curr Opin Gastroenterol* 2006;22(5):546–50.

32. O'Keefe SJ, Foody W, and Gill S. Transnasal endoscopic placement of feeding tubes in the intensive care unit. *JPEN* 2003;27(5):349–54.

33. Fang JC, Hilden K, Holubkov R, and DiSario JA. Transnasal endoscopy vs. fluoroscopy for the placement of nasoenteric feeding tubes in critically ill patients. *Gastrointest Endosc* 2005;62(5): 661–6.

34. Wiggins TF and DeLegge MH. Evaluation of a new technique for endoscopic nasojejunal feeding-tube placement. *Gastrointest Endosc* 2006;63(4):590–5.

35. Bankhead RR, Fisher CA, and Rolandelli RH. Gastrostomy tube placement outcomes: Comparison of surgical, endoscopic, and laparoscopic methods. *Nutr Clin Pract* 2005;20(6):607–12.

36. Gauderer MW, Ponsky JL, and Izant RJ, Jr. Gastrostomy without laparotomy: A percutaneous endoscopic technique. *J Pediatr Surg* 1980;15(6):872–5.

37. Ponsky JL and Gauderer MW. Percutaneous endoscopic gastrostomy: Indications, limitations, techniques, and results. *World J Surg* 1989;13(2):165–70.

38. Russell TR, Brotman M, and Norris F. Percutaneous gastrostomy. A new simplified and cost-effective technique. *Am J Surg* 1984;148(1):132–7.

39. Kim CY, Patel MB, Miller MJ, Jr., Suhocki PV, Balius A, and Smith TP. Gastrostomy-to-gastrojejunostomy tube conversion: Impact of the method of original gastrostomy tube placement. *J Vasc Interv Radiol* 2010;21(7):1031–7.

40. Petsas T, Kraniotis P, Spyropoulos C, Katsanos K, Karatzas A, and Kalfarentzos F. The role of CT-guided percutaneous gastrostomy in patients with clinically severe obesity presenting with complications after bariatric surgery. *Surg Laparosc Endosc Percutan Tech* 2010;20(5):299–305.

41. Ponsky JL and Aszodi A. Percutaneous endoscopic jejunostomy. *Am J Gastroenterol* 1984;79(2):113–6.

42. Simon T and Fink AS. Recent experience with percutaneous endoscopic gastrostomy/jejunostomy (PEG/J) for enteral nutrition. *Surg Endosc* 2000;14(5):436–8.

43. DeLegge MH, Patrick P, and Gibbs R. Percutaneous endoscopic gastrojejunostomy with a tapered tip, nonweighted jejunal feeding tube: Improved placement success. *Am J Gastroenterol* 1996;91(6):1130–4.

44. Berger WL, Shaker R, and Dean RS. Percutaneous endoscopic gastrojejunal tube placement. *Gastrointest Endosc* 1996;43(1):63–6.

45. Parasher VK, Abramowicz CJ, Bell C, Delledonne AM, and Wright A. Successful placement of percutaneous gastrojejunostomy using steerable glidewire—A modified controlled push technique. *Gastrointest Endosc* 1995;41(1):52–5.

46. Adler DG, Gostout CJ, and Baron TH. Percutaneous transgastric placement of jejunal feeding tubes with an ultrathin endoscope. *Gastrointest Endosc* 2002;55(1):106–10.

47. DeLegge MH. Small bowel endoscopic enteral access. *Gastrointest Endosc Clin N Am* 2007;17(4):663–86.

48. Baron TH. Direct percutaneous endoscopic jejunostomy. *Am J Gastroenterol* 2006;101(7):1407–9.

49. Foutch PG, Talbert GA, Waring JP, and Sanowski RA. Percutaneous endoscopic gastrostomy in patients with prior abdominal surgery: Virtues of the safe tract. *Am J Gastroenterol* 1988;83(2):147–50.

50. Varadarajulu S and DeLegge MH. Use of a 19-gauge injection needle as a guide for direct percutaneous endoscopic jejunostomy tube placement. *Gastrointest Endosc* 2003;57(7):942–5.

51. Grant JP. and Percutaneous endoscopic gastrostomy. Initial placement by single endoscopic technique and long-term follow-up. *Ann Surg* 1993;217(2):168–74.

52. McClave SA and Chang WK. Complications of enteral access. *Gastrointest Endosc* 2003;58(5):739–51.

53. George DL, Falk PS, Umberto Meduri G et al. Nosocomial sinusitis in patients in the medical intensive care unit: A prospective epidemiological study. *Clin Infect Dis* 1998;27(3):463–70.

54. McClave SA, DeMeo MT, DeLegge MH et al. North American Summit on aspiration in the critically Ill patient: Consensus statement. *JPEN* 2002;26(Suppl 6):S80–5.

55. Rabeneck L, Wray NP, and Petersen NJ. Long-term outcomes of patients receiving percutaneous endoscopic gastrostomy tubes. *J Gen Intern Med* 1996;11(5):287–93.

56. Amann W, Mischinger HJ, Berger A et al. Percutaneous endoscopic gastrostomy (PEG). 8 years of clinical experience in 232 patients. *Surg Endosc* 1997;11(7):741–4.

57. Larson DE, Burton DD, Schroeder KW, and DiMagno EP. Percutaneous endoscopic gastrostomy. Indications, success, complications, and mortality in 314 consecutive patients. *Gastroenterology* 1987;93(1):48–52.

58. Gossner L, Keymling J, Hahn EG, and Eil C. Antibiotic prophylaxis in percutaneous endoscopic gastrostomy (PEG): A prospective randomized clinical trial. *Endoscopy* 1999;31(2):119–24.

59. Lockett MA, Templeton ML, Byrne TK, and Norcross ED. Percutaneous endoscopic gastrostomy complications in a tertiary-care center. *Am Surg* 2002;68(2):117–20.

60. Jain NK, Larson DE, Schroeder KW et al. Antibiotic prophylaxis for percutaneous endoscopic gastrostomy. A prospective, randomized, double-blind clinical trial. *Ann Intern Med* 1987;107(6):824–8.

61. Akkersdijk WL, van Bergeijk JD, van Egmond T, et al. Percutaneous endoscopic gastrostomy (PEG): Comparison of push and pull methods and evaluation of antibiotic prophylaxis. *Endoscopy* 1995;27(4):313–6.

62. Chung RS and Schertzer M. Pathogenesis of complications of percutaneous endoscopic gastrostomy. A lesson in surgical principles. *Am Surg* 1990;56(3):134–7.

63. Henderson JM, Strodel WE, and Gilinsky NH. Limitations of percutaneous endoscopic jejunostomy. *JPEN* 1993;17(6):546–50.

# 14 Transition to Enteral Nutrition

*Julie E. Bines and Eva S. Nagy*

## CONTENTS

## 14.1 INTRODUCTION

Although parenteral nutrition (PN) provides the essential fluid, electrolytes, and nutrients essential to sustain life in patients with intestinal failure, it is also associated with potential life-threatening complications such as infection, loss of central venous line sites, and PN-associated liver disease (see Chapters 20 and 21). This stark reality has prompted the development of new therapeutic approaches aimed at improving enteral feeding tolerance to limit the duration and dependence on PN therapy while still ensuring adequate nutrition to support a good quality of life. However, due to the diversity of clinical characteristics in this complex and heterogeneous patient population, the management of intestinal failure still remains largely individualized and requires an understanding of normal gastrointestinal physiology and the changes in gastrointestinal morphology and function anticipated in the setting of disease or following surgical resection.

## 14.2 INTESTINAL ADAPTATION: THE KEY TO THE TRANSITION FROM PN TO ENTERAL TOLERANCE AND ORAL DIET

An insight into the pathophysiology of intestinal failure has been provided by the study of short bowel syndrome—one of the major causes of intestinal failure in children and adults. Following massive (>75%) small bowel resection, a series of complex changes in intestinal morphology, mucosal function, gastrointestinal motility, and hormones occur in an effort to compensate for the loss of bowel length [1]. The site of maximal adaptation following a proximal small intestinal resection occurs distal to the anastomosis and is stimulated in response to luminal exposure to nutrients and pancreatico-biliary secretions that normally do not reach the distal intestine [2]. However, changes are also observed in the proximal jejunum following a distal resection and in studies involving fistula models, suggesting that a humoral factor or factors may also play a role [3]. The extent of adaptive response is influenced by the site and length of resection, the integrity of the remaining bowel and temporal relationship to the date of surgery [4]. However, minimal, or no structural or functional features of adaptation are observed following massive resections resulting in an end-jejunostomy [5]. Features of the adaptive response are seen as early as 24 h following intestinal resection. Maximal adaptation is usually complete within 12 months although may continue beyond the second year.

The adaptive response following small intestinal resection is aided by the underlying regenerative capacity of the normal intestine. This can be accentuated in infants, in whom the natural process of growth and maturation of the gastrointestinal tract favors the promotion of adaptation. All layers of the bowel are involved, although the changes in the mucosa are more fully characterized. Intestinal epithelium is continually renewed by balanced cell proliferation, migration, differentiation, and death. Crypt cell proliferation is increased after resection of a segment of the small intestine and as a result, crypts become deeper. In rodent resection models, evidence of increased epithelial proliferation is seen as early as 12–16 h following resection. Initially, the crypt stem cells direct differentiation to secretory cells, specifically goblet and Paneth cells. This is observed within 12 h in rodents and may last for up to 4 weeks following resection, suggesting a potential role for the secretory cells in initiating the early phase of the adaptive response. Apoptosis is also increased and may assist in the regulation of cell numbers and proportions [6]. Increased rates of enterocyte proliferation and migration to the villus tip further increases the villus diameter and length resulting in a greater potential for absorption [7]. The intensity of the adaptive response appears to be proportional to the length and the specific region of intestine resected. Mucosal features of adaptation are greater in the distal small intestine following a proximal resection, compared with that observed in the proximal small intestine after a distal resection [8]. Adaptive hyperplasia of colonic mucosa occurs after jejunal and/or ileal resection [9].

The clinical observation that patients with intestinal failure who are totally PN dependent may successfully wean from PN due to a gradual improvement in enteral tolerance supports the concept of functional adaptation. These changes are observed on an organ as well as a cellular level. The absorption of glucose, galactose, amino acids, and fat per unit of length of small intestine increases following resection [10]. Although this was initially thought to reflect the increase in intestinal surface area associated with morphological adaptation, it now appears that brush border enzyme activity, modification of brush border membrane permeability and the expression of enterocyte-specific genes involved in nutrient trafficking are also altered in response to adaptation [11,12]. Changes in the expression of apical membrane sodium/hydrogen exchangers (NHE2 and NHE3), sodium–glucose cotransporters including the apical sodium-dependent transporter (SGLT1) and the basolateral glucose transporter (GLUT2) have also been observed in rodent models of resection and may contribute to enhanced fluid and electrolyte absorption following resection [13].

Early after a massive small intestinal resection, small intestinal transit is rapid due to a loss in intestinal length as well as altered motor activity [14]. Not only does the resection disrupt neural pathways isolating the distal bowel from proximal pacemakers, but it also may remove the jejunal, ileal, or colonic "brake" that normally provides feedback to the proximal intestine to slow intestinal transit [15]. The impact of this change is manifested as watery diarrhea, malabsorption, and fluid and electrolyte imbalance—all clinical hallmarks of intestinal failure. In a patient with successful adaptation, intestinal transit, and gastroduodenal motility slows and the cycling fasting pattern, the migrating motor complex may return to normal within 6 months of surgery [16]. These likely reflect adaptive changes involving nerves, muscles, and enterochromaffin cells in parallel to those observed in the epithelium in animal models of intestinal adaptation.

Since the ability to transition from PN to enteral nutrition and oral diet appears to be closely linked to successful intestinal adaptation, the management of patients with intestinal failure should take into consideration factors that may enhance or accelerate the adaptive response and limit those factors known to limit this response (Figure 14.1). The timing of specific interventions at critical phases in the adaptive response has the potential to optimize the adaptation and improve clinical outcome. The luminal environment is a key factor in defining the adaptive response following

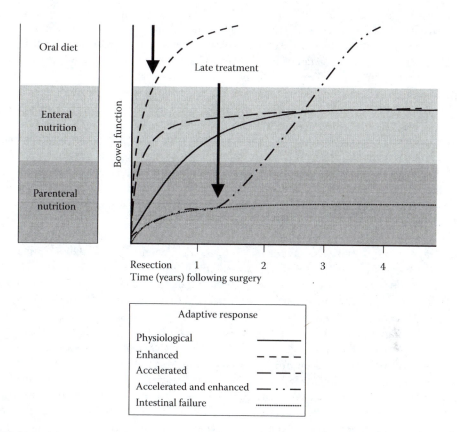

**FIGURE 14.1** The potential impact of specific interventions aimed at accelerating and/or enhancing the intestinal adaptive following small bowel resection. [Adapted from Jeppesen, P.B. *Drugs* 2006;66(5):581–9. With permission.]

intestinal resection. Luminal nutrition influences the bowel directly by maintaining functional workload on the epithelium. In addition, nutrients indirectly stimulate the mucosa by the release of salivary, gastric, and pancreatico-biliary secretions and gastrointestinal hormones that are trophic to the intestine [17]. Not all enteral nutrients exert the same trophic effect. The nature of the presentation of nutrients (liquid vs. solid diet), the macro- and micronutrient composition and dietary complexity (amino acid vs. whole protein; short-chain/medium-chain triglycerides vs. long-chain triglycerides; monosaccharides vs. complex carbohydrates), can influence the adaptive response [3,18]. Specific nutrients, such as glutamine, have been associated with trophic effects in the small and/or large intestine have been targeted in strategies aimed at enhancing adaptation [19]. Short-chain fatty acids exert trophic effects on enterocytes and colonocytes and may assist in enhancing the colonic response to small intestinal resection or disease. Colostrum supplementation of polymeric formula was associated with improved clinical outcome and enhanced morphological and functional features of adaptation following massive small bowel resection compared to polymeric formula alone, in a preclinical pig model of short bowel syndrome in children [20].

## 14.3 PRINCIPLES OF TARGETING THERAPY TO THE REMAINING INTESTINE

Whereas knowledge of the underlying disease and length of bowel resected is essential information for the management of patients with intestinal failure, the approach to the transition to enteral nutrition is primarily dependent on understanding the characteristics of the remaining intestine and the potential for adaptation. Historically, the clinical outcome in patients with short bowel syndrome has been linked to the length of bowel resected or the length of bowel remaining at the time of initial resection [21–23]. However, accurate measurement of length of small intestine is notoriously difficult. Estimation of bowel length can be performed radiologically, surgically, or using functional markers such as serum or urinary citrulline but there is large variability between methodologies and observers. Also there is considerable individual variation between normal subjects. The normal adult small intestine ranges from 260 to 800 cm, with male subjects generally having a longer small intestine than female subjects [24,25]. The intestine also grows significantly during the third trimester and throughout childhood, so that a 100 cm resection has quite different implications for a 26-week preterm infant when compared to a 3-month old infant [26]. Therefore, some prefer to refer to the length of remaining intestine as a proportion of total intestinal length rather than as a direct linear measurement [27]. In adults, disease that results in <25–30% original small intestinal length or 200 cm of viable small intestine usually places the patient at risk for developing intestinal failure [21]. However, this will also depend on the site of the resection and functional integrity of the remaining intestine.

There are significant differences in macroscopic, microscopic, and ultrastructural morphology of the intestine moving distally from the stomach to the duodenum onto the ileum. This results in segmental differences in the capacity for digestion, absorption, secretion of enzymes and co-enzymes, hormones, and motility. Hypergastrinemia and increased gastric acid secretion occurs in about half of patients following extensive small intestinal resection and is more common after a jejunal resection compared with an ileal resection [28]. Increased gastric acid has been associated with peptic ulceration, impaired fat absorption due to inactivation of pancreatic enzymes and bile salt precipitation, and stimulation of jejunal motility. However, the increase in gastric acid secretion usually does not persist beyond the first weeks following resection [29]. The jejunum represents 40% of the total small intestinal length, however, has a sevenfold greater absorption capacity than the ileum due to increased surface area. This increase in absorptive surface is not only important for the absorption of ingested fluid and food but also for the reabsorption of gastrointestinal secretions and hormones. In the normal adult about 6 L of chyme and 4 L of endogenous secretions pass the duodeno-jejunal flexure per day [30] (Table 14.1). Therefore, 100 cm beyond the duodenojejunal flexure the net luminal fluid volume is greater than the ingested volume. It is not surprising that a patient with a jejunostomy sited within 100 cm of the duodeno-jejunal junction has a high jejunal output and problems with fluid and balance during enteral feeding. Even in the fasting state there is an obligatory loss of intestinal secretions produced along with the migrating myoelectric complex [31]. The mucosa of the proximal jejunum is highly specialized. The enterocytes are highly efficient for the absorption of carbohydrates and protein, whereas intracellular permeability is increased so that the jejunal contents are isotonic and fluid and electrolyte absorption is less efficient than in the ileum (jejunum 44% vs. ileum 72%). By 1 m distal to the duodeno-jejunual junction and the volume becomes equivalent to the oral intake but now comprises of a combination of ingested intake and gastrointestinal secretions [32,33]. Pancreatic exocrine function is not impacted directly by small intestinal resection if the colon is left intact, but function may decline in the setting of fasting or

**TABLE 14.1**

**Mean Daily Volume and Composition of Small Intestinal Secretions in Response to Food in Adults**

| Secretion | Volume (L) | pH | Na | K | $HCO_3$ |
|---|---|---|---|---|---|
| Saliva | 0.5 | 7 | 45 | 20 | 60 |
| Gastric secretions | 2.0 | 2 | 10 | 10 | 0 |
| Pancreatic secretions | 0.6 | 8 | 140 | 10 | 110 |
| Hepatic bile | 0.9 | 7 | 145 | 5 | 28 |
| Total small intestinal secretions | 1.8 | 7 | 138 | 6 | <5 |
| Serum | | 7.4 | 140 | 4 | 24 |

malnutrition association with intestinal failure [34]. The stimulation of cholecystokinin and secretin can be decreased following jejunal resection and may impact on gall bladder contraction and exocrine pancreatic secretion.

The potential for macro- and micronutrient deficiencies and electrolyte and mineral imbalance in patients with intestinal failure reflect the absorptive function of specific regions of the intestine. Most water-soluble vitamins are absorbed in the proximal jejunum, therefore, it is unusual for deficiencies to develop in patients following a mid- or distal-jejunal resection, except in those with a high output jejunostomy [21]. Iron deficiency is uncommon unless there is disturbance of duodenal and proximal jejunal absorptive function or chronic inflammation [35]. Folate is mainly absorbed in the proximal jejunum so folate deficiency can occur following extensive jejunal resection [36].

The ileum, particularly terminal ileum, has a distinct villus and crypt structure, cellular proportions within the mucosa and cellular content of the lamina propria. As a result, the terminal ileum plays a key role in the absorption of fat, fat-soluble vitamins (A, D, E), vitamin $B_{12}$, calcium, and magnesium. The entero-hepatic circulation of bile salts is essential to provide sufficient quantities of bile acids required for effective fat digestion and absorption which cannot be sustained by *de novo* synthesis alone [37]. Following resection of the terminal ileum, the jejunum is unable to compensate for these functions, in particular the absorption of vitamin $B_{12}$ and bile salts. The ileum also plays an important role in the absorption of fluid and electrolytes. In the normal bowel, small intestinal motility is 3 times slower in the ileum than in the jejunum, allowing more time for absorption. This normal variation in motility is disturbed following resection but will depend on the extent and site of resection. Loss of 100 cm of terminal ileum usually results in fat malabsorption, large-volume diarrhea, and loss of other micronutrients in the effluent such as zinc, copper, and selenium [38]. The ileocecal valve slows the emptying of chyme into the colon and helps to prevent reflux of colonic bacteria into the small intestine. The presence of the ileocecal valve has been defined as a predictor of patients with short bowel syndrome who will successfully wean from PN [39].

As a consequence of small intestinal resection, the colon receives a larger load of fluids and electrolytes as well as unabsorbed nutrients and secretions. The dehydroxylation of excess bile salts into potentially toxic bile acids induces water secretion and may act as a carcinogen [40]. Following small intestinal resection the colon becomes important not only in water, magnesium, calcium, and electrolyte conservation but also in reducing fecal volume and fecal energy loss [41]. The normal small intestine absorbs only 2–20% of dietary starch so that the remaining starch becomes available for bacterial fermentation in the large intestine along with dietary fiber, sloughed epithelial cells, mucins, and intestinal enzymes [42]. The colonic bacteria ferment the 60–80 g/day of unabsorbed complex carbohydrates into short-chain fatty acids, in particular acetate, butyrate, and proprionate [43]. These short-chain fatty acids have several important actions including enhancing water and electrolyte absorption, providing trophic stimulation to the colonocytes and are a rich source of energy [43]. Due to slow colonic intestinal transit time (normally between 24 and 150 h) and the tight intracellular junctions within the colon, the efficiency of water and sodium absorption can exceed 90%. This equates to ~3–4 L of isotonic saline solution per day [44,45]. Gastric emptying and gastrointestinal transit is significantly slower in short bowel syndrome patients with colon in continuity and is similar to normal individuals. The loss of inhibition on gastric emptying and intestinal transit in patients without colon in continuity is associated with a significant decrease in peptide YY, glucagon-like peptide −1 and neurotensin [46]. Peptide YY is normally released from L cells in the ileum and colon when stimulated by unabsorbed nutrients or bile salts is involved in to slowing intestinal motility via the "ileal brake" and "colonic brake" [47]. The colonic brake alone can salvage up to 0.5–1.5 L of fluid each day [43,48]. However, the normal complement of L cells will be missing in patients who have had a distal ileal and colonic resection. There is evidence of neural feedback in motility that is interfered by resection or disease. Short bowel syndrome patients without a colon in continuity, generally have rapid gastric emptying associated with enhanced intestinal transit [49]. Patients with a short or dysfunctional small intestine but a normal colon in continuity can often maintain fluid and electrolyte balance due effective colonic absorption.

The underlying disorder necessitating treatment including surgical resection may influence the potential of the remaining intestine to recover from surgery or injury and the ability to adapt and compensate for loss of bowel length. Acute malrotation and volvulus usually involves a segment of the bowel defined the distribution of the superior mesenteric artery. The remaining, unaffected intestine would be expected to be healthy and recover following surgery. This is in contrast to a diffuse ischemic lesion such as necrotizing enterocolitis, where ischemic, but not infarcted, bowel may be left *in situ* in an effort to preserve intestinal length. Similarly, resection required for the management of Crohn's disease may target a severely inflamed segment of bowel, leaving segments of sub-acute inflammation or segments of bowel that may become inflamed in the future. Perhaps the best example of the importance of remaining bowel function is seen in patients with functional disorders, such as chronic intestinal pseudo-obstruction or long-segment Hirschsprung's disease, where there is complete or sufficient bowel length but the bowel functions poorly and patients develop symptoms characteristic of short bowel syndrome. Unfortunately for patients with extensive functional abnormalities, the potential for intestinal rehabilitation is usually limited.

## 14.4  THE APPROACH TO IMPROVING ENTERAL FEEDING TOLERANCE

A major obstacle in the management of patients with intestinal failure is the limited number of controlled trials on which to base recommendations across this heterogeneous patient population. The management of patients with short bowel syndrome was described by Piena-Spoel and colleagues, as more often based on "gut feeling" rather than an evidence-based approach [50]. However, despite these limitations, insight can be gained from the understanding of normal gastrointestinal physiology and from studies in animal models.

The approach to enteral feeding in patients with intestinal failure is guided by the following aims:

1. Promote gut "health" and the recovery of intestinal function.
2. Promote the adaptation response and optimize the potential to achieve intestinal autonomy.
3. Minimize the risk of complications associated with PN therapy.
4. Reduce the risk of oral aversion in infants.
5. Improve the quality of life of patients and their families.

The treatment of a patient following massive small intestinal resection may be considered as occuring in three key phases. Therefore, during the course of an individual patient's therapy the relative priority each of these aims may vary. The *acute phase* occurs during the immediate postoperative period. This phase is marked by poor absorption of almost all nutrients, including water, electrolytes, protein, carbohydrates, fats, vitamins, and trace elements. Gastrointestinal fluid loss tends to be greatest during the first days following resection and stomal output can be up to 5 L/day, particularly in patients with a proximal or mid-jejunostomy. Therefore, initial management is focused on maintaining fluid and electrolyte balance. PN will usually be required to maintain nutritional status until enteral feeding can be introduced or provided to a volume sufficient to meet nutritional requirements. The *adaptation phase* generally commences within 24–48 h after resection and may continue for years. Clinical markers of successful adaptation include the stabilization of gastrointestinal fluid loss and gradual improvement in enteral feeding or oral tolerance resulting in reduction in PN requirement. The *maintenance phase* is defined as when the period when the potential for further adaptation has passed and the value of therapeutic strategies aimed at stimulating the adaptive response may be expected to have limited or short-term benefit. In this phase, treatment efforts are based on limiting the risk of complications and resolving any ongoing practical issues associated with nutritional management, with a focus on improving quality of life and promoting nutritional interventions that are compatible with the individual's lifestyle requirements—whether this be school, work, or other activities.

---

**TABLE 14.2**

**Factors Influencing the Approach to Enteral Nutrition Management in Patients with Intestinal Failure**

**Patient Factors**

Age

Developmental stage (if infant)

Barriers to oral nutrition such as oral aversion, orophageal inco-ordination

Complications of PN therapy such as loss of venous access sites, PN-associated liver disease

Comorbidities and their treatment

**Gastrointestinal Factors**

Primary gastrointestinal pathology

Extent of small and large intestine disease or resection

Site of disease or resection

Extent of residual disease or intestinal dysfunction following resection and/or treatment

Time elapsed from surgical resection

Presence of ileocecal valve

Presence of a stoma and site of stoma

Presence of colon

Gastric disease or dysfunction

Liver and/or pancreatic disease or dysfunction

Bacterial overgrowth

Site of enteral access

---

## 14.5   PLANNING FOR ENTERAL NUTRITION ADMINISTRATION

When commencing enteral nutrition a number of factors are considered including formula composition and complexity, route of delivery and method of administration. Management decisions are made in the context of individual patient factors including age, disease status, and comorbidities as well the status of the gastrointestinal tract considering the anatomy and function (Table 14.2). Enteral feeds are often commenced as a continuous infusion via a gastric or jejunal feeding tube. The choice of the site of the tube depends on the gastrointestinal anatomy and function and is discussed in more detail in Chapter 14. Continuous enteral infusion enables for maximal saturation of carrier proteins and use of the remaining surface area to maximize the potential for absorption [50]. In the first days to weeks following a surgical resection continuous enteral infusion is often better tolerated than intermittent feeding and has been associated with markers indicative of improved absorption [3]. Graduating to bolus feeds allows a more physiological feeding pattern and preparation for advancement to oral diet.

## 14.6   FORMULA COMPOSITION AND COMPLEXITY

A range of commercial formulae is available for use in adults and children with intestinal failure. These formulae differ according to their macro- and micronutrient content, the presentation of the macronutrients (e.g., whole proteins vs. chemically derived amino acids, disaccharides vs. monosaccharides, long-chain fats vs. short-chain fats), osmolality and specific additives (e.g., fiber, glutamine, omega-3 fatty acids). In the adaptive phase it is preferable, if possible, to use a complex formula or diet as it has been associated with a greater adaptive response compared with elemental formulae [20]. The choice of formula is initially based on anatomy and function of the remaining gastrointestinal tract.

Tolerance to feeding is assessed clinically by monitoring stool output, emesis, abdominal pain and distension, and weight gain. Stool microscopy for fat globules, fatty acid crystals and cells, and biochemistry for pH, reducing substances, osmolality, and electrolytes provides a simple and helpful parameter to monitor absorptive status and to guide nutritional interventions aimed at reducing stool output and improving absorption. As the adaptive phase progresses, formulae that were not initially tolerated may be better absorbed as a reflection of the dynamic process of adaptation.

For the neonate and the young infant with intestinal failure, enteral feeding options include breast milk or infant formulae. In addition to the full complement of macro- and micronutrients required for the growing infant, breast milk also contains growth factors, nucleotides and essential amino acids that promote normal gastrointestinal development and may enhance adaptation in infants following intestinal resection. Breast milk immunoglobulin contributes to mucosal barrier function and protection against luminal pathogens and antigens. Breast milk also promotes the colonization of the lumen with lactobacilli and bifidobacteria. Interestingly, bovine colostrum protein concentrate supplementation of a polymeric infant formula in a preclinical pig model of short bowel syndrome in children was associated with improved clinical outcome and morphological and functional features of the adaptive response, when compared to polymeric infant formula alone [51]. However, the impact of this supplement in patients with intestinal failure has not yet been reported. The provision of breast milk to a sick infant also has other psychological, but often under-appreciated benefits for mothers and their babies. Based on the potential benefits of breast milk it is not altogether surprising that the duration of breast-feeding has been linked to the duration of PN dependence. For infants who do have access to breast milk or do not tolerate breast milk, a range of infant formulae is available.

Elemental formula has been used extensively in patients with intestinal failure and food intolerance. Use of a chemically derived amino acid formula in long-term PN-dependent children with intestinal failure was associated with a reduction in chronic inflammation in the small intestine, improved intestinal permeability and enteral nutrition tolerance resulting in cessation of PN in all four patients studied [52]. The authors postulated that increased intestinal permeability resulted in non–IgE-mediated food sensitivity that responded to protein antigen restriction. However, some researchers argue that there is no significant difference in caloric absorption, stomal output, or electrolyte losses among elemental, polymeric, and normal diets in patients with short bowel syndrome [53]. Furthermore, elemental diets may be unpalatable, and some are hyper-osmolar and therefore may contribute to increased diarrhea in some patients.

Nitrogen absorption is the least affected by decreased intestinal surface area compared to the other macronutrients [25,54]. However, conditions that result in intestinal loss of protein, such as protein losing enteropathy, may require an increased protein intake that may exceed the ability of a shortened intestine to absorb enterally provided protein. Excluding this clinical scenario, decisions concerning protein provided in enteral formulations for patients with intestinal failure usually relate more to the presentation of the nitrogen source (whole protein, peptide, or amino acid) than the absolute quantity of nitrogen [20]. Formulas containing whole proteins are considered to promote a greater adaptive stimulus relative to amino acids-based formulae [55]. Whether a polymeric or a small peptide-based diets is the most appropriate formula for patients with a high jejunostomy remains controversial.

Early exposure to dietary fat is considered important in stimulating adaptation following massive small intestinal resection [52,56]. Long-chain fatty acids, in particular omega-3 and omega-6 and polyunsaturated fats, exert a greater effect on adaptation when compared to medium-chain fatty acids or carbohydrates [57]. A diet high in unsaturated fat was associated with increased mucosal weight, DNA content, and bowel protein content after resection in an animal model and supplementation with linoleic acid increased the mucosal protein content in rats following resection [58]. In short bowel syndrome patients with a colon in continuity, medium-chain fatty acids can become a significant energy source [9]. Medium-chain fatty acids are absorbed by the enterocytes directly into the portal vein without the need for digestion by bile salts or micellar formation. Medium-chain fatty acids are more energy dense (8.3 kcal/g) than carbohydrates (4 kcal/g) and unabsorbed fats are generally associated with less diarrhea than an equivalent amount of unabsorbed carbohydrates. Unabsorbed medium-chain fatty acids can also be absorbed by colonocytes to provide an additional source of energy. In short bowel syndrome patients with the colon in continuity, higher energy absorption was achieved when patients received a diet containing long-chain fatty acids supplemented with medium-chain fatty acids compared to a diet containing exclusively long-chain fatty acids [21]. This may provide a critical source of energy in patients with intestinal failure in whom bacterial overgrowth and decreased levels of bile salts interfere with long-chain fat absorption. However, long-chain fatty acids are an important source of essential fatty acids and therefore should not be totally substituted by medium-chain fatty acids. Excessive consumption of medium-chain fatty acids can cause nausea, vomiting, and ketosis [54]. There is usually no benefit in terms of energy absorption by restricting dietary fat, especially in those patients without a colon [54]. In a crossover study comparing a high fat (60% of calories as fat) diet with a low fat (20% of calories as fat) diet, no difference in electrolyte loss and stool volume was observed between the two diets [45]. Since fat is a richer source of energy compared with carbohydrates, restricting fat from the diet may be more harmful depriving the patient of an important energy source as well as decreasing the palatability of the diet [37].

For patients with colon in continuity suffering diarrhea on a high-fat diet, a reduction of the lipid–carbohydrate ratio and/or treatment with a conjugated bile acid that is resistant to bacterial conjugation, such as Chylosarcosine (Diamalt AG, Munich, Germany) may aid in the absorption of long-chain fatty acids and improve steatorrhea [9,58,59]. However, the modification of the dietary fat-to-carbohydrate ratio and supplementation of the diet with medium-chain fatty acids tends to be less effective in patients without a functioning colon [21,60].

Carbohydrates are a key source of energy in enteral formulae. Diets containing disaccharides (saccharose, maltose, or lactose) tend to be associated with greater stimulation of adaptive response than diets containing predominantly monosaccharides [21]. Because disaccharidases are well represented in the proximal jejunum most patients with short bowel syndrome that did not involve resection of this region, can tolerate a lactose-containing diet [61]. However, mucosal inflammation due to bacterial overgrowth or protein sensitivity may result in secondary disaccharide intolerance. Unabsorbed carbohydrates can be metabolized by bacteria into osmotically active organic acids resulting in diarrhea. The colon can play an important role in the salvaging energy from unabsorbed carbohydrates [62]. Approximately 75 mmol of short-chain fatty acids are produced from 10 g of unabsorbed carbohydrates and there is a potential to increase this amount in patients receiving a high carbohydrate diet [63]. In short bowel syndrome patients with a functioning colon, the loss of fecal energy can be reduced by 30–40% with treatment with a diet rich in carbohydrates compared to a low carbohydrate, high-fat diet [9]. Jeppesen et al. compared the energy balance of an iso-caloric, high-carbohydrate, low-fat (60% carbohydrates: 20% fat) diet to a low carbohydrate, high-fat (20% carbohydrates: 60% fat) diet in short bowel syndrome patients with and without a colon [42]. In patients with a colon receiving the high carbohydrate, low-fat diet there was a decrease in fecal energy loss of up to 500 per kcal/day associated with an increase in energy absorption from 49% to 69% ($p < 0.001$) compared to the low carbohydrate, high-fat diet [64].

Insoluble fiber, such as pectin and guar gum, can be fermented in the colon and act as a precursor for short-chain fatty acids. Apart from the ability of the colon to produce and absorb short-chain fatty acids from a fiber-containing diet, fiber can also delay gastric emptying and transit time, and increase intragastric viscosity in children with short bowel syndrome. Furthermore, short-chain fatty acids increase nitrogen and oxygen uptake in the colon and thereby may assist in the maintenance of gut integrity [65]. In infants with protracted diarrhea, pectin supplementation was associated with improved electrolyte absorption and mucosal permeability [21,66]. Because insoluble fiber undergoes minimal digestion it increases stool bulk and can improve colonic motility. However, the use of insoluble fiber has also been associated with some adverse effects, including increased nitrogen, calcium, zinc, iron, and fat excretion and therefore caution should be given to avoid overuse.

Patients with intestinal failure are often sensitive to the osmotic load within the lumen. This is an important but often under-recognized cause of diarrhea and may result in secondary malabsorption due to rapid intestinal transit. Unfortunately the advantages of an elemental or predigested formula may be outweighed by an increase in osmolality of the formula as the protein source moves to a higher proportion of amino acids. Patients with diarrhea driven by a hyperosmolar formula will have a reduction in stool output when the formula is ceased or the volume is reduced. This can be confirmed on stool examination.

Other considerations that may improve enteral feeding tolerance include the administration of gastrointestinal growth factors, therapies aimed at modifying gastrointestinal secretion and motility, and modifying the luminal environment. These are the focus of discussion in other chapters.

## 14.7   MAKING THE TRANSITION FROM PN TO ENTERAL NUTRITION AND ORAL DIET

The transition from PN to enteral nutrition in patients with intestinal failure often requires patience and perseverance by staff and patients alike, as progress is often peppered by periods of feeding intolerance and setbacks. A program of a small but steady increase in volume of enteral infusion (10 mL/kg/day depending on the patient age and size) each day or every other day is usually more successful than advancing in large volumes. This is usually done via a continuous infusion initially, advancing to bolus feeds combining the previous 1–3 h volume together in one feed as enteral tolerance improves. As the proportion of nutritional intake delivered via the gastrointestinal tract becomes nutritionally significant, PN volume and/or concentration can be reduced. This is done by either reducing the PN volume infused over a 24-h period or by cycling the PN solution over specific periods of the day, such as a 12-h overnight infusion. An interim program may include daily bolus enteral feeds supplemented by a continuous enteral infusion overnight with PN delivered as a 12-h infusion to supplement the enteral intake nightly or less frequently (2–3 nights/week). Depending on the individual clinical scenario, successful transition often is best achieved with gradual transition if the balance between the nutritional requirement and intake is to be met and weight loss avoided. However, fluid shifts associated with PN administration and changes in body composition can make the assessment of weight difficult during this transition period. Measurement of body composition by any of the range of methodologies including anthropometry, dexa scan, bioelectrical impedance, total body potassium and nitrogen, and isotopic analysis may assist clinical decision making during in this period.

Oral electrolyte replacement solutions can be used alone or in conjunction with enteral formula, especially for those patients with a high output jejunostomy or high stool losses [66,67]. Hypotonic solutions, such as water, can increase gastrointestinal sodium losses and should be limited [67]. Oral rehydration solutions take advantage of the sodium–glucose cotransporters including the apical SGLT1 and the GLUT2 to maximize water and electrolyte absorption [68]. The current recommended, and the least expensive, oral solution is that recommended by the World Health Organization for the treatment of acute infectious diarrhea. The adequacy of electrolyte intake can be easily monitored using urinary electrolyte measurements. Urinary sodium concentration <10 mEq/L is suggestive of a deficit in total body sodium, even in the presence of a normal serum sodium level. If enteral rehydration strategies are inadequate to prevent fluid and electrolyte imbalance, intravenous supplementation may be required. Significant sodium or water imbalance is less common in short bowel syndrome patients with a colon as the colon has the capacity to absorb water and electrolytes against a steep electrochemical gradient [38]. Magnesium, zinc, and selenium are lost in significant quantities in patients with a high output stoma or large volume diarrhea [69,45]. Supplementation is indicated in these patients, as serum measures can be poor indicators of body status. Supplementation of magnesium may also assist in the maintenance of calcium balance [70]. In patients with fat malabsorption, the absorption of fat-soluble vitamins may also be suboptimal and a supplement should be provided. In patients with extensive ileal resection or atresias, supplemental vitamin B12 will be required.

## 14.8  STRATEGIES TO IMPROVE TRANSITION TO AN ORAL DIET

The administration of PN, enteral formula, and oral diet should not be considered mutually exclusive, even though the proportion of total nutrition obtained from the enteral or oral route may initially be limited. Once gastrointestinal function has stabilized and enteral nutrition has been introduced, a plan for advancement to oral diet should be considered. Often oral diet is better tolerated if initially introduced as frequent small meals, gradually increasing in size, and complexity as tolerated. However, as some patients with intestinal failure only absorb 30% of ingested nutrients a higher than normal oral intake will need to be consumed, if body weight is to be maintained. There is no obvious physiological benefit with respect to macronutrient, electrolyte and mineral absorption, fecal volume, or body weight in separating liquids from solid diet [71].

Oral diet has many indirect social benefits and progression to a diet based on solid food is associated with improved quality of life (see Chapter 35, Oral Aversion). In infants, early oral stimulation is critical even if the prospects for oral independence seem optimistic. Oral aversion is a major barrier to achieving a successful transition to oral diet in children who have missed early stages of oral development due to illness and learned behaviors in response to adverse early oral experiences associated with nasogastric intubation. Involvement of a speech pathologist in promoting oral skills in infants with intestinal failure receiving PN or enteral nutrition can make a major impact on the ability to successfully progress to oral diet once gastrointestinal function has improved. Even in PN-dependent children with intestinal failure, solid food can still be introduced at about 6 months to encourage the development of feeding skills and avoid oral aversion. The choice of foods is based more of an understanding the foods less likely to result in significant osmotic load or to be associated with food protein sensitivity. Therefore appropriate early choices include rice cereal and low-starch vegetables, followed by meats. Foods are introduced one at a time so that any intolerance to a specific food can be easily identified.

## 14.9  STRATEGIES AIMED AT LIMITING COMPLICATIONS OF PN AND ENTERAL NUTRITION THERAPY

PN-associated liver disease occurs more frequently in those children who are unable to tolerate any enteral nutrition compared with children who receive some nutrition via the enteral route [72]. Enteral feeding induces hormonal stimulation of bile flow, gall bladder emptying, and hepatobiliary development. Serum cholecystokinin, glucagon, enteroglucagon, gastrin, motilin, gastric inhibitory polypeptide, and secretin levels differ markedly between infants who are enterally fed compared with infants receiving total PN [73,74]. In the absence of enteral feeding, intestinal motility, and the enterohepatic circulation of bile acids are decreased [75]. Luminal nutrients also assist in the maintenance of the function of the mucosal barrier. Villus atrophy occurs in the absence of luminal nutrition and may increase the risk of bacterial translocation and sepsis. Recurrent sepsis is an important cause of mortality in patients with intestinal failure as well as one of the most important risk factors for the development of PN-associated liver disease [76].

The treatment of small bowel bacterial overgrowth is often challenging in patients with intestinal failure and gastrointestinal dysmotility, (see Chapter 24, Bacterial Overgrowth of the Small Intestine). The presence of a high concentration of bacterial species not normally present in the small intestine can cause distension, abdominal pain, diarrhea, malabsorption, and sometimes altered mental state. The lack of an ileocecal valve and disturbed motility are important predisposing factors. Formula composition and excess enteral macronutrients may increase the risk of bacterial overgrowth [77]. Antibiotic treatment is effective, however, it can have unwanted effects such as alteration of bacterial flora toward antibiotic resistant species and the eradication of colonic flora required for the production of short-chain fatty acids. Prebiotics and probiotics may have a role in the future management in patients with intestinal failure (Chapter 29).

Dietary oxalate is absorbed in only limited amounts in the small intestine and in the colon. However, in the presence of significant fat malabsorption, dietary calcium preferentially binds to free fatty acids, rendering the oxalate free to pass into the colon where it is absorbed by coloncytes. The kidneys filter oxalate, where it may bind to calcium, resulting in hyperoxaluria and calcium oxalate renal stones. Therefore, dietary oxalate is usually restricted in short bowel syndrome patients with colon in continuity. Oral calcium supplements may be of value for prevention of calcium-oxalate renal stone formation [78]. As hyperoxaluria may develop in patients receiving PN due to metabolism of vitamin C in the presence of light, PN solutions containing vitamin C should be shielded from ultraviolet light [1].

## 14.10   CONCLUSION

Effective enteral nutrition administration in patients with intestinal failure is challenging and requires consideration of the underlying intestinal pathophysiology, the characteristics of the remaining intestinal morphology and function and coexisting problems. If intestinal failure occurs as a result of a surgical bowel resection then the time interval from surgery, site of resection, extent of residual disease, and the age and gestation in infants are important considerations in defining the enteral nutrition strategy. The approach to enteral feeding in patients with intestinal failure include strategies aimed at promoting gut "health," promoting the adaptation response and optimize the potential to achieve intestinal autonomy, minimizing the complications of PN therapy and improving the quality of life of patients and their families. With patience and perseverance significant progress can be made toward achieving enteral independence without comprising nutritional status, growth, and development in children.

## REFERENCES

1. Jeppesen, P.B. and P.B. Mortensen, Enhancing bowel adaptation in short bowel syndrome. *Curr Gastroenterol Rep*, 2002; 4(4): 338–47.
2. Weser, E., R. Heller, and T. Tawil, Stimulation of mucosal growth in the rat ileum by bile and pancreatic secretions after jejunal resection. *Gastroenterology*, 1977; 73(3): 524–9.
3. Bines, J.E., R.G. Taylor, F. Justice, M.C.V. Paris, M. Sourial, E. Nagy, S. Emselle, A.G. Catto-Smith, and P. J. Fuller, Influence of diet complexity on intestinal adaptation following massive small bowel resection in a preclinical model. *J Gastroenterol Hepatol*, 2002; 17(11): 1170–9.
4. Hanson, W.R., J.W. Osborne, and J.G. Sharp, Compensation by the residual intestine after intestinal resection in the rat. II. Influence of postoperative time interval. *Gastroenterology*, 1977; 72(4 Pt 1): 701–5.
5. Cisler, J.J. and A.L. Buchman, Intestinal adaptation in short bowel syndrome. *J Investig Med*, 2005; 53(8): 402–13.
6. Hall, P.A., P.J. Coates, B. Ansari, and D. Hopwood, Regulation of cell number in the mammalian gastro-intestinal tract: The importance of apoptosis. *J Cell Sci*, 1994; 107( Pt 12): 3569–77.
7. Wolvekamp, M.C., E. Heineman, R.G. Taylor, and P.J. Fuller, Towards understanding the process of intestinal adaptation. *Dig Dis*, 1996; 14(1): 59–72.
8. Hanson, W.R., J.W. Osborne, and J.G. Sharp, Compensation by the residual intestine after intestinal resection in the rat. I. Influence of amount of tissue removed. *Gastroenterology*, 1977; 72(4 Pt 1): 692–700.
9. Jeppesen, P.B. and P.B. Mortensen, The influence of a preserved colon on the absorption of medium chain fat in patients with small bowel resection. *Gut*, 1998; 43(4): 478–83.
10. Althausen, T.L. and P.B. Mortensen, Digestion and absorption after massive resection of the small intestine. II. Recovery of the absorptive function as shown by intestinal absorption tests in two patients and a consideration of compensatory mechanisms. *Gastroenterology*, 1950; 16(1): 126–39.
11. O'Connor, T.P., M.M. Lam, and J. Diamond, Magnitude of functional adaptation after intestinal resection. *Am J Physiol*, 1999; 276(5 Pt 2): R1265–75.
12. Rubin, D.C., Enterocyte gene expression in intestinal adaptation: Evidence for a specific cellular response. *Am J Physiol*, 1996; 270: G143–52.
13. Musch, M.W., C. Bookstein, F. Rocha, A. Lucioni, H. Rea, J. Daniel, Y. Xie et al., Region-specific adaptation of apical Na/H exchangers after extensive proximal small bowel resection. *Am J Physiol Gastrointest Liver Physiol*, 2002; 283(4): G975–85.

14. Scolapio, J.S., M. Camilleri, and C.R. Fleming, Gastrointestinal motility considerations in patients with short-bowel syndrome. *Dig Dis*, 1997; 15(4–5): 253–62.

15. Yanagida, H., H. Yanase, K.M. Sanders, and S.M. Ward, Intestinal surgical resection disrupts electrical rhythmicity, neural responses, and interstitial cell networks. *Gastroenterology*, 2004; 127(6): 1748–59.

16. Remington, M., J.-R. Malagelada, A. Zinsmeister, and C.R. Fleming, Abnormalities in gastrointestinal motor activity in patients with short bowels: Effect of a synthetic opiate. *Gastroenterology*, 1983; 85(3): 629–36.

17. Altmann, G.G., Influence of bile and pancreatic secretions on the size of the intestinal villi in the rat. *Am J Anat*, 1971; 132(2): 167–77.

18. Vanderhoof, J.A., C.J. Grandjean, S.S. Kaufman, K.T. Buckley, and D.L. Antonson, Effect of high percentage medium-chain triglyceride diet on mucosal adaptation following massive bowel resection in rats. *JPEN J Parenter Enteral Nutr*, 1984; 8(6): 685–9.

19. Scolapio, J.S., Effect of growth hormone and glutamine on the short bowel: Five years later. *Gut*, 2000; 47(2): 164.

20. Nagy, E.S., M.C.V. Paris, R.G. Taylor, P.J. Fuller, M. Sourial, F. Justice, and J.E. Bines, Colostrum protein concentrate enhances intestinal adaptation after massive small bowel resection in juvenile pigs. *J Pediatr Gastroenterol Nutr*, 2004; 39(5): 487–92.

21. Buchman, A.L., J. Scolapio, and J. Fryer, AGA technical review on short bowel syndrome and intestinal transplantation. *Gastroenterology*, 2003; 124(4): 1111–34.

22. Carbonnel, F., L. Beaugerie, Y. Ngo, M. Malafosse, Y. Le Quintec, and J.P. Gendre, The role of anatomic factors in nutritional autonomy after extensive small bowel resection. *JPEN J Parenter Enteral Nutr*, 1996; 20(4): 275–80.

23. Messing, B., P. Crenn, P. Beau, M.C. Boutron-Ruautt, J.-C. Rambaud, and C. Matuchansky, Long-term survival and parenteral nutrition dependence in adult patients with the short bowel syndrome. *Gastroenterology*, 1999; 117(5): 1043–50.

24. Lennard-Jones, J.E., Indications and need for long-term parenteral nutrition: Implications for intestinal transplantation. *Transplant Proc*, 1990; 22(6): 2427–9.

25. Weser, E., Nutritional aspects of malabsorption: Short gut adaptation. *Clin Gastroenterol*, 1983; 12(2): 443–61.

26. Touloukian, R.J. and G.J. Smith, Normal intestinal length in preterm infants. *J Pediatr Surg*, 1983; 18(6): 720–3.

27. Sondheimer, J.M., M. Cadnapaphornchai, M. Sontag, and G.O. Zerbe, Predicting the duration of dependence on parenteral nutrition after neonatal intestinal resection. *J Pediatr*, 1998; 132(1): 80–4.

28. Williams, N.S., P. Evans, and R.F. King, Gastric acid secretion and gastrin production in the short bowel syndrome. *Gut*, 1985; 26(9): 914–9.

29. Windsor, C.W., J. Fejfar, and D.A. Woodward, Gastric secretion after massive small bowel resection. *Gut*, 1969; 10(10): 779–86.

30. Buchman, A.L., K. Iyer, and J. Fryer, Parenteral nutrition-associated liver disease and the role for isolated intestine and intestine/liver transplantation. *Hepatology*, 2006; 43(1): 9–19.

31. Vantrappen, G.R., T.L. Peeters, and J. Janssens, The secretory component of the interdigestive migrating motor complex in man. *Scand J Gastroenterol*, 1979; 14(6): 663–7.

32. Fordtran, J.S. and T.W. Locklear, Ionic constituents and osmolality of gastric and small-intestinal fluids after eating. *Am J Dig Dis*, 1966; 11(7): 503–21.

33. Borgstrom, B., A. Dahlqvist, G. Lundh, and J. Sjovall, Studies of intestinal digestion and absorption in the human. *J Clin Invest*, 1957; 36(10): 1521–36.

34. Remington, M., C.R. Fleming, and J.R. Malagelada, Inhibition of postprandial pancreatic and biliary secretion by loperamide in patients with short bowel syndrome. *Gut*, 1982; 23(2): 98–101.

35. Muir, A. and U. Hopfer, Regional specificity of iron uptake by small intestinal brush-border membranes from normal and iron-deficient mice. *Am J Physiol*, 1985; 248(3 Pt 1): G376–9.

36. Denburg, J., W. Bensen, M.A. Ali, J. McBride, and J. Ciok, Megaloblastic anemia in patients receiving total parenteral nutrition without folic acid or vitamin B12 supplementation. *Can Med Assoc J*, 1977; 117(2): 144–6.

37. Heydorn, S., P.B. Jeppesen, and P.B. Mortensen, Bile acid replacement therapy with cholylsarcosine for short-bowel syndrome. *Scand J Gastroenterol*, 1999; 34(8): 818–23.

38. Wolman, S.L., G.H. Anderson, E.B. Marliss, and K.N. Jeejeebhoy, Zinc in total parenteral nutrition: Requirements and metabolic effects. *Gastroenterology*, 1979; 76(3): 458–67.

39. Wilmore, D.W., Factors correlating with a successful outcome following extensive intestinal resection in newborn infants. *J Pediatr*, 1972; 80(1): 88–95.

40. Bernstein, H. and H.S. Wiggins, Bile acids as carcinogens in human gastrointestinal cancers. *Mutat Res*, 2005; 589(1): 47–65.

41. Cummings, J.H., W.P. James, and H.S. Wiggins, Role of the colon in ileal-resection diarrhoea. *Lancet*, 1973; 1(7799): 344–7.

42. Nordgaard, I., B.S. Hansen, and P.B. Mortensen, Importance of colonic support for energy absorption as small-bowel failure proceeds. *Am J Clin Nutr*, 1996; 64(2): 222–31.

43. Nordgaard, I., What's new in the role of colon as a digestive organ in patients with short bowel syndrome. *Nutrition*, 1998; 14(5): 468–9.

44. Hylander, E., K. Ladefoged, and S. Jarnum, Calcium absorption after intestinal resection. The importance of a preserved colon. *Scand J Gastroenterol*, 1990; 25(7): 705–10.

45. Woolf, G.M., C. Miller, R. Kurian, and K.N. Jeejeebhoy, Nutritional absorption in short bowel syndrome. Evaluation of fluid, calorie, and divalent cation requirements. *Dig Dis Sci*, 1987; 32(1): 8–15.

46. Nightingale, J.M., M.A. Kamm, J.R. van der Sijp, G.P. Morris, M.A. Ghatel, S.R. Bloom, and J.E. Lennard-Jones, Gastrointestinal hormones in short bowel syndrome. Peptide YY may be the "colonic brake" to gastric emptying. *Gut*, 1996; 39(2): 267–72.

47. Savage, A.P., T.E. Adrian, G. Carolan, V.K. Chatterjee, and S.R. Bloom, Effects of peptide YY (PYY) on mouth to caecum intestinal transit time and on the rate of gastric emptying in healthy volunteers. *Gut*, 1987; 28(2): 166–70.

48. Nightingale, J.M., M.A. Kamm, J.R. van der Sijp, G.P. Morris, E.R. Walker, S.J. Mather, K.E. Britton, and J.E. Lennard-Jones, Disturbed gastric emptying in the short bowel syndrome. Evidence for a "colonic brake." *Gut*, 1993; 34(9): 1171–6.

49. Piena-Spoel, M., M. Sharman-Koendijaiharle, T. Yamanouchi, and D. Tibboel, "Gut-feeling" or evidence-based approaches in the evaluation and treatment of human short-bowel syndrome. *Pediatr Surg Int*, 2000; 16(3): 155–64.

50. Weizman, Z., A. Schmueli, and R.J. Deckelbaum, Continuous nasogastric drip elemental feeding. Alternative for prolonged parenteral nutrition in severe prolonged diarrhea. *Am J Dis Child*, 1983; 137(3): 253–5.

51. Bines, J., D. Francis, and D. Hill, Reducing parenteral requirement in children with short bowel syndrome: Impact of an amino acid-based complete infant formula. *J Pediatr Gastroenterol Nutr*, 1998; 26(2): 123–8.

52. Sukhotnik, I., A.G. Coram, A. Kramer, E. Shiloni, and J.G. Mogliner, Advances in short bowel syndrome: An updated review. *Pediatr Surg Int*, 2005; 21(12): 947–53.

53. Jeejeebhoy, K.N., Management of short bowel syndrome: Avoidance of total parenteral nutrition. *Gastroenterology*, 2006; 130(2 Suppl 1): S60–6.

54. Woolf, G.M., C. Miller, R. Krian, and K.N. Jeejeebhoy, Diet for patients with a short bowel: High fat or high carbohydrate? *Gastroenterology*, 1983; 84(4): 823–8.

55. Sukhotnik, I., N. Mor-Vaknin, R.A. Drongowski, I. Miselevich, A.G. Coran, and C.M. Harmon, Effect of dietary fat on early morphological intestinal adaptation in a rat with short bowel syndrome. *Pediatr Surg Int*, 2004; 20(6): 419–24.

56. Maxton, D.G., E.U. Cynk, A.P. Jenkins, and R.P. Thompson, Effect of dietary fat on the small intestinal mucosa. *Gut*, 1989; 30(9): 1252–5.

57. Mascioli, E.A., B.R. Bistrian, V.K. Babaya, and G.L. Blackburn, Medium chain triglycerides and structured lipids as unique nonglucose energy sources in hyperalimentation. *Lipids*, 1987; 22(6): 421–3.

58. Jeppesen, P.B. and P.B. Mortensen, Colonic digestion and absorption of energy from carbohydrates and medium-chain fat in small bowel failure. *JPEN J Parenter Enteral Nutr*, 1999; 23(5 Suppl): S101–5.

59. Haderslev, K.V., P.B. Jeppesen, P.M. Mortensen, and M. Staun, Absorption of calcium and magnesium in patients with intestinal resections treated with medium chain fatty acids. *Gut*, 2000; 46(6): 819–23.

60. Weser, E., J. Babbitt, M. Hoban, and A. Van deventer, Intestinal adaptation. Different growth responses to disaccharides compared with monosaccharides in rat small bowel. *Gastroenterology*, 1986; 91(6): 1521–7.

61. Bond, J.H., B.E. Currier, H. Buchwald, and M.D. Levitt., Colonic conservation of malabsorbed carbohydrate. *Gastroenterology*, 1980; 78(3): 444–7.

62. Cummings, J.H., G.R. Gibson, and G.T. Macfarlane, Quantitative estimates of fermentation in the hind gut of man. *Acta Vet Scand Suppl*, 1989; 86: 76–82.

63. Nordgaard, I., B.S. Hansen, and P.B. Mortensen, Colon as a digestive organ in patients with short bowel. *Lancet*, 1994; 343(8894): 373–6.

64. Finkel, Y., G. Brown, H.L. Smith, E. Buchanan, and I.W. Booth, The effects of a pectin-supplemented elemental diet in a boy with short gut syndrome. *Acta Paediatr Scand*, 1990; 79(10): 983–6.

65. Rabbani, G.H., T. Teka, S.K. Saha, B. Zaman, N. Majid, M. Khatun, M.A. Wahed, and G.J. Fuchs, Green banana and pectin improve small intestinal permeability and reduce fluid loss in Bangladeshi children with persistent diarrhea. *Dig Dis Sci*, 2004; 49(3): 475–84.

66. Nightingale, J.M., J.E. Lennerd-Jones, E.R. Walker, and M.J. Farthing, Oral salt supplements to compensate for jejunostomy losses: Comparison of sodium chloride capsules, glucose electrolyte solution, and glucose polymer electrolyte solution. *Gut*, 1992; 33(6): 759–61.

67. Fordtran, J.S., Stimulation of active and passive sodium absorption by sugars in the human jejunum. *J Clin Invest*, 1975; 55(4): 728–37.

68. Fordtran, J.S., F.C. Rector, Jr., and N.W. Carter, The mechanisms of sodium absorption in the human small intestine. *J Clin Invest*, 1968; 47(4): 884–900.

69. Ladefoged, K., P. Nicolaidou, and S. Jarnum, Calcium, phosphorus, magnesium, zinc, and nitrogen balance in patients with severe short bowel syndrome. *Am J Clin Nutr*, 1980; 33(10): 2137–44.

70. Carter, B.A. and R.J. Shulman, Mechanisms of disease: Update on the molecular etiology and fundamentals of parenteral nutrition associated cholestasis. *Nat Clin Pract Gastroenterol Hepatol*, 2007; 4(5): 277–87.

71. Lucas, A., S.R. Bloom, and A. Aynsley-Green, Metabolic and endocrine consequences of depriving preterm infants of enteral nutrition. *Acta Paediatr Scand*, 1983; 72(2): 245–9.

72. Levinson, S., M. Bhasker, T.R. Gibson, R. Morin, and W.J. Snape, Comparison of intraluminal and intravenous mediators of colonic response to eating. *Dig Dis Sci*, 1985; 30(1): 33–9.

73. Matsui, J., R.G. Cameron, R. Kurian, and G.C. Kuo, Nutritional, hepatic, and metabolic effects of cachectin/tumor necrosis factor in rats receiving total parenteral nutrition. *Gastroenterology*, 1993; 104(1): 235–43.

74. Candusso, M., D. Faraguna, D. Sperli, and N. Dodaro, Outcome and quality of life in paediatric home parenteral nutrition. *Curr Opin Clin Nutr Metab Care*, 2002; 5(3): 309–14.

75. Gracy, M., The contaminated short bowel syndrome: Pathogenesis, diagnosis and treatment. *Am J Clin Nutr*, 1979; 32: 234–43.

76. Barilla, D.E., C. Notz, D. Kennedy, and C.Y.C. Pak, Renal oxalate excretion following oral oxalate loads in patients with ileal disease and with renal and absorptive hypercalciurias. Effect of calcium and magnesium. *Am J Med*, 1978; 64(4): 579–85.

77. Rockwell, G.F., T. Campfield, B.C. Nelson, and P.C. Uden, Oxalogenesis in parenteral nutrition solution components. *Nutrition*, 1998; 14(11–12): 836–9.

78. Buchman, A.L., ed. *Clinical Nutrition in Gastrointestinal Disease*. 2006, Slack Incorporated: Thorofare, New Jersey.

79. Jeppesen, P.B., The use of growth factors in the treatment of patients with short bowel syndrome. *Drugs* 2006;66(5):581–9.

# 15 Drug Dosing and Pharmacokinetics

*Kathleen M. Gura*

## CONTENTS

## 15.1 INTRODUCTION

Patients in whom significant amounts of small bowel is resected or nonfunctional, managing drug therapy with orally administered medication is a critical but often overlooked component of patient care. As per a report by the American Gastrointestinal Association, "Oral medication absorption is often impaired and larger doses, intravenous, or sublingual (SL) delivery may be required; significant interpatient variability may be observed" [1, p. 1116]. To further complicate matters, even in a healthy individual without intestinal failure (IF), the exact location within the intestinal tract where a medication is absorbed is not known nor are the specific factors that can impact it, making it even more challenging to determine drug response in a patient with dysmotility or an intestinal resection. The function of the remaining bowel, the presence (or absence) of terminal ileum, and the pH within the intestine can all be altered, further influencing the extent of medication absorption.

By definition, pharmacokinetics involves the study of drug absorption, distribution, metabolism, and excretion and the interrelationship of these processes with the therapeutic and toxicologic properties of the medication (i.e., what the body does to a drug) [2]. In contrast, pharmacodynamics is the study of the biochemical and physiological effects of drugs and the mechanisms of their actions (i.e., what the drug does to the body) [2]. Bioavailability refers to the fraction of the total dose of a medication that reaches the general circulation; it characterizes the rate and extent of systemic absorption of the active drug [2]. The goal of this chapter is to discuss how IF can impact these properties and what approaches should be used to optimize drug therapies impacted by IF [3].

## 15.2   OVERVIEW OF GASTROINTESTINAL PHYSIOLOGY
##          AND DRUG ABSORPTION

The gastrointestinal (GI) tract is comprised of the mouth, stomach, small intestine, and large intestine (colon). The small intestine, where the majority of drug absorption occurs, is further divided into the duodenum, jejunum, and ileum. The site of intestinal resection may therefore impact on drug absorption, as well as the well-known effects on macro- and micronutrient absorption.

Very little drug absorption actually occurs in the mouth as the contact time with the oral mucosa and medication is limited. SL administration obviates this and is useful for drugs that undergo extensive first past hepatic metabolism, such as nitroglycerin.

With normal gastric emptying, the role of the stomach in drug absorption is modest at best since it is primarily an organ of physical and chemical digestion. In various experimental models, weakly acidic drugs, such as aspirin, or nonionized drugs and lipophilic substances can be extensively absorbed by the stomach, although low gastric pH tends to degrade most medications, thereby decreasing their bioavailability. Table 15.1 summarizes the site of absorption within the GI tract of several commonly used oral medications.

The rate of gastric emptying of its contents into the intestine helps determine the rate of drug delivery to the systemic circulation. Slowing the rate of *gastric* emptying will decrease the rate of *intestinal* absorption. For this reason, many medications are administered on an empty stomach so as to increase the rate of passage from the stomach into the intestine. In some patients with dysmotility, decreased intestinal transit time may reduce the amount of drug absorbed; thus higher than recommended doses are often needed to compensate for this [3].

The small intestine is the most important site for drug absorption. The absorption of weak bases, which constitute the majority of commonly used medications, is particularly dependent on the speed with which they reach the intestine. Due to its large surface area and abundant blood supply, the upper portion of the small intestine, comprised of the duodenum and jejunum, is the site of the majority of drug absorption [3]. Following a concentration gradient, dissolved drug moves from the intestine into the systemic circulation where it is subjected to first-pass metabolism by the liver. Typical ways in which drugs are absorbed include passive diffusion, pore transport, vesicular transport, and carrier-mediated transport. Bile and pancreatic enzymes (i.e., carboxypeptidase, lipase, and trypsin) are secreted into the duodenum allowing for otherwise insoluble drugs to be dissolved.

The primary role of the colon is to reabsorb water and sodium. Drugs that are not absorbed in the small intestine may be absorbed in the colon. Medications such as metoprolol and nifedipine are primarily absorbed in the colon. In patients with jejunocolic anastomosis with an intact colon, drug absorption should not be impacted [3].

Many factors can impact the passive processes of drug absorption (Table 15.2). The concentration of the drug and its solubility characteristics can determine the extent of absorption. Other factors that can influence the extent of absorption include the pharmacokinetic properties of the drug, the formulation of the medication, the presence of other substances in the GI tract, and patient characteristics (Table 15.3). Chapter 27, Medication Administration in the Enterally Fed Patient, discusses the impact of medication formulations on drug absorption in greater detail.

## 15.3   IMPACT OF INTESTINAL RESECTION ON DRUG ABSORPTION

Owing to its large surface area, and more permeable membranes in comparison to the stomach, the small intestine is the primary site of drug absorption. Depending on the amount and location of the bowel resected, the number of carriers, channels, or pores used to transport a drug into the systemic circulation will be reduced [3]. Similarly, the amount of drug that can be absorbed via active transport across a cell membrane becomes limited. Furthermore, in situations of reduced blood flow

## TABLE 15.1
## Examples of Sites of Absorption of Commonly Used Oral Medications

| Medication | Site of Absorption |
| --- | --- |
| Acetaminophen | Small intestine—jejunum distal from the duodenojejunal flexure (dependent on the rate of gastric emptying) |
| Amytriptyline | Stomach and small intestine |
| Aspirin | Stomach |
| Cimetidine | Ileum |
| Cyclosporine | Duodenum and jejunum |
| Digoxin | Duodenum and proximal jejunum |
| Diltiazem (controlled release) | Duodenum—high rate of absorption |
| | Ileum—medium rate |
| | Colon—low rate |
| Gabapentin | Maximally in duodenum–jejunum; some in ileum and cecum |
| Hydrochlorothiazide | Duodenum and upper jejunum |
| Ibuprofen | GI tract (small intestine, usually jejunum) |
| Loperamide | Acts locally (minimally absorbed) |
| Mesalamine (coated with a pH-sensitive enteric soluble film) | Limited absorption in the colon |
| Metoprolol | Colon |
| Nifedipine | Colon |
| Omeprazole (enteric coated) | Jejunum (if ≥0.5 m remaining) |
| Oral contraceptives | Small intestine |
| Procainamide | Small intestine |
| Propranolol | Small intestine |
| Ranitidine | Proximal GI tract |
| Tacolimus | Greater absorption in the jejunum than in the ileum or colon; better absorption in resected patients with a closed stoma |
| Ursodiol | Solubilized in proximal jejunum reabsorbed in distal ileum |
| Warfarin | Stomach and proximal small intestine |

*Source:* Adapted from Severijnen R. et al., *Clin Pharmacokinet* 2004;43(14):951–62; Nightingale JMD. et al., *Gut* 1993;34:1171–6; Blackman L, Beerman B, and Groschinsky-Grind M. *Clin Pharmacokinet* 1979;4:63–8; Hoffman AF and Poley R. *Gastroenterology* 1972;62:918–34; Frieri G. et al., *Am J Gastroenterol* 2000;95:1486–90; Ehrenpreis ED. et al., *Ann Pharmacother* 1994;28:1239–40; Vetticaden SJ. et al., *Clin Pharmacokinet* 1986;62–4; Victor A, Odlind V, and Kral JG. *Gastroenterol Clin North Am* 1987;16:483–91.

## TABLE 15.2
## Factors that May Impact the Bioavailability and Pharmacokinetic Properties of a Drug

Solubility characteristics

Does the drug undergo transformation? (i.e., is it a prodrug?)

Method of drug release from its dosage form

pH required for absorption

Rate of drug release from its dosage form

Site of drug absorption

Site of distribution

Site of drug release from its dosage form

Route of excretion

---

**TABLE 15.3**

**Patient Characteristics Impacting Drug
Absorption from the GI Tract**

Bile salt content
Extent of intestinal surface area
Gastric emptying time
Gastric motility
Intestinal transit time
Intraluminal pH
Mesenteric blood supply

---

(e.g., shock), the concentration gradient of drug across the intestinal mucosa is lowered which further reduces the amount of drug absorbed by passive diffusion.

Dysmotility can often occur as a result of resection of the small intestine. Normally, motility in the ileum is three times slower than the jejunum [3]. Depending on the area removed, transit time will vary. Following a jejunal resection, gastric emptying is more rapid; however, intestinal transit time may remain normal due to the ileal brake [4]. In patients with residual bowel in continuity, gastric emptying is slower and similar to normal controls. In patients with ileal or colonic resection, cells that release peptide YY are missing resulting in a loss of inhibition on gastric emptying and intestinal transit time [4]. Adults with less than 100 cm of residual jejunum demonstrate the most rapid gastric emptying. Blackman et al. reported a 50% decrease in hydrochlorothiazide uptake in patients who had undergone jejunoilesotomy and ileocaecostomy procedures after intestinal shunt surgeries for obesity. They theorized that this was due to malabsorption of the hydrochlorothiazide due to shortened transit time [5]. Drug response may be altered depending on the location of the resection because of impaired bile salt reabsorption. For example, if more than 100 cm of ileum is removed, the use of cholestyramine may actually worsen steatorrhea because of binding to dietary lipid [6].

The type of resection can also impact drug absorption. Patients treated with mesalamine for Crohn's disease may have different drug concentrations depending on the type of anastomosis. This medication, formulated as a tablet containing a pH-sensitive enteric coating, is designed to release the active drug in the colon. In patients with a small bowel resection, the type of anastomosis (side to side vs. end to end) influences its effectiveness. In a study by Frieri et al., patients with end-to-end anastomosis had lower mucosal concentrations of drug and more frequent disease recurrence [7]. The authors concluded that side-to-side anastomosis increased segmental transit time that results in improved absorption and higher concentrations of mesalamine in the mucosa.

In addition to the type of resection, the type of dosage formulations can impact drug response in an IF patient. For example, if an IF patient is prescribed a sustained release dosage form, drug response tends to be unreliable due to the variability in drug absorption which is both unpredictable and erratic [1]. To circumvent this, the medication should be converted into the equivalent immediate-release dosage forms.

## 15.3.1 Impact of Resection on Absorption Capacity

As noted in Chapter 2, Pathophysiology of Intestinal Failure, the degree of nutrient malabsorption will vary after GI resection. In cases where more than 50% of the small intestine is resected, malabsorption of macro- and micronutrients can occur and may similarly alter the drug absorption process.

Within hours after intestinal resection, the remaining bowel will start to undergo physiological and structural changes. If the jejunum is resected, the ileum will begin to adapt and acquire the functional and structural characteristics of the jejunum. This is possible because the ileum has superficial crypts and shorter villi. The jejunum, however, is less able to adapt and cannot assume the functions of the ileum in the event of an ileal resection.

Studies investigating digoxin therapy in IF patients have demonstrated that the colon can compensate and is able to absorb sufficient digoxin to achieve therapeutic levels in patients who have undergone complete small bowel resection. In one case report, a patient with only 18 cm of jejunum and without continuity of the small intestine and bowel had severe digoxin malabsorption such that only intravenous administration of the agent was able to achieve adequate serum levels [8]. Conversely, in another patient with an end jejunostomy and only 12–15 cm remaining jejunum, adequate serum levels were achieved despite reduced digoxin absorption when the liquid formulation was used [9].

Patients receiving oral contraceptive steroids are also at risk for treatment failure as these agents are primarily absorbed in the small intestine. In patients receiving levonorgestrel, the lowest levels were seen in patients with the largest amount of small bowel resected. Moreover, jejunoileal bypass may result in reduced bioavailability of both norethindrone and levonorgestrel [10].

## 15.3.2 IMPACT OF RESECTION ON MUCOSAL ENZYME ACTIVITY

Whenever there is a major resection of the small intestine, there may be a significant loss of activity of the mucosal enzymes and those enzymes produced by bacteria. Ester prodrugs (i.e., chloramphenicol and erythromycin) and steroids may have reduced biotransformation to their active form [11]. Dosage adjustments may be necessary to compensate, and therapeutic substitution to a medication that is not a prodrug should be considered.

## 15.4 BACTERIAL OVERGROWTH AND DRUG ABSORPTION

In addition to altering transit time, small bowel resection may increase the risk of bacterial overgrowth in the remaining intestine. Furthermore, if the ileocecal valve is resected, colonic bacteria can backwash into the small bowel and colonize it. Bacterial overgrowth may damage intestinal mucosa directly through bacterial adherence and translocation and by producing enterotoxins to alter absorption [11]. As discussed in Chapter 24, Bacterial Overgrowth of the Small Intestine, bacterial overgrowth can alter the physical environment within the intestinal lumen that can impact drug solubility within lipid membranes (Table 15.4). For example, lactobacilli present within the intestine have metabolic activity that can become altered in patients with IF. Increased production of lactic acid can impact intraluminal pH and thus alter the ionization of the drug molecule [12]. The enteral uptake of drugs that must be protonated in order to improve their hydrophilicity may be affected because of the lactic acid production [13]). Drugs that are weak acids (i.e., penicillin, phenobarbital, phenytoin, and zidovudine) are protonated, unionized, and lipid soluble, whereas drugs that are weak bases (i.e., morphine, erythromycin, and zalcitabine) are unprotonated, ionized, and water soluble. Any changes in pH can impact these absorption requirements.

Bacterial flora can influence the intestinal absorption of drugs in other ways. Heterolactic lactobacilli (e.g., *Lactobacillus fermentum*) can produce carbon dioxide and ethanol which can increase motility and result in diarrhea [14]. Conversely, in an animal model, germ-free mice showed decreased gut motility which can also impact drug absorption [15]. Similarly, using a rat model, Wu et al. [16] demonstrated that bacterial overgrowth increased intestinal transit time which could potentially increase drug absorption.

Gut microflora may also have some metabolic effect on a drug within the GI tract. Some medications require colonic bacteria to metabolize it to its active moiety (Table 15.4). For example,

**TABLE 15.4**

**Medications That Are Metabolized by Intestinal Bacteria**

Balsalazide

Chloramphenicol

Colchicine

Conjugated estrogens

Digoxin

Levodopa

Morphine

Rifampin

Sulfasalazine

*Source:*    Adapted from Ilett  KF. et al., *Pharmacol Ther* 1990;46(1):67–93.

sulfasalazine is metabolized by colonic intestinal flora to sulfapyridine and 5-aminosalicylic acid (5-ASA). Other medications that require bacterial transformation include metronidazole which is metabolized to acetamide and *N*-(2-hydroxyethyl)-oxamic acid by intestinal flora [17]. Bacterial overgrowth may also impact drug response by changing the type and amount of flora present in the small bowel. In a study by Giuliano et al. [18], the authors initially theorized that the amount of flora responsible for vitamin K synthesis may interfere with the anticoagulant effect of warfarin, thus affecting the individual dose requirement. They subsequently found that rather than altering the synthesis of vitamin K by the increased amount of flora, vitamin K absorption was enhanced due to the damage intestinal mucosa, resulting in an increased warfarin requirement to produce the desired level of anticoagulation. Conversely, Scarpellini et al. [19] reported that the weekly mean dosage of warfarin was found to be significantly lower in adult patients with overgrowth in comparison to those without. They suggested that this is due to the extent of intestinal damage and that only some species of the gut microflora are able to produce vitamin K, while other bacteria compete for its utilization.

## 15.5   ENTEROHEPATIC RECIRCULATION

Many medications undergo biliary excretion in the unchanged form. Drugs eliminated in the bile may also be absorbed in the GI tract. Enterohepatic recirculation occurs by biliary excretion and intestinal reabsorption of a medication, prolonging its effect or that of its metabolites. To determine the extent of enterohepatic recirculation of a medication, one must compare the fraction of drug in the systemic circulation that is excreted in the bile with the fraction of drug reabsorbed from the gut that reaches the systemic circulation in each enterohepatic cycle [20]. The bioavailability of any drug that undergoes any enterohepatic recirculation will be decreased. However, some medications may remain in the enterohepatic circulation for a prolonged period of time, which may actually result in an increase in effect as well as a greater risk for hepatotoxicity due to higher hepatic concentrations. Furthermore, drugs that are converted into their active metabolites in the liver, such as loperamide and digoxin, will have their metabolism disrupted and require dosage adjustments. If the ileum is resected, the enterohepatic absorption of intact bile acids will be further reduced [21]. After ileal resection or diversion, there is reduced enterohepatic recirculation which will likewise alter bioavailability [13].

   As previously mentioned, gut microflora may be an important factor in the intestinal reabsorption as they are necessary for the hydrolysis of the drug conjugate. For example, some opioids form glucuronidated metabolites, which are converted by intestinal flora from certain metabolites back to the parent drug. This is the result of deconjugation of the metabolite within the gut lumen [22]. A

---

**TABLE 15.5**

**Examples of Drugs That Undergo Enterohepatic Recirculation**

Ampicillin

Buprenorphine

Ceftriaxone

Clindamycin

Digoxin

Doxycyline

Erythromycin

Indomethacin

Loperamide

Metronidazole

Morphine

Mycophenolate mofetil

Radiologic contrast media

Warfarin

---

second peak in its plasma-concentration/time profile may occur due to enterohepatic recirculation. Furthermore, if the drug has active metabolites, enterohepatic recycling can produce a "depot" effect. This can potentially result in a delayed but stronger pharmacologic response such as seen with the opiods morphine and buprenorphine [23]. Similarly, the loop diuretic furosemide undergoes enterohepatic cycling, followed by hydrolysis that results in a second and slow elimination phase with a half-life of 20–30 h [24]. Another example of this process involves the immunosuppressant agent myophenolate mofetil. This drug undergoes significant enterohepatic recirculation as shown by secondary peaks of mycophenolic acid [25]. Table 15.5 lists examples of medications that undergo enterohepatic recirculation.

## 15.6   IMPACT OF HEPATIC DYSFUNCTION ON PHARMACOKINETICS

Since many IF patients at some point during their clinical course develop some form of hepatic dysfunction, it is important to consider its impact on drug therapy, including drug interactions. In patients with hepatic disease, biliary excretion of drugs may be altered by the decreased uptake into hepatocytes and impaired distribution and metabolism within the hepatocytes. Liver disease may also decrease the transfer of a drug into the bile. It is known that the hepatic expression of cytochrome P (CYP) enzymes can be decreased in patients with cholestasis, possibly through bile salt retention. Bile salts have been shown to inhibit CYP *in vitro*, which may lead to hypertrophy of the smooth endoplasmic reticulum [26]. Furthermore, in patients with cirrhosis, CYP450 activity in the small intestine has been shown to be reduced [27]. Hepatic disease results in blood shunting around hepatocytes, which has the effect of reducing the delivery of drugs to the metabolizing enzymes. Moreover, cirrhosis may alter the ability of hepatocytes to uptake drug, perhaps via active transporters. This could influence the magnitude of a drug interaction as the concentration of an enzyme inhibitor in the hepatocyte would be reduced. For example, in patients with cirrhosis, the effect of fluvoxamine, a CYP1A2 inhibitor, on the metabolism of lidocaine, a CYP1A2 substrate, was recently evaluated [28]. In healthy individuals, the normal expectation is that the fluoxamine would decrease the metabolism of lidocaine, thus increasing the risk of lidocaine toxicity. In patients with cirrhosis, however, fluvoxamine had a diminished response as an inhibitor of lidocaine metabolism as there was less CYP1A2 to inhibit. The reduced magnitude of effect of CYP450 inhibitors in the presence of hepatic disease appears to be similar to that in patients who are genetically poor metabolizers [29]. Moreover, in the aforementioned example, despite the interaction with fluox-amine being blunted due to liver disease, cirrhotic patients would still be at risk for lidocaine toxic-ity because of reduced hepatic clearance. Thus, when considering drug interactions and drug clearance in patients with hepatic dysfunction, it is important to evaluate the impact on both enzyme inducers as well as the substrates (i.e., object drugs) that are hepatically cleared.

## 15.7 IMPACT OF MEDICATIONS COMMONLY USED IN IF PATIENTS

### 15.7.1 ACID BLOCKERS

In patients with short bowel syndrome, gastric hypersecretion commonly occurs in the first several months following surgery due to decreased gastrin activity coupled with decreased levels of intestinal hormones responsible for inhibiting gastrin activity. H-2 receptor antagonists such as cimetidine, famotidine, and ranitidine are absorbed in the ileum. Due to rapid transit time that is often seen in IF patients, it may be necessary to slow gastric emptying to improve overall H-2 blocker bioavailability. Moreover, higher doses might be required to compensate for the decreased drug absorption. H-2 blockers also decrease the acid load delivered to the duodenum. This may help reduce the amount of fecal loss in patients with massive ileal resection.

Proton pump inhibitors (PPIs) such as omeprazole are often used in IF. Like H-2 antagonists, PPIs slows acid secretion. PPIs work by targeting the terminal step in acid production by irreversibly blocking the hydrogen/potassium adenosine triphosphatase enzyme system (i.e., the gastric proton pump) within the parietal cells, resulting in a class of medications that are significantly more effica-cious than H-2 antagonists in reducing gastric acid secretion. Furthermore, unlike H-2 antagonists, PPIs have a longer half-life, allowing for less frequent dosing, and patients are not prone to becom-ing tolerant to them. In patients with IF, orally administered PPIs may not be effective because of insufficient contact time with the intestinal mucosa, a fact that may be further complicated by the lower pH in the duodenum and upper jejuneum resulting from gastric acid hypersecretion. In such cases, parenteral therapy may be preferred.

Unfortunately, by increasing gastric pH and decreasing gastric secretions, the use of acid block-ers may predispose patients to bacterial overgrowth (see Chapter 24, Bacterial Overgrowth of the Small Intestine).

### 15.7.2 ANTIDIARRHEAL AGENTS

Patients who experience diarrhea often have a deranged state of absorption than can impact on the bioavailability of nutrients and many medications [30]. Antidiarrheal agents are a mainstay of ther-apy in the management of IF patients. Given that both hypersecretion and accelerated propulsion are present in diarrhea, both antimotility and antisecretory agents have a role. In addition to decreasing fecal fluid losses, they slow down intestinal transit time that may be beneficial in enhancing drug absorption [30]. Conversely, antisecretory agents, such as octreotide, however, can also inhibit intes-tinal absorption by decreasing intestinal blood flow and altering fat absorption. For example, octreo-tide can decrease the absorption of the immunosuppressant cyclosporine from the gut and require that increased doses of cyclosporine be used [31].

The opioids are the largest class of nonantibacterial antidiarrheal agents. They inhibit intesti-nal motility both centrally and peripherally. These medications act by increasing intestinal transit time and by inhibiting the net secretion of electrolytes and fluid. Loperamide is commonly used since it is largely devoid of the adverse effects seen with the morphine line analgesics. It exerts antidiarrheal effects on the intestinal smooth muscle as well as possesses antisecretory proper-ties. Loperamide appears to have a predominately peripheral action but possesses other pharma-cokinetic properties that include enterohepatic recirculation and local deposition within the gut wall [32].

Moreover, loperamide appears to be active when the intestine is in a secretory diarrheal state, exerting its action at sites below the epithelium or at the level of the basolateral membranes of secretory epithelial cells [33].

Drugs such as antidiarrheal agents and others that decrease GI motility may also influence the absorption of other orally administered drugs. For example, digoxin absorption can be enhanced due to increased contact time with the intestine when patients are treated with propantholine, an antispasmodic agent with antimotility properties [34].

### 15.7.3 ALTERNATIVE ROUTES OF ADMINISTRATION

It is often better to consider routes other than the oral one to ensure consistent drug delivery. Transmucosal routes of medication administration (i.e., SL, buccal, intranasal, rectal, vaginal, and ocular) offer several advantages over the oral route for systemic drug delivery. These advantages include avoidance of hepatic first-pass metabolism, minimizing presystemic elimination within the GI tract, and, depending on the particular drug, improved absorption. Other commonly used methods of medication administration include the parenteral routes such as intramuscular, subcutaneous, and intravenous injections. A classic example of the use of alternative methods of medication is cyanobalamin supplementation. This B vitamin is absorbed only in the distal 100 cm of the ileum. In patients with IF, supplementation is especially important in whom there is >100 cm of terminal ileum resected [35]. Although available as a tablet, it is typically administered as a monthly intramuscular injection. Weekly application of a nasal gel, however, may be even more effective and is associated with fewer fluctuations in B12 levels [36].

The buccal and SL routes of administration are often used as they offer the convenience of oral administration with very few disadvantages. Buccal administration involves placement of a tablet between the cheek and gum, whereas SL administration involves placing the medication under the tongue. Drugs are absorbed through the oral mucosa which is relatively permeable and possesses a rich blood supply. Of these two routes, the SL delivery is by far the most widely studied. The SL mucosa is relatively permeable, allowing for rapid absorption of many medications. It is convenient and generally well accepted. SL dosage forms are available in two different designs those consisting of soft gelatin capsules filled with liquid drug and those composed of rapidly disintegrating tablets. These formulations create a very high drug concentration in the SL region before they are absorbed across the mucosa. Medications that have been formulated for this route of administration include nitroglycerin and mirtazapine. In patients with IF, the SL is sometimes used for medications not traditionally administered using this route. For example, morphine, in its liquid form, can be administered sublingually in patients with unpredictable absorption and have poor venous access [37]. The buccal mucosa is considerably less permeable than the SL area, and is generally not able to provide the rapid absorption and similar bioavailability properties seen with the SL route. One medication, testosterone, has a special buccal delivery system that allows for controlled release of drug over a prolonged period of time.

Another route that is sometimes used is the nasal route. Like other routes of administration, factors influencing intranasal drug absorption are related to nasal physiology, the physicochemical characteristics of the medication, and the properties of the specific formulation [38]. Nasally administered medications do not undergo first-pass metabolism. Table 15.6 lists medications that may be given via the nasal route. Limitations with this route of administration include volume and drug particle size. In adults, volumes >1 mL are difficult to deliver. Typical volumes of administration should be 0.3–0.5 mL. Particles of 10–50 μm are able to adhere best to the nasal mucosa, whereas smaller particles become nebulized and pass on to the lungs and particles >50 μm simply form droplets and run out of the nose. Nasal mucosa characteristics must also be considered. Nasal congestion, bloody nose, or mucous discharge can prevent the drug from coming in contact with the nasal mucosa, thus limiting absorption. Cocaine use can prevent absorption secondary to vasoconstriction and its chronic use lead to destruction of the nasal mucosa.

**TABLE 15.6**

**Examples of Medications That Can Be Given Intranasally**

Calcitonin

Cyanocobalamin

Fentanyl

Midazolam

Naloxone

The rectal route is another consideration but should be avoided in patients with diarrhea or dumping syndrome. Because of the partial bypass of the first-pass effect, the bioavailability of drugs given rectally is often improved. Due to the reduced mucosal surface area in the rectum, absorption is not as rapid or as complete as after oral administration. Depending on the actual site of absorption within the rectum, bioavailability may be impacted. Drugs that are absorbed into the upper hemorroidal veins will undergo first-pass hepatic metabolism before entering the general circulation, whereas drugs that are absorbed in the area of either the lower or the middle hemorroidal veins will bypass the liver and have improved bioavailability [39]. Not all medications, however, are available in a form suitable for this route. The drug must have some degree of lipid solubility in addition to water solubility in order to be absorbed across the mucous lining of the rectum. Medications with poor solubility will take longer to dissolve into the surrounding tissue and the overall rate of absorption will be reduced. Any condition that may increase the amount of fluid within the rectum (e.g., diarrhea and enema use) can impact rectal drug absorption. Increased colonic motility may result in early expulsion of a suppository from the rectum and decrease the amount of drug absorbed due to the reduced contact time. Drug inactivation may occur if the suppository is placed too high up in the rectal cavity and is absorbed in the area of the upper hemorroidal veins only, thus increasing the amount of drug that can undergo first-pass hepatic metabolism and reducing the amount of drug reaching the systemic circulation.

Transdermal drug delivery systems (TDDSs) and other topical formulations are often used in IF patients. The use of the topical route is not a new concept in this patient population. Prior to the availability of parenteral lipid emulsions, patients often received topical applications of canola and safflower oils in order to meet their essential fatty acid requirements [40]. TDDSs are polymeric formulations that are applied to the skin to deliver a medication at a predetermined rate across the dermis to achieve systemic effects [41]. Transdermal patches are becoming popular because of their unique advantages, although they are typically more expensive in comparison to conventional formulations. Improved bioavailability, needle-free delivery, along with more uniform plasma levels, make their use popular with both patients and clinicians. Drug administration simply ends upon removal of the patch. There are several different product designs, each consisting of a polymer matrix, that controls the release of the medication from the reservoir device. Membrane-controlled patches have a five-layer general structure (i.e., the protective peel strip, adhesive layer, membrane, drug reservoir, and backing). Liquid medication is released from the reservoir via the rate-controlling membrane to the skin. The amount of drug in the reservoir is significantly greater than the amount delivered to the patient over the labeled lifespan of the patch. For this reason, membrane-controlled patches must not be cut, since damage to the membrane may affect the rate of drug release, and/or allow the drug to leach out of the opening onto the skin, potentially resulting in toxic effects. Partial doses are delivered by covering a portion of the patch with an impermeable bandage prior to applying the patch. The dose delivered will be equivalent to the amount of the patch that is in direct contact with the skin. Solid monolithic transdermal systems use a copolymer or matrix system to control drug delivery. The amount of medication released is directly proportional to the surface area of the patch and does not rely on a membrane to control the rate of delivery. For smaller doses, these types of patches can be cut. Table 15.7 lists medications that are available as a TDDS.

---

**TABLE 15.7**

**Medications Available as a TDDS**

Buprenorphine

Clonidine

Diclofenac epolamine

Estrogen

Fentanyl

Granisetron

Lidocaine

Methylphenidate

Nicotine

Scopolamine

Selegiline

Testosterone

---

## 15.8   CONCLUSIONS/RECOMMENDATIONS

Patients in whom significant amounts of small bowel is resected, drug therapy is often a challenge. Absorption is altered and variable due to accelerated intestinal transit time, decreased contact time, and/or gastric hypersecretion. Each regimen must be individualized; rather than using a "standard" dose, dosing should be determined by the pharmacokinetic profile specific for the patient's weight and organ function, preferably using the evidence-based literature. If such data do not exist, the pharmacokinetic profile of each medication should be reviewed and empiric dosage adjustments should be made. As previously mentioned, certain dosage forms, such as sustained released products, should be avoided in this patient population due to the erratic absorption patterns seen in IF patients. Patients/caregivers should be educated on the importance of not changing formulations without first discussing with their healthcare team. In some cases, therapeutic substitutions may be preferable.

## REFERENCES

1. American Gastroenterological Association. Medical position statement: Short bowel syndrome and intestinal transplantation. *Gastroenterology* 2003;124:1105–10.
2. Janada SM and Fagan NL. Practical review of pharmacology concepts. *Urol Nurs* 2010;1:15–20.
3. Severijnen R, Bayat N, Bakker H. et al. Enteral drug absorption in patients with short small bowel: A review. *Clin Pharmacokinet* 2004;43(14):951–62.
4. Nightingale JMD, Kamm MA, van der Sljp J. et al. Disturbed gastric emptying in the short bowel syndrome. Evidence for a colonic brake. *Gut* 1993;34:1171–6.
5. Blackman L, Beerman B, and Groschinsky-Grind M. Malabsorption of hydrochlorothiazide following intestinal shunt surgery. *Clin Pharmacokinet* 1979;4:63–8.
6. Hoffman AF and Poley R. Role of bile acid malabsorption in pathogenesis of diarrhea and steatorrhea in patients with ileal resection. *Gastroenterology* 1972;62:918–34.
7. Frieri G, Pimpo MT, Palumbo G. et al. Anastomotic configuration and mucosal 5-aminosalicyclic acid (5-ASA) concentrations in patients with Crohn's disease: A GISC study. Gruppo Italiano per lo Studio del Colon e del Retto. *Am J Gastroenterol* 2000;95:1486–90.
8. Ehrenpreis ED, Guerriero S, Nogueras JJ. et al. Malabsorption of digoxin tablets, gel caps, and elixir in a patient with an end jejuostomy. *Ann Pharmacother* 1994;28:1239–40.
9. Vetticaden SJ, Lehman ME, Barnhart GR. et al. Digoxin absorption in a patient with short bowel syndrome. *Clin Pharmacokinet* 1986;5:62–4.
10. Victor A, Odlind V, and Kral JG. Oral contraceptive absorption and sex hormone binding globulins in obese women: Effects of jejuoileal bypass. *Gastroenterol Clin North Am* 1987;16:483–91.

11. Ilett KF, Tee LB, Reeves PT, and Minchin RF. Metabolism of drugs and other xenobiotics in the gut lumen and wall. *Pharmacol Ther* 1990;46(1):67–93.

12. Saltzman JR and Russell RM. Nutritional consequences of intestinal bacteria overgrowth. *Comp Ther* 1994;20:523–30.

13. Bongaerts G, Severijnen R, Tangerman A. et al. Bile acid deconjugation by lactobacilli and its effects in patients with a short small bowel. *J Gastroenterol* 2000;35:801–4.

14. Bongaerts G, Bakkeren J, Severijnen R. et al. Lactobacilli and acidosis in children with short small bowel. *J Pediatr Gastroenterol Nutr* 2000;30(3):288–93.

15. Abrams GD and Bishop JE. Effect of the normal microbial flora on gastrointestinal motility. *Proc Soc Exp Biol Med* 1967;126:301–4.

16. Wu WC, Zhao W, and Li S. Small intestinal bacteria overgrowth decreases small intestinal motility in the NASH rats. *World J Gastroenterol* 2008;14(2):313–7.

17. Rowland IR. Reduction by the gut microflora of animals and man. *Biochem Pharmacol* 1986; 35:27–32.

18. Giuliano V, Bassotti G, Mourvaki E. et al. Small intestinal bacterial overgrowth and warfarin dose requirement variability. *Thromb Res* 2010; [Epub ahead of print]

19. Scarpellini E, Gabrielli M, Za T. et al. The Interaction between small intestinal bacterial overgrowth and warfarin treatment. *Am J Gastroenterol* 2009;104:2364–5.

20. Plusquellec Y and Houin G. Drug recirculation model with multiple cycles occurring at unequal time intervals. *J Biomed Eng* 1992;14:521–6.

21. Roberts MS, Magnusson BM., Burczynski FJ, and Weiss M. Enterohepatic circulation: Physiological pharmacokinetic and clinical implications. *Clin Pharmacokinet* 2002;41(10):751–90.

22. Gonzalez FJ and Tukey, RH. Drug metabolism. In: Brunton LL, Lazo JS, and. Parker KL editors. *Goodman & Gilman's The Pharmacological Basis of Therapeutics*. New York, NY: The McGraw-Hill Companies, Inc.; 2006. pp. 71–92.

23. Cowan A, Friderichs E, Straßburger W. et al. Basic pharmacology of buprenorphine. In: Budd K, and Raffa RB, editors. *Buprenorphine—The Unique Opioid Analgesic: Pharmacology and Clinical Application. Stuttgart*. Germany: Thieme Medical Publishing; 2005. pp. 3–21.

24. Vree T and Ven AVD. Clinical consequences of the biphasic elimination kinetics for the diuretic effect of furosemide and its acyl glucuronide in humans. *J Pharm Pharmacol* 1999;51(3): 239–48.

25. Bullingham R, Nicholls A, and Kamm B. Clinical pharmacokinetics of mycophenolate mofetil. *Clin Pharmacokinet* 1998;34(6):429–55.

26. Reichen J. Mechanisms of cholestasis. In: Tavoloni N, and Berk P editors. *Hepatic Transport and Bile Secretion: Physiology and Pathophysiology*. New York: Raven Press, 1993. pp. 665–72.

27. McConn II DJ, Lin YS, Mathisen TL. et al. Reduced duodenal cytochrome P450 3A protein expression and catalytic activity in patients with cirrhosis. *Clin Pharmacol Ther* 2009;85:387–393.

28. Orlano R, Piccoli P, De Martin S, Piccoli P, and Palatini P. Cytochrome P450 1A2 is a major determinant of lidocaine metabolism *in vivo*: Effects of liver function. *Clin Pharmacol Ther* 2004;75:80–8.

29. Horn JR and Hansten PD. Understanding an important variable in patient response. *Pharmacy Times* 2006;72:84.

30. Dressman JB, Bass P, Rtschel WA. et al. Gastrointestinal parameters that influence oral medications. *J Pharm Sci* 1993;82:857–2.

31. Rosenberg L, Dafoe DC, Schwartz R. et al. Administration of somatostatin analog (SMS 201–995) in the treatment of a fistula occurring after pancreas transplantation. *Transplantation* 1987;43:764–6.

32. Ooms LAA, DeGryse AD, and Janssen P. Mechanism of action of loperamide. *Scand J Gastroenterol* 1984;19(Suppl 96):145–55.

33. Baird AW, Taylor CT, and Brayden DJ. Non-antibiotic anti-diarrhoeal drugs: Factors affecting oral bioavailability of berbine and loperamide in intestinal tissue. *Adv Drug Deliv Rei* 1997;23:111–20.

34. Kumer KP, Nwangwu JT, and Nwangwu PU. Perspectives on digoxin absorption from small bowel resections. *Drug Intell Clin Pharm* 1983;17:121–3.

35. Okuda K. Discovery of vitamin B12 in the liver and its absorption factor in the stomach: A historical review. *J Gastroenterol Hepatol* 1999;14:301–8.

36. Romeo VD, Sileno A, and Wenig DN. Intranasal cyanocobalamin. *JAMA* 1992;268:1268–9.

37. Harris D and Robinson JR. Drug delivery via the mucous membranes of the oral cavity. *J Pharm Sci* 1992;81:1–10.

38. Pires A, Fortuna A, Alves G, and Falcão A. Intranasal drug delivery: How, why and what for? *J Pharm Pharm Sci* 2009;12:288–311.

39. Song Y, Wang Y, Thakur R. et al., Mucosal drug delivery: Membranes, methodologies, and applications. *Crit Rev Ther Drug Carrier System* 2004;21:195–256.
40. Yurdakök M and Yurdakök K. Topical vegetableoil therapy for premature infants. *J Pediatr* 1997;130:330–2.
41. Tanner T and Marks R. Delivering drugs by the transdermal route: Review and comment. *Skin Res Technol* 2008;14:249–60.

# 16 Autologous Intestinal Reconstruction Surgery

*Melissa A. Hull, Kristina M. Potanos, Brian A. Jones, and Heung Bae Kim*

## CONTENTS

## 16.1   INTRODUCTION

The development of parenteral nutrition (PN) by Wilmore and Dudrick in 1968[1] enabled infants and children with short-bowel syndrome (SBS) to survive more than a few days postoperatively. Unfortunately, deleterious effects of PN, most notably intestinal failure-associated liver disease (IFALD) and complications related to central venous catheters, make its long-term use undesirable. The goal of intestinal rehabilitation programs to transition patients with intestinal failure to complete enteral nutrition has been met with variable success. While patients with adequate bowel length may achieve enteral autonomy prior to the development of PN complications, patients with extreme SBS may never wean from PN, or may develop serious complications of PN during the process.

The transition from parenteral to enteral nutrition is dependent on several factors. These include the length of remnant bowel, the intrinsic motility of the bowel, the presence or absence of ileocecal valve,[2] and the degree of adaptation. Adaptation refers to the process by which the surface area of the intestine increases following a massive bowel resection. This change in surface area can be observed on both macroscopic and microscopic levels. The remnant intestine dilates radially and lengthens, the muscular wall hypertrophies, and intestinal mucosal villous height and crypt depth increase. In the years following massive bowel resection, this increase in surface area leads to increased absorptive capacity.

Improving the ability of children to progress to enteral autonomy following massive bowel resection is desirable to prevent PN-associated complications. Additional benefits of enteral nutrition are improved quality of life and decreased cost of care. Autologous intestinal reconstruction surgery (AIRS) has been used as an adjunct to medical management for SBS. Techniques of autologous reconstruction are varied but have the common goal of using surgical manipulation of existing bowel in an attempt to improve intestinal absorption and facilitate enteral autonomy.

## 16.2   HISTORY OF AUTOLOGOUS RECONSTRUCTION

### 16.2.1   PROCEDURES TO INCREASE TRANSIT TIME

The field of AIRS encompasses a wide variety of procedures. The first procedures were designed to prolong intestinal transit time, thus increasing enterocyte exposure to vital nutrients, which might otherwise remain unabsorbed due to rapid transit. This group of procedures included intestinal valves, vagotomy, antiperistaltic segments, and recirculating loops.

John Hammer conducted a series of experiments in the 1950s to examine the effect of antiperistaltic ileal segments in a canine model. An antiperistaltic segment just 2 in. in length resulted in maintenance of weight and improved survival compared with those who underwent massive intestinal resection alone. The dogs with reversed segments developed proximal intestinal dilatation and had delayed transit time through the small bowel on fluoroscopic imaging.[3] Keller further investigated antiperistaltic segments by comparing single versus paired reversed segments. Dogs with two reversed segments survived longer and lost less weight than those with a single reversed segment, and both groups fared significantly better than 90% bowel resection alone, which was uniformly fatal. Keller also looked at the effect of truncal vagotomy and ileocecal valve bypass in the setting of massive bowel resection. Truncal vagotomy slowed weight loss and improved survival, while the functional loss of the ileocecal valve was fatal when combined with 75% bowel resection.[2] Another study in rats found that a single reversed segment resulted in weight maintenance and higher vitamin B12 levels than bowel resection alone.[4] Recirculating loops to increase transit time have also been described.[5] In 1967, Budding and Smith[6] published results of a comparison between reversed segments and various types of recirculating loops in a canine model. The simplest procedure (5 cm reversed ileal segment following a 90% bowel resection) was also the best tolerated procedure, minimizing weight loss and improving survival when compared with the other experimental groups. Intestinal valves, gastric pouches,[5] and isoperistaltic segmental colon transposition have also been attempted with the goal of slowing transit, thus improving absorption following massive intestinal resection. A notable finding in the colon transposition experiments was that experimental dogs had more bacteria in the remnant small bowel.[7] In fact, an unforeseen complication of procedures designed to prolong intestinal transit was bacterial overgrowth within dilated intestinal loops. Due to multiple complications including bowel obstructions and stagnation of intestinal contents, these procedures are rarely used and cannot be recommended.

### 16.2.2   INTESTINAL PLICATION AND TAPERING

Tapering enteroplasty[8] and intestinal plication[9] were designed to correct the dysmotility and size discrepancy that occurs with a dilated proximal loop in intestinal atresias. Both procedures avoid the problem of bacterial overgrowth which was seen with procedures to prolong the transit time. Tapering enteroplasty removes a portion of the dilated blind loop to narrow its caliber and facilitate anastamosis between a dilated proximal segment and decompressed distal segment. The main disadvantage is the loss of mucosal surface area, which may be undesirable in a patient with minimal remnant bowel.[8] Plication involves folding the bowel wall in on itself at the antimesenteric border, then securing this with a longitudinal suture line, resulting in normal external intestinal caliber, with the infolded mucosa protruding into the lumen. This maintains intestinal absorptive surface area.[9] Tapering enteroplasty and plication are often used in infants and children with intestinal atresia and a proximal dilated segment, although an intestinal lengthening procedure may be preferred when a patient has only a short length of remnant bowel.[10]

### 16.2.3 Intestinal Lengthening

Although several procedures designed to increase intestinal transit time or lengthen remnant intestine in children with SBS have been described, the primary procedures used clinically today are the longitudinal intestinal lengthening and tailoring (LILT) and serial transverse enteroplasty (STEP). The goal of both procedures is to capitalize on existing bowel dilation to create a longer, narrower segment of intestine. These procedures may improve stasis and bacterial overgrowth in a dilated segment while sparing precious intestinal surface area. Although infrequently used, the Iowa II (Kimura) procedure merits further discussion because of its potential to be used when other lengthening procedures are infeasible. This procedure, along with the LILT and STEP procedures, is discussed in detail in a later section.

## 16.3 INDICATIONS FOR AIRS

Although there are no absolute indications for AIRS, three primary uses for these procedures include failure to progress toward enteral autonomy in a patient with SBS, neonatal atresia with a dilated proximal segment and marginal bowel length, and refractory bacterial overgrowth. SBS with failure to progress toward enteral autonomy is the most common indication for AIRS today. The ability to wean from PN is dependent on bowel length, function, absorptive capacity, and adaptation. There is no set length below which a child cannot wean from PN[11], although a bowel length of less than 35 cm or citrulline level <12 µmol/L have been shown to be associated with failure to tolerate full enteral nutrition.

Intestinal atresia in a neonate who has marginal small bowel length is another indication for AIRS.[10,12–14] Both jejunal and ileal atresias typically occur in the first trimester of gestation, and thus the proximal segment is often quite dilated at birth. A tapering enteroplasty has been the standard technique for anastamosis of a dilated proximal segment to a decompressed distal segment. A tapering enteroplasty, while effective, reduces existing enterocyte mass. In neonates with a very short length of remnant intestine, preserving enterocyte mass is crucial. An alternative to tapering enteroplasty is a bowel-lengthening procedure on the proximal dilated segment at the time of the initial surgery. This will create a better size match between the proximal and distal bowel. Although this may result in only a modest increase in length, optimizing bowel width and length while maintaining enterocyte mass may increase the likelihood that a neonate with SBS will be able to achieve enteral autonomy.

A third indication for AIRS is refractory bacterial overgrowth in a patient with one or more dilated segments of intestine.[15] Bacterial overgrowth can develop in a dilated poorly motile segment of the intestine, and its complications can be life threatening. Bacterial overgrowth in children with SBS can lead to D-lactic acidosis, electrolyte imbalances, feeding intolerance, and bacteremia. Effective treatment of bacterial overgrowth is a key component of intestinal rehabilitation. Most patients with bacterial overgrowth can be treated effectively with rotating courses of antibiotics, but other patients may have overgrowth-related complications despite oral antibiotic therapy. In these refractory patients, bacterial overgrowth is frequently due to stasis in one or more dilated segments of the intestine. Decreasing the caliber of the bowel with an intestinal lengthening procedure may result in decreased bacterial overgrowth while maintaining enterocyte mass.[16]

In order for a patient to benefit from an intestinal lengthening procedure, the remnant bowel must be dilated. Both LILT and STEP procedures narrow the bowel caliber. The LILT procedure decreases the bowel circumference to half the original, regardless of the degree of dilation. The STEP procedure allows the surgeon to determine bowel caliber by the position of the staple lines, thus allowing the STEP to be performed on a patient with varying degrees of bowel dilation.

Although the pre-STEP caliber of the bowel may vary, doing the procedure on a patient without significant dilation will result in minimal increase in length.

Finally, the overall condition and prognosis of the patient is of critical importance in determining whether a patient will benefit from AIRS. A patient with end-stage liver disease is unlikely to achieve significant benefit from autologous reconstruction surgery. The risk–benefit ratio must be carefully weighed for each operative candidate. Careful assessment by a multidisciplinary team, including surgeons and gastroenterologists, with experience in the treatment of children with intestinal failure is an important component of the overall management of these children.[17]

## 16.4   CONTRAINDICATIONS FOR AIRS

The overall condition of the patient is of utmost importance when considering AIRS. Infants and children with SBS frequently have multiple comorbidities, often related to therapy for SBS, such as IFALD or central venous catheter infections. Prematurity is common in this patient population, as are chronic lung disease and congenital cardiac disease. Both LILT and STEP require a patient to be able to tolerate a major abdominal procedure and prolonged general anesthesia. Any comorbid condition may complicate an intestinal lengthening procedure, and these issues should be further investigated in the preoperative planning period. Intraoperatively, patients may have large fluid requirements due to prolonged open abdominal surgery, often with extensive adhesiolysis and bowel manipulation. Fluid shifts in the postoperative period may cause electrolyte imbalances. Thus, patients with chronic heart or lung disease may require prolonged mechanical ventilation, putting them at increased risk for ventilator-associated pneumonia.

Many patients undergoing AIRS have some degree of liver dysfunction. Children being evaluated for these procedures often have a history of prolonged PN dependence with associated liver dysfunction. The spectrum of liver dysfunction ranges from cholestasis with direct bilirubin and transaminase elevations to decompensated cirrhosis with thrombocytopenia, coagulopathy, and ascites. Although attaining enteral autonomy is the most effective means of reversing IFALD, patients with a prior history of PN exposure may still have liver dysfunction. While direct bilirubin normalizes a median of 4 months after cessation of PN, transaminase elevations may persist much longer. Because direct bilirubin is an insensitive marker of the degree of liver damage, some children have histologic evidence of liver injury, even cirrhosis, with normal liver function tests.[18] Any benefits of an intestinal lengthening procedure are not usually seen immediately, thus patients evaluated for AIRS with the goal of enteral autonomy must be expected to survive to the point of realizing a benefit. The average time to wean from PN in patients undergoing an intestinal lengthening procedure for SBS ranges from 9 to 19 months. Even if able to survive the procedure and recovery period, a patient with end-stage liver disease would be unlikely to survive to reach full enteral nutrition without prior liver transplantation.[19] Patients with decompensated end-stage liver disease should be considered for primary liver and small bowel transplantation rather than AIRS.

An intestinal lengthening procedure may have limited benefits in a patient with extremely short bowel, or one who is able to tolerate minimal enteral nutrition. Benefits of decreased infections and reversal of IFALD have been seen with attainment of full enteral nutrition. Although there is no absolute minimum length requirement for a lengthening procedure, a patient who is unlikely to reach full enteral autonomy with an intestinal lengthening procedure may best benefit from small bowel transplantation.

## 16.5   PRE- AND POSTOPERATIVE MANAGEMENT

The benefits of a bowel lengthening procedure are rarely realized in the immediate postoperative period, thus, every effort should be made to optimize nutritional and clinical status in the preoperative period.[20] Intake of adequate calories and protein, often in the form of PN, is necessary to maximize weight gain and optimize growth. Patients with evidence of liver disease should be considered for an Ω-3-based lipid emulsion at 1 g/kg/day,[21] which is associated with diminution of the hepatotoxic effects of PN. Any electrolyte imbalance and vitamin or micronutrient deficiency should be corrected in the preoperative period. Anemia, coagulation disorders, and thrombocytopenia should be thoroughly evaluated and treated.[20] If metabolic derangements are due to underlying liver disease, serious consideration should be given to whether the patient is best served by a bowel lengthening procedure. Careful patient selection and optimization of clinical and nutritional status preoperatively will maximize the likelihood that a patient will survive and perhaps benefit from an intestinal lengthening procedure.

Preoperative imaging studies including upper gastrointestinal (GI) series with small bowel follow through and barium enema can serve several functions. They may assist with operative planning by giving a general idea of the amount of remnant intestine and the degree of dilation. They may also reveal another reason for feeding intolerance, such as poor gastric emptying or stricture. If another reason for feeding intolerance is found, it is generally advisable to correct that problem prior to performing an intestinal lengthening procedure. In general, patients being considered for an intestinal lengthening procedure for PN dependence should have remnant bowel in continuity. If not, restoration of bowel continuity alone may increase the absorptive surface area enough to permit weaning from PN.

The surgeon should also consider which procedures, if any, should be done concurrently with AIRS. Establishment of enteral feeding access to facilitate enteral advancement postoperatively is often beneficial, and a liver biopsy may give invaluable information about the presence and severity of liver disease.[20]

Any type of bowel lengthening procedure typically results in prolonged ileus due to extensive adhesiolysis and manipulation of the bowel. This delay in return of bowel function necessitates that most patients remain on PN postoperatively.[22] Nasogastric decompression and acid-blocking medications are important during this time. Often, a fluoroscopic study to evaluate the bowel and rule out leak or obstruction is performed prior to initiating feeds. Antibiotics to cover bowel flora are used in the initial postoperative period, as there is extensive manipulation of the bowel and disruption of bowel mucosal integrity with any intestinal lengthening procedure.

## 16.6 PROCEDURAL DETAILS

Although numerous procedures have been described to increase intestinal transit time or lengthen remnant intestine in children with SBS, the two primary procedures used in this patient population are the longitudinal intestinal lengthening and tailoring (LILT) and serial transverse enteroplasty (STEP) procedures. The Iowa Model (Kimura procedure) is also discussed because it has the potential for use in situations where other intestinal lengthening procedures are not technically feasible.

### 16.6.1 LILT PROCEDURE

The first autologous intestinal lengthening procedure was described by Bianchi in 1980.[23] In the initial porcine model, intestinal segments of 10–30 cm were isolated from the remainder of the bowel. The mesentery of the isolated segment was bluntly split into two peritoneal leaves. A stapler was fired sequentially along the antimesenteric border to create two hemiloops which were half the diameter of the original. These hemiloops were anastamosed in an isoperistaltic direction to create a segment of bowel which was double its original length (Figure 16.1). In the first experiments, the LILT segments were self-emptying blind loops.[23]

The first human case of the LILT technique was described in 1981 in a 4-year-old with gastroschisis and midgut necrosis with massive bowel dilation. This child attained enteral autonomy 10 weeks postoperatively.[24] Because the circumference is halved, the LILT requires a relatively uniformly dilated segment of bowel. After the dilated segment is separated from the rest of the bowel, the mesentery is then bluntly split into two peritoneal leaves. This step is critical, as each leaf of the

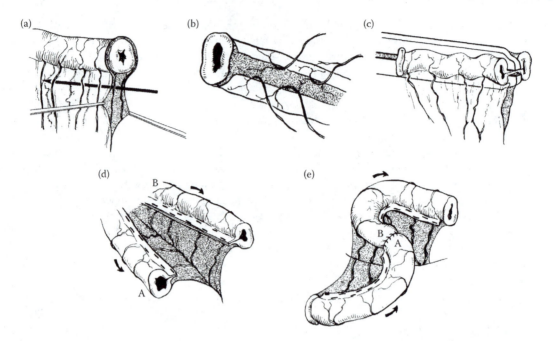

**FIGURE 16.1**   Longitudinal intestinal lengthening and tailoring. (a, b): Creation of the mesenteric tunnel. (c, d) Division of the dilated bowel into two hemiloops. (e) Reanastomosis in an isoperistaltic fashion.

mesentery will provide the sole blood supply to a segment of bowel, and failure to carefully split the mesentery results in a devascularized segment of bowel. After stapling along the antimesenteric border, the two hemiloops are anastamosed in an isoperistaltic fashion, and this narrowed segment is then reanastamosed with the remainder of the bowel.[14]

The original LILT procedure required three bowel anastamoses—one to connect the two hemiloops, and two more to connect the hemiloops to the nondilated bowel at proximal and distal ends. Subsequent modifications to the original procedure have been developed,[25,26] with the goal of reducing the number of anastamoses. Rather than isolating the dilated segment of intestine from the rest of the bowel, Chahine and Ricketts[25] angled the first staple line obliquely to the bowel, then proceeded parallel to the mesentery, finishing with a staple line angled obliquely toward the opposite side. This kept both proximal and distal ends of the segment to be lengthened attached to the remainder of the bowel. The two blind ends were sewn together into a single wide anastamosis. A case series of five infants and children found that fat balance, carbohydrate absorption, and intestinal transit time improved following LILT.[27]

Complications of the LILT procedure are not uncommon and include a leak along the staple line or at the anastamosis(es), and devascularized bowel with division of the mesenteric leaves.[20] Although devascularization is generally evident at the time of the procedure, a leak along the staple line or at an anastamosis may present late as an abscess. Sepsis and/or bacteremia have also been reported.[20] Long-term complications include recurrent dilation and dysmotility, bacterial overgrowth and D-lactic acidosis,[20] anastamotic stricture,[28] cholelithiasis, and urolithiasis.[20,28]

## 16.6.2   IOWA MODEL (KIMURA)

A two-stage method of bowel elongation is the Iowa model. Although it has not gained widespread use in children with SBS, it has several key features that may make it useful when other bowel-lengthening procedures may be impossible. In the original Iowa I model,[29] a laparotomy is performed, with creation of an isolated bowel segment and enteropexy between the abdominal wall and the antimesenteric side of the bowel segment. During the interval between the first and second

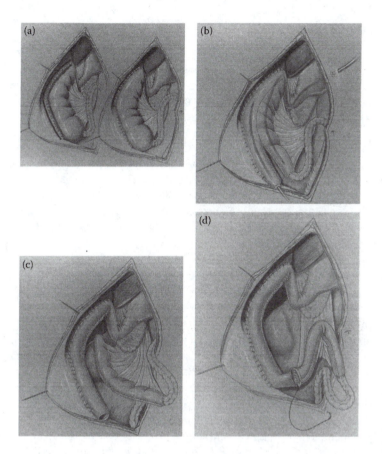

**FIGURE 16.2**   Iowa procedure. (a) Approximation of the dilated duodenum to the liver and abdominal wall with one row of sutures. The creation of seromyotomies is then followed by the second row of sutures to create the hepatomyoenteropexy. (b, c) Division of the bowel into two hemiloops. (d) Reanastomosis in an isoperistaltic fashion.

stages of the procedure, collaterals form between the liver margin and the attached loop of intestine. It then becomes possible to divide the mesentery from the isolated bowel segment, which remains viable due to neovascularization. This procedure was subsequently modified (Iowa II)[30] so that the isolated bowel loop was coapted to the liver margin, rather than to the abdominal wall (Figure 16.2). While developing these models in rats, they identified 6 weeks as the minimum duration between first and second stages of the procedure, in order to allow adequate collateral blood flow to sustain the segment of bowel after mesenteric attachments were removed. Studies of the Iowa II model in rats showed that glucose and leucine absorption were preserved,[31] and motility was unchanged[30,32] following division of the mesentery. Subsequent studies found that mucosal mass, DNA content, sucrose activity, and villous height/crypt depth were maintained following division of the mesentery when the bowel remained in continuity.[33] The Iowa II model was subsequently adapted for use in an infant with extreme SBS due to intrauterine midgut volvulus. Because he was left with only remnant duodenum and his mesentery was essentially absent, he was not a candidate for the LILT procedure. In this infant, the initial hepatomyoenteropexy was performed at 6 weeks of age, with the second stage 8 weeks later. Rather than removing the mesentery from the coapted bowel segment, the intestinal segment was divided into two hemiloops—one with vascular supply from the mesentery and the other with collaterals from the liver. The two loops were anastamosed to restore bowel continuity.[34] This model has been extended to use enteroenteropexy (Iowa III), with similar motility and absorption.[35,36]

### 16.6.3   STEP Procedure

The STEP procedure was first described in a porcine model by Kim et al. in 2003.[37] This procedure uses sequential stapler application from alternating directions perpendicular to the mesentery to create a zig-zag channel. The initial porcine model induced bowel dilation by creating a partial obstruction using an antiperistaltic jejunal segment. This was followed by resection of the reversed segment and STEP of the remaining bowel 5 weeks later.[37] This model was later modified to include 90% bowel resection, including the reversed segment, to create a porcine model of SBS. Studies utilizing this porcine SBS model showed that STEP improved weight retention, carbohydrate and fat absorption, as well as serum citrulline, while decreasing bacterial overgrowth.[16] More recent porcine studies used strain gauge monitors implanted at intervals from gastric antrum to terminal ileum distal to the STEP segment to evaluate intestinal motility. This study demonstrated normal MMCs within the small intestine and an equal number of phase III contractions in control and STEP animals; manometry also showed no differences between groups.[38] In addition, animals who underwent STEP were found to have higher postoperative serum levels of citrulline, a nonprotein amino acid which correlates with small bowel enterocyte mass.[39] Though the STEP procedure does not create new bowel, it is hypothesized that by tapering and lengthening the previously dilated bowel, the process of adaptation is facilitated, thus allowing enterocyte mass to increase. Increased levels of the gut growth factor GLP-2 have been noted in rodents that have undergone a modified STEP operation.[40]

The first human STEP was performed on a 2-year-old with gastroschisis and midgut volvulus who had undergone a prior LILT procedure. Following the procedure, his carbohydrate absorption improved and enteral tolerance increased from 10% to 50% in the first 6 months postoperatively.[41] The STEP procedure begins with laparotomy and adhesiolysis, which can be extensive in the setting of prior surgical procedures. The bowel is measured along the antimesenteric border, which is marked to facilitate stapler application perpendicular to the mesentery. A small mesenteric window is created, large enough to allow passage of a surgical stapler. A surgical stapler is inserted through the mesenteric defect at a 90° angle to the mesentery and the stapler is fired. This is repeated at intervals, with each staple line approaching the bowel from the opposite direction of the prior one, creating a zig-zag channel (Figure 16.3). The distance between staple firings and the degree to which each staple line crosses the mesentery is determined by the degree of intestinal dilation and desired channel width. The channel width is typically 1–2 cm, based on age and normal bowel caliber. As the bowel becomes less dilated, there is decreased overlap of staple firings. A suture is placed at the crotch of the staple line to decrease the risk of leak from the weakest area. The STEP procedure was subsequently described for the initial management of neonates with a dilated segment due to intestinal atresia[10,12,13] and for refractory D-lactic acidosis.[15]

Advantages of the STEP procedure include less technical complexity than the LILT or the Iowa II, less potential to compromise intestinal vascular supply,[13] no intestinal anastamosis, and the ability to apply to bowel with varying degrees of dilation. Due to its straightforward technical approach the use of the STEP has spread rapidly. One clear surgical advantage of the STEP is that a uniform bowel diameter can be created in variably dilated bowel.

Similar complications have been reported with both the STEP and LILT, including staple line leaks. Although there are no anastamoses with the STEP, bowel obstruction (sometimes requiring reoperation) and prolonged ileus have been reported.[42] Sepsis, abscess formation, catheter-related bacteremia, and gastrointestinal bleeding as a result of portal hypertension have also been described.[42,43] Finally, as with the LILT procedure, redilation of the intestine is common.

## 16.7   SEQUENTIAL INTESTINAL LENGTHENING PROCEDURES

Redilation following an intestinal lengthening procedure may present as worsening bacterial overgrowth, enteral intolerance, or growth failure. Due to prior manipulation of the mesenteric blood

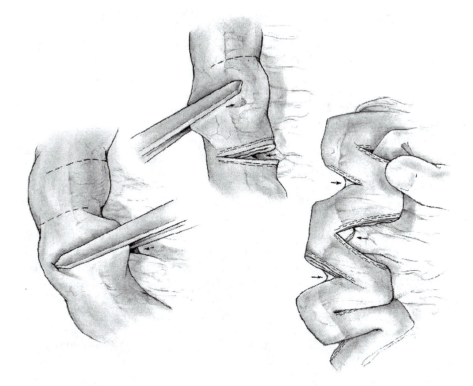

**FIGURE 16.3**    Serial transverse enteroplasty. The dilated bowel is flattened, and the stapler is applied perpendicular to the long axis of the bowel, from alternating sides. A small defect in the mesentery was created at each point of stapler application. The end result is a zig-zag pattern to the lengthened bowel.

supply, repeat LILT is not feasible. One option for addressing intestinal redilation following an intestinal lengthening procedure is to perform a STEP. In fact, the first human case of a STEP was described in a patient who had a prior LILT.[41] The feasibility of a second STEP when bowel redilation occurs post-STEP was first described in a porcine model in 2006.[44] In 2007, a second STEP was reported in two children who had an initial STEP procedure for intestinal atresia and gastroschisis as infants, but failed to adequately progress in their tolerance of enteral nutrition and experienced redilation of the intestine. At 8 and 6.5 months post-STEP, each patient underwent laparotomy and repeat STEP for additional bowel lengthening. The first patient increased from 15% to 39% enteral nutrition 13 months after repeat STEP and is doing well; the other increased from 20% to 50% enteral nutrition following repeat STEP, but ultimately succumbed to liver failure.[45] In 2008, Andres et al. reported 14 patients with a prior intestinal lengthening procedure (LILT = 7 patients, STEP = 7 patients) who underwent STEP. Two of the patients in the series developed redilation after their second STEP, and underwent a third procedure. The overall survival in this series was 100% with a median follow-up of 14.5 months. Six of the 14 patients (43%) were able to achieve enteral autonomy after the second STEP.[46]

The Kimura procedure has also been described for redilation following LILT in a patient with extreme SBS due to gastroschisis and volvulus. This child's enteral tolerance improved from 5% to 55%, and he remained alive 4 years after the procedures.[47] This patient was part of a case series of nine patients who had sequential procedures performed. Six of these patients had intestinal dilation induced by creation of an intestinal valve, followed by LILT procedure. Two patients died, two reached enteral autonomy, and enteral autonomy averaged 50% for patients followed more than 1 year.[47]

## 16.8   OUTCOMES OF INTESTINAL LENGTHENING PROCEDURES

Both LILT and STEP procedures have shown promise in transitioning patients who would otherwise be dependent on PN to full enteral nutrition. Controlled studies in animals have shown improved nutritional status following AIRS, however, there are no human trials comparing rate of PN weaning and time to reach enteral nutrition with AIRS versus nonsurgical intestinal rehabilitation.

A retrospective analysis of 20 LILT procedures performed for dilated dysfunctional jejunum found that long-term survivors were more likely to have >40 cm remnant small bowel, intact ileocecal valve, and longer colon length preoperatively. They also tended to have minimal hepatic dysfunction,[28] and procedures were performed at a later age. A subsequent study of 49 patients with a median age of 25 months who underwent LILT for SBS reported nine patient deaths. All occurred in the late postoperative period, and over three-quarters of the deaths were attributable to end-stage liver disease or sepsis. Of the 16 who weaned from PN, the median time to reach full enteral nutrition was 9 months.[20] Finally, a single-center study of 19 patients undergoing LILT reported a long-term survival rate of 79%, with 60% of the survivors eventually requiring small bowel transplantation. The 42% of patients who achieved enteral autonomy without transplantation tended to be older at the time of the initial procedure, and were more likely to have an intact ileocecal valve.[48]

Because the STEP is a relatively new procedure, long-term follow up data is limited. A single-center case series of five patients undergoing STEP for SBS and PN-dependence reported no postoperative complications and an increase in mean enteral tolerance from 49% to 80% with median follow-up of 17 months. In this study, both of the children who had pre-STEP D-xylose tests normalized D-xylose levels within 12 months of STEP, indicating improved carbohydrate absorption.[49] Growth analysis of post-STEP patients showed statistically significant increases in weight for age Z score, weight for height, and upper arm anthropomorphic tests.[50] Subsequent follow-up from this single institution study included 16 patients who had undergone STEP procedure with a median follow-up of 23 months.[43] They found that 38% of patients had reached enteral autonomy in a median time of 20 months.

In order to better track the STEP outcomes worldwide, a web-based International Data Registry for patients undergoing STEP was established in 2004 (http://www.stepoperation.org). Early reports of the voluntary registery (median follow-up 12.6 months) found an 8% mortality and an increase in mean enteral tolerance from 31% to 67%.[42] Jones et al. presented the most recent report from this registry in 2010, summarizing the largest experience to date of the STEP procedure, in 111 patients from 50 centers in 14 countries. The underlying disease was gastroschisis ($n = 50$), intestinal atresia ($n = 38$), or NEC ($n = 9$) in 87% of patients. Of the 97 patients with adequate follow-up, 55 were male. Median age at STEP was 7 (0–241) months with median pre-STEP bowel length and width of 49 (inter-quartile range 28–85) cm and 5 (IQR 4–7) cm, respectively. Median follow-up time was 16.7 months. Analyses of 78 patients who were greater than 7 days of age and dependent on PN at the time of STEP revealed that 47% had achieved enteral autonomy, 19% had an improved percentage of enteral nutrition, and 8% had an unchanged or decreased percentage of enteral nutrition. Median time to reach enteral autonomy was 21 months (95% CI: 12–30). As with LILT, deaths ($n = 11$) following STEP were secondary to concomitant liver disease and sepsis (31,44–46). Five patients progressed to combined liver–intestine transplantation; overall transplant-free survival was 84%. Multivariate analysis identified higher direct bilirubin and shorter bowel length as pre-STEP risk factors for progression to transplant or death.[51]

When outcomes from 43 LILT and 34 STEP procedures from a single institution were compared, survival rates were slightly higher for STEP (95% vs. 88%) but STEP procedures had a shorter duration of follow-up. Sixty-nine percent of patients reached enteral autonomy, including eight patients who received intestinal transplantation. Overall, 10% of patients had surgical complications and 14% progressed to intestinal transplantation.[52] Based on these studies, an intestinal lengthening procedure facilitates transition to full enteral nutrition in approximately 50% of patients. It is difficult to quantify the contribution of AIRS to the weaning from PN in these patients because the natural history of enteral advancement without operation has not been well studied. The process of bowel adaptation following a lengthening procedure that allows transition to enteral nutrition is a gradual one. Further research is needed to determine those patients most likely to benefit from an intestinal lengthening procedure. The leading causes of mortality following STEP and LILT procedures are end-stage liver disease, followed by sepsis. This suggests that patients with hepatic decompensation who have failed medical therapy for SBS and are being considered for AIRS may be better served by transplantation. In addition, evaluation of long-term outcomes, including gastrointestinal motility, is needed.

## 16.9 FUTURE STUDIES

While autologous reconstruction, particularly bowel lengthening procedures, have allowed many children with SBS to wean from PN, other children remain dependent on PN or progress to transplantation. Recent advances in tissue engineering and mechanical lengthening devices have shown the potential to eventually help some of these children achieve better outcomes.

Advances in tissue-engineered small intestine have been made in the past decade.[53] Vacanti and colleagues created tissue-engineered small intestine with organoid units derived from neonatal rat intestine and implanted on a scaffold.[54] These cyst-like structures have been shown to contain smooth muscle, IAP (a brush border protein found only in differentiated enterocytes), and villin (an actin-binding protein important for apical microvilli). When these cysts were anastamosed with remnant intestine, weight gain, B12 levels, and IAP all increased,[54] although it is unclear if these improvements were due to stasis at that segment or an increase in absorptive surface area.[55] More recently, implantation of vascular endothelial growth factor (VEGF) microspheres into the construct were shown to increase epithelial proliferation and microcapillary density.[56]

Mechanical means of increasing intestinal length have also been studied in animal models. Two types of mechanical implants include screws[57–59] and hydraulic pistons.[59] Using mechanical devices, an isolated segment of small intestine can be lengthened up to 240% of its original length[58] and still maintain contractility,[60] although some shrinkage may occur following removal of the mechanical expander. In order to apply a longitudinal lengthening force, current device prototypes require the bowel be removed from continuity during the lengthening process, thus necessitating a second surgery for reanastamosis of the lengthened segment.[59] Potential risks include dislodgement of the device and perforation. To date, these devices have been used to lengthen only short segments of the bowel.

## 16.10 CONCLUSION

SBS remains a complex problem with substantial mortality. When a child fails to reach enteral autonomy despite maximal medical management or develops refractory bacterial overgrowth due to a dilated segment, AIRS provides a surgical option that may help infants and children with SBS wean from PN.

## REFERENCES

1. Wilmore DW, Dudrick SJ. Growth and development of an infant receiving all nutrients exclusively by vein. *JAMA*. 1968;203(10):860–864.
2. Keller JWS, William RC, Westerheide R, Pace WG. Prolonged survival with paired reversed segment after massive intestinal resection. *Arch Surg*. 1965;91:174–179.
3. Hammer JM, Seay PH, Johnston RL, Hill EJ, Prust FH, Campbell RJ. The effect of antiperistaltic bowel segments on intestinal emptying time. *Arch Surg*. 1959 Oct;79:537–541.
4. Venables CW, Ellis H, Smith AD. Antiperistaltic segments after massive intestinal resections. *Lancet*. 1966 Dec 24;2(7478):1390–1394.
5. Poth EJ. Use of gastrointestinal reversal in surgical procedures. *Am J Surg*. 1969 Dec;118(6):893–899.

6. Budding JS, Smith CC. Role of recirculating loops in the management of massive resection of the small intestine. *Surg Gynecol Obstet.* 1967;125(2):243–249.
7. Hutcher NE, Salzberg AM. Pre-ileal transposition of colon to prevent the development of short bowel syndrome in puppied with 90 percent small intestinal resection. *Surgery.* 1971 Aug;70(2):189–197.
8. Weber TR, Vane DW, Grosfeld JL. Tapering enteroplasty in infants with bowel atresia and short gut. *Arch Surg.* 1982 May;117(5):684–688.
9. de Lorimier AA, Harrison MR. Intestinal plication in the treatment of atresia. *J Pediatr Surg.* 1983 Dec;18(6):734–737.
10. Wales PW, Dutta S. Serial transverse enteroplasty as primary therapy for neonates with proximal jejunal atresia. *J Pediatr Surg.* 2005 Mar;40(3):E31–34.
11. Kosloske AM, Jewell PF. A technique for preservation of the ileocecal valve in the neonatal short intestine. *J Pediatr Surg.* 1989 Apr;24(4):369–370.
12. Ismail A, Alkadhi A, Alnagaar O, Khirate A. Serial transverse enteroplasty in intestinal atresia management. *J Pediatr Surg.* 2005 Feb;40(2):E5–E6.
13. Cowles RA, Lobritto SJ, Stylianos S, Brodlie S, Smith LJ, Jan D. Serial transverse enteroplasty in a newborn patient. *J Pediatr Gastroenterol Nutr.* 2007 Aug;45(2):257–260.
14. Bianchi A. Intestinal lengthening: An experimental and clinical review. *J R Soc Med.* 1984;77Suppl 3:35–41.
15. Modi BP, Langer M, Duggan C, Kim HB, Jaksic T. Serial transverse enteroplasty for management of refractory D-lactic acidosis in short-bowel syndrome. *J Pediatr Gastroenterol Nutr.* 2006 Sep;43(3):395–397.
16. Chang RW, Javid PJ, Oh JT, Andreoli S, Kim HB, Fauza D, and Jaksic T. Serial transverse enteroplasty enhances intestinal function in a model of short bowel syndrome. *Ann Surg.* 2006 Feb;243(2):223–228.
17. Andorsky DJ, Lund DP, Lillehei CW, Jaksic T, Dicanzio J, Richardson DS, Collier SB, Lo C, and Duggan C. Nutritional and other postoperative management of neonates with short bowel syndrome correlates with clinical outcomes. *J Pediatr.* 2001 Jul;139(1):27–33.
18. Fitzgibbons SC 2009. The relationship between biopsy proven parenteral nutrition associated liver disease and biochemical cholestasis in children with short bowel syndrome. Paper presented at the American Pediatric Surgical Association 40th Annual Meeting, Fajardo, Puerto Rico.
19. Bianchi A. Longitudinal intestinal lengthening and tailoring: Results in 20 children. *J R Soc Med.* 1997 Aug;90(8):429–432.
20. Hosie S, Loff S, Wirth H, Rapp HJ, von Buch C, Waag KL. Experience of 49 longitudinal intestinal lengthening procedures for short bowel syndrome. *Eur J Pediatr Surg.* 2006 Jun;16(3):171–175.
21. Alwayn IP, Gura K, Nose V, Zausche B, Javid P, Garza J, Verbesey J et al. Omega-3 fatty acid supplementation prevents hepatic steatosis in a murine model of nonalcoholic fatty liver disease. *Pediatr Res.* 2005 Mar;57(3):445–452.
22. Bianchi A. Lengthening a baby's gut. *Lancet.* 1985 Apr 6;1(8432):819.
23. Bianchi A. Intestinal loop lengthening—A technique for increasing small intestinal length. *J Pediatr Surg.* 1980 Apr;15(2):145–151.
24. Boeckman CR, Traylor, R. Bowel lengthening for short gut syndrome. *J Pediatr Surg.* 1981 Dec;16(6):996–997.
25. Chahine AA Ricketts RR. A modification of the Bianchi intestinal lengthening procedure with a single anastomosis. *J Pediatr Surg.* 1998 Aug;33(8):1292–1293.
26. Aigrain Y, Cornet D, Cezard JP, Boureau M. Longitudinal division of small intestine: A surgical possibility for children with the very short bowel syndrome. *Z Kinderchir.* 1985 Aug;40(4):233–236.
27. Weber TR, Powell MA. Early improvement in intestinal function after isoperistaltic bowel lengthening. *J Pediatr Surg.* 1996 Jan;31(1):61–63; discussion 63–64.
28. Bianchi A. Experience with longitudinal intestinal lengthening and tailoring. *Eur J Pediatr Surg.* 1999 Aug;9(4):256–259.
29. Ienaga T, Kimura K, Hashimoto K, Lee SC, Brakstad M, Soper RT. Isolated bowel segment (Iowa Model 1): Technique and histological studies. *J Pediatr Surg.* 1990 Aug;25(8):902–904.
30. Yamazato M, Kimura K, Yoshino H, Soper RT. The isolated bowel segment (Iowa model II) created in functioning bowel. *J Pediatr Surg.* 1991 Jul;26(7):780–783.
31. Yoshino H, Kimura K, Yamazato M, Scott DH, Soper RT. The isolated bowel segment (Iowa Model II): Absorption studies for glucose and leucine. *J Pediatr Surg.* 1991 Dec;26(12):1372–1375.
32. Yamazato M, Kimura K, Yoshino H, Murr M, Ellsbury D, Soper RT. The isolated bowel segment (Iowa model II): motility across the anastomosis with or without mesenteric division. *J Pediatr Surg.* 1992 Jun;27(6):691–695.

33. Bishop WP, Kim SI, Yamazato M, Yoshino H, Kimura K. Mucosal morphology in isolated bowel segments: Importance of exposure to luminal contents. *J Pediatr Surg.* 1992 Aug;27(8):1061–1065.
34. Kimura K, Soper RT. A new bowel elongation technique for the short-bowel syndrome using the isolated bowel segment Iowa models. *J Pediatr Surg.* 1993 Jun;28(6):792–794.
35. el-Murr M, Kimura K, Ellsberg D, Yamazato M, Yoshino H, Soper RT. Motility of isolated bowel segment Iowa model III. *Dig Dis Sci.* 1994 Dec;39(12):2619–2623.
36. Murr M, Kimura K, Ellsbury D, Yoshino H, Yamazato M, Soper R. Absorption in the isolated bowel segment. *J Pediatr Gastroenterol Nutr.* 1993 Aug;17(2):182–185.
37. Kim HB, Fauza D, Garza J, Oh JT, Nurko S, Jaksic T. Serial transverse enteroplasty (STEP): A novel bowel lengthening procedure. *J Pediatr Surg.* 2003 Mar;38(3):425–429.
38. Modi BP, Ching YA, Langer M, Donovan K, Fauza D, Kim HB, Jaksic T, and Nurko S. Preservation of intestinal motility after the serial transverse enteroplasty procedure in a large animal model of short bowel syndrome. *J Pediatr Surg.* 2009 Jan;44(1):229–235; discussion 235.
39. Crenn P, Coudray-Lucas C, Thuillier F, Cynober L, Messing B Postoperative plasma citrulline concentration is a marker of absorptive enterocyte mass and intestinal failure in humans. *Gastroenterology.* 2000:119(6):1496–1505.
40. Kaji T, Tanaka H, Sigalet D, Wallace LE, Kravarusic D, Hoist J, and Sigalet DL. Nutritional effects of the serial transverse enteroplasty procedure in experimental short bowel syndrom. *J Pediatr Surg.* 2009 Aug;44(8):1552–1559.
41. Kim HB, Lee PW, Garza J, Duggan C, Fauza D, Jaksic T. Serial transverse enteroplasty for short bowel syndrome: A case report. *J Pediatr Surg.* 2003 Jun;38(6):881–885.
42. Modi BP, Javid PJ, Jaksic T, Piper H, Langer M, Duggan C, Kamin D, and Kim HB. First report of the international serial transverse enteroplasty data registry: Indications, efficacy, and complications. *J Am Coll Surg.* 2007 Mar;204(3):365–371.
43. Ching YA, Fitzgibbons S, Valim C, Zhou J, Duggan C, Jaksic T, and Kim HB. Long-term nutritional and clinical outcomes after serial transverse enteroplasty at a single institution. *J Pediatr Surg.* 2009 May;44(5):939–943.
44. Piper H, Modi BP, Kim HB, Fauza D, Glickman J, Jaksic T. The second STEP: The feasibility of repeat serial transverse enteroplasty. *J Pediatr Surg.* 2006 Dec;41(12):1951–1956.
45. Ehrlich PF, Mychaliska GB, Teitelbaum DH. The 2 STEP: An approach to repeating a serial transverse enteroplasty. *J Pediatr Surg.* 2007 May;42(5):819–822.
46. Andres AM, Thompson J, Grant W, Botha J, Sunderman B, Antonson D, Langnas A, and Sudan D. Repeat surgical bowel lengthening with the STEP procedure. *Transplantation.* 2008;85(9):1294–1299.
47. Georgeson K, Halpin D, Figueroa R, Vincente Y, Hardin W, Jr. Sequential intestinal lengthening procedures for refractory short bowel syndrome. *J Pediatr Surg.* 1994 Feb;29(2):316–320; discussion 320–311.
48. Walker SR, Nucci A, Yaworski JA, Barksdale EM, Jr. The Bianchi procedure: A 20-year single institution experience. *J Pediatr Surg.* 2006 Jan;41(1):113–119; discussion 113–119.
49. Javid PJ, Kim HB, Duggan CP, Jaksic T. Serial transverse enteroplasty is associated with successful short-term outcomes in infants with short bowel syndrome. *J Pediatr Surg.* 2005 Jun;40(6):1019–1023; discussion 1023–1014.
50. Duggan C, Piper H, Javid PJ, Valim C, Collier S, Kim HB, and Jaksic T. Growth and nutritional status in infants with short-bowel syndrome after the serial transverse enteroplasty procedure. *Clin Gastroenterol Hepatol.* Oct 2006;4(10):1237–1241.
51. Jones BA, Hull MA, Zurakowski D, McGuire MM, Fitzgibbons SC, Ching YA, Duggan C, Jaksic T, and Kim HB. Report of 111 consecutive patients enrolled in the international serial transverse enteroplasty (STEP) data registry. Presented at the American Academy of Pediatrics National Conference and Exhibition, San Francisco, CA, Oct 3, 2010:11276.
52. Sudan D, Thompson J, Botha J, Grant W, Antonson D, Raynor S, and Langnas A. Comparison of intestinal lengthening procedures for patients with short bowel syndrome. *Ann Surg.* 2007 Oct;246(4):593–601; discussion 601–594.
53. Javaid Ur R, Waseem T. Intestinal tissue engineering: Where do we stand? *Surg Today.* 2008;38(6):484–486.
54. Grikscheit TC, Siddique A, Ochoa ER, Srinivasan A, Aisberg E, Hodin RA, and Vacanti JP. Tissue-engineered small intestine improves recovery after massive small bowel resection. *Ann Surg.* 2004 Nov;240(5):748–754.
55. Warner BW. Tissue engineered small intestine: A viable clinical option? *Ann Surg.* 2004 Nov;240(5):755–756.

56. Rocha FG, Sundback CA, Krebs NJ, Leach JK, Mooney DJ, Ashley SW, Vacanti JP, and Whang EE. The effect of sustained delivery of vascular endothelial growth factor on angiogenesis in tissue-engineered intestine. *Biomaterials.* 2008 Jul;29(19):2884–2890.
57. Chang PC, Mendoza J, Park J, Lam MM, Wu B, Atkinson JB, and Dunn JC. Sustainability of mechanically lengthened bowel in rats. *J Pediatr Surg.* 2006 Dec;41(12):2019–2022.
58. Shekherdimian S, Scott A, Chan A, Dunn JC. Intestinal lengthening in rats after massive small intestinal resection. *Surgery.* 2009 Aug;146(2):291–295.
59. Luntz J, Brei D, Teitelbaum D, Spencer A. Mechanical extension implants for short-bowel syndrome. *Proc Soc Photo Opt Instrum Eng.* 2006;6173:617309.
60. Mendoza J, Chang CY, Blalock CL, Atkinson JB, Wu BM, Dunn JC. Contractile function of the mechanically lengthened intestine. *J Surg Res.* 2006 Nov;136(1):8–12.

# 17 Intestinal Transplantation

*Margaret McGuire, Daniel S. Kamin, and Heung Bae Kim*

## CONTENTS

## 17.1   INTRODUCTION

Intestinal transplantation was first described in an animal model in 1951 by Mueller et al. [1]. However, it was not until 1967 that the first attempt at intestinal transplantation in humans was reported [2]. With the introduction of parenteral nutrition (PN) in 1968 by Dudrick, patients with intestinal failure (IF) had a new treatment which provided them life-saving nutrition [3]. Because of this major advance, and the unacceptably poor transplant outcomes in the precalcineurin inhibitor era, clinical intestinal transplantation was not reconsidered until the introduction of cyclosporine (the first calcineurin inhibitor) in 1980 [4–6]. The first successful combined liver–intestine transplant in a patient with short bowel syndrome (SBS) was reported in 1990 [7]. Despite the clear demonstration of the technical feasibility of intestinal transplantation, posttransplant survival still remained comparatively poor until the introduction of tacrolimus in 1990 [8]. Results of intestinal transplantation slowly improved through the 1990s due to a combination of technical improvements as well as a better understanding of the management of intestinal rejection. The 2001 American Society of Transplantation position paper established intestinal transplantation as an option for those who could no longer be sustained on PN [9]. In 2001, the Centers for Medicare and Medicaid Services approved Medicare coverage of intestinal transplantation for patients with complications from irreversible IF. Data from the Intestinal Transplant Registry show that between 1985 and 2009 there were 2291 intestine transplants in 2061 patients at 86 centers [10].

## 17.2   IF IN CONTEXT

IF is defined as an inability to absorb adequate enteral nutrition to sustain normal growth and function. This can be a result of either loss of intestinal mass (short bowel syndrome) or impaired intestinal function (motility disorders, malabsorption syndromes, etc.). The causes of IF differ between children and adults. IF in adults is secondary to ischemia (23%), Crohn's disease (14%), and trauma (10%) [11]. Children most often have IF secondary to gastroschisis (21%), volvulus (17%), and necrotizing enterocolitis (12%) [11]. With the use of PN many children with IF successfully grow and achieve enteral autonomy after intestinal adaptation. According to Howard, et al., 63% of patients with congenital bowel disorders achieve complete rehabilitation and 94% survive 1 year on PN [12]. However, weaning off PN is unlikely if the patient remains on therapy for over 2 years despite maximal attempts for medical and surgical rehabilitation [13]. The survival rates associated with long-term PN in SBS patients is 86% and 75% at 2 and 5 years respectively [14].

## 17.3   INDICATIONS

The decision to pursue intestinal transplant depends on the comparative survival of continuing non-transplant therapy versus survival posttransplantation. However, this simple statement belies the serious methodologic concerns hampering efforts to achieve valid risk assessments, and does not take comparative quality of life into account. Small numbers, heterogeneous diagnoses, and practice variation between institutions and over time account for the mainly retrospective studies in the literature.

Intestinal Failure Associated Liver Disease (IFALD) is the strongest predictor of mortality in patients with IF, and has been the most important indication for combined liver/intestine transplantation. Adult patients with advanced IFALD fair poorly, and nearly all succumb to the complications of liver disease within 1 year of onset [15]. In the 1990s, the prevalence of IFALD was reported to be approximately 40–60% in infants on long-term PN [16]. More recent reports have demonstrated a decrease in IFALD to approximately 20% in children on home PN [17]. The introduction of alternate types of lipid emulsions has also improved the rate of IFALD [18]. The degree of IFALD in children with SBS is partially related to early, recurrent episodes of catheter-related sepsis, lack of enteral feeding, and continuous, high glucose and lipid infusion rates [16]. Early referral for transplant evaluation is important as Kaufman et al. showed that the probability of overt life-threatening liver failure from IFALD was at least 36% in patients 6–9 months of age who had a total bilirubin level of 6.0 mg/dL or greater [19]. Lopushinsky et al. predicted, using a Markov analysis, that survival posttransplantation was favorable (compared with continued PN) when the risk for developing IFALD was greater than 11% per year, based on data from Canadian life tables adjusted for disease-related mortality from 1995 to 1997 [20].

Unfortunately, it remains difficult to predict which patients will fail to achieve independence from PN and/or develop life-threatening complications from its use. Optimal timing of referral for intestinal transplantation is thus poorly defined. Through the use of a multidisciplinary team approach, medical and surgical therapies can be employed optimally and expeditiously, with organ replacement as the next appropriate treatment when more conservative measures are unsuccessful. Consensus groups, government bodies, and insurance companies have developed indications for intestinal transplantation [9,21,22]. All are relatively similar in structure, with minor variations, such as the detail offered when characterizing the qualifying complications from PN. Table 17.1 is

**TABLE 17.1**

**Pediatric Criteria for Referral for Transplant Evaluation**

Children with massive small bowel resection

Children with severely diseased bowel or motility disorders

Continuing prognostic and diagnostic uncertainty

Microvillous inclusion disease or intestinal epithelial dysplasia

Persistent hyperbilirubinemia (>6 mg/dL)

Thrombosis of two upper body central veins

The request of the patient or family

*Source:*   Adapted from Beath, S et al. *Transplantation* 2008;85:1378–84.

adapted from the most recent consensus statement, which identifies reasons for referring patients for transplant evaluation [21].

## 17.4   PREOPERATIVE EVALUATION

The intestine transplant evaluation involves a multidisciplinary team including physicians, coordinators, nutritionists, pharmacists, psychologists, and social workers. Medical evaluation includes: (1) assessing fulfillment of criteria for intestinal transplant; (2) deliberation over the type of graft needed (e.g., isolated intestine, multivisceral, and/or liver-inclusive grafts); and (3) evaluation of other comorbidities that are common in this patient population including chronic lung disease, renal insufficiency, cardiac anomalies, neurodevelopmental delay, and chronic pain issues. Surgical evaluation should include: (1) assessment of abdominal vasculature and anatomy; (2) review of surgical history including central venous access; (3) vascular/gastrointestinal (GI) imaging as indicated; and (4) assessment of perioperative risks by a transplant anesthesiologist.

Education and counseling are an important part of preparing the patient and family for life post-transplantation. A thorough review of current survival statistics and potential complications is critical, so that parents and patients can make fully informed decisions regarding transplantation versus remaining on PN. Explication of the criteria for transplant listing and national organ allocation policy is essential. Parents and patients may find it useful to talk to other transplant families who have already been through the process.

## 17.5   TYPES OF GRAFTS

Intestinal transplantation can be done alone using an isolated intestine graft (ITx) or with other organs as part of a combined liver–intestine (LITx) or multivisceral graft (MVTx). The choice of transplant type can depend on many factors, both medical and surgical.

ITx is indicated for patients who suffer from permanent IF without significant liver disease. In this type of transplant, any residual dysfunctional native small intestine is replaced with the donor small intestine graft (Figure 17.1). The proximal donor jejunum is anastomosed to the recipient jejunum to restore intestinal continuity and an end ileostomy is created to allow for close monitoring of the graft by visual inspection as well as by serial biopsies. In most cases, a gastrojejunostomy tube is placed as well. Arterial inflow for this graft is usually obtained directly from the aorta and venous drainage can be either into the portal system or directly into the inferior vena cava. Due to technical considerations, systemic drainage is most commonly used today.

Combined liver–intestine transplantation is indicated when IF is complicated by IFALD. Combined liver–intestine transplantation was first described in 1990 and in the original technique, only the liver and intestine were transplanted with removal of the donor duodenum and pancreas. However, the current method for combined liver–intestine transplantation involves the en-bloc transplantation of the donor liver, duodenum, pancreas, and small intestine (Figure 17.2). This method originally described by the Omaha group, has the advantage of no donor portal dissection or biliary anastomosis [23]. In this type of transplant, the recipient jejunum is anastomosed end-to-side to the donor jejunum to achieve upper intestinal continuity. Interestingly, the recipient ends up with both the native and transplanted duodenum and pancreas which is important to remember should there be any complications involving these organs such as pancreatitis. Arterial inflow for the entire graft is usually achieved via the infrarenal aorta and outflow is via piggybacked anastomosis to the suprahepatic inferior vena cava (IVC). The native stomach, duodenum, pancreas, and spleen are drained via a native portosystemic shunt [7].

MVTx is indicated in cases where the stomach or duodenopancreatic complex requires replacement. In addition, MVTx is sometimes required due to vascular involvement with specific types of tumors or in cases of complete portomesenteric thrombosis. The MVTx graft is similar to the LITx graft but also includes the stomach and in some cases the spleen (Figure 17.3). When there is a

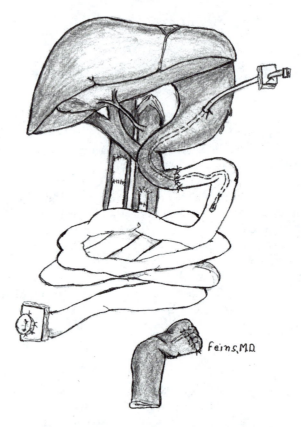

**FIGURE 17.1** Graphical depiction of an implanted isolated intestinal allograft.

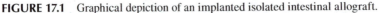

significant donor–recipient size discrepancy, the MVTx may be preferable over the LITx as it allows removal of more native organs and therefore creates more space. This is particularly true for very small infants. In a MVTx, the proximal gastrointestinal anastomosis is between the donor and recipient gastric fundus and a pyloroplasty must be performed as the stomach lacks vagal innervation. Vascular anastomoses are similar to those found in the LITx.

In the very select group of patients with IFALD who are close to achieving enteral autonomy, one can consider performing an isolated liver transplant. In some cases, portal hypertension secondary to end-stage liver disease may impair intestinal function and prevent weaning from PN. Botha et al. [24] describe liver transplantation alone in a cohort of 23 SBS children with partial enteral tolerance but end-stage liver disease secondary to IFALD. The children considered had enteral tolerance of at least 50%, age <2 years, no less than 25 cm of small bowel and no underlying intestinal mucosal or motility disorder. The reported patient and graft survival following isolated liver transplantation were 82%/75% at 1 year, and 72%/60% at 5 years, respectively. Fourteen of the 17 children alive at a median follow-up of 54 months had achieved enteral autonomy on average 3 months posttransplantation.

## 17.6  ORGAN ALLOCATION

In the United States, the deceased donor organ allocation system is managed by the United Network for Organ Sharing (UNOS). Patients are placed on each organ-specific allocation list and ranked according to specific national policies. For potential liver transplant recipients, the rank order is determined by an objective scoring system that estimates 3-month mortality risk based on the severity of liver disease. For adolescents and adults, the MELD (Model for End-Stage Liver Disease)

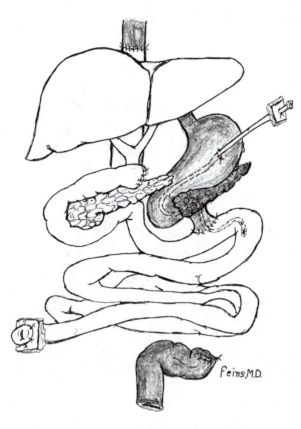

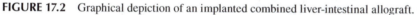

**FIGURE 17.2**  Graphical depiction of an implanted combined liver-intestinal allograft.

score is determined using three laboratory values: bilirubin, creatinine, and international normalized ratio (INR). For children <12 years old, the PELD (Pediatric End-Stage Liver Disease) score is calculated based on bilirubin, albumin, and INR values with a factor for growth impairment in children <1 year old.

The majority of patients in the United States listed for liver and intestine transplantation (83.1%) are in the pediatric age group [25]. Patients awaiting combined liver and intestine transplantation have one of the highest waitlist mortality rates of any organ. Chung et al. reported a waitlist mortality of 8.8% for those awaiting intestine only versus 29.8% for liver and intestine [25]. This mortality seems to be driven by the severity of the liver disease and is significantly more than that seen in children requiring isolated liver transplants at the equivalent PELD score. Therefore, when children are listed for both a liver and an intestine transplant, they are automatically granted an additional 23 PELD points which allows them a greater opportunity to be transplanted in a timely fashion. Those awaiting an isolated intestine transplant have a low mortality compared to liver–intestine patients. Since there is no scoring system for prioritizing intestine alone patients, the waitlist rank is determined by waiting time. Wait time has improved from a median of 313 days in 1999 to a median of 142 days in 2008 [26]. Pediatric patients have a longer wait time than adults [26].

## 17.7   POSTOPERATIVE MANAGEMENT

1. *Surgical Complications.* Potential technical complications after intestinal transplantation include bleeding, thrombosis, anastomotic leaks, bowel perforation, or loss of domain requiring temporary abdominal wall closure. Kato et al. found that 74 patients

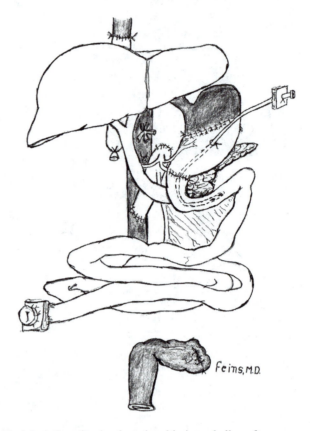

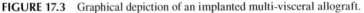

**FIGURE 17.3**    Graphical depiction of an implanted multi-visceral allograft.

of their group of 141 transplants required 107 reexplorations [27]. More recently a review of 500 transplants at one program reported a technical complication rate of 7.6% [28]. While technical complications were a significant source of morbidity and mortality in the early development of intestinal transplantation, recent improvements in surgical management have minimized the impact of technical problems on overall patient outcomes.

2. *Immunosuppression and Rejection.* The introduction of cyclosporine made intestinal rejection following transplantation manageable but there remained a very high rate of rejection with associated complications and mortality. Currently, most patients receive a tacrolimus-based maintenance immunosuppression regimen with or without additional agents including mycophenolate mofetil or steroids. Induction therapy with IL-2 receptor blockade or antithymocyte preparations have been shown to improve the 1-year patient and graft survival and are used by most programs [29]. Most recently, some centers have used Alemtuzumab (Campath) successfully as an induction agent or for treatment of acute rejection.

Acute cellular rejection (ACR) is one of the most common causes of patient death after intestinal transplantation [29]. It occurs most commonly in the first year after transplantation. ACR can develop rapidly and often presents with diarrhea or increased stomal output, fever, dehydration, nausea, and vomiting. Early diagnosis is crucial for graft salvage and many programs perform surveillance endoscopies and biopsies two to three times per week in the early postoperative period. Histologic criteria for the diagnosis of rejection have been established by Wu et al. [30] (Table 17.2). Mild-to-moderate

**TABLE 17.2**

**Histological Grade of Intestinal Allograft Rejection**

| Grade | Findings |
|---|---|
| Indeterminate | Changes insufficient for the diagnosis of mild acute rejection: minimal inflammatory infiltrate or crypt epithelial injury, increased crypt epithelial apoptosis (<6 apoptotic bodies/10 crypts), no mucosal ulceration |
| Mild ACR | Mild inflammatory infiltrate, mild crypt epithelial injury, increased crypt apoptosis (>6 apoptotic bodies/10 crypts) |
| Moderate ACR | Wide inflammatory infiltrate, diffuse crypt epithelial injury, increased crypt apoptosis, possible intimal arteritis |
| Severe ACR | Mucosal ulceration, possible severe intimal arteritis |

*Source:* Adapted from Wu T et al. *Transplantation* 2003;75:1241–8.

rejection is treated with high-dose steroids for 3–5 days and an increase in maintenance of immunosuppression. Severe rejection or episodes that have failed to respond to steroid pulse may receive antilymphocyte antibody therapy which has been shown to improve graft survival [31]. ACR is seen in 79% of intestine only patients versus 71% in liver–intestine recipients and 56% in multivisceral recipients, suggesting a beneficial effect from the liver [32]. Chronic rejection is not as common as ACR but the prevalence of this problem seems to have increased recently and may be related to improvements in overall graft survival. Isolated intestinal grafts appear to be at higher risk for chronic rejection, accounting for the observation that late isolated graft losses are more common in this group [33]. The hallmark of chronic rejection is microscopic evidence for arterial intimal hyperplasia with resultant ischemia and fibrosis that leads to the clinical inability of the bowel to perform its absorptive function [34].

As of yet there is no noninvasive clinical marker of acute or chronic rejection, although several potential markers are being actively investigated including fecal calprotectin, granzyme B, and perforin [35,36]. Citrulline, a serum marker of small bowel enterocyte mass, has shown some promise as such a noninvasive marker for ACR. David et al. reported decreased citrulline levels in patients with moderate or severe acute rejection [37].

3. *Infections.* Intestinal transplant patients appear to require higher levels of maintenance immunosuppression than other organ transplant recipients. Unfortunately, the result of this increased immunosuppression requirement is an increased incidence of bacterial, fungal, viral, and opportunistic infections [38]. Infection and sepsis continue to be the leading causes of death in intestinal transplant recipients [32]. In addition, pediatric patients have an increased risk of viral infections which is inversely related to their age, likely due to lack of prior exposure or development of immunity [39]. Most programs actively screen for cytomegalovirus (CMV), and some prophylactically treat with antiviral medication. In the past, most programs avoided CMV-positive donors but with the use of gancyclovir and other antiviral drugs CMV can now be successfully treated more than 90% of the time [38]. Other viral infections that are commonly seen in intestinal transplant patients include adenovirus and Epstein–Barr virus (EBV). Adenovirus can infect the intestinal graft resulting in diarrhea that can be difficult to distinguish from acute rejection. In some cases, even the pathology on intestinal biopsies can be misleading. Adenovirus can now be detected using polymerase chain reaction (PCR)

technology in both blood and stool specimens to assist in this differentiation so that appropriate treatment may be initiated.

EBV associated posttransplant lymphoproliferative disorder (PTLD) is a significant cause of morbidity and mortality in intestinal transplant patients. Doak et al. first described lymphoma after transplantation in a renal transplant recipient in 1968 [40]. The term PTLD was first used in 1984 by Starzl et al. [41]. PTLD encompasses a range of disease from Epstein–Barr virus proliferation to more aggressive proliferations which resemble lymphomas [42]. PTLD is usually associated with EBV but has been seen in EBV-negative patients. PCR monitoring for EBV replication is an effective method for early screening and detection of PTLD. Newly positive results or a significant increase in viral replication usually warrants additional evaluation for PTLD which can present as a mass in either donor or host organs. Presenting symptoms vary widely and can range from chronic diarrhea, weight loss, and nausea to low-grade fevers, lymphadenopathy, or a palpable mass [43]. Central nervous system involvement carries a poor prognosis and often presents with vague neurologic symptoms. Diagnosis often involves radiographic imaging studies including magnetic resonance imaging (MRI), computerized tomography (CT), or positron emission tomography (PET) scans. Treatment consists of reduction of immunosuppression and in cases with a predominance of CD20+ cells, monoclonal antibody therapy with rituximab may be beneficial [44]. PTLD that is unresponsive to these measures, or, which presents clinically or histologically like that of aggressive lymphoma may be more appropriately treated with chemotherapy [45].

4. *Graft versus Host Disease (GVHD)*. GVHD is not very common after intestinal transplantation despite the large amount of lymphoid tissue that is transplanted, although it is still more common than in other solid organ transplants. A recent series reported clinical GVHD in 8% and histologically confirmed GVHD in 6% of intestinal transplant recipients [28]. Although GVHD following bone marrow transplantation is often clinically significant, most cases of GVHD following solid organ transplantation are transient and easily treated. One of the differences in intestine transplant patients is that the target organs with the most morbidity have often been transplanted and are no longer potential targets for GVHD. Any transplanted intestine is not subject to injury by GVHD, but residual native stomach, intestine, or colon can be affected. In liver–intestine or multivisceral patients, the liver is also spared from GVHD. The diagnosis can often be made definitively by biopsy of native rectum. Skin is most commonly involved, manifest by papulo-macular rash on the hands, feet, trunk, and extremities [46]. GVHD can also target the lungs and bone marrow [46]. Treatment of mild GVHD with increased immunosuppression and bolus steroids is usually successful. Unfortunately, some cases are resistant to steroid treatment and may result in significant morbidity or mortality usually related to opportunistic infections associated with treatment for GVHD.

## 17.8   OUTCOMES

Short-term graft and patient survival have markedly improved since the early era of intestinal transplantation. In 1998, 1-year adjusted graft and patient survival was 52% and 69% respectively, while in 2007, the comparable values were 75% and 79% [26]. Multiple factors may be responsible for improvement, including donor selection, technical/graft preserving advances, the use of "induction" immunosuppression, and improved opportunistic infection monitoring and treatment. In comparison, long-term survival has not enjoyed similar improvements. The 2009 Organ Procurement and Transplantation Network report (based on US data) found that 10-year patient

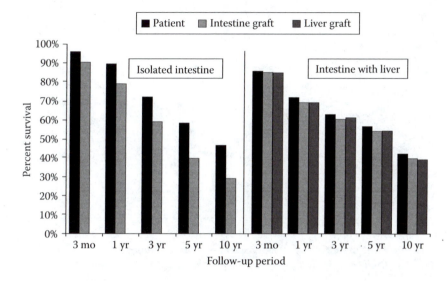

**FIGURE 17.4** Unadjusted patient and graft survival for isolated and combined liver-intestine transplant recipients. [Reprinted from Mazariegos GV et al. *Am J Transpl* 2010;10(4 Pt 2):1020–34. With permission.]

and graft survival for isolated intestinal transplants were 46%/29%, respectively, and 42%/39% for liver-inclusive grafts (Figure 17.4) [26]. Prior 10-year epochs have yielded similar survival statistics [10].

Single-center experiences demonstrate similar outcomes. The Pittsburgh group recently reported its work on 500 intestinal transplants, spanning 25 years and three "eras," defined by major shifts in the approach to immunosuppression. Patient survival during the latest era (2001–2008) was approximately 90% at 1-year, dropping to 80% at 3 years, and 70% by 5-years posttransplantation. The Pittsburgh pediatric experience is generally similar, with near 80% 5-year patient survival for combined liver/intestine recipients under the rATG protocol. Importantly, in this pediatric group, 5-year graft survival for isolated intestinal grafts appears qualitatively different: while 5-year patient survival is preserved (near 80%), graft survival is markedly lower at 56% [33]. The preponderance of chronic rejection in the isolated grafts may account for this difference, although this distinction was not observed in the overall experience [28].

Potential pretransplant factors that might be expected to predict outcomes include diagnosis, age at transplant, presence or absence of significant comorbidities, graft-type, and strategy for immunosuppression. In a multivariable analysis using these factors and typical demographic data, workers at the Intestinal Transplant Registry (2291 transplants during 1985–2009 and an estimated >95% of cases worldwide) found that center volume, out of hospital at time of match, and presence of a liver in graft predicted improved survival, while other factors were not predictive [10]. Abu-Elmagd et al. [28] have also reported a protective effect of the liver on graft survival. However, a similar analysis of UNOS data for pediatric transplants between 1991 and 2008 found that children who received liver-inclusive grafts may fare worse. Interestingly children with volvulus were significantly more likely to have improved long-term survival compared with other diagnoses (Figure 17.5) [47].

## 17.9  FINANCIAL CONSIDERATIONS

When outcomes on long-term PN and after intestinal transplantation become reasonably comparable, costs of therapy become more relevant. There is limited published data on this topic of interest to payers interested in maximizing benefit while attempting to control costs.

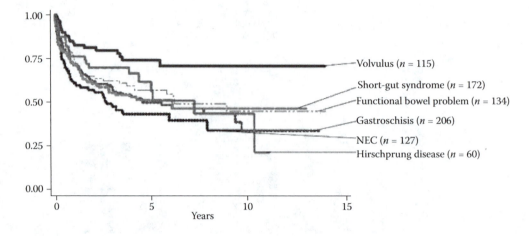

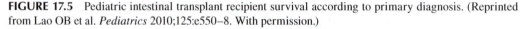

**FIGURE 17.5**  Pediatric intestinal transplant recipient survival according to primary diagnosis. (Reprinted from Lao OB et al. *Pediatrics* 2010;125:e550–8. With permission.)

In 2006, Sudan examined the costs associated with care at her institution. The estimated cost of an ITx is $132,285–135,000, LITx is $207,000–214,716, and MVTx is $219,098 [13]. Readmission after transplantation costs an average of $9792–23,500 per year and immunosup-pression medications are estimated at $12,000 per year. When comparing the cost of transplant versus continued PN therapy it appeared that with a functioning graft transplant was less costly after the initial year. Importantly, many recipients (up to 20% [ITR-2010 data]) do not have fully functioning grafts, meaning that they may be receiving intravenous (IV) supplementation; total costs after transplant would certainly be higher when including these recipients. The annual cost of PN therapy ranges from $75,000 to $150,000. This does not include the added cost of supplies, nursing, and hospitalizations that might be required for the treatment of PN-associated complications [13].

## 17.10  CONCLUSION

Intestinal transplantation has slowly evolved over the past 50 years. While intestinal transplantation has been viewed by many as an option of last resort for patients with IF, improved outcomes with both home PN and intestine transplant will result in more refined indications for these treatments. At this point, patients with IF should be carefully evaluated by a multidisciplinary group with a special interest in intestinal rehabilitation. Collaboration with and/or referral to an intestinal transplantation center should be considered early, so that the best decisions can be made after careful evaluation.

## REFERENCES

1. Mueller CB and Fischer HW. Transplantation of the ileum: An experimental study. *Surgery* 1951; 30:477–83.
2. Lillehei RC, Idezuki Y, Feemster JA et al. Transplantation of stomach, intestine, and pancreas: Experimental and clinical observations. *Surgery* 1967;62:721–41.
3. Dudrick SJ, Wilmore DW, Vars HM, and Rhoads JE. Long-term total parenteral nutrition with growth, development, and positive nitrogen balance. *Surgery* 1968;64:134–42.
4. Diliz-Perez HS, McClure J, Bedetti C et al. Successful small bowel allotransplantation in dogs with cyclosporine and prednisone. *Transplantation* 1984;37:126–9.
5. Pritchard TJ and Kirkman RL. Small bowel transplantation. *World J Surg* 1985;9:860–7.
6. Starzl TE, Weil R III, Iwatsuki S et al. The use of cyclosporin A and prednisone in cadaver kidney transplantation. *Surg Gynecol Obstet* 1980;151:17–26.

7. Grant D, Wall W, Mimeault R et al. Successful small-bowel/liver transplantation. *Lancet* 1990;335:181–4.

8. Todo S, Tzakis AG, Abu-Elmagd K et al. Cadaveric small bowel and small bowel-liver transplantation in humans. *Transplantation* 1992;53:369–76.

9. Kaufman SS, Atkinson JB, Bianchi A et al. Indications for pediatric intestinal transplantation: A position paper of the American Society of Transplantation. *Pediatr Transplant* 2001;5:80–7.

10. Registry IT. Intestine Transplant Registry: 25 Years of follow up. In: XI International Small Bowel Transplant Symposium. 2009; Bologna, Italy.

11. Abu-Elmagd KM. Intestinal transplantation for short bowel syndrome and gastrointestinal failure: Current consensus, rewarding outcomes, and practical guidelines. *Gastroenterology* 2006;130(2 Suppl 1):S132–7.

12. Howard L and Hassan N. Home parenteral nutrition. 25 years later. *Gastroenterol Clin North Am* 1998;27:481–512.

13. Sudan D. Cost and quality of life after intestinal transplantation. *Gastroenterology* 2006;130(2 Suppl 1):S158–62.

14. DeLegge M, Alsolaiman MM, Barbour E et al. Short bowel syndrome: Parenteral nutrition versus intestinal transplantation. Where are we today? *Dig Dis Sci* 2007;52:876–92.

15. Chan S, McCowen KC, Bistrian BR et al. Incidence, prognosis, and etiology of end-stage liver disease in patients receiving home total parenteral nutrition. *Surgery* 1999;126:28–34.

16. Kelly DA. Liver complications of pediatric parenteral nutrition–epidemiology. *Nutrition* 1998;14:153–7.

17. Colomb V, Dabbas-Tyan M, Taupin P et al. Long-term outcome of children receiving home parenteral nutrition: A 20-year single-center experience in 302 patients. *J Pediatr Gastroenterol Nutr* 2007;44:347–53.

18. Goulet O, Joly F, Corriol O, and Colomb-Jung V. Some new insights in intestinal failure-associated liver disease. *Curr Opin Organ Transplant* 2009;14:256–61.

19. Kaufman SS, Pehlivanova M, Fennelly EM et al. Predicting liver failure in parenteral nutrition-dependent short bowel syndrome of infancy. *J Pediatr* 2010;156:580–5 e1.

20. Lopushinsky SR, Fowler RA, Kulkarni GS et al. The optimal timing of intestinal transplantation for children with intestinal failure: A Markov analysis. *Ann Surg* 2007;246:1092–9.

21. Beath S, Pironi L, Gabe S et al. Collaborative strategies to reduce mortality and morbidity in patients with chronic intestinal failure including those who are referred for small bowel transplantation. *Transplantation* 2008;85:1378–84.

22. Buchman AL, Scolapio J, and Fryer J. AGA technical review on short bowel syndrome and intestinal transplantation. *Gastroenterology* 2003;124:1111–34.

23. Sudan DL, Iyer KR, and Deroover A. A new technique for combined liver/small intestinal transplantation. *Transplantation* 2001;72:1846–8.

24. Botha JF, Grant WJ, Torres C et al. Isolated liver transplantation in infants with end-stage liver disease due to short bowel syndrome. *Liver Transpl* 2006;12:1062–6.

25. Chungfat N, Dixler I, Cohran V et al. Impact of parenteral nutrition-associated liver disease on intestinal transplant waitlist dynamics. *J Am Coll Surg* 2007;205:755–61.

26. Mazariegos GV, Steffick DE, Horslen S et al. Intestine transplantation in the United States, 1999–2008. *Am J Transpl* 2010;10(4 Pt 2):1020–34.

27. Kato T, Tzakis AG, Selvaggi G et al. Intestinal and multivisceral transplantation in children. *Ann Surg* 2006;243:756–64; discussion 764–6.

28. Abu-Elmagd KM, Costa G, Bond GJ et al. Five hundred intestinal and multivisceral transplantations at a single center: Major advances with new challenges. *Ann Surg* 2009;4:567–81 [Epub ahead of print].

29. Vianna RM and Mangus RS. Present prospects and future perspectives of intestinal and multivisceral transplantation. *Curr Opin Clin Nutr Metab Care* 2009;12:281–6.

30. Wu T, Abu-Elmagd K, Bond G et al. A schema for histologic grading of small intestine allograft acute rejection. *Transplantation* 2003;75:1241–8.

31. Selvaggi G, Gaynor JJ, Moon J et al. Analysis of acute cellular rejection episodes in recipients of primary intestinal transplantation: A single center, 11-year experience. *Am J Transpl* 2007;7:1249–57.

32. Fryer JP. The current status of intestinal transplantation. *Curr Opin Organ Transplant* 2008;13:266–72.

33. Nayyar N, Mazariegos G, Ranganathan S et al. Pediatric small bowel transplantation. *Semin Pediatr Surg* 2010;19:68–77.

34. Tryphonopoulos P, Weppler D, Nishida S et al. Mucosal fibrosis in intestinal transplant biopsies correlates positively with the development of chronic rejection. *Transpl Proc* 2006;38:1685–6.

35. Altimari A, Gruppioni E, Capizzi E et al. Blood monitoring of granzyme B and perforin expression after intestinal transplantation: Considerations on clinical relevance. *Transplantation* 2008;85:1778–83.
36. Akpinar E, Vargas J, Kato T et al. Fecal calprotectin level measurements in small bowel allograft monitoring: A pilot study. *Transplantation* 2008;85:1281–6.
37. David AI, Gaynor JJ, Zis PP et al. An association of lower serum citrulline levels within 30 days of acute rejection in patients following small intestine transplantation. *Transpl Proc* 2006;38:1731–2.
38. Hauser GJ, Kaufman SS, Matsumoto CS, and Fishbein TM. Pediatric intestinal and multivisceral transplantation: A new challenge for the pediatric intensivist. *Intensive Care Med* 2008;34:1570–9.
39. Kato T, Gaynor JJ, Selvaggi G et al. Intestinal transplantation in children: A summary of clinical outcomes and prognostic factors in 108 patients from a single center. *J Gastrointest Surg* 2005;9:75–89; discussion 89.
40. Doak PB, Duke AJ, Maclaurin CH et al. Two years experience with renal transplantation. *N Z Med J* 1968;68:221–7.
41. Starzl TE, Nalesnik MA, Porter KA et al. Reversibility of lymphomas and lymphoproliferative lesions developing under cyclosporin-steroid therapy. *Lancet* 1984;1:583–7.
42. Bakker NA, van Imhoff GW, Verschuuren EA, and van Son WJ. Presentation and early detection of post-transplant lymphoproliferative disorder after solid organ transplantation. *Transpl Int* 2007;20:207–18.
43. Selvaggi G and Tzakis AG. Intestinal and multivisceral transplantation: Future perspectives. *Front Biosci* 2007;12:4742–54.
44. Svoboda J, Kotloff R, and Tsai DE. Management of patients with post-transplant lymphoproliferative disorder: The role of rituximab. *Transpl Int* 2006;19:259–69.
45. Parker A, Bowles K, Bradley JA et al. Management of post-transplant lymphoproliferative disorder in adult solid organ transplant recipients - BCSH and BTS guidelines. *Br J Haematol* 2010;149:693–705.
46. Mazariegos GV, Abu-Elmagd K, Jaffe R et al. Graft versus host disease in intestinal transplantation. *Am J Transpl* 2004;4:1459–65.
47. Lao OB, Healey PJ, Perkins JD et al. Outcomes in children after intestinal transplant. *Pediatrics* 2010;125:e550–8.

# 18 Critical Care Management

*Nilesh M. Mehta*

## CONTENTS

## 18.1 INTRODUCTION

Children with intestinal failure (IF) may require admission to the pediatric intensive care unit (PICU) at various times during their illness course. With the advent of intestinal and multivisceral transplants at major centers in the United States, pediatric intensivists will frequently care for patients with intestinal and liver failure. More than 200 intestinal transplants are performed in the United States every year (Organ Procurement and Transplantation Website: http://www.optn.org/latestData/step2.asp), and many children are listed and awaiting transplantation in various stages of their illness. Table 18.1 describes the common scenarios when patients with IF require admission to the PICU.

Management in the critical care unit, including during the rehabilitation process or in the pre- or posttransplantation settings, is complex or requires a multidisciplinary effort to achieve favorable outcomes. The pediatric intensivist is an important member of the IF and the multivisceral transplant team. The liaison between the transplant team and the intensivist is critical and must be initiated in advance. This chapter describes some of the common management scenarios and approach to managing a child with IF in the PICU.

**TABLE 18.1**

**Common Scenarios Where Children with Intestinal Failure Require Admission to the PICU**

1. Management of complications in children with intestinal failure awaiting intestinal transplantation—for example, stomal bleeding, fluid and electrolyte imbalance, respiratory insufficiency.
2. Children with liver failure presenting with neurologic, hemorrhagic (GI bleeding) complications.
3. Sepsis, catheter-related blood stream infection (CRBSI) or multisystem failure.
4. Recovery from autologous reconstructive gastrointestinal surgical procedures.
5. Management of peritransplantation complications following intestinal or multivisceral transplantation.

## 18.2  THE PRETRANSPLANTATION PERIOD

### 18.2.1  PREOPERATIVE MANAGEMENT OF CHILDREN AWAITING INTESTINAL TRANSPLANTATION

Despite rising number of intestinal and multivisceral transplants being performed every year, there remains a deficiency of suitable donors to meet the number of children requiring transplants. As a result, a significant number of children at various stages of organ failure are listed and await transplantation. A significant proportion of children die on the transplant wait list, the majority of whom are less than 1 year old and weigh less than 10 kg.[1] These patients are characterized by marginal organ function with morbidity acquired due to long-term reliance on parenteral nutrition (PN), malnutrition, liver failure, and underlying chronic respiratory insufficiency. Thus, they are frequent consumers of the PICU services, where they present for a myriad of reasons requiring multidisciplinary support (Table 18.1).

The challenge for the intensive care team is to support compromised organ function and manage complications during this prolonged wait for a suitable graft. Principles of management include optimization of respiratory status, minimization of ventilator-induced lung injury, careful attention to fluid and electrolyte balance and maintenance of adequate perfusion, preservation of residual liver function, and maintenance of hemodynamic stability in the setting of capillary leak while avoiding edema due to fluid overload and hypoalbuminemia.

### 18.2.2  BLEEDING FROM STOMA

Many infants with IF have surgical stoma sites and are at risk of bleeding from these sites. Parenteral nutrition associated liver disease (PNALD)[2] with portal hypertension and thrombocytopenia, predisposes them to the risk of bleeding from the mucocutaneous junction of gastrostomy, ileostomy, or entero-cutaneous fistulae. Stomal bleeding is addressed by prudent stoma care in liaison with the general surgical team. Commonly used techniques for cessation of stomal bleeding include application of direct pressure and the use of chemical or electrical cauterization. Chronic stoma blood loss may result in fluid shifts, anemia, and hypovolemic shock. Ongoing stomal bleeding may necessitate frequent transfusions of blood products with all their associated complications, including sodium and volume overload as well as pulmonary hypertension. These complications must be promptly assessed and managed as they can progress to multisystem failure and require intensive care.

### 18.2.3  UPPER GASTROINTESTINAL BLEEDING

Acute variceal bleeding remains relatively uncommon in patients with isolated IF. However, in patients with advanced liver disease, bleeding from large esophagogastric, gastric, or peristomal varices can be devastating. Jaundice, easy bruising, and changes in stool color may signal underlying liver disease. Emergent management of severe upper gastrointestinal (GI) bleeding involves prompt rehydration and volume support. Blood transfusion must be provided while attempting to stem the source of bleeding. In patients with bleeding and hemodynamic instability, access with two large-bore intravenous catheters must be obtained as a priority. When venous access is difficult, either due to hemodynamic collapse or peripheral vasoconstriction, access to the intraosseus space must be promptly obtained using a special intraosseous needle or an intraosseous gun. Airway protection with endotracheal intubation must be provided early, and is often difficult in the setting of acute bleeding. Consultation with the gastroenterologist must be sought for consideration of upper gastrointestinal endoscopy. Endoscopic visualization of the bleeding site and hemostasis may be life saving but its application may be limited during severe ongoing bleeding. Gastroenterologists may be able to achieve endoscopic control of active hemorrhage with sclerotherapy or with elastic ligature. Occasionally a transjugular intrahepatic portosystemic shunt (TIPS) procedure may be considered.[3] If endoscopic procedure is not feasible due to the massive bleeding, special upper gastroenterology devices such as the Sengstaken–Blakemore balloon may be placed for temporary tamponade.[4] The device is not available in smaller sizes and hence its use is limited to older children.

Medical management of upper GI bleeding includes acid suppressive therapies and hormonal analogues. Combination of acid-suppressing drugs is used to neutralize gastric acidity and increases pH of stomach and duodenal bulb. Ranitidine inhibits histamine stimulation of H2 receptor in gastric parietal cells, which reduces gastric acid secretion, gastric volume, and hydrogen ion concentrations. Famotidine competitively inhibits histamine at H2 receptor of gastric parietal cells. Proton pump inhibitors (PPI) such as pantoprazole have been used as a continuous infusion with some success for upper GI bleeding, especially in patients with gastric bleeding.[5] In patients with acute bleeding from peptic ulcer, PPI treatment initiated prior to endoscopy in upper GI bleeding significantly reduces the proportion of patients with stigmata of recent hemorrhage at index endoscopy but does not reduce mortality, rebleeding or the need for surgery. For bleeding from esophageal varices, pharmacologic treatment to reduce portal pressure is important. Although propranolol has been studied in adults for both primary and secondary prophylaxis of esophageal varices, studies in children are limited. In addition, vasopressin had been used as a splanchnic vasoconstrictor, but its many adverse effects (e.g., bowel-wall or cutaneous ischemia, hypertension, abdominal pain) have made it less desirable than other options, even when tempered with the vaso-dilatory effects of nitroglycerin. As a result, octreotide has emerged as the recommended treatment, especially in conjunction with sclerotherapy for patients with variceal bleeding. Octreotide is a synthetic polypeptide, which acts as a natural somatostatin and has the added advantage of being more resistant to enzymatic degradation and therefore has a longer half-life in circulation than somatostatin.[6] Some early literature suggests that, for GI bleeds a dose of 1 μg/kg IV bolus, then 1 μg/kg/h continuous IV infusion is reasonable. The infusion rate should be titrated to response with the dose tapered by 50% every 12 h when no active bleeding occurs for 24 h. The medication can be discontinued when the dose reaches 25% of the initial dose and bleeding has ceased.

Other modalities of treatment for severe esophageal varices that are not commonly used include fibrin sealants or tissue glues such as cyanoacrylate, as well as electrocoagulation with argon plasma coagulation. When significant GI bleeding cannot be controlled by the use of the previously mentioned medical or endoscopic techniques, surgical intervention including laparoscopy may be required. Of note, slow GI bleeding may remain occult in the pediatric population and careful monitoring of hematocrit levels will allow early detection of blood loss.

## 18.2.4  FLUID AND ELECTROLYTE IMBALANCE

The major problems following established short bowel syndrome are related to fluid or electrolyte imbalance; deficiencies in calcium, magnesium, zinc, and vitamins A, D, E, K, and B$_{12}$;

hypergastrinemia; bile salt depletion, protein-calorie malnutrition; pancreatic maldigestion; and oxalate nephrolithiasis. Patients with ileal resection and ileostomies lose large amounts of fecal sodium (85–180 mmol/day), inevitably resulting in chronic sodium depletion, dehydration, and hyperaldosteronism.[7] Diuretics and supplemental electrolytes are frequently required during the management of children with IF. Acute renal failure may complicate the course of some of these patients due to sodium and fluid depletion or sepsis. Metabolic acidosis may arise from excessive GI bicarbonate loss (normal anion gap or hyperchloremic metabolic acidosis) and is compounded by impaired renal homeostasis caused by profound salt and water depletion. D-lactic metabolic acidosis (a raised anion gap metabolic acidosis) is caused by malabsorption of carbohydrate in the small intestine, which is then fermented and leads to accumulation of the D-isomer of lactic acid. Furthermore, disturbances of calcium and magnesium homeostasis have been reported.[8]

Management of fluid and electrolyte losses may require intravenous replacement of fluids and sodium. Intravascular fluid status can be difficult to assess in the setting of inflammation and capillary leak. Daily weights, careful monitoring of fluid balance, and serum chemistry allows judicious fluid and electrolyte replacement strategy. Judicious supplementation of sodium and isotonic fluids will help correct sodium homeostasis; urine sodium concentrations lower than 10 mEq/L suggest sodium depletion. Intravenous replacement is invariably required initially, but in the long term oral sodium supplements (tablets or solutions) usually suffice. In some cases long-term parenteral therapy is required. Antimotility agents such as loperamide may help reduce fecal losses of water and electrolytes. In a subset of patients with sepsis presenting with shock, management involves prompt and aggressive rehydration with crystalloids and often requires vasoactive drugs to maintain mean arterial pressure and preserve organ perfusion.

## 18.2.5   VENTILATOR SUPPORT FOR RESPIRATORY INSUFFICIENCY

Infants with IF may present in frank respiratory failure or are dependent on ventilatory support for chronic lung disease of prematurity. Management of acute respiratory insufficiency in this population involves the use of prudent ventilator strategy for optimal oxygenation and ventilation, while preventing ventilator-induced lung injury (VILI). Prolonged ventilation is associated with complications such as ventilator-associated pneumonia and ventilator-induced lung injury. On the one hand, patients must be weaned from the ventilator as soon as it is feasible. However, premature extubation is associated with significantly higher mortality. Centers must review their mechanical ventilation practice and adopt evidence-based prudent strategies to minimize harm. Respiratory care is a complex and interdisciplinary process, which is fraught with variability in practice. Development of protocols based on evidence or consensus for benefit may reduce variability in practice, optimize coordinated care, and potentially improve patient outcomes. For example, nonrespiratory interventions such as sedation protocols have been shown to decrease duration of mechanical ventilation, length of stay, and complications in adults.[9]

Acute lung injury affects over 150,000 adults in the United States each year, with mortality close to 50%. In the PICU, approximately 17% of all admissions require mechanical ventilation with overall mortality much lower than adults, at 1.6%. However, mortality is much higher in a subgroup of children with acute respiratory distress syndrome (ARDS) especially in high-risk patient groups. Recently, lung-protective ventilatory strategies have been adopted with the goal of minimizing lung damage secondary to mechanical ventilation. In 1999, a landmark trial in critically ill adults with ARDS, showed a dramatic decrease in mortality in patients with low-tidal volume (6 mL/kg) ventilation compared to those with high tidal volumes (12 mL/kg).[10] Low tidal volume ventilation strategy decreased mortality by 22% in this study, which has significantly influenced pediatric mechanical ventilation strategies. The principle behind lung protective ventilation is to prevent or minimize VILI secondary to high tidal volumes (volutrauma) by using low tidal volumes; and due to repeated shear forces during opening and complete collapse of lungs (atelectrauma) by applying prudent positive end expiratory pressure (PEEP).[11] Optimal PEEP remains elusive and the intensivist uses surrogates such as oxygenation to determine an optimal level. The aim is to open the lung (recruitment) and then to keep it open (prevent lung collapse with PEEP application).

Patients with IF may require high frequency oscillatory ventilation (HFOV). HFOV allows the use of low tidal volumes with enhanced lung recruitment and prevents biotrauma (from alveolar shear injury). There are limited data on HFOV use in the pediatric population and its mortality benefits have not been shown.[12] The use of HFOV remains center specific and in some centers, up to one-third of mechanically ventilated children are exposed to HFOV.[13]

### 18.2.6 SEPSIS/SHOCK

Children with IF may present with distributive shock secondary to infections, especially catheter-related blood stream infections. Children with IF are also more susceptible to hypovolemic shock due to chronic and severe obligatory GI fluid losses; intercurrent GI or other infections can commonly result in life-threatening hypovolemia. Tissue perfusion is critically altered due to an imbalance between oxygen supply and oxygen demand in shock. Reduced delivery of oxygen and other nutrients to the tissue beds results in cellular dysfunction, which manifests as organ dysfunction. The decreased substrate delivery to the tissues may be due to low cardiac output as seen in hemorrhagic or cardiogenic shock, or due to maldistribution of blood volume as seen in vasodilatory or septic shock. The expedient recognition and correction of tissue dysoxia may limit organ dysfunction, reduce complications, and improve outcome.[14]

Recently, the concept of early goal-directed therapy has been adopted with the aim of improving outcomes in patients. In an emergency department-based therapeutic protocol, Rivers et al. randomized 263 adult patients with features of systemic inflammatory response syndrome (SIRS) and hypotension to receive either standard hemodynamic support (control group) or goal-directed therapy (intervention group) aimed at optimizing blood pressure and mixed venous oxygen saturation (cvSO2) during the first 6 h after presentation.[15] In-hospital mortality in the intervention group was 30% versus 46.5% in the control group. Central venous saturation ($ScvO_2$) substituted for mixed venous saturation, was used as an end-point, and patients received packed red cell transfusion to maintain $ScvO_2$ >70%. In a review of randomized control trials examining the role of goal-directed therapy in shock, studies were divided into groups based on the timing of the implementation of goals— "Early" (8–12 h postoperative or before organ failure was expected) versus "Late" (after onset of organ failure).[16] Increase in cardiac index (CI) and oxygen delivery ($DO_2$) with pulmonary artery occlusion pressure (PAOP) <18 were commonly used goals for increasing oxygen delivery in these studies. When implemented early and aggressively, goal-directed therapy was associated with reduced mortality and the prevalence of organ failure rates in acute posttrauma and postoperative states.

Goal-directed therapy for shock is ineffective in the late stages after onset of organ failure, and may even be harmful. Oxygen debt may be irreversible at this stage and attempts at increasing $O_2$ transport are futile. Thus, it appears that early optimization of hemodynamic parameters in critically ill patients with shock may improve outcomes if implemented before the onset of organ failure. Figure 18.1 shows a timeline for intervention in patients with shock.[17] Clinicians aiming to optimize tissue perfusion at the bedside have to take into account (a) the available inotropic or vasopressor drugs and their individual effects, (b) the available monitoring parameters and their application as end points of resuscitation, and finally (c) the evidence base for benefits of providing hemodynamic support.

Vasopressors are drugs that induce vasoconstriction and elevate arterial blood pressure. Although pure vasopressors do not increase cardiac contractility (inotropy), certain drugs possess both a vasopressor and inotropic effect. Vasopressors are indicated in maldistributive shock where hypotension persists despite adequate fluid resuscitation, associated with global indices of tissue hypoperfusion. Hypovolemia must be corrected before the institution of vasopressor therapy. Inotropes are drugs that

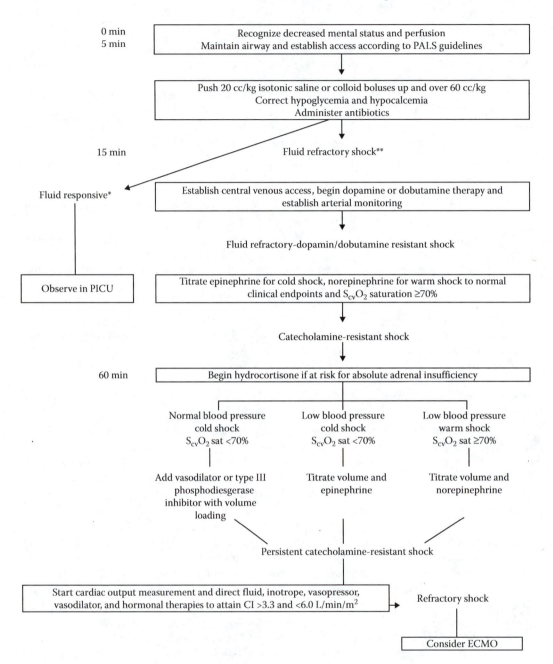

**FIGURE 18.1** Recommendations for step-wise hemodynamic support in critically ill infants and children with shock. (Adapted from Carcillo JA, Fields AI. *Crit Care Med.* 2002;30:1365–78.)

increase stroke volume by altering the contractile state of the ventricle. Cardiac muscle has the ability to alter its inotropy (contractility) and effect a change in stroke volume, independent of preload. The two main groups of inotropic drugs are: (a) sympathomimetic amines and (b) phosphodiesterase inhibitors. Many commonly available drugs have properties of both inotropy and vasopressor effect. The choice of an appropriate drug will depend on the etiology of shock (Table 18.2). Common drugs used in pediatric shock include norepinephrine, epinephrine, dopamine, dobutamine, phenylephrine, and vasopressin.

**TABLE 18.2**

**Commonly Used Drugs for Management of Shock in the PICU**

| Drug Class | Properties | Dopamine | Dobutamine | Epinephrine | Norepinephrine | Milrone | Vasopressin |
|---|---|---|---|---|---|---|---|
| Inotropes | Increase cardiac contractility and often heart rate | ++ | ++ | ++ | + | | |
| Vasopressors | Increase vascular resistance and blood pressure | + | | ++ | ++ | | + |
| Inodilators | Increase cardiac contractility and reduce afterload | | | | | + | |

Due to the complexity of pathophysiology of the heterogeneous group of shock states, few clear recommendations for monitoring end points and selection of appropriate therapies can be made. In hemorrhagic, hypovolemic, or vasodilatory shock, initial resuscitation must focus on adequate fluid resuscitation, which improves preload and hence cardiac output. Optimal fluid replacement, guided by traditional cardiac-filling measures such as central venous pressure must be achieved as a priority. In patients not responsive to fluid resuscitation, inotropes and/or vasopressor agents may be employed. Adequate fluid resuscitation is a prerequisite for the successful use of vasopressors. The current pediatric advanced life support (PALS) guidelines recommend a bolus volume of 20 mL/kg, which may be given rapidly (over 5–10 min) in cases of severe hypovolemic shock. If severe myocardial dysfunction is suspected, as in cases of toxicity (calcium channel blocker, beta adrenergic blocker) 5–10 mL/kg boluses may be given at a slower rate. In all cases, the clinician must assess the child's response to the fluid bolus and consider repeating as required. The nature of fluid (crystalloid vs. colloid) used for resuscitation has been debated and a recently conducted trial comparing the two showed no significant differences in outcome.[18] In hemorrhagic shock, 2–3 boluses of crystalloid (40 mL/kg) may be followed by blood transfusion for further fluid replacement. In septic shock, vascular tone alterations are heterogeneous and ideally, drugs that improve microcirculation in select regions are desirable. Commonly used vasopressors in the pediatric intensive care include dopamine, norepinephrine, epinephrine, and more recently, vasopressin. These drugs are administered intravenously in an infusion and titrated to the desired effect.

In summary, clinicians utilize a variety of vasomodulatory and inotropic drugs to improve cardiac output with an aim to maintain critical tissue perfusion. Prompt and prudent fluid resuscitation is a prerequisite for using these drugs and each intervention must be evaluated for patient responsiveness. Using available markers of tissue perfusion in combination with clinical end points, therapy is titrated with an aim to optimize tissue perfusion parameters. The timing of achieving these hemodynamic goals is likely to be critical in influencing outcomes and achieving supraphysiological levels may be harmful. In resistant cases, other supportive therapies such as corticosteroids and extracorporeal membrane oxygenation (ECMO) support may be useful.

### 18.2.7 Catheter-Related Infections in Children with Intestinal Failure in the PICU

Catheter related blood stream infection (CRBSI) increases cost and the length of stay in the hospital. CRBSI is a major cause of morbidity and mortality in patients with IF, which is potentially preventable.[19] Children with IF require extended periods of PN during the process of intestinal adaptation or when awaiting intestinal transplant. Surgically placed central venous catheters facilitate home administration of PN and are crucial for supportive therapy during posttransplant rehabilitation. However, these catheters need to be accessed with great care using strict sterile precautions to avoid the complication of CRBSI.[20] Catheters may become colonized with pathogenic bacteria, and result in bacteremia, sepsis, multiorgan dysfunction, and even death. The treatment of CRBSI involves prolonged courses of antimicrobial therapy and in some cases, removal of the catheter.

Hermans et al.[21] suggested that the risk factor for further liver damage in the cholestatic PN-dependent patient is increased when septicemia occurs before 4 or 6 weeks of life. The endotoxins released with a bacterial infection cause an inflammatory response that leads to scarring and liver fibrosis. A risk factor may be related to an initial infection with Gram-negative *Bacillus*. Sondheimer et al.[22] also reported that cholestasis was developed shortly after the first infection in 90% of PN-dependent patients with IF. Cholestasis was most common in the Gram-negative, pneumococcal, and *Candida* infections. Hence, a comprehensive approach to the prevention of CRBSI is warranted in the IF patient dependent on PN for survival. Although some CRBSIs result from translocation of microorganisms from the intestine into the bloodstream, most infections are acquired due to lack of sterile precautions during insertion or are related to contamination during the process of accessing the catheters. Strict aseptic precautions and standardized procedures for placement and access of catheters are critical. Preventive interventions, demonstrated to be effective in preventing CRBSI, include training all persons involved in central venous catheter (CVC) placement, care, and catheter access along with monitoring of adherence to established guidelines.[23]

## 18.2.8 Prevention of CRBSI in the PICU

Prevention of CRBSI is one the most important goals of critical care. Implementation of education programs to train those who insert and maintain catheters is a key intervention in any PICU. Evidence-based catheter practices promote the use of increased sterile barrier precautions during insertion with the use of chlorhexedine for skin disinfection prior to insertion. The Centers for Disease Control and Prevention (CDC) guidelines recommend dressing changes every 7 days or when soiled or loosened. Intravenous tubing should be changed within 24 h of starting infusion of lipids or blood products. Staff education on best practice with CVC care and maintenance has proven to reduce complications and improve patient outcomes.[24]

Selection of the CVC site could be an important factor in reducing CRBSIs as well. There are limited data for site selection for catheter placement in the pediatric population, as compared with the adult population. Advantages for use of the femoral site include easily identifiable landmarks and avoidance of pneumothorax, hemothorax, and carotid artery perforation. Arterial puncture, hematoma, leg edema, and thrombosis are the most common complications of femoral-line placement.[25] In children, there is a lower incidence of mechanical complication in the femoral site. Although placing a CVC in the femoral site may be easier and safer especially in the ICU setting when access of often need emergently, higher rates of bacterial colonization are noted when compared with subclavian or internal jugular sites.[26]

CRBSI may be reduced with certain antibiotic- or antiseptic-impregnated catheters in adult patients.[25] The first-generation catheters are externally impregnated with chlorhexidine/silver sulfadiazine. Second-generation catheters contain chlorhexidine coating on the internal and external surfaces. These catheters have been approved for use in infants and children weighing 3 kg or more by the Food and Drug Administration (FDA). Minocycline- and rifampin-internally and externally impregnated catheters are now commercially available and may lower the incidence of infection when compared to the first-generation antibiotic-impregnated catheters.[24] The antimicrobial effects, however, last no more than 28 days and therefore would offer little advantage to IF patients who require long-term catheter placement.

The use of a chlorhexidine-impregnated sponge dressing at the insertion site also showed a three-fold reduction in CRBSIs. These dressings can cause irritation at the site for very low birth-weight neonates but were found to be helpful in the pediatric and high-risk adult patients. Antibiotic ointments applied to the catheter site have shown an increase in catheter colonization by fungi and promote the incidence of antibiotic-resistant bacteria. The use of antibiotic ointment has not shown to decrease the incidence or CRBSIs. At our institution the use of chlorhexidine-impregnated sponge is standard and antibiotic ointments are discouraged.

Ethanol-lock and antibiotic-lock techniques have been used to prevent and treat CRBSIs. The use of ethanol-lock technique with systemic antibiotics was compared to the use of systemic antibiotics alone in 28 pediatric oncology patients with CVC infection.[27] Sixty-seven percent of those treated with the combined therapy had no infectious relapse in a 4-week period after treatment as compared to 47% of those treated with only systemic antibiotics. Onland et al.[28] used an ethanol-lock treatment with systemic antibiotics in 40 children with long-term CVC use for diverse reasons. Their retrospective report demonstrates 88% clearance without recurrence in a 30-day period after therapy. Jones et al.[29] have also demonstrated the safety and efficacy of ethanol lock therapy administered three days per week in reducing the rate of CVC infections in PN-dependent children with IF. Onder et al.[30] reported that tobramycin and tissue-plasminogen activator as prophylactic CVC treatment decreased the episodes of CRBSIs.

In summary, it is imperative to prevent CRBSI in the PN-dependent child. Key factors include consistently following the CDC guidelines for catheter placement, care, and maintenance. This requires education at multiple levels, including the hospital staff and home-care teams. Serious consideration of CVC site with regards to severity of illness, age of the patient, and presence of body secretions with avoidance of the femoral site is warranted. The use of prophylactic ethanol-lock techniques and medication-impregnated hubs appear promising to prevent CRBSI and require further multicenter clinical trials. Continual reassessment of the need for the CVC is an important strategy for limiting the duration of CVC use in this population.

### 18.2.9   MANAGEMENT OF A CHILD WITH END-STAGE LIVER FAILURE

Children with liver cell failure who are admitted to the PICU may require medical management to preserve residual function, or have advanced liver failure necessitating transplant.[31] Acute liver failure is characterized by the onset of hepatic encephalopathy within 8 weeks after the development of jaundice in a patient with no underlying liver disease. The incidence of fulminant liver failure in children requiring liver transplantation is approximately 10–15% in most transplant centers. Without transplantation, the outcome of fulminant liver failure in children is uniformly fatal, secondary to neurologic complications or multiorgan failure.[32] Criteria used for predicting outcome in adult patients with acute liver failure (ALF) are not applicable in children as it is not practical.[33] Children < 2 years old have a poorer prognosis in acute liver failure and also after transplantation compared with older children and adults.

Irreversible neurological disease remains a major cause of death in children with ALF. The importance of protecting and supporting the patient medically to avoid irreversible neurological changes until transplantation remains a major consideration in their outcome. While delayed development of encephalopathy is recognized as a bad prognostic indicator in acute liver failure, encephalopathy in children can be difficult to assess, especially in the infant and toddler age group. Physicians may be lulled into a false sense of security when the child seems neurologically normal despite very poor liver function tests.

### 18.2.10   HEPATOPULMONARY SYNDROME

Hepatopulmonary syndrome (HPS) is characterized by the triad of liver disease, arterial hypoxemia due to abnormalities in pulmonary gas exchange, and widespread pulmonary vascular dilatation.[34] The prevalence of HPS in children with liver disease is reported between 2% and 8%.[35] Formerly, a contraindication to liver transplant (LT), HPS is now considered a relative indication for orthotopic LT. The condition must be suspected in children with liver disease manifesting with clinical signs and symptoms of hypoxemia, such as cyanosis, digital clubbing, and dyspnea. This presentation can be confused with reactive airway disease or exercise-induced asthma and hence a high index of suspicion is necessary to make the diagnosis. Arterial blood $PaO_2$ in room air at rest, cutaneous oxygen saturation ($SaO_2$) and cardiopulmonary assessment (chest x-ray, electrocardiogram, and echocardiogram) assist in determining the degree of hypoxemia. Measurement of $SaO_2$ is a simple, reliable, and painless method to evaluate blood oxygenation, so it is a useful noninvasive way for early detection of HPS particularly useful in small children. Initial cardiopulmonary assessment must be performed to detect causes of hypoxemia. The pathogenesis of intrapulmonary vasodilatation and shunting in HPS is poorly understood although increased levels of circulating vasoactive substances, such as nitric oxide are seen in the presence of portal hypertension and liver injury.[36] The management of hypoxemia in the ICU for patients with HPS may involve oxygen supplementation or mechanical ventilatory support. In patients with severe hypoxemia, the use of inhaled nitric oxide may redress the ventilation perfusion mismatch and improve oxygenation post-LT.[37] A variety of pharmacologic agents have been tried in patients with HPS without strong evidence of consistent benefit. Thus, the only definitive treatment for HPS is orthotopic liver transplantation. The data to support this is incontrovertible although the mechanism of pulmonary vasculature remodeling after transplantation is not clearly understood. Transcatheter coil embolization of the arteriovenous pulmonary fistulas may reduce morbidity of HPS before and after liver transplantation.[38] Embolotherapy may be a reasonable first line of bridging therapy in such patients.

## 18.2.11   THE PREOPERATIVE ICU MANAGEMENT OF THE DONOR

The outcome of transplantation depends to a large extent on the preoperative clinical management of the potential donor. In addition to continuing measures to treat the donor's primary condition, there is a shift away from cerebral resuscitation and intravascular volume contraction to safeguarding cellular oxygenation and perfusion, and anticipating the normal physiologic sequelae of brain death. The most common cardiovascular system changes encountered during the clinical management of the organ donor are hypertension, dysrhythmias, and hypotension, in addition to alterations in metabolic and electrolyte homeostasis.

By far the most common cardiovascular system anomaly in the organ donor is hypotension (MAP < 60 mm Hg). Hypotension regularly occurs before or soon after brain death occurs, and its etiology is multifactorial. Hypovolemia, left ventricular dysfunction, loss of vasomotor control, and endocrine changes either alone or in combination with each other contribute to the hypotension seen in the organ donor. Hypovolemia is the most common cause of hypotension in the organ donor. The hypovolemia may be absolute due to a reduction in intravascular volume. Intravascular volume depletion may have been instituted therapeutically to avoid central nervous system edema, or a consequence of inadequate replacement of essential and third-space fluid losses, polyuria from diabetes insipidus, osmotic diuresis, or the residual effects of diuretic drugs. Hypovolemia may also be relative—that is, the vascular space is abnormally dilated, from the loss of central vasomotor control. Often the hypotension is a combination of absolute and relative hypovolemia. Additionally, the hypotension may be further compounded by left ventricular dysfunction from myocardial contusion, electrolyte disturbances, injury to the heart during the progression of brain death, or acute pulmonary hypertension.

Regardless of the cause of the hypotension, the goal is to stabilize and improve the donor's hemodynamic status in order to ensure optimal end-organ perfusion. Aggressive therapy aimed at restoring and maintaining intravascular volume will usually improve the hemodynamic status of many donors. The choice of fluids used for volume expansion is based on the type of fluid lost, the hemoglobin levels, and serum electrolytes. Crystalloids, colloids, and blood products should be used as required. Inadequate fluid resuscitation as well as overly aggressive fluid resuscitation can lead to a complete loss of organs and/or a reduction in the quality of organs transplanted. Despite the evidence of adequate rehydration or during the initial stages of fluid resuscitation, potential organ donors may require vasopressor support to maintain an adequate blood pressure. On the basis of its pharmacology, dopamine is the vasopressor of choice. Additional vasopressors may also be necessary to support the blood pressure of the unstable organ donor. Regardless of the type and rate of the vasopressor(s) infusions, every effort should be made to keep them at the lowest rate possible while still maintaining an adequate blood pressure and, if possible, titrated off all together.

Hypertension may be encountered during the final stages of brain herniation. The hypertension in this situation results from the intense catecholamine storm seen during herniation and is usually self-limiting and requires no treatment. If hypertension persists after declaration of brain death, vasopressor infusions, if present, should be titrated downward. If treatment is considered necessary, a quick-acting agent with a short half-life, such as nitroprusside, is preferred.

Atrial or ventricular dysrhythmias and various degrees of conduction block occur with varying frequency in the organ donor. The use of high-dose vasopressors, acid–base abnormalities, electro-lyte disorders, hypothermia, and myocardial injury will increase the incidence of dysrhythmias in the organ donor, and timely therapeutic intervention must be implemented as dysrhythmias may be difficult to treat in the organ donor.

Coupled with the treatment of a potential donor's fluid volume deficit is the treatment of electro-lyte, hormones, and glucose abnormalities. These abnormalities are usually a result of the treatment given during patient care prior to brain death or from the effects of brain death.

## 18.3   THE POSTTRANSPLANT ICU PERIOD

### 18.3.1   POSTOPERATIVE MANAGEMENT AFTER INTESTINAL TRANSPLANT

After the transplant surgery, children are admitted for recovery in the PICU. A detailed hand-off between the surgical transplant team, the IF medical team, and the intensivist is mandatory. A mul-tidisciplinary team participates in the postoperative care in the PICU, and includes the intensivist, the bedside nurse, respiratory therapist, pharmacist, and nutritionist. The immediate postoperative period is characterized by frequent laboratory tests, intense monitoring of vital signs, urine and stool output, and close attention to fluid balance and hydration. PN with intralipids is often used to provide nutrient support and allow the GI tract to recover. Multiple catheters and lines, including intravenous catheters, arterial catheter, urinary bladder catheter, nasogastric tube, and endotracheal tube, are commonly placed to facilitate monitoring.

The principles of postoperative care include ensuring adequate oxygenation and ventilation (using prudent ventilator strategy when mechanical support is required), attention to organ perfu-sion, hemodynamic monitoring and support with fluids and/or vasopressor as required, close moni-toring of fluid balance and intravascular fluid volume, analgesia, sedation, and monitoring of serum electrolyte and other laboratory parameters. Some of the potential complications during the postop-erative period and after and management strategies are described in the following section.

### 18.3.2   INTESTINAL TRANSPLANT REJECTION IN THE ICU

As regards intestinal transplants, the early and most significant complication is certainly rejection in its various forms. During the postoperative period, the ileostomy allows endoscopic access to the trans-planted intestine in order to monitor for intestinal health and to look for signs of rejection. During endoscopy, the intestine is visualized, and intestinal biopsies are obtained to examine for histopatho-logical features of rejection. Since there is no specific blood test for rejection, endoscopy remains an important diagnostic test and is performed weekly for the first month after surgery. Additional ileosco-pies may be performed for other signs of rejection, such as (a) increased stool output, (b) fever or signs of infection, (c) changes in stoma or tissue color, and (d) blood-stained ostomy output. Close collabo-ration between the gastroenterologist and the intensivist will facilitate the judicious use of short-acting sedatives, analgesics and anxiolytics during the bedside endoscopy procedure.

High doses of immunosuppressive drugs are required owing to the large lymphatic component present in the ileum. The immunosuppression strategies require careful monitoring of drug levels.

Because of a fine balance that needs to be maintained between suboptimal immunosuppressant level and the adverse effects of immunosuppressant toxicity, close coordination between the intensive care team and the transplant team is mandatory when titrating doses to reach desired target ranges. In the case of biopsy- and clinically proven signs of rejection, intensification of immunosuppression is the usual remedy. Failure of medical therapy requires the early removal of the graft.

Strict policies for asepsis during patient care, sterile precautions during access to the various lines and catheters, restricted visitation from the lay public and special precautions to screen and avoid contact with anyone who has been exposed to communicable diseases or who is ill (cold, flu, etc.) are essential during this period. Visits from family members are coordinated with the PICU nurse. This also allows for planning quiet time with the patient during the visit.

### 18.3.3    FLUID AND ELECTROLYTE IMBALANCE

Children with IF may have underlying hyponatremia and are at risk of postoperative rapid changes in electrolytes, glucose, and osmolarity. The need to infuse plasma for hemocoagulation support and the failure to use prudent crystalloid infusion strategy can rapidly increase the sodium values in the postoperative period. The sodium balance is further altered due to the inappropriate renal response to atrial natriutretic hormone. Excessive intestinal losses in this population also contributes to fluid imbalance and careful attention to hemodynamic parameters is necessary in the postoperative period.[39] The prompt management of fluid and electrolyte imbalances is essential in order to prevent rapid alterations that have repercussions for graft perfusion.[40] In intestinal transplants, the most frequent nutritional complication is metabolic acidosis due to systematic consumption and loss of bases.[41] The therapy consists of intravenous or oral bicarbonate administration. Preserving the trophism of the transplanted intestine is one of the main objectives. The integrity of the mucosal and villi requires a continuous supply of nutrients.[42] In the early posttransplant phase nutritional support is represented by PN with clears (5% glucose) administered through the port of the gastrostomy tube. Enteral nutrition is gradually introduced and advanced as tolerated.

### 18.3.4    NEUROLOGICAL COMPLICATIONS

Devastating neurological insult from pontine myelinosis secondary to a rapid alteration in the plasma osmolarity is rare. Encephalopathy (11.8%) is the most frequent complication followed by convulsions (8.2%), neurotoxicity due to immunosuppressants (5.6%), as well as cerebral hemorrhage and stroke (2.3%) in this population. Neurotoxicity of immunosuppressant drugs (in particular cyclosporine and tacrolimus) remains an important cause of morbidity following transplant. In these patients it is necessary to follow the response to the immunosuppression endoscopically and with serial biopsies in order to identify the minimum level of immunosuppression compatible with a lack of rejection. Peripheral neuropathies secondary to prolonged suboptimal posture during surgical interventions and psychiatric complications are some of the other neurologic issues in this population.

## 18.4    LIVER TRANSPLANT: POSTOPERATIVE MANAGEMENT

A majority of the complications resulting in morbidity and mortality following pediatric liver transplant is observed in the weeks after the procedure, during the stay in the PICU.[43–45] Thus prudent management in the PICU, along with better timing of transplantation and surgical technique, are important factors associated with survival in this cohort. The essential priciples of ICU management after pediatric liver transplantation include: (a) diligent monitoring of the quality and function of the graft, (b) the maintenance of adequate perfusion with close monitoring of fluid balance and prompt fluid resuscitation in the setting of hypovolemia, (c) maintenance of adequate oxygenation and ventilation, using prudent ventilatory strategies, (d) early detection and management of thrombotic and infectious complications, and (e) prevention, detection, and management of graft rejection.

Improvements of the postoperative monitoring and a high standard of interdisciplinary intensive care management have significantly contributed to an improved survival of the recipient and of the graft. Data from international centers indicate that 1-year survival after pediatric LTx may be as high as 90%.[46] Information regarding graft perfusion is obtained from the intraoperative Doppler ultrasound examination, which is subsequently performed daily. Some of the issues in the postoperative period after liver transplantation are described here.

### 18.4.1 Mechanical Ventilation Posttransplant

The presence of preexisting HPS, failure of the transplanted liver to metabolize vasoactive substances, and restrictive syndrome due to ascites, pleural effusions, and/or pulmonary infections are all factors that may contribute to respiratory insufficiency in the posttransplant period. In adult liver recipients, prolonged mechanical ventilation time is correlated with increased morbidity and mortality.[47] Mechanical ventilation negatively impacts hemodynamics of the transplanted organ, especially when a high positive end-expiratory pressure is required. Excessive intraoperative blood loss, hypotension, and oliguria are related to a complicated postoperative course and longer mechanical ventilation time.[48] Judicious intra-operative fluid management may allow early extubation of patients. Shorter mechanical ventilation decreases postoperative incidence of pneumonia and may decrease the stay in the PICU.

### 18.4.2 Infections after Liver Transplantation

Infections strongly influence morbidity and mortality after liver transplantation[49] and have been reported to be the commonest complication following this procedure.[50] Bacterial and fungal infections, often related to central venous catheter insertion, percutaneous catheter drainage, or mechanical ventilation, are frequent problems. There has been a reduction in life-threatening systemic infections resulting from close monitoring and early therapy. The relatively lower incidence of PICU acquired infections in recent years parallels a shortened stay in the PICU. Cytomegalovirus (CMV) disease usually occurs $4 \pm 6$ weeks posttransplant and hence is not commonly encountered in the PICU.[51] The incidence of major infectious complications in this patient population is similar in most centers. Attempts to remove central venous lines and abdominal drains as early as possible have not reduced the incidence of infectious episodes. This may be explained by the mandatory need for high immunosuppression in the early postoperative period and by an increasing incidence of multiresistant bacterial pathogens in the ICU environment.

### 18.4.3 Rejection

The overall incidence of rejection episodes is 30–60%.[52] Almost one-third of the episodes occur during the stay in the ICU. The diagnosis is assumed by clinical and laboratory findings, and confirmed by histological examination. Fever and rising levels of bilirubin, alkaline phosphatase, aspartate, and alanine transaminases may be signs of an acute rejection. Percutaneous needle biopsy allows histopathological confirmation of rejection. Recently, interleukin-1 receptor antagonist was found to be an additional early marker of acute cellular rejection in drained ascitic fluid.[53] The declining incidence of rejection episodes in the ICU paralleled the shortened duration of time in the ICU, whereby the overall incidence of rejections declined only slightly over duration of our study.

## 18.5 CARE BUNDLES IN THE PICU

Children with intestinal and liver failure represent a high-risk population admitted to the PICU where every effort to reduce complications must be made. Ventilator-associated pneumonia (VAP) and CRBSI are examples of acquired conditions in the PICU, which result in significant increase in costs and morbidity. The concept of the care "bundle" was developed by the Institute for Healthcare Improvement (IHI) as a tool to facilitate the application of best practices and evidence-based care at the bedside. A bundle is "a structured way of improving the processes of care and patient outcomes: a small, straightforward set of practices—generally three to five—that, when performed collectively and reliably, have been proven to improve patient outcomes" (Institute for Healthcare Improvement: *What Is a Bundle?* http://www.ihi.org/IHI/Topics/CriticalCare/IntensiveCare/ ImprovementStories/WhatIsaBundle.htm). Sustained and reliable performance of the bundle tasks requires a high level of teamwork and collaboration, an important step in developing an organizational culture of patient safety and quality improvement (QI).

Reductions in the incidence of intensive care unit (ICU)-acquired infections, specifically VAP and CRBSI, can be achieved with a collaborative multiple-intervention strategy to improve adherence with evidence-based practices using the bundle approach. A large multiple-intervention QI study showed a sustained 66% reduction in the rate of CRBSI across 103 ICUs in the state of Michigan associated with implementation of a central line bundle.[54]

In conclusion, the care of the child with IF in the ICU requires interdisciplinary effort, meticulous monitoring and prudent supportive therapy. Intensivists are routinely required to care for children with IF at various stages of their disease. The intensivist is a critical part of the IF team. The challenge for the intensive care team is to support and improve marginal organ function and manage complications during the pretransplant and posttransplant period. Principles of management include optimization of respiratory status, minimization of VILI, careful attention to fluid and electrolyte balance, maintenance of adequate perfusion, preservation of residual liver function, maintenance of hemodynamic stability in the setting of capillary leak while avoiding edema due to fluid overload and hypoalbuminemia, meticulous posttransplant monitoring for signs of rejection and titration of immunomodulation. With the application of prudent ventilator strategies, bundles of care for the prevention of hospital-acquired infections and improving communication between the transplant and intensive care teams, the outcomes for children with IF admitted to the PICU may be improved.

## REFERENCES

1. Fryer J, Pellar S, Ormond D, Koffron A, Abecassis M. Mortality in candidates waiting for combined liver-intestine transplants exceeds that for other candidates waiting for liver transplants. *Liver Transpl.* 2003;9:748–53.
2. Kaufman SS, Gondolesi GE, Fishbein TM. Parenteral nutrition associated liver disease. *Semin Neonatol.* 2003;8:375–81.
3. Bleeding oesophageal varices: IST, EVL, or TIPS. *Lancet.* 1992;340:515–6.
4. Pasquale MD, Cerra FB. Sengstaken-Blakemore tube placement. Use of balloon tamponade to control bleeding varices. *Crit Care Clin.* 1992;8:743–53.
5. Tsibouris P, Zintzaras E, Lappas C et al. High-dose pantoprazole continuous infusion is superior to somatostatin after endoscopic hemostasis in patients with peptic ulcer bleeding. *Am J Gastroenterol.* 2007;102:1192–9.
6. Chanson P, Timsit J, Harris AG. Clinical pharmacokinetics of octreotide. Therapeutic applications in patients with pituitary tumours. *Clin Pharmacokinet.* 1993;25:375–91.
7. Ladefoged K, Olgaard K. Sodium homeostasis after small-bowel resection. *Scand J Gastroenterol.* 1985;20:361–9.
8. Banerjee A, Warwicker P. Acute renal failure and metabolic disturbances in the short bowel syndrome. *QJM.* 2002;95:37–40.
9. Brook AD, Ahrens TS, Schaiff R et al. Effect of a nursing-implemented sedation protocol on the duration of mechanical ventilation. *Crit Care Med.* 1999;27:2609–15.
10. Ventilation with lower tidal volumes as compared with traditional tidal volumes for acute lung injury and the acute respiratory distress syndrome. The Acute Respiratory Distress Syndrome Network. *N Engl J Med.* 2000;342:1301–8.
11. Levy MM. Optimal peep in ARDS. Changing concepts and current controversies. *Crit Care Clin.* 2002;18:15–33, v–vi.

12. Arnold JH, Hanson JH, Toro-Figuero LO, Gutierrez J, Berens RJ, Anglin DL. Prospective, randomized comparison of high-frequency oscillatory ventilation and conventional mechanical ventilation in pediatric respiratory failure. *Crit Care Med.* 1994;22:1530–9.

13. Arnold JH, Anas NG, Luckett P et al. High-frequency oscillatory ventilation in pediatric respiratory failure: A multicenter experience. *Crit Care Med.* 2000;28:3913–9.

14. Han YY, Carcillo JA, Dragotta MA et al. Early reversal of pediatric-neonatal septic shock by community physicians is associated with improved outcome. *Pediatrics.* 2003;112:793–9.

15. Rivers E, Nguyen B, Havstad S et al. Early goal-directed therapy in the treatment of severe sepsis and septic shock. *N Engl J Med.* 2001;345:1368–77.

16. Kern JW, Shoemaker WC. Meta-analysis of hemodynamic optimization in high-risk patients. *Crit Care Med.* 2002;30:1686–92.

17. Carcillo JA, Fields AI. Clinical practice parameters for hemodynamic support of pediatric and neonatal patients in septic shock. *Crit Care Med.* 2002;30:1365–78.

18. Finfer SR, Boyce NW, Norton RN. The SAFE study: A landmark trial of the safety of albumin in intensive care. *Med J Aust.* 2004;181:237–8.

19. Drews BB, Sanghavi R, Siegel JD, Metcalf P, Mittal NK. Characteristics of catheter-related bloodstream infections in children with intestinal failure: Implications for clinical management. *Gastroenterol Nurs.* 2009;32:385–90; quiz 91–2.

20. Colomb V, Dabbas-Tyan M, Taupin P et al. Long-term outcome of children receiving home parenteral nutrition: A 20-year single-center experience in 302 patients. *J Pediatr Gastroenterol Nutr.* 2007;44:347–53.

21. Hermans D, Talbotec C, Lacaille F, Goulet O, Ricour C, Colomb V. Early central catheter infections may contribute to hepatic fibrosis in children receiving long-term parenteral nutrition. *J Pediatr Gastroenterol Nutr.* 2007;44:459–63.

22. Sondheimer JM, Asturias E, Cadnapaphornchai M. Infection and cholestasis in neonates with intestinal resection and long-term parenteral nutrition. *J Pediatr Gastroenterol Nutr.* 1998;27:131–7.

23. O'Grady NP, Alexander M, Dellinger EP et al. Guidelines for the prevention of intravascular catheter-related infections. *Am J Infect Control.* 2002;30:476–89.

24. Byrnes MC, Coopersmith CM. Prevention of catheter-related blood stream infection. *Curr Opin Crit Care.* 2007;13:411–5.

25. Kline AM. Pediatric catheter-related bloodstream infections: Latest strategies to decrease risk. *AACN Clin Issues.* 2005;16:185–98; quiz 272–4.

26. Gowardman JR, Robertson IK, Parkes S, Rickard CM. Influence of insertion site on central venous catheter colonization and bloodstream infection rates. *Intensive Care Med.* 2008;34:1038–45.

27. Dannenberg C, Bierbach U, Rothe A, Beer J, Korholz D. Ethanol-lock technique in the treatment of bloodstream infections in pediatric oncology patients with broviac catheter. *J Pediatr Hematol Oncol.* 2003;25:616–21.

28. Onland W, Shin CE, Fustar S, Rushing T, Wong WY. Ethanol-lock technique for persistent bacteremia of long-term intravascular devices in pediatric patients. *Arch Pediatr Adolesc Med.* 2006;160:1049–53.

29. Jones BA, Hull MA, Richardson DS et al. Efficacy of ethanol locks in reducing central venous catheter infections in pediatric patients with intestinal failure. *J Pediatr Surg.* 2010;45(6):1287–93.

30. Onder AM, Kato T, Simon N et al. Prevention of catheter-related bacteremia in pediatric intestinal transplantation/short gut syndrome children with long-term central venous catheters. *Pediatr Transplant.* 2007;11:87–93.

31. Ee LC, Shepherd RW, Cleghorn GJ et al. Acute liver failure in children: A regional experience. *J Paediatr Child Health.* 2003;39:107–10.

32. Devictor D, Tahiri C, Rousset A, Massenavette B, Russo M, Huault G. Management of fulminant hepatic failure in children—An analysis of 56 cases. *Crit Care Med.* 1993;21:S348–9.

33. Anand AC, Nightingale P, Neuberger JM. Early indicators of prognosis in fulminant hepatic failure: An assessment of the King's criteria. *J Hepatol.* 1997;26:62–8.

34. Rodriguez-Roisin R, Krowka MJ. Hepatopulmonary syndrome—A liver-induced lung vascular disorder. *N Engl J Med.* 2008;358:2378–87.

35. Noli K, Solomon M, Golding F, Charron M, Ling SC. Prevalence of hepatopulmonary syndrome in children. *Pediatrics.* 2008;121:e522–7.

36. Rolla G, Brussino L, Colagrande P et al. Exhaled nitric oxide and impaired oxygenation in cirrhotic patients before and after liver transplantation. *Ann Intern Med.* 1998;129:375–8.

37. Durand P, Baujard C, Grosse AL et al. Reversal of hypoxemia by inhaled nitric oxide in children with severe hepatopulmonary syndrome, type 1, during and after liver transplantation. *Transplantation.* 1998;65:437–9.

38. White RI, Jr, Lynch-Nyhan A, Terry P et al. Pulmonary arteriovenous malformations: Techniques and long-term outcome of embolotherapy. *Radiology.* 1988;169:663–9.

39. Kumar N, Grant D. Gastrointestinal transplantation: An update. *Liver Transpl.* 2000;6:515–9.

40. Farmer DG, McDiarmid SV, Edelstein S et al. Improved outcome after intestinal transplantation at a single institution over 12 years. *Transplant Proc.* 2004;36:303–4.

41. Fishbein TM, Kaufman SS, Florman SS et al. Isolated intestinal transplantation: Proof of clinical efficacy. *Transplantation.* 2003;76:636–40.

42. Masetti M, Cautero N, Lauro A et al. Three-year experience in clinical intestinal transplantation. *Transplant Proc.* 2004;36:309–11.

43. Singh N, Gayowski T, Wagener MM. Intensive care unit management in liver transplant recipients: Beneficial effect on survival and preservation of quality of life. *Clin Transplant.* 1997;11:113–20.

44. Hauser GJ, Kaufman SS, Matsumoto CS, Fishbein TM. Pediatric intestinal and multivisceral transplantation: A new challenge for the pediatric intensivist. *Intensive Care Med.* 2008;34:1570–9.

45. Ganschow R, Nolkemper D, Helmke K et al. Intensive care management after pediatric liver transplantation: A single-center experience. *Pediatr Transplant.* 2000;4:273–9.

46. Van der Werf WJ, D'Alessandro AM, Knechtle SJ et al. Infant pediatric liver transplantation results equal those for older pediatric patients. *J Pediatr Surg.* 1998;33:20–3.

47. Glanemann M, Langrehr JM, Muller AR et al. Incidence and risk factors of prolonged mechanical ventilation and causes of reintubation after liver transplantation. *Transplant Proc.* 1998;30:1874–5.

48. Sun CK, Chen CL, Kuo YC, Chen YS. Intensive care after orthotopic liver transplantation. *Transplant Proc.* 1994;26:2246–7.

49. Saint-Vil D, Luks FI, Lebel P et al. Infectious complications of pediatric liver transplantation. *J Pediatr Surg.* 1991;26:908–13.

50. Beath SV, Brook GD, Kelly DA et al. Successful liver transplantation in babies under 1 year. *BMJ.* 1993;307:825–8.

51. Gane E, Saliba F, Valdecasas GJ et al. Randomised trial of efficacy and safety of oral ganciclovir in the prevention of cytomegalovirus disease in liver-transplant recipients. The Oral Ganciclovir International Transplantation Study Group [corrected]. *Lancet.* 1997;350:1729–33.

52. Murphy MS, Harrison RF, Hubscher S, Mayer AD, Buckels JA, Kelly DA. Liver allograft rejection is less common in children transplanted in the first year of life. *Transplant Proc.* 1994;26:157–8.

53. Ganschow R, Baade B, Hellwege HH, Broering DC, Rogiers X, Burdelski M. Interleukin-1 receptor antagonist in ascites indicates acute graft rejection after pediatric liver transplantation. *Pediatr Transplant.* 2000;4:289–92.

54. Pronovost P, Needham D, Berenholtz S et al. An intervention to decrease catheter-related bloodstream infections in the ICU. *N Engl J Med.* 2006;355:2725–32.

# Part III

Prevention and Treatment of
Complications of Intestinal Failure

# 19 Central Venous Catheter Infections

## Prevention and Treatment

*Mary Petrea Cober and Daniel H. Teitelbaum*

## CONTENTS

## 19.1 EPIDEMIOLOGY AND ETIOLOGY

Sepsis is one of the most frequent and serious complications of centrally infused parenteral nutrition (PN) in adults and children [1]. In fact, of the greater than 150 million intravenous catheters placed in the United States each year, approximately 80,000 central venous catheter (CVC)-associated infections develop [2]. Worldwide it is estimated that 250,000–500,000 cases of CVC-associated bloodstream infections (BSI) occur annually. The estimated cost to the healthcare system ranges from 12,000 to 56,000 U.S. dollars per episode, with an estimated total cost of approximately $2.3 billion annually in the United States [3–5]. Care includes a mean length of stay of up to 6 days in an intensive care unit, and up to 21 days at the hospital [5,6]. The mortality associated with major CVC-associated infection is estimated between 12% and 35% per infection [5]. Additionally, the Center for Medicare and Medicaid Services 2008 reimbursement guidelines consider infections which are the result of a vascular catheter to be a preventable hospital-acquired condition which will no longer be reimbursed [7]. Interestingly, those patients with intestinal failure (IF) are at the highest risk in developing CVC-associated infections [8]. Additionally, of those patients with IF on home parenteral nutrition (HPN), half of all hospitalizations were due to proven CVC-associated infections [8]. Most series report an incidence of 0.5–2.0 infections per 1000 catheter-days for a nonimmunosuppressed patient with a CVC [9,10]. For immunosuppressed patients (e.g., hematology or oncology patients), a rate of 2–3 infections per 1000 catheter-days is generally reported [11,12]. A considerably higher rate of infection is found in children with the short-bowel syndrome with rates ranging from 2.1 to 9 infections per 1000 catheter-days [8,13–17]. The mean rate of CVC infections in adult IF patients may be lower, with one group reporting a rate of 0.48 infections/1000 catheter-days [18].

Catheter infections may occur from one of three sources: the insertion site, the catheter hub, or seeded via the bloodstream. The hub has often been considered the most common source of CVC infections, and great care must be used to protect this site when gaining access to these catheters [19–21]. Infections secondary to bacteria from around the entrance site include skin contaminants such as *Staphylococci* or *Streptococci* [9]. These organisms can colonize the fibrin sleeve that develops around the catheter tip and start proliferating. Other infections are a result of seeding from other foci, such as bacterial translocation, and may be Gram-negative or enteric in nature. Although tunneling of the catheter was initially thought to reduce the rate of CVC infections, this does not appear to be the case; and CVC infection rates are similar between tunneled and nontunneled silicone lines [20]. Polyurethane and silicone catheters appear to be superior materials for reducing CVC infections, and are now the standard of care [22].

## 19.2  CLINICAL MANIFESTATIONS OF CVC-ASSOCIATED INFECTIONS

Fever and sudden glucose intolerance are suggestive of sepsis. Persistent hyperglycemia has been shown to increase infection rates and intensive control is recommended in adult surgical intensive care patients [23]. Other signs of CVC infection may include chills, or may be as extreme as septic shock. One of the more insidious manifestations in infants with a CVC infection may be a fairly rapid rise in the child's C-reactive protein (CRP), serum bilirubin levels, or a sudden thrombocytopenia [24–26].

## 19.3  DIAGNOSIS OF CVC-ASSOCIATED INFECTIONS

The usual workup of a patient on PN who develops an acute, unexplained fever should include a comprehensive set of blood cultures. The clinical practice guidelines for the diagnosis and management of intravascular catheter-related infection by the Infectious Diseases Society of America (IDSA) have been updated and recommend paired blood culture samples should be drawn from the suspected catheter and a peripheral vein [27]. If a blood sample cannot be drawn from a peripheral vein, then two blood samples should be drawn from different catheter lumens. A definitive diagnosis of catheter-related bloodstream infection (CRBSI) should be based on the findings of the same organism growing from at least one percutaneous blood culture and from a catheter tip culture (should the CVC be removed), or two blood samples one drawn from the catheter hub and the other from a peripheral vein; so when cultured, they meet the CRBSI criteria for quantitative blood cultures (ratio of > 3:1 colony forming units/mL of blood; catheter:peripheral) or differential time to positivity (growth in a blood culture obtained through a catheter hub is detected by an automated blood culture system at least 2 h prior to a peripheral culture of an equal volume of blood obtained simultaneously) [27].

Microbial culturing of PN should be performed if PN is suspected as a source of microbial contamination, though this is a rare occurrence with the use of strict sterile compounding techniques and increased glucose concentrations. CVC infections remain the main cause of sepsis in patients receiving PN. The most important factors in reducing the incidence of septic complications are placement of catheters under strict aseptic conditions and meticulous care of the catheter sites.

## 19.4  TREATMENT GUIDELINES

Treatment guideline recommendations from IDSA published in 2009 are summarized in this section, additionally see Figure 19.1 [27]. In general, nonpermanent, polyvinyl chloride lines should be removed with catheter sepsis [2,3]. However, up to 80% of patients with a silastic catheter (e.g., Broviac or Hickman) may be able to have the infection cleared with intravenous antibiotics. The most critical decision is the medical stability of the patient. Seriously septic patients should undergo

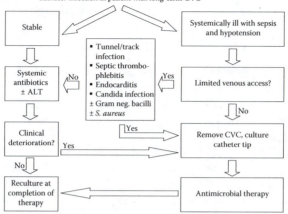

**FIGURE 19.1** Suggested approach to a patient with a CVC-associated infection. Antibiotic lock therapy, ALT; *Staphyloccocus aureus, S. aureus*; Negative, neg. (Adapted from Mermal LA et al. *Clin Infect Dis* 2009;49:1–45.)

prompt cultures, and have the CVC removed, should no other source be identified. Patients who are only moderately ill, but lack evidence of hypotension or organ failure, should be cultured, and should clinical suspicion strongly suggest a CVC-associated infection, be started on antimicrobials until blood cultures come back. In general, most IF patients should be started on a combination of vancomycin for methicillin-resistant *Staphylococcus aureus* (MRSA) and a fourth-generation cephalosporin or a β-lactam/β-lactamase inhibitor with or without an aminoglycoside for Gram-negative enteric coverage. Significantly septicemic patients should also be started on anti-Candida therapy, typically fluconazole. Once patient-specific culture results are available, therapy should be tailored to the specific organism(s) and sensitivity pattern.

For those patients where there is an attempt at CVC salvage, additional cultures need to be obtained 72 h after initiation of antimicrobials. Should the patient fail antimicrobial therapy, the CVC should be removed. For those IF patients with limited access, one could consider guide-wiring of the CVC, with replacement with a fresh CVC. CVCs should also be removed should patients show signs of suppurative thrombophlebitis or endocarditis. As well, cultures growing *Mycobacteria, S. aureus,* or *Pseudomonas aeruginosa* should be an indication for CVC removal.

Most patients with fungal infections should also have the catheter removed due to reports of fatalities and high failure rates with attempts at trying to salvage the line with antifungal therapy [28]. Attempting to maintain a catheter with a Candidal infection is associated with a mortality of up to 25% and the low chance of clearing the infection with the catheter remaining in place (13%) [29]. Only a relatively short course of antifungal agents needs to be given after the catheter is removed (14 days); however, the results of blood cultures must be negative [27,30]. Patients should be screened for evidence of thrombophlebitis via echocardiography, as this would indicate a much longer course after CVC removal. For unusual cases in which central venous access is limited because of previous placement of several catheters, a trial of antifungal agents with the catheter in place may be attempted. An uncommon fungal organism associated with PN is *Malassezia furfur*. This organism thrives in a lipid-rich environment, but as long as lipids are withheld, it generally responds to antifungal treatment without catheter removal. Antifungal therapy should continue for 4–6 weeks in such cases.

Two other types of CVC infections include exit site infections. The site should be cultured, and initial therapy can begin with local care and topical antibiotic ointments. Should this fail, systemic antibiotics may be used. A more severe infection comprises the subcutaneous tunnel or track of the

CVC. These infections can be severe in nature, and are not responsive to systemic antibiotic therapy. CVC tunnel infections should be approached with prompt catheter removal [31].

## 19.5 PREVENTION OF CVC-ASSOCIATED INFECTIONS

Prevention of CVC-associated infections is important in conserving limited central venous access sites particularly in pediatric patients, decreasing life-threatening infections, and optimizing quality of life. Many routine techniques have been attributed to improvements [22]. Such actions include proper catheter selection, with a lower incidence of infections being associated with the use of a sub-cutaneously implanted port [31]. Routine care is also indicated, including good hand washing, use of a 2% chlorhexidine with 70% isopropyl alcohol (or just chlorhexidine for those patients with an intolerance to alcohol) for dressing changes, and meticulous cleansing of the hub with alcohol prior to accessing the CVC device [22,31]. Use of commercial dressing products with a chlorhexidine-impregnated sponge may offer an advantage of a simple occlusive polyurethane dressing. These products have only been examined on a limited basis; however, one prospective randomized controlled trial did show a benefit [32]. These dressings have not been studied in long-term CVC patients receiving home PN infusions; however, they have been shown to be beneficial in chronic hemodialysis lines [33]. Additionally, standardization of catheter care is essential. Intravenous tubing should be changed every 24 h if they contain intravenous lipid emulsions, and every 72 h without lipid emulsions. In-line filters have also been associated with a reduction in CVC-associated infections [31]. Use of CVCs for multiple drugs and blood sampling, as well as, PN has been shown to increase infectious complications [34,35]. In fact, when a formal protocol for catheter insertion and care is instituted, a dramatic reduction in catheter infections can be seen. In one prospective study, the rate of catheter infections declined from 11.3/1000 catheter-days to 1.6/1000 catheter-days over the 4-year period in which these methods were used [21]. It appears multiple central venous lumens may predispose patients to a higher risk of infection, but this association is not proven [36]. Peripherally inserted central venous catheters (PICCs) have not been shown to have a significantly lower incidence of infection; however, PICCs have been associated with higher rates of thrombophlebitis [37].

## 19.6 ANTIMICROBIAL-COATED CATHETER DEVICES

Over the past 20 years, a number of CVC devices have been advanced with some type of antimicrobial coating, either internally, externally, or both. This has recently afforded very detailed analyses of the outcome of the use of these catheters in two recent publications [38,39]. Meta-analysis showed externally impregnated catheters with either chlorhexidine or silver sulfadiazine resulted in a modest reduction in CVC infections compared to uncoated catheters. Even more effective are catheters coated with minocycline and rifampicin, which provided significant reductions compared to chlorhexidine and silver sulfadiazine-treated catheters. No significant reduction in CVC infections was found for heparin-coated catheters compared to silver-impregnated catheters. One concern that arises in the care of IF patients is the potential development of antibiotic resistance with the use of these catheters. Additionally, no antibiotic-impregnated CVC catheters currently exist for small infants (less than 3 kg body weight).

## 19.7 ANTIBIOTIC LOCK THERAPY

Treatment with systemic antimicrobial agents usually lasts between 7 and 14 days for uncomplicated infections with a success rate between 60% and 91%. The most common reason for failure of systemic therapy is lack of eradication of the organisms in the biofilm [40]. Plasma proteins, leukocytes, platelets, and fibrin all coalesced together to form a fibrin sheath that forms the foundation for bacteria to produce a biofilm which impedes the penetration of phagocytes or antimicrobials [41]. CVC infections related to biofilm formation are extremely difficult to eradicate. A technique to treat and then ultimately prevent such infections is the antibiotic-lock technique (ALT). This

**TABLE 19.1**

**Commonly Used Antimicrobial Locks**

| Medication | Concentration (mg/mL) | Heparin (U/mL) |
|---|---|---|
| Amphotericin B | 1 | None |
| Cefazolin | 0.5 | 10 |
| Fluconazole | 2 | None |
| Gentamicin | 0.02 | 10 |
| Gentamicin | 0.02 | 1000[a] |
| Linezolid | 1.8 | 10 |
| Vancomycin | 0.025 | 10 |
| Vancomycin | 0.025 | 1000[a] |

[a] For use in hemodialysis catheters.

technique consists of filling and closing a CVC lumen with an antibiotic solution to prevent or treat CVC infections. This allows markedly higher antibiotic concentrations to be maintained within the internal surface of the CVC for prolonged period of times (hours to days) in order to penetrate the biofilm layer [42–44]. This approach also allows use of antibiotics that would normally have such high minimal inhibitory concentrations (MIC) that systemic use would result in potential renal failure (e.g., nafcillin or vancomycin for a staphylococcal line infection). The use of ALT has gained popularity over the past decade and is now a more recognized treatment and prevention option in the updated 2009 guidelines for the management of catheter-related infections by IDSA [27]. If used for the treatment of CVC infection, ALT should be used in combination with systemic antibiotics, leading to improved catheter salvage rates [27]. Table 19.1 lists commonly used antimicrobial locks.

Issues with ALT remain. ALT lacks activity against organisms at distant sites or those involved in tunneled site infections due to a lack of antibiotic presence at the infection site. In addition, standardized concentrations and stability with and without heparin for various antibiotic locks exist but sometimes involve conflicting reports [45].

## 19.8 ETHANOL LOCK THERAPY

Unfortunately, ALT is dependent on knowing the organism causing the CVC infection or most likely to cause a future CVC infection in the patient. Additionally, with the increasing rates of resistant organisms, concern has arisen regarding possible antibiotic resistance [40]. In order to avoid the development of antibiotic resistance, a similar technique involving ethanol has recently been used to prevent or treat CVC infections, resulting in a dramatic reduction in the rate of CVC infections and the ability to salvage many infected CVCs. This has had special importance in pediatric populations with limited access sites [46–51]. Similar to ALT, ethanol-lock therapy (ELT) consists of filling and closing a CVC lumen with an ethanol solution to prevent or treat CVC infections. This therapy was previously used for lipid precipitate in CVCs from 3-in-1 PN solutions [52]. An advantage of ELT is the elimination of the offending organism that does not depend on the sensitivity of the organisms to an antimicrobial agent. This may be of particular value for infections with multi-drug-resistant organisms. Another advantage of ELT is the lack of selection of resistant organisms which may reduce the use of broad-spectrum antibiotics [44]. A 70% ethanol-lock solution is adequate for treatment or prevention of infection because an ethanol concentration greater than 40% inhibits bacterial growth in established biofilms. A 70% ethanol-lock solution must dwell in the CVC lumen for a minimum of 2 h in order to be effective [46]. The IDSA's current guidelines for CVC infections feel insufficient data exist regarding ELT to make an official recommendation of its use at this time [27].

When ELT is considered for patients many considerations must be addressed prior to initiation of therapy often necessitating an institutional policy/protocol for use. Education to patients, caregivers, staff, and other healthcare providers is of utmost importance. Unlike ALT, ELT cannot be used in all CVC catheters. Due to potential weakening of the catheter leading to breakage, ELT is recommended for silicone-based catheters only [53,54]. Thus, it is of extreme importance to confirm the composition of the catheter prior to initiation of ELT. Additionally, 70% ethanol used most commonly for ELT is not compatible with heparin or citrate solutions and will form a precipitate if mixed with either solution [55]. Instead, patients will have their catheters flushed with saline. The first dose of ELT should be withdrawn from the catheter following the prescribed dwell time period to prevent introduction of bacteria into the body of the patient after disruption of the biofilm layer by the ethanol. For pediatric patients, concerns have been raised about the potential exposure of systemic ethanol to the developing central nervous system [17]. For this reason, certain pediatric institutions recommend determining the catheter lumen volume to personalize the dose to the patient's catheter, as well as removing the ethanol solution from the catheter lumen following each prescribed dwell time period [17]. Finally, a 70% ethanol-lock solution can be made by adding 98% dehydrated alcohol injection, USP, to sterile water for injection, USP, and the resulting solution is stable for up to 14 days at room temperature [55].

## 19.9 CONCLUSIONS

CVC infections dramatically impact the lives of IF patients. Special attention should be given to prevent CVC infections, but if they occur, treatment should be initiated immediately. Potentially, the only sign of infection in the patient may be fever or an increase in bilirubin levels. However, without treatment, CVC infections can lead to life-threatening sepsis in a matter of hours. Therefore, it is important for patients to contact their healthcare providers at the first sign of potential infection and start therapy immediately after blood cultures (both from a peripheral source and from the catheter lumen) are drawn. Therapy should be based on the infection patterns of the institution and the patient's previous infection history and may include antibiotic-lock therapy in addition to systemic antimicrobials. In the hope of decreasing the impact of CVC infections, newer techniques such as ethanol-lock therapy have shown dramatic reductions in the rates of CVC infections among the IF patient population.

## REFERENCES

1. Donnell S, Taylor N, van Saene H, Magnall V, Pierro A, Lloyd D. Infection rates in surgical neonates and infants receiving parenteral nutrition: A five-year prospective study. *J Hosp Infect* 2002;52:273–80.
2. Mermel LA. Prevention of catheter-related infections. *Ann Intern Med* 2000;132:391–402.
3. O'Grady NP, Alexander M, Dellinger EP, Gerberding JL, Heard SO, Maki DG et al. Guidelines for the prevention of intravascular catheter-related infections. Centers for disease control and prevention. *MMWR Recomm Rep* 2002;51:1–29.
4. Rodriguez-Paz JM, Pronovost P. Prevention of catheter-related bloodstream infections. *Adv Surg* 2008;42:229–48.
5. Zack J. Zeroing in on zero tolerance for central line-associated bacteremia. *Am J Infect Control* 2008;36:S176 e1–2.
6. Safdar N, Mermel L, Maki D. The epidemiology of catheter-related infection in the critically ill. In: O'Grady N, Pittet D editors. *Catheter Related Infections in the Critically Ill*. New York: Kluwer; 2004. pp. 1–23.
7. Brown J, Doloresco Iii F, Mylotte JM. "Never events": Not every hospital-acquired infection is preventable. *Clin Infect Dis* 2009;49:743–6.
8. Colomb V, Jobert-Giraud A, Lacaille F, Goulet O, Fournet JC, Ricour C. Role of lipid emulsions in cholestasis associated with long-term parenteral nutrition in children. *JPEN* 2000;24:345–50.
9. King DR, Komer M, Hoffman J, Ginn-Pease ME, Stanley ME, Powell D et al. Broviac catheter sepsis: The natural history of an iatrogenic infection. *J Pediatr Surg* 1985;20:728–33.

10. Wurzel CL, Halom K, Feldman JG, Rubin LG. Infection rates of Broviac-Hickman catheters and implantable venous devices. *AJDC* 1988;142:536–40.

11. Dawson S, Pai MKR, Smith S, Rothney M, Ahmed K, Barr RD. Right atrial catheters in children with cancer: A decade of experience in the use of tunnelled, exteriorized devices at a single institution. *Am J Pediatr Hematol/Oncol* 1991;13:126–9.

12. Johnson PR, Decker MD, Edwards KM, Schaffner W, Wright PF. Frequency of broviac catheter infections in pediatric oncology patients. *J Infect Dis* 1986;154:570–8.

13. Caniano DA, Starr J, Ginn-Pease ME. Extensive short-bowel syndrome in neonates: Outcome in the 1980s. *Surgery* 1989;105:119–24.

14. Kurkchubasche AG, Smith SD, Rowe MI. Catheter sepsis in short-bowel syndrome. *Arch Surg* 1992;127:21–5.

15. Moukarzel AA, Haddad I, Ament ME, Buchman, AL, Reyen L, Maggioni A et al. 230 patient years of experience with home long-term parenteral nutrition in childhood: Natural history and life of central venous catheters. *J Pediatr Surg* 1994;29:1323–7.

16. Piedra PA, Dryja DM, LaScolea LJ, Jr. Incidence of catheter-associated gram-negative bacteremia in children with short bowel syndrome. *J Clin Microbiol* 1989;27:1317–9.

17. Cober M, Teitelbaum D, Kovacevich D. Ethanol-lock therapy for the prevention of central venous access device infections in pediatric intestinal failure patients. *JPEN* 2011 Jan;35(1):67–73.

18. Wasa M, Takagi Y, Sando K, Harada T, Okada A. Long-term outcome of short bowel syndrome in adult and pediatric patients. *JPEN* 1999;23:S110–2.

19. Sitges-Serra A, Puig P, Linares J, Perez JL, Farrero N, Jaurrieta, E et al. Hub colonization as the initial step in an outbreak of catheter-related sepsis due to coagulase negative staphylococci during parenteral nutrition. *JPEN* 1984;8:668–72.

20. Sitges-Serra A, Linares J. Tunnels do not protect against venous-catheter-related sepsis [letter]. *Lancet* 1984;1:459–60.

21. Berenholtz S, Pronovost P, Lipsett P, Hobson D, Earsing K. Eliminating catheter-related bloodstream infections in the intensive care unit. *Crit Care Med* 2004;32:2014–20.

22. Pittiruti M, Hamilton H, Biffi R, MacFie J, Pertkiewicz M. ESPEN Guidelines on Parenteral Nutrition: Central venous catheters (access, care, diagnosis and therapy of complications). *Clin Nutr* 2009;28:365–77.

23. van den Berghe G, Wouters P, Weekers F, Verwaest C, Bruyninckx F, Schetz M et al. Intensive insulin therapy in the critically ill patients. *N Engl J Med* 2001;345:1359–67.

24. Beath SV, Davies P, Papadopoulou A, Khan AR, Buick RG, Corkery JJ et al. Parenteral nutrition-related cholestasis in postsurgical neonates: Multivariate analysis of risk factors. *J Pediatr Surg* 1996;31:604–6.

25. Warris A, Semmekrot BA, Voss A. Candidal and bacterial bloodstream infections in premature neonates: A case–control study. *Med Mycol* 2001;39:75–9.

26. Clare A, Teubner A, Shaffer JL. What information should lead to a suspicion of catheter sepsis in HPN? *Clin Nutr* 2008;27:552–6.

27. Mermel LA, Allon M, Bouza E, Craven DE, Flynn P, O'Grady NP et al. Clinical practice guidelines for the diagnosis and management of intravascular catheter-related infection: 2009 Update by the Infectious Diseases Society of America. *Clin Infect Dis* 2009;49:1–45.

28. Clarke DE, Raffin TA. Infectious complications of indwelling long-term central venous catheters. [Review] [48 refs]. *Chest* 1990;97:966–72.

29. Eppes SC, Troutman JL, Gutman LT. Outcome of treatment of candidemia in children whose central catheters were removed or retained. *Pediatr Infect Dis J* 1989;8:99–104.

30. Donowitz LG, Hendley JO. Short-course amphotericin B therapy for candidemia in pediatric patients. *Pediatrics* 1995;95:888–91.

31. Guidelines for the use of parenteral and enteral nutrition in adult and pediatric patients. *JPEN* 2002;26:1SA–138SA.

32. Levy I, Katz J, Solter E, Samra Z, Vidne B, Birk E et al. Chlorhexidine-impregnated dressing for prevention of colonization of central venous catheters in infants and children: A randomized controlled study. *Pediatr Infect Dis J* 2005;24:676–9.

33. Onder AM, Chandar J, Coakley S, Francoeur D, Abitbol C, Zilleruelo G. Controlling exit site infections: Does it decrease the incidence of catheter-related bacteremia in children on chronic hemodialysis? *Hemodial Int* 2009;13:11–8.

34. Faubion WC, Wesley. JR, Khalidi N, Silva J. Total parenteral nutrition catheter sepsis: Impact of the team approach. *JPEN* 1986;10:642–5.

35. Reed CR, Sessler CN, Glauser FL, Phelan BA. Central venous catheter infections: Concepts and controversies. *Intensive Care Med* 1995;21:177–83.
36. Dezfulian C, Lavelle J, Nallamothu B, Kaufman S, Saint S. Rates of infection for single-lumen versus multilumen central venous catheters: A meta-analysis. *Crit Care Med* 2003;31:2385–90.
37. Cowl C, Weinstock J, Al-Jurf A. Complications and cost associated with parenteral nutrition delivered to hospitalized patients through either subclavian or peripherally-inserted central catheters. *Clin Nutr* 2000;19:237–43.
38. Ramritu P, Halton K, Collignon P, Cook D, Fraenkel D, Battistutta D et al. A systematic review comparing the relative effectiveness of antimicrobial-coated catheters in intensive care units. *Am J Infect Control* 2008;36:104–17.
39. Gilbert R, Harden M. Effectiveness of impregnated central venous catheters for catheter related blood stream infection: A systematic review. *Curr Opin Infect Dis* 2008;21:235–45.
40. Bagnall-Reeb H. Evidence for the use of the antibiotic lock technique. *J Infus Nurs* 2004;27:118–22.
41. Costerton W, Veeh R, Shirtliff M, Pasmore M, Post C, Ehrlich G. The application of biofilm science to the study and control of chronic bacterial infections. *J Clin Invest* 2003;112:1466–77.
42. Cowan CE. Antibiotic lock technique. *J Intraven Nurs* 1992;15:283–7.
43. Messing B, Peitra-Cohen S, Debure A, Beliah M, Bernier JJ. Antibiotic-lock technique: A new approach to optimal therapy for catheter-related sepsis in home-parenteral nutrition patients. *JPEN* 1988;12:185–9.
44. von Eiff C, Jansen B, Kohnen W, Becker K. Infections associated with medical devices: Pathogenesis, management and prophylaxis. *Drugs* 2005;65:179–214.
45. Bestul MB, Vandenbussche HL. Antibiotic lock technique: Review of the literature. *Pharmacotherapy* 2005;25:211–27.
46. Metcalf S, Chambers S, Pithie A. Use of ethanol locks to prevent recurrent central line sepsis. *J Infect* 2004;49:20–2.
47. Dannerberg C, Bierbach U, Rothe A, Beer J. Ethanol-lock technique in the treatment of bloodstream infections in pediatric oncology patients with broviac catheter. *J Pediatr Hematol Oncol* 2003;25:616–21.
48. Onland W, Shin C, Fustar S, Rushing T, Wong W. Ethanol-lock technique for persistent bacteremia of long-term intravascular devices in pediatric patients. *Arch Pediatr Adolesc Med* 2006;160:1049–53.
49. Mouw E, Chessman K, Lesher A, Tagge E. Use of an ethanol lock to prevent catheter-related infections in children with short bowel syndrome. *J Pediatr Surg* 2008;43:1025–9.
50. Sanders J, Pithie A, Ganly P, Surgenor L, Wilson R, Merriman E et al. A prospective double-blind randomized trial comparing intraluminal ethanol with heparinized saline for the prevention of catheter-associated bloodstream infection in immunosuppressed haematology patients. *J Antimicrob Chemother* 2008;62:809–15.
51. Opilla MT, Kirby DF, Edmond MB. Use of ethanol lock therapy to reduce the incidence of catheter-related bloodstream infections in home parenteral nutrition patients. *JPEN* 2007;31:302–5.
52. Pennington CR, Pithie AD. Ethanol lock in the management of catheter occlusion. *JPEN* 1987;11:507–8.
53. McHugh GJ, Wild DJ, Havill JH. Polyurethane central venous catheters, hydrochloric acid and 70% ethanol: A safety evaluation. *Anaesth Intensive Care* 1997;25:350–3.
54. Crnich C, Halfmann J, Crone W, Maki DG. The effects of prolonged ethanol exposure on the mechanical properties of polyurethane and silicone catheters used for intravascular access. *Infect Control Hosp Epidemiol* 2005;26:708–14.
55. Cober M, Johnson C. Stability of 70% alcohol solutions in polypropylene syringes for use in ethanol-lock therapy. *Am J Health Syst Pharm* 2007;64:2480–2.

# 20 Intestinal Failure–Associated Liver Disease

*Ivan R. Diamond and Paul W. Wales*

## CONTENTS

## 20.1 INTRODUCTION

Parenteral nutrition (PN) is a lifesaving therapy for patients with intestinal failure who are unable to receive sufficient calories enterally, and its development in the late 1960s can be regarded as a significant advance in modern medicine. However, no sooner was PN developed, did reports of the association between PN administration and cholestatic liver disease emerge, with the first publication occurring in 1971 [1]. This liver disease, being variously known as parenteral nutrition associated liver disease (IFALD) or parenteral nutrition associated cholestasis, is one of the most common complications experienced by patients on long-term PN and is a significant contributor to morbidity and mortality in this patient population.

While it may be debatable whether the term intestinal failure associated liver disease (IFALD) is entirely synonymous with IFALD, this term has recently emerged as the most commonly used term to describe the cholestatic liver disease that occurs in patients with intestinal failure who are on long-term PN. The term IFALD recognizes the multitude of factors at play in the development of this liver disease. Given the multiple etiologic factors, we favor the term IFALD, when discussing liver disease in our intestinal failure patients.

This chapter will consider the clinical presentation, epidemiology, pathogenesis of IFALD, as well as potential treatment strategies. While the review will focus primarily on the pediatric patient, given that this population is most at risk of IFALD, the issues for adult patients are quite similar although the overall risk and incidence of IFALD is lower in adults.

## 20.2 CLINICAL PRESENTATION

The clinical spectrum of IFALD ranges from mild cholestasis to hepatic fibrosis and resultant liver failure. The initial biochemical features are that of an elevated conjugated serum bilirubin and gamma-glutamyl transferase (GGT), which rise within 1–4 weeks of initiating therapy [2,3]. There are age related differences in the presentation of IFALD, with children demonstrating a predominantly cholestatic picture with relatively rapid progression to advanced liver disease, with the predominant finding in adults being that of steatosis [4,5]. Biochemically, in adults, transaminitis is the earliest indicator of the disease [6] with jaundice a late and concerning sign [7]. Both adults and children develop evidence of biliary sludge and cholelithiasis related to the duration of PN use [8–10]. It is likely that these processes contributes to IFALD, with evidence that flushing of the biliary system via percutaneous cholangiography improves time to resolution of hyperbilirubinemia [11].

As IFALD progresses, other features of liver disease develop such as synthetic dysfunction and hypersplenism resulting in thrombocytopenia and coagulopathy. We have demonstrated a serum conjugated bilirubin of 100 μmol/L (6.7 mg/dL) in neonates to have a sensitivity of 94% and specificity of 87% for end-stage liver disease [12]. However, the marker occurred late in the disease course and as such was an inappropriate to be utilized as a referral criterion for transplantation. Aside from the risk to life posed by progressive IFALD; the disease likely also significantly impairs quality of life in children by hindering intestinal adaptation and the chance that the child may ultimately be able to be weaned from PN [13]. Given the close resemblance of IFALD to other cholestatic and steatotic liver diseases, it is advisable to adequately investigate any patient with suspected IFALD for other causes of liver disease prior to attributing the hepatic dysfunction to PN [14].

Although in our experience liver biopsy is infrequently done, the histopathological findings are variable but the key features include intracellular and intracanalicular cholestasis, steatosis, and periportal fibrosis [5]. Hepatic steatosis is more common in adults and may occur without associated inflammation, cholestasis, or necrosis; in contrast, infants present with centrilobular cholestasis, portal inflammation and necrosis with steatosis being less prevalent. Other histological features may include signs of hepatocellular injury such as balloon degeneration and multinucleated giant cells.

## 20.3 EPIDEMIOLOGY OF IFALD

Descriptions of the epidemiology of IFALD are challenging to interpret as no consistent definitions exist to characterize this condition. While some studies have defined the condition on the basis of consistent elevations in various liver enzymes, recently definitions based purely on the serum-conjugated bilirubin have become more frequent [6,7,15–18]. Definition of liver disease will alter the incidence of the disorder with one study showing an incidence of liver disease of 57% based on a panel of abnormal liver function tests, with the incidence declining to 12% if only the serum-conjugated bilirubin is considered [19]. Yang et al., also recently demonstrated persistent and prolonged elevations in the transaminase levels in patients with IFALD following achievement of full enteral tolerance despite normalization of serum conjugated bilirubin. This demonstrates that hepatic pathology may occur in the absence of hyperbilirubinemia [20]. Depending on definition, the incidence of IFALD lies between 40% and 60% of infants on long-term PN and 15–40% of adults on home PN [5]. The risk of end-stage liver disease approaches 25% in pediatric patients with short-bowel syndrome [21] and up to 15% in adult patients on home PN [7]. In pediatric patients, the end-stage liver disease is frequently fatal due to a relative unavailability of size appropriate allografts particularly when an intestinal transplant is required; with up to 1.4% of deaths in children <4 years attributable to short-bowel syndrome, with most of these deaths being related to hepatic disease [4,15,21–23].

Cohort studies have also been utilized to define demographic risk factors for IFALD, with premature infants, particularly those <500 g, having the greatest risk of this condition [2,16,24]. Preterm infants, with short-bowel syndrome, have a significant risk of developing end-stage liver disease from IFALD with incidences as high as 90% in those on PN for >3 months [25]. While short-bowel syndrome is a substantial predictor for the development of IFALD, a study from France demonstrated the greatest risk in those with intractable diarrhea of infancy [26]. A diagnosis of gastroschisis or jejunal atresia is also associated with an increased risk of IFALD [24]. In adult patients, demographic risk factors for IFALD are related to residual small intestinal length, comorbid liver disease, female gender, and the absence of the colon in continuity [6,17,19,27].

## 20.4 PATHOGENESIS OF IFALD

In addition to defining demographic risk factors for IFALD, animal models and cohort studies have also elucidated some of the pathophysiologic processes underlying the development of IFALD. The pathophysiology of IFALD can be thought to be related to aspects of the PN as well as those related to host factors (Table 20.1).

**TABLE 20.1**
**Pathogensis of IFALD**

**PN-Associated Factors**

- Hypercaloric feeds with excess macronutrients
  - Amino acid
    - Deficiencies of
    - Taurine
    - Cysteine
    - Carnitine
    - Choline
  - Excess methionine
- Lipids
  - Phospholipid accumulation
  - Phytosterols
  - ω-6LCPUFA
  - Antioxidant imbalance
- Minerals and trace elements
  - Manganese
  - Chromium
  - Copper

**Host Factors**

- Prematurity
  - Immaturity of hepatic pathways
- Intestinal failure
  - Deranged enterohepatic circulation
  - Stasis
  - Sepsis
    - Catheter related
    - Translocation related

## 20.4.1  PN-Related Factors

Hypercaloric feeds, with excess of any of the macronutrients of PN can result in steatosis as well as chronic cholestasis [28–30]. The mechanism underlying this phenomenon is thought to be related to increased hepatic oxygen demand resulting in relative ischemia [31]. However, specific macronutrient effects also likely result in the development of IFALD as do effects of certain minerals and trace elements.

### 20.4.1.1  Glucose

While glucose is not inherently hepatoxic, excess glucose administration results hyperinsulinism. This results in an upregulation of enzymes involved in fatty acid synthesis leading to hepatic steatosis [32]. This issue was particularly germane early in the experience with PN prior to the development of adequate intravenous lipid preparations. However, with an increased focus on the role of lipid in the development of IFALD and strategies to limit lipid use, the issue deserves renewed consideration as calories lost due to lipid minimization are frequently made up by increasing the glucose load.

### 20.4.1.2  Amino Acids

Excessive administration of parenteral amino acids has been demonstrated to result in cholestatic jaundice in neonates. This is thought to be related both to cumulative exposure, as well as dose with premature infants who received daily amino acids of 3.6 g/kg/day having a more rapid rise in bilirubin levels than those who received 2.5 g/kg/day [18,33]. However, the notion of amino acid dose-related toxicity is not uniformly accepted [34].

At physiologic doses, it is possible that hepatotoxicity is related to a deficiency of taurine or cysteine. These are considered conditionally essential amino acids in neonates because of the low levels of hepatic cystathionase and cysteine sulfinic decarboxylase which allow for their synthesis from methionine [35–37]. Taurine deficiency leads to the inability to form taurine-conjugated bile acids resulting in increased formation of toxic glycine-conjugated bile acids. While taurine supplementation has been shown to improve bile secretion in an animal model, clinical efficacy is limited with taurine-containing PN solutions not altering the risk of IFALD [38,39]. Neonates, also have a limited ability to convert lysine and methionine into carnitine which is important for mitochondrial fatty-acid oxidation [40]. Although carnitine deficiency has been demonstrated in those on PN, normalization of serum carnitine levels have not been demonstrated to result in improvement of IFALD [41]. It has also been suggested that choline deficiency may exacerbate steatosis, with a pilot study demonstrating reduction in steatosis in adults with choline supplementation [42].

A consequence of immaturity of the pathways of methionine metabolism, is accumulation of toxic metabolites of this amino acid such as 3-methyl propionic acid in the neonate [43,44]. These metabolites are thought to contribute to the development of IFALD with inappropriate methionine load being regarded as important contributor to the development of IFALD in infants.

### 20.4.1.3  Lipids

Lipids have been demonstrated to play a significant role in the development of IFALD in both children and adults. In adults, a lipid dose in excess of 1 g/kg/day is related to the development of IFALD [17]. In children, Colomb et al., demonstrated that episodes of cholestasis were correlated with lipid concentrations [45]. A recent multiple variable study by our group examining risk factors for severe IFALD (serum-conjugated bilirubin >100 μmol/L) demonstrated that each day of parenteral lipid >2.5 g/kg/day was associated with a 1.04 increase in the odds of developing this outcome [46]. While this risk may seem trivial, it is important to recognize that the risk is expressed per day of lipid, with the odds of severe IFALD approaching 10 with 60 days of PN lipid use at this dose.

The mechanism whereby lipids contribute to IFALD, is likely multifactorial relating to accumulation of phospholipids [17], excess phytosterols [47–49], predominance of omega-6 long-chain polyunsaturated fatty acids (ω-6LCPUFA) leading to a proinflammatory state [50–52] and also antioxidant imbalance [53,54].

Plant-based, particularly soy, lipid emulsions have been the mainstay of PN to date, with at present no nonplant-based lipid emulsions having regulatory approval in North America. These emulsions have a high phytosterol and ω-6LCPUFA content and low antioxidant content. Therefore it is likely that intravenous lipid emulsions play a significant role in the development of IFALD. Serum levels of phytosterols have been demonstrated to be elevated in patients with IFALD, with correlation between these levels and the severity of IFALD [48,49]. The mechanism whereby phytosterols contribute to IFALD may be related to increased lithogenicity of bile or alterations in the canalicular membrane affecting canalicular flow [47]. More recently a molecular mechanism has been described whereby phytosterols antagonize messenger RNA for critical bile acid homeostatic proteins [55,56].

Long-chain polyunsaturated fatty acids (LCPUFA) contained in lipid emulsions, are readily incorporated in a dose-dependent manner into cell phospholipid membranes and other tissues, where they are involved in cell signaling, the production of eicosanoids involved in inflammation, blood vessel tone, platelet aggregation, and modulation of the immune system [57]. LCPUFA also directly affect gene transcription and lipid metabolism [58]. LCPUFA provide the substrate for systemic eicosanoid production, with eicosanoids arising from ω-6LCPUFA (Thromboxane A2, Leukotrienes B4, C4, D4, Prostaglandins D2, E2, and F2, and Prostacyclin I2) having a primarily proinflammatory effect which is thought to contribute to the development of IFALD [50–52]. In addition to being proinflammatory, ω-6LCPUFA also impair bile flow in an animal model of IFALD [47] and induce steatosis [59,60].

The final mechanism whereby, intravenous lipid emulsions may contribute to the development of IFALD relates to imbalance of antioxidants. Antioxidants, such as α-tocopherol are an important addition to lipid emulsions as they prevent lipid peroxidation and free radical generation. However, soy-based lipid emulsions have limited antioxidant concentration, particularly when considering the most biologically active form, α-tocopherol. This may result in a reduction of this substance in plasma lipoproteins and a resultant decrease in antioxidant defenses [14,61]. In clinical studies of lipid emulsions containing α-tocopherol, improved antioxidant measures were associated with improvements in liver function [53,54]. An additional approach for provision of antioxidants is addition of zinc and selenium to the PN solution [62–64].

#### 20.4.1.4 Minerals and Trace Elements

Trace elements, particularly manganese, have been implicated in the development of IFALD [65–67]. In a study of 57 children on long-term PN, 45 had evidence of excess blood manganese levels. This is particularly concerning the given adverse neurological effects of manganese accumulation within the basal ganglia. There was also a correlation between the degree of hypermanganesemia and IFALD. Furthermore, liver disease improved following reduction or elimination of the manganese from the PN. Since manganese is excreted in bile, accumulation of this substance is particularly important in the setting of a cholestatic liver disease such as IFALD. For this reason, we do not add manganese to our PN solutions for infants at risk of IFALD. While aluminum toxicity has been associated with PN induced bone disease, there is no evidence of an association with IFALD [31,68]. Similarly, while chromium toxicity, secondary to PN, has been reported in animals there has been no relation to IFALD in humans although there is evidence of intrahepatic accumulation of this trace element [69,70]. Copper is also potentially hepatotoxic and since its elimination is biliary, it is suggested that monitoring of blood concentrations is justified to prevent hepatic injury [14].

## 20.4.2   HOST FACTORS

### 20.4.2.1   Prematurity

Children are at a greater risk of developing IFALD, with the youngest and smallest children being most vulnerable. Beath et al. [71] found the highest incidence of IFALD in infants <34-week gestation weighing <2 kg. It is logical to assume that this finding relates to immaturity of the liver, with infants having diminished hepatic synthesis and uptake of bile salts and reduced enterohepatic circulation [72]. This may be due to developmental differences in the regulation of genes involved in this process [73,74]. Other hepatic functions are also immature with evidence of cystathionase deficiency [37], glutathione deficiency [75] and a decreased ability for transulfuration of toxic bile salts such as lithocholic acid [76].

### 20.4.2.2   Intestinal Failure

Patients receiving PN for intestinal failure are at much greater risk of IFALD than those who receive PN for other reasons. Stanko et al. demonstrated in a group of patients who received identical PN infusions, that only those with short-bowel syndrome developed liver disease [77]. Other studies have shown an increased risk with absence of the colon [27,78]. Children who are not able to tolerate any enteral feeds are at greater risk of IFALD than those who are partially enteraly fed [71,78,79]. Degree of bowel loss is also related to outcome, with children with <50 cm of small bowel being at greatest risk of death from liver failure [4,80].

The reason why patients with intestinal failure are at increased risk for IFALD likely relates to both the negative impact of absence of feeds, impaired enterohepatic circulation, as well as an increased risk for sepsis related to deficiencies in gastrointestinal mucosal integrity and immunity. Absence of enteral feeds, results in alterations in release of gastrointestinal hormones which may affect biliary and intestinal motility [81]. Reduced bile flow is exacerbated by fasting and is a primary factor in the development of biliary sludge and gall stones. Reduced enteral intake also contributes to intestinal hypomotility which may result in bacterial overgrowth due to stasis. Particularly in the setting of a compromised intestine, with increased mucosal permeability, this overgrowth may result in translocation of bacteria resulting in sepsis [82]. Intraluminal bacteria have also been implicated in the conversion of chenodeoxycholic acid into the hepatotoxin lithocholic acid [83].

### 20.4.2.3   Sepsis

IFALD has been demonstrated to be associated with recurrent episodes of sepsis in numerous series [4,16,78,80,84]. Key sources of sepsis in patients on PN relate to both the need for a central venous catheter for PN administration as well as bacterial translocation from bacterial overgrowth [85]. Sepsis is frequently contributory to death in patients with advanced IFALD [4]. Proinflammatory cytokines elaborated following endotoxin exposure from a septic insult have been shown to downregulate the molecular mechanisms underlying bile acid transport [86,87]. Short-bowel syndrome is believed to represent a proinflammatory state, with an exaggerated inflammatory response including hepatitis arising from a septic insult [88]. The fact that the ω-6LCPUFA may result in enhanced levels of proinflammatory mediators is intriguing and leads one to speculate whether traditional lipid emulsions potentiate the adverse hepatic response to endotoxin mediated cholestasis.

## 20.5   TREATMENT AND PREVENTION OF IFALD

Table 20.2 provides a summary of the various possible treatments that can be utilized for IFALD.

## 20.5.1   NUTRITIONAL STRATEGIES

The key principle in the nutritional management of a child on PN, is to minimize the risk of IFALD by avoiding aspects of the PN that have been associated with this outcome such as avoiding

---

**TABLE 20.2**

**Possible Treatment Strategies for IFALD**

- *Nutritional Strategies*
  - Encourage enteral autonomy
    - Restore continuity
    - Intestinal lengthening
  - Multidisciplinary intestinal rehabilitation
  - Appropriate PN macronutrients and additives
  - Cycling of PN
  - Lipid strategies
    - ω-3 lipid preparations
    - Lipid minimization

- *Sepsis Prevention*
  - Line-related sepsis prevention
    - Multidisciplinary care and patient education
    - Appropriate catheter care
    - Antibiotic and ethanol locks
  - Bacterial overgrowth prevention
    - Gut decontamination with cyclical antibiotics
    - Bulk forming enteral agents
    - Glutamine
    - Probiotics

- *Pharmacologic Therapies*
  - Ursodeoxycholic acid
  - *N*-acetylcysteine
  - Choline
  - Antioxidants
    - α-Tocopherol
    - Zinc, selenium

- *Percutaneous Cholangiography*
- *Transplantation*

---

overfeeding of parenteral calories as well as addition of detrimental elements to the PN such as manganese. However with data that IFALD may be reversible if enteral feeding can be resumed prior to the establishment of significant fibrosis or cirrhosis [89], encouragement of enteral autonomy is essential; and may be facilitated by multidisciplinary intestinal rehabilitation [21,90]. Restoration of gastrointestinal continuity in those who have proximal enterostomies [91] as well as surgical lengthening procedures [92], may play a role. There is evidence of biochemical normalization following a surgical lengthening procedure even in the setting of fibrosis [93,94]. However, re-establishment of enteral feeds was important in achieving this outcome with five out of eight patients who remained PN dependent after the operation having ongoing cholestasis [94].

For those patients with limited capacity to adapt, or in whom a prolonged period of adaptation is anticipated, cyclic infusions of PN may be protective. These infusions result in lower insulin levels, less hepatomegally and improved biochemistry [95,96]. Cyclic PN permits a period of free fatty acid mobilization from body stores during the noninfusion period and are thought to protect the liver by promoting more efficient energy utilization, which is important in the setting of hepatotoxic stresses [14,97].

Given the importance that lipid likely plays in the pathogenesis of IFALD, there has been a effort to employ lipid minimization strategies for the treatment of IFALD. Colomb et al., demonstrated improvement in serum bilirubin and thrombocytopenia in patients with IFALD with temporary cessation of parenteral lipids [45]. Similarly, Rollins demonstrated improvement or resolution of hyperbilirubinaemia with lipid reduction or elimination [98]. Ultimately, controlled studies are needed to assess both the safety and efficacy of lipid restriction protocols.

Although the subject will be covered in more detail in Chapter 21, Use of Paretneral Fish Oil in the Management of Intestinal Failure-Associated Liver Disease, no review of IFALD will be complete without mentioning the exciting data suggesting that IFALD may be treated by substitution of the ω-6LCPUFA containing soy-based lipid emulsion with Omegaven (Fresenius Kabi, Bad Hamburg, Germany) a lipid emulsion derived from fish oil with substantial omega-3 long-chain polyunsaturated fatty acids (ω-3LCPUFA). The initial clinical reports of the use of this emulsion originated from Children's Hospital Boston with a case report published in 2006 of two children with severe end-stage liver IFALD who demonstrated complete reversal of their liver disease after starting Omegaven [99]. Most recent published data from that group demonstrated resolution of IFALD in 45% (19 of 42 cases) while receiving PN compared with 5% in a historic control group who received a soy-based lipid emulsion [100].

Our experience has been similar, with our most recent analysis demonstrating resolution in 63% while receiving PN (14 of 22 cases) [101]. While the group from Boston have advocated suggested sole Omegaven use at 1 g/kg/day; we have adopted an approach whereby the Omegaven is initially dosed together with Intralipid (each at 1 g/kg/day). Our practice is based on the belief that this approach should allow for improved nutrition and energy balance, while still providing the antiinflammatory effect of the ω-3 lipid. We also have significant concerns as to potential adverse long-term neurocognitive outcomes with fat restriction in developing infants. However, in selected instances, the Intralipid is discontinued due to concern as to the severity of IFALD or as the parenteral lipid is weaned with improved enteral tolerance. We believe that the optimal dosing strategy for Omegaven, both from an efficacy and safety perspective, is still to be determined.

Also, while lipid restriction, whether affected by of lipid minimization or dosing Omegaven at 1 g/kg/day, may be appropriate in a child with advanced liver disease, it may not be appropriate in one with more mild disease where the goal of treatment is more preventative. We have held that despite the potential for intravenous lipid emulsions containing ω-3LCPUFA, at present their use remains investigational and should only be used in those with severe IFALD unless in the context of a randomized trial examining their safety and efficacy as a preventative strategy [102,103]. These preventative randomized trials are ongoing, with one examining Omegaven [104] and the other SMOFlipid (a composite lipid emulsion comprised of 30% soybean oil, 30% medium-chain triglycerides, 25% olive oil, and 15% fish oil) (Fresenius Kabi, Bad Hamburg, Germany) [105].

### 20.5.2  PREVENTION OF SEPSIS

Given the key role that sepsis has been shown to play in the development of IFALD, it is logical to assume that prevention of sepsis should be an important factor in the prevention and treatment of IFALD. Sepsis reduction should focus on both care of the central catheter as well as prevention of bacterial overgrowth and resultant translocation.

Prevention of central catheter infections requires individual and team efforts, with data supporting a reduced incidence of catheter infection with dedicated infusion therapy teams [106,107]. In the home setting education of parents is critical. A meta-analysis has shown that chlorhexidine was superior to povidoneiodine for the prevention of catheter-related infections [108]. Also, there is evidence to suggest that antibiotic and ethanol locks may also be useful [109,110]. The potential impact that enhanced line care may have, is highlighted by the fact that there is a substantial difference between the incidence and the age of development of liver disease in children whose central line catheter care was managed by a team experienced in this setting [111]. As well, there is a case report of a child with IFALD who demonstrated improvement in their liver disease with change of caregiver presumably secondary to a reduction in the rate of line infection [112].

Treatment of bacterial overgrowth with cycled antibiotics has also been suggested to have a beneficial impact in reducing the risk of sepsis and resultant IFALD [113]. A randomized trial of prophylactic erythromycin in 182 very low-birth weight neonates demonstrated a significant reduction in liver disease and sepsis, but since the primary objective was to examine this drug as a motility agent its not clear as to whether the results were due to the effects on motility or as an antimicrobial [114]. Given the high prevalence of rapid transit in our patient population, we do not believe that erythromycin is an optimal drug in patients with short-bowel syndrome. We generally, do not use antibiotics prophylactically but do so for the treatment of clinically significant bacterial overgrowth.

Another strategy that may hold promise are animal models suggesting that bulk-forming enteral agents may limit bacterial translocation [115,116]. Glutamine supplementation has also been demonstrated in animal models to limit translocation [117,118]. In rats, glutamine reverses the inhibition of hepatocyte mitochondrial metabolism observed following endotoxemia [119]. However, a randomized trial of glutamine supplementation in infants did not show substantial benefit [120]. Finally, the role of probiotics in preventing bacterial overgrowth and translocation needs to be examined further [113].

### 20.5.3 Pharmacologic Strategies

Pharmacologic treatments for IFALD are limited. Ursodeoxycholic acid is commonly suggested for IFALD [121,122]. A recent randomized trial demonstrated reduction in GGT but not serum bilirubin with its use [123]. Also, in our experience diarrhea related to its use limits is applicability in many patients with short-bowel syndrome. We recently reported some success with N-acetylcysteine demonstrating normalization of red-cell glutathione concentrations [124]. This therapy requires further evaluation, although we generally employ it in patients with moderate to advanced IFALD given the lack of other options. As discussed earlier there is also evidence that choline supplementation may limit steatosis in adults [42]. Other treatments suggested to be beneficial for IFALD that have been proven not to be effective, in controlled studies, have included cholecystokinin [125,126] and tauroursodeoxycholic acid [127]. The fact that these therapies demonstrated promise in the noncontrolled setting highlights the importance of adequately powered controlled studies when evaluating therapies for IFALD.

### 20.5.4 Transplantation

Transplantation can be an effective and lifesaving therapy for patients with IFALD refractory to other therapies. However, transplantation, in infants, poses a significant challenge because of the shortage of size appropriate grafts particularly when attempting combined liver-intestinal transplantation with significant waitlist mortality [4,15,21–23]. As well, although the outcomes continue to improve, the long-term survival of patients receiving an intestinal transplant remains suboptimal. One and 5 year graft survival for this procedure are 80% and 50% respectively with the poor outcomes primarily related to the significant medical complications associated with small bowel transplantation [128]. This has led some to suggest that for patients who are likely to achieve independence from PN once that their liver disease is treated, that isolated liver transplantation be performed [129,130]. While we have adopted this approach occasionally, we believe it is only appropriate in carefully selected patients in whom there is a very high likelihood that the child will achieve nutritional independence.

## 20.6 CONCLUSION

IFALD is the most common complication arising from prolonged PN use and has the potential for significant morbidity and mortality. Its etiology is related to both components of the PN as well as host factors. Understanding of the etiology of IFALD provides targets for intervention with exiting developments in terms of the use of novel ω-3LCPUFA enriched emulsions that have the potential to have a significant impact on the management of patients with IFALD. As well, given the central role of sepsis in the pathogenesis of this condition, optimal patient care to prevent this complication should allow for the best outcome of patients on prolonged PN.

## DISCLOSURE

The authors have received Investigator Initiated Trial funding from Fresenius Kabi, the manufacturer of both Omegaven and Intralipid to evaluate SMOFlipid for the prevention of IFALD.

## ACKNOWLEDGMENTS

The authors wish to acknowledge the following members of the GIFT team, our multidisciplinary intestinal rehabilitation program, for their contributions to our experience with and understanding of IFALD: J. Darch, J. Brennan-Donnan, J. Bowers, M. Carricato, K. Cormier, G. Courtney-Martin, L. Coxson, N. D'Amato, M. De Angelis, N. de Silva, A. Fecteau, D. Fierheller, D. Grant, A. Gold, D. Harrison, J. Hawes, L. Ives-Baine, P. Kean, C. Kosar, C. Koziolek, K. Lang, S. Ling, J. Maxwell, A. Moore, K. Murch, C. Newman, V. Ng, C. Patterson, P. Pencharz, A. Rogers, M. Rugg, S. So.

Ivan Diamond was supported by a Fellowship award from the Canadian Institutes of Health Research with additional support from the Surgeon Scientist Training Program, Department of Surgery, University of Toronto.

## REFERENCES

1. Peden VH, Witzleben CL, Skelton MA. Total parenteral nutrition. *J Pediatr.* 1971;78:180–1.
2. Beale EF, Nelson RM, Bucciarelli RL, Donnelly WH, Eitzman DV. Intrahepatic cholestasis associated with parenteral nutrition in premature infants. *Pediatrics.* 1979;64:342–7.
3. Black DD, Suttle EA, Whitington PF, Whitington GL, Korones SD. The effect of short-term total parenteral nutrition on hepatic function in the human neonate: A prospective randomized study demonstrating alteration of hepatic canalicular function. *J Pediatr.* 1981;99:445–9.
4. Sondheimer JM, Asturias E, Cadnapaphornchai M. Infection and cholestasis in neonates with intestinal resection and long-term parenteral nutrition. *J Pediatr Gastroenterol Nutr.* 1998;27(2):131–7.
5. Kelly DA. Intestinal failure-associated liver disease: What do we know today? *Gastroenterology.* 2006;130:S70–7.
6. Luman W, Shaffer JL. Prevalence outcome and associated factors of deranged liver function tests in patients on home parenteral nutrition. *Clin Nutr.* 2002;21:337–43.
7. Chan S, McCowen KC, Bistrian BR et al. Incidence, prognosis, and etiology of end-stage liver disease in patients receiving home total parenteral nutrition. *Surgery.* 1999;126:28–34.
8. Messing B, Bories C, Kunstlinger F, Bernier JJ. Does total parenteral nutrition induce gallbladder sludge formation and lithiasis? *Gastroenterology.* 1983;84:1012–9.
9. Pitt HA, King W, Mann LL et al. Increased risk of cholelithiasis with prolonged total parenteral nutrition. *Am J Surg.* 1983;145:106–12.
10. Roslyn JJ, Berquist WE, Pitt HA et al. Increased risk of gallstones in children receiving total parenteral nutrition. *Pediatrics.* 1983;71:784–9.
11. Wales PW, Brindle M, Sauer CJ, Patel S, de Silva N, Chait P. Percutaneous cholangiography for the treatment of parenteral nutrition-associated cholestasis in surgical neonates: Preliminary experience. *J Pediatr Surg.* 2007;42:1913–8.
12. Nasr A, Avitzur Y, Ng VL, De Silva N, Wales PW. The use of conjugated hyperbilirubinemia greater than 100 micromol/L as an indicator of irreversible liver disease in infants with short bowel syndrome. *J Pediatr Surg.* 2007;42:359–62.
13. Weber TR, Keller MS. Adverse effects of liver dysfunction and portal hypertension on intestinal adaptation in short bowel syndrome in children. *Am J Surg.* 2002;184:582–6.
14. Goulet O, Joly F, Corriol O, Colomb-Jung V. Some new insights in intestinal failure-associated liver disease. *Curr Opin Organ Transplant.* 2009;14:256–61.
15. Wales PW, de Silva N, Kim J, Lecce L, To T, Moore A. Neonatal short bowel syndrome: Population-based estimates of incidence and mortality rates. *J Pediatr Surg.* 2004;39:690–5.

16. Wales PW, de Silva N, Kim JH, Lecce L, Sandhu A, Moore AM. Neonatal short bowel syndrome: A cohort study. *J Pediatr Surg*. 2005;40:755–62.

17. Cavicchi M, Beau P, Crenn P, Degott C, Messing B. Prevalence of liver disease and contributing factors in patients receiving home parenteral nutrition for permanent intestinal failure. *Ann Intern Med*. 2000;132:525–32.

18. Steinbach M, Clark RH, Kelleher AS et al. Demographic and nutritional factors associated with prolonged cholestatic jaundice in the premature infant. *J Perinatol*. 2008;28:129–35.

19. Salvino R, Ghanta R, Seidner DL, Mascha E, Xu Y, Steiger E. Liver failure is uncommon in adults receiving long-term parenteral nutrition. *JPEN*. 2006;30:202–8.

20. Yang CF, Lee M, Valim C et al. Persistent alanine aminotransferase elevations in children with parenteral nutrition-associated liver disease. *J Pediatr Surg* 2009;44:1084–7.

21. Diamond IR, de Silva N, Pencharz PB, Kim JH, Wales PW. Neonatal short bowel syndrome outcomes after the establishment of the first Canadian multidisciplinary intestinal rehabilitation program: Preliminary experience. *J Pediatr Surg*. 2007;42:806–11.

22. Teitelbaum DH, Tracy T. Parenteral nutrition-associated cholestasis. *Semin Pediatr Surg*. 2001;10:72–80.

23. Fecteau A, Atkinson P, Grant D. Early referral is essential for successful pediatric small bowel transplantation: The Canadian experience. *J Pediatr Surg*. 2001;36:681–4.

24. Christensen RD, Henry E, Wiedmeier SE, Burnett J, Lambert DK. Identifying patients, on the first day of life, at high-risk of developing parenteral nutrition-associated liver disease. *J Perinatol*. 2007;27:284–90.

25. Carter BA, Shulman RJ. Mechanisms of disease: Update on the molecular etiology and fundamentals of parenteral nutrition associated cholestasis. *Nat Clin Pract Gastroenterol Hepatol*. 2007;4:277–87.

26. Colomb V, Dabbas-Tyan M, Taupin P et al. Long-term outcome of children receiving home parenteral nutrition: A 20-year single-center experience in 302 patients. *J Pediatr Gastroenterol Nutr*. 2007;44:347–53.

27. Lloyd DA, Zabron AA, Gabe SM. Chronic biochemical cholestasis in patients receiving home parenteral nutrition: Prevalence and predisposing factors. *Aliment Pharmacol Ther*. 2008;27:552–60.

28. Sheldon GF, Peterson SR, Sanders R. Hepatic dysfunction during hyperalimentation. *Arch Surg*. 1978;113:504–8.

29. Mashima Y. Effect of calorie overload on puppy livers during parenteral nutrition. *J Parenter Enteral Nutr*. 1979;3:139–45.

30. Messing B, Colombel JF, Heresbach D, Chazouilleres O, Galian A. Chronic cholestasis and macronutrient excess in patients treated with prolonged parenteral nutrition. *Nutrition*. 1992;8:30–6.

31. Nightingale JM. Hepatobiliary, renal and bone complications of intestinal failure. *Best Pract Res Clin Gastroenterol*. 2003;17:907–29.

32. Kaminski DL, Adams A, Jellinek M. The effect of hyperalimentation on hepatic lipid content and lipogenic enzyme activity in rats and man. *Surgery*. 1980;88:93–100.

33. Vileisis RA, Inwood RJ, Hunt CE. Prospective controlled study of parenteral nutrition-associated cholestatic jaundice: Effect of protein intake. *J Pediatr*. 1980;96:893–7.

34. Blau J, Sridhar S, Mathieson S, Chawla A. Effects of protein/nonprotein caloric intake on parenteral nutrition associated cholestasis in premature infants weighing 600–1000 grams. *JPEN*. 2007;31:487–90.

35. Rigo J, Senterre J. Is taurine essential for the neonates? *Biol Neonate*. 1977;32:73–6.

36. Zlotkin SH, Anderson GH. The development of cystathionase activity during the first year of life. *Pediatr Res*. 1982;16:65–8.

37. Vina J, Vento M, Garcia-Sala F. L-Cysteine and glutathione metabolism are impaired in premature infants due to cystathionase deficiency. *Am J Clin Nutr*. 1995;61:1067–9.

38. Guertin F, Roy CC, Lepage G et al. Effect of taurine on total parenteral nutrition-associated cholestasis. *JPEN*. 1991;15:247–51.

39. Hata S, Kubota A, Okada A. A pediatric amino acid solution for total parenteral nutrition does not affect liver function test results in neonates. *Surg Today*. 2002;32:800–3.

40. Shenai JP, Borum PR. Tissue carnitine reserves of newborn infants. *Pediatr Res*. 1984;18:679–82.

41. Bowyer BA, Miles JM, Haymond MW, Fleming CR. L-Carnitine therapy in home parenteral nutrition patients with abnormal liver tests and low plasma carnitine concentrations. *Gastroenterology*. 1988;94:434–8.

42. Buchman AL, Ament ME, Sohel M et al. Choline deficiency causes reversible hepatic abnormalities in patients receiving parenteral nutrition: Proof of a human choline requirement: A placebo-controlled trial. *JPEN*. 2001;25:260–8.

43. Dever JT, Elfarra AA. L-Methionine-DL-sulfoxide metabolism and toxicity in freshly isolated mouse hepatocytes: Gender differences and inhibition with aminooxyacetic acid. *Drug Metab Dispos*. 2008;36:2252–60.

44. Dever JT and Elfarra AA. L-Methionine toxicity in freshly isolated mouse hepatocytes is gender-dependent and mediated in part by transamination. *J Pharmacol Exp Ther.* 2008;326:809–17.

45. Colomb V, Jobert-Giraud A, Lacaille F, Goulet O, Fournet JC, Ricour C. Role of lipid emulsions in cholestasis associated with long-term parenteral nutrition in children. *JPEN.* 2000;24(6):345–50.

46. Diamond IR, de Silva NT, Tomlinson GA, Pencharz PB, Feldman BM, Moore AM, Ling SC, Wales PW. The role of parenteral lipids in the development of advanced intestinal failure associated liver disease in infants—a multiple variable analysis. *JPEN*, in press.

47. Van Aerde JE, Duerksen DR, Gramlich L et al. Intravenous fish oil emulsion attenuates total parenteral nutrition-induced cholestasis in newborn piglets. *Pediatr Res.* 1999;45:202–8.

48. Llop JM, Virgili N, Moreno-Villares JM et al. Phytosterolemia in parenteral nutrition patients: Implications for liver disease development. *Nutrition.* 2008;24:1145–52.

49. Clayton PT, Bowron A, Mills KA, Massoud A, Casteels M, Milla PJ. Phytosterolemia in children with parenteral nutrition-associated cholestatic liver disease. *Gastroenterology.* 1993;105:1806–13.

50. Heller A, Koch T, Schmeck J, van Ackern K. Lipid mediators in inflammatory disorders. *Drugs.* 1998;55:487–96.

51. Broughton KS, Wade JW. Total fat and (n-3):(n-6) fat ratios influence eicosanoid production in mice. *J Nutr.* 2002;132:88–94.

52. Grimm H, Tibell A, Norrlind B et al. Immunoregulation by parenteral lipids: Impact of the n-3 to n-6 fatty acid ratio. *JPEN.* 1994;18(5):417–21.

53. Antebi H, Mansoor O, Ferrier C et al. Liver function and plasma antioxidant status in intensive care unit patients requiring total parenteral nutrition: Comparison of 2 fat emulsions. *JPEN.* 2004;28:142–8.

54. Grimm H, Mertes N, Goeters C et al. Improved fatty acid and leukotriene pattern with a novel lipid emulsion in surgical patients. *Eur J Nutr.* 2006;45:55–60.

55. Carter BA, Karpen SJ. Intestinal failure-associated liver disease: Management and treatment strategies past, present, and future. *Semin Liver Dis.* 2007;27:251–8.

56. Carter BA, Taylor OA, Prendergast DR et al. Stigmasterol, a soy lipid-derived phytosterol, is an antagonist of the bile acid nuclear receptor FXR. *Pediatr Res.* 2007;62:301–6.

57. Calder PC. n-3 Polyunsaturated fatty acids, inflammation, and inflammatory diseases. *Am J Clin Nutr.* 2006;83:1505S–19S.

58. Deckelbaum RJ, Worgall TS, Seo T. n-3 Fatty acids and gene expression. *Am J Clin Nutr.* 2006;83:1520S–5S.

59. Beckh K, Kneip S, Arnold R. Direct regulation of bile secretion by prostaglandins in perfused rat liver. *Hepatology.* 1994;19:1208–13.

60. Zaman N, Tam YK, Jewell LD, Coutts RT. Effects of intravenous lipid as a source of energy in parenteral nutrition associated hepatic dysfunction and lidocaine elimination: A study using isolated rat liver perfusion. *Biopharm Drug Dispos.* 1997;18:803–19.

61. Steephen AC, Traber MG, Ito Y, Lewis LH, Kayden HJ, Shike M. Vitamin E status of patients receiving long-term parenteral nutrition: Is vitamin E supplementation adequate? *JPEN.* 1991;15:647–52.

62. Huston RK, Jelen BJ, Vidgoff J. Selenium supplementation in low-birthweight premature infants: Relationship to trace metals and antioxidant enzymes. *JPEN.* 1991;15:556–9.

63. Huston RK, Shearer TR, Jelen BJ, Whall PD, Reynolds JW. Relationship of antioxidant enzymes to trace metals in premature infants. *JPEN.* 1987;11:163–8.

64. Pironi L, Ruggeri E, Zolezzi C et al. Lipid peroxidation and antioxidant status in adults receiving lipid-based home parenteral nutrition. *Am J Clin Nutr.* 1998;68:888–93.

65. Fell JM, Reynolds AP, Meadows N et al. Manganese toxicity in children receiving long-term parenteral nutrition. *Lancet.* 1996;347:1218–21.

66. Reynolds AP, Kiely E, Meadows N. Manganese in long term paediatric parenteral nutrition. *Arch Dis Child.* 1994;71:527–8.

67. Kafritsa Y, Fell J, Long S, Bynevelt M, Taylor W, Milla P. Long-term outcome of brain manganese deposition in patients on home parenteral nutrition. *Arch Dis Child.* 1998;79:263–5.

68. Moreno A, Dominguez C, Ballabriga A. Aluminum in the neonate related to parenteral nutrition. *Acta Paediatr.* 1994;83:25–9.

69. Bougle D, Bureau F, Deschrevel G et al. Chromium and parenteral nutrition in children. *J Pediatr Gastroenterol Nutr.* 1993;17:72–4.

70. Moukarzel AA, Song MK, Buchman AL et al. Excessive chromium intake in children receiving total parenteral nutrition. *Lancet.* 1992;339:385–8.

71. Beath SV, Davies P, Papadopoulou A et al. Parenteral nutrition-related cholestasis in postsurgical neonates: Multivariate analysis of risk factors. *J Pediatr Surg.* 1996;31:604–6.

72. Watkins JB, Szczepanik P, Gould JB, Klein P, Lester R. Bile salt metabolism in the human premature infant. Preliminary observations of pool size and synthesis rate following prenatal administration of dexamethasone and phenobarbital. *Gastroenterology.* 1975;69:706–13.

73. Karpen SJ. Nuclear receptor regulation of hepatic function. *J Hepatol.* 2002;36:832–50.

74. Zollner G, Marschall HU, Wagner M, Trauner M. Role of nuclear receptors in the adaptive response to bile acids and cholestasis: Pathogenetic and therapeutic considerations. *Mol Pharm.* 2006;3:231–51.

75. Heyman MD, Tseng HC, Thaler MM. Total parenteral nutrition (TPN) decreases hepatic glutathione concentration in weaning rats. *Hepatology.* 1984;416:9.

76. Watkins JB. Placental transport: Bile acid conjugation and sulfation in the fetus. *J Pediatr Gastroenterol Nutr.* 1983;2:365–73.

77. Stanko RT, Nathan G, Mendelow H, Adibi SA. Development of hepatic cholestasis and fibrosis in patients with massive loss of intestine supported by prolonged parenteral nutrition. *Gastroenterology.* 1987;92:197–202.

78. Andorsky DJ, Lund DP, Lillehei CW et al. Nutritional and other postoperative management of neonates with short bowel syndrome correlates with clinical outcomes. *J Pediatr.* 2001;139:27–33.

79. Kaufman SS. Prevention of parenteral nutrition-associated liver disease in children. *Pediatr Transplant.* 2002;6:37–42.

80. Sondheimer JM, Cadnapaphornchai M, Sontag M, Zerbe GO. Predicting the duration of dependence on parenteral nutrition after neonatal intestinal resection. *J Pediatr.* 1998;132:80–4.

81. Greenberg GR, Wolman SL, Christofides ND, Bloom SR, Jeejeebhoy KN. Effect of total parenteral nutrition on gut hormone release in humans. *Gastroenterology.* 1981;80:988–93.

82. Lichtman SN, Sartor RB, Keku J, Schwab JH. Hepatic inflammation in rats with experimental small intestinal bacterial overgrowth. *Gastroenterology.* 1990;98:414–23.

83. Fedorowski T, Salen G, Tint GS, Mosbach E. Transformation of chenodeoxycholic acid and ursodeoxycholic acid by human intestinal bacteria. *Gastroenterology.* 1979;77:1068–73.

84. Bell RL, Ferry GD, Smith EO et al. Total parenteral nutrition-related cholestasis in infants. *JPEN.* 1986;10:356–9.

85. O'Brien DP, Nelson LA, Kemp CJ et al. Intestinal permeability and bacterial translocation are uncoupled after small bowel resection. *J Pediatr Surg.* 2002;37:390–4.

86. Ghose R, Zimmerman TL, Thevananther S, Karpen SJ. Endotoxin leads to rapid subcellular re-localization of hepatic RXRalpha: A novel mechanism for reduced hepatic gene expression in inflammation. *Nucl Recept.* 2004;2:4.

87. Trauner M, Arrese M, Lee H, Boyer JL, Karpen SJ. Endotoxin downregulates rat hepatic ntcp gene expression via decreased activity of critical transcription factors. *J Clin Invest.* 1998;101:2092–100.

88. Aprahamian CJ, Chen M, Yang Y, Lorenz RG, Harmon CM. Two-hit rat model of short bowel syndrome and sepsis: Independent of total parenteral nutrition, short bowel syndrome is proinflammatory and injurious to the liver. *J Pediatr Surg.* 2007;42:992–7.

89. Dahms BB, Halpin TC, Jr. Serial liver biopsies in parenteral nutrition-associated cholestasis of early infancy. *Gastroenterology.* 1981;81:136–44.

90. Modi BP, Langer M, Ching YA et al. Improved survival in a multidisciplinary short bowel syndrome program. *J Pediatr Surg.* 2008;43:20–4.

91. Diamond IR, Wales PW. Advantages of the distal sigmoid colostomy in the management of infants with short bowel syndrome. *J Pediatr Surg.* 2008;43:1464–7.

92. Wales PW. Surgical therapy for short bowel syndrome. *Pediatr Surg Int.* 2004;20:647–57.

93. Iyer KR, Horslen S, Torres C et al. Functional liver recovery parallels autologous gut salvage in short bowel syndrome. *J Pediatr Surg.* 2004;39:340–4.

94. Reinshagen K, Zahn K, Buch C et al. The impact of longitudinal intestinal lengthening and tailoring on liver function in short bowel syndrome. *Eur J Pediatr Surg.* 2008;18:249–53.

95. Maini B, Blackburn GL, Bistrian BR et al. Cyclic hyperalimentation: An optimal technique for preservation of visceral protein. *J Surg Res.* 1976;20:515–25.

96. Hwang TL, Lue MC, Chen LL. Early use of cyclic TPN prevents further deterioration of liver functions for the TPN patients with impaired liver function. *Hepatogastroenterology.* 2000;47:1347–50.

97. Morikawa N, Suematsu M, Kyokane T et al. Discontinuous total parenteral nutrition prevents postischemic mitochondrial dysfunction in rat liver. *Hepatology.* 1998;28:1289–99.

98. Rollins MD, Book LS, Meyers RL. Elimination of soybean lipid emulsion in total parenteral nutrition improves parenteral nutrition associated liver disease in infants with short bowel syndrome. *Pacific Association of Pediatric Surgeons.* Grand Teton, Wyoming, 2008.

99. Gura KM, Duggan CP, Collier SB et al. Reversal of parenteral nutrition-associated liver disease in two infants with short bowel syndrome using parenteral fish oil: Implications for future management. *Pediatrics.* 2006;118:e197–201.

100. Puder M, Valim C, Meisel JA et al. Parenteral fish oil improves outcomes in patients with parenteral nutrition-associated liver injury. *Ann Surg.* 2009;250:395–402.

101. Diamond IR, Grant RC, de Silva NT, Pencharz PB, Wales PW. Combination therapy with Omegaven and Intralipid in children with intestinal failure and advanced parenteral nutrition associated liver disease (IFALD). *XI International Small Bowel Transplant Symposium.* Bologna, Italy, 2009.

102. Diamond IR, Pencharz PB, Wales PW. Omega-3 lipids for intestinal failure associated liver disease. *Semin Pediatr Surg.* 2009;18:239–45.

103. Diamond IR, Pencharz PB, Wales PW. What is the current role for parenteral lipid emulsions containing omega-3 fatty acids in infants with short bowel syndrome? *Minerva Pediatr.* 2009;61:263–72.

104. Efficacy of an omega-3 enriched intravenous fat emulsion in the prevention of parenteral nutrition induced injury in infants. ClinicalTrials.gov—U.S. National Institutes of Health. http://www.clinicaltrials.gov/ct2/show/NCT00512629 (accessed February 24, 2009).

105. Can SMOFlipid, a composite parenteral nutrition lipid emulsion, prevent progression of parenteral nutrition associated liver disease in infants? ClinicalTrials.gov—U.S. National Institutes of Health. http://www.clinicaltrials.gov/ct2/show/NCT00793195 (accessed February 24, 2009).

106. Hadaway LC. Best-practice interventions: Keeping central line infection at bay. *Nursing.* 2006;36:58–63.

107. O'Grady NP, Alexander M, Dellinger EP et al. Guidelines for the prevention of intravascular catheter-related infections. *CDC MMWR Recomm Rep.* 2002;51:1–29.

108. Chaiyakunapruk N, Veenstra DL, Lipsky BA, Saint S. Chlorhexidine compared with povidone-iodine solution for vascular catheter-site care: A meta-analysis. *Ann Intern Med.* 2002;136:792–801.

109. Messing B, Peitra-Cohen S, Debure A, Beliah M, Bernier JJ. Antibiotic-lock technique: A new approach to optimal therapy for catheter-related sepsis in home-parenteral nutrition patients. *JPEN.* 1988;12:185–189.

110. Opilla MT, Kirby DF, Edmond MB. Use of ethanol lock therapy to reduce the incidence of catheter-related bloodstream infections in home parenteral nutrition patients. *JPEN.* 2007;31:302–305.

111. Beath SV, Booth IW, Murphy MS et al. Nutritional care and candidates for small bowel transplantation. *Arch Dis Child.* 1995;73:348–50.

112. Wu PA, Kerner JA, Berquist WE. Parenteral nutrition-associated cholestasis related to parental care. *Nutr Clin Pract.* 2006;21:291–5.

113. Vanderhoof JA, Young RJ, Murray N, Kaufman SS. Treatment strategies for small bowel bacterial overgrowth in short bowel syndrome. *J Pediatr Gastroenterol Nutr.* 1998;27:155–60.

114. Ng PC, Lee CH, Wong SP et al. High-dose oral erythromycin decreased the incidence of parenteral nutrition-associated cholestasis in preterm infants. *Gastroenterology.* 2007;132:1726–39.

115. Spaeth G, Gottwald T, Hirner A. Fibre is an essential ingredient of enteral diets to limit bacterial translocation in rats. *Eur J Surg.* 1995;161:513–8.

116. Spaeth G, Specian RD, Berg RD, Deitch EA. Bulk prevents bacterial translocation induced by the oral administration of total parenteral nutrition solution. *JPEN.* 1990;14:442–7.

117. Alverdy JA, Aoys E, Weiss-Carrington P, Burke DA. The effect of glutamine-enriched TPN on gut immune cellularity. *J Surg Res.* 1992;52:34–8.

118. Ding LA, Li JS. Effects of glutamine on intestinal permeability and bacterial translocation in TPN-rats with endotoxemia. *W J Gastroenterol.* 2003;9:1327–32.

119. Markley MA, Pierro A, Eaton S. Hepatocyte mitochondrial metabolism is inhibited in neonatal rat endotoxaemia: Effects of glutamine. *Clin Sci.* 2002;102:337–44.

120. Albers MJ, Steyerberg EW, Hazebroek FW et al. Glutamine supplementation of parenteral nutrition does not improve intestinal permeability, nitrogen balance, or outcome in newborns and infants undergoing digestive-tract surgery: Results from a double-blind, randomized, controlled trial. *Ann Surg.* 2005;241:599–606.

121. De Marco G, Sordino D, Bruzzese E et al. Early treatment with ursodeoxycholic acid for cholestasis in children on parenteral nutrition because of primary intestinal failure. *Aliment Pharmacol Ther.* 2006;24:387–94.

122. Spagnuolo MI, Iorio R, Vegnente A, Guarino A. Ursodeoxycholic acid for treatment of cholestasis in children on long-term total parenteral nutrition: A pilot study. *Gastroenterology* 1996;111:716–9.

123. Arslanoglu S, Moro GE, Tauschel HD, Boehm G. Ursodeoxycholic acid treatment in preterm infants: A pilot study for the prevention of cholestasis associated with total parenteral nutrition. *J Pediatr Gastroenterol Nutr.* 2008;46:228–31.

124. Mager DR, Marcon M, Wales P, Pencharz PB. Use of *N*-acetyl cysteine for the treatment of parenteral nutrition-induced liver disease in children receiving home parenteral nutrition. *J Pediatr Gastroenterol Nutr.* 2008;46:220–3.

125. Tsai S, Strouse PJ, Drongowski RA, Islam S, Teitelbaum DH. Failure of cholecystokinin-octapeptide to prevent TPN-associated gallstone disease. *J Pediatr Surg.* 2005;40:263–7.

126. Teitelbaum DH, Tracy TF, Jr, Aouthmany MM et al. Use of cholecystokinin-octapeptide for the prevention of parenteral nutrition-associated cholestasis. *Pediatrics* 2005;115:1332–40.

127. Heubi JE, Wiechmann DA, Creutzinger V et al. Tauroursodeoxycholic acid (TUDCA) in the prevention of total parenteral nutrition-associated liver disease. *J Pediatr.* 2002;141:237–42.

128. Abu-Elmagd KM, Costa G, Bond GJ et al. Five hundred intestinal and multivisceral transplantations at a single center: Major advances with new challenges. *Ann Surg.* 2009;250:567–81.

129. Diamond IR, Wales PW, Grant DR, Fecteau A. Isolated liver transplantation in pediatric short bowel syndrome: Is there a role? *J Pediatr Surg.* 2006;41:955–9.

130. Horslen SP, Sudan DL, Iyer KR et al. Isolated liver transplantation in infants with end-stage liver disease associated with short bowel syndrome. *Ann Surg.* 2002;235:435–9.

# 21 Use of Parenteral Fish Oil in the Management of IF-Associated Liver Disease

*Erica M. Fallon and Mark Puder*

## CONTENTS

## 21.1 INTRODUCTION

As discussed in Chapters 10 and 11, parenteral nutrition (PN) is typically administered with an intravenous lipid emulsion (ILE) to provide a calorically dense source of nonprotein calories, and to supply the essential omega-3 and omega-6 fatty acids needed for biologic membranes and the maintenance of immune function [1,2]. Currently, the only Food and Drug Administration (FDA)-approved lipid emulsions in the United States are comprised of soybean oil (i.e., Intralipid, manufactured by Fresenius Kabi, Stockholm, Sweden) or a combination of soybean and safflower oils (i.e., Liposyn II, Hospira Inc., Lake Forest, IL). These oils are rich in omega-6 fatty acids and phytosterols (e.g., stigmasterol, β-sitosterol, campesterol) that are associated with impaired biliary secretion and may contribute to liver injury [3]. Omega-6 polyunsaturated fatty acids (PUFAs), in particular linoleic acid (LA) and arachidonic acid (AA), are proinflammatory agents. LA increases the production of inflammatory mediators, such as interleukin-6 (IL-6) and tumor necrosis factor-alpha (TNF-α) [4,5]. AA is a substrate for proinflammatory mediators, and is thought to initiate or worsen inflammatory states [6]. Past and recent studies have hypothesized that phytosterols may be the hepatotoxic or cholestatic component within soybean oil-based emulsions. In particular, lipid emulsions derived from soybean oil have been shown to cause liver injury in rodent models, and immunosuppressive effects *in vitro* and in clinical studies [7–10].

Other ILEs that are approved for use in Europe include SMOFLipid (Fresenius Kabi, Austria GmbH; Graz, Austria), Lipoplus (B Braun; Melsungen, Germany), and Omegaven (Fresenius Kabi AG, Bad Homburg VDH, Germany). These formulations utilize the potential anti-inflammatory benefit of omega-3 fatty acids. See Table 21.1 for compositions of different parenteral fish oil emulsions.

**TABLE 21.1**

**Comparison and Characteristics of Parenteral Fish Oil Emulsions**

| Product Manufacturer | Lipoplus B Braun (20%) | SMOF® Fresenius Kabi (10%) | Omegaven Fresenius Kabi (10%) |
|---|---|---|---|
| Oil source (g/100 mL) | | | |
| Soybean | 8 | 3 | 0 |
| Safflower | 0 | 0 | 0 |
| MCT | 10 | 3 | 0 |
| Olive oil | 0 | 2.5 | 0 |
| Fish oil | 2 | 1.5 | 10 |
| α-tocopherol (mg/L) | 190 ± 30 | 200 | 150–296 |
| Phytosterols (mg/L) | NR | 47.6 | 0 |
| Fat composition (g) | | | |
| Linoleic | 4.44 | 2.9 | 0.1–0.7 |
| α-linolenic | 0.66 | 0.3 | <0.2 |
| EPA | 0.56 | 0.3 | 1.28–2.82 |
| DHA | 0.26 | 0.05 | 1.44–3.09 |
| Oleic | 1.96 | 2.8 | 0.6–1.3 |
| Palmitic | 1.08 | 0.9 | 0.25–1 |
| Stearic | 0.34 | 0.3 | 0.05–0.2 |
| Arachidonic | 0.04 | 0.05 | 0.1–0.4 |

*Note:* Values in Omegaven group represent means. Data provided by each manufacturer.
DHA, docosahexaenoic acid; EPA, eicosapentaenoic acid; MCT, Medium-chain triglyceride; NR, not reported.

## 21.2  FISH OIL AS A NOVEL STRATEGY TO PREVENT AND MANAGE PNALD

Based on recent evidence, the etiology of PNALD appears to be, in part, related to the composition of the ILE administered with PN. Fish-oil-based emulsions have only recently been introduced as an alternative to soybean oil in the United States, despite being available in Europe and Asia for over 10 years [11,12]. The recent studies involving fish oil are based on its anti-inflammatory properties and hepatoprotective effects. Fish oil contains omega-3 PUFAs, including alpha-linolenic acid (ALA), eicosapentaenoic acid (EPA), and docosahexaenoic acid (DHA); see Figure 21.1. Based on the high concentration of EPA and DHA, the anti-inflammatory potential of fish oil is attributed to interference of the AA pathway and production of the eicosanoids prostaglandin $E_3$, leukotriene $B_5$, and thromboxane $A_3$ [13–17]. Despite its potential beneficial effects, the use of fish oil was initially met with uncertainty, particularly involving its ability to provide adequate essential fatty acids to prevent essential fatty acid deficiency (EFAD) and growth impairment [18].

Following these concerns, subsequent studies have investigated alternatives for the conventional soybean-based lipid emulsions. Yeh et al. [19] demonstrated that omega-3 PUFAs reduced superoxide dismutase and glutathione peroxidase levels in rats receiving PN. These results suggested that omega-3 FAs could suppress the inflammatory pathway, a finding consistent with subsequent studies which demonstrated that fish oil modulates inflammation through the inhibition of TNF-α and reduction of cytokines that trigger proinflammatory reactions [20–23]. Furthermore, Alwayn et al. [24,25] showed that a fish-oil-based lipid emulsion attenuated fatty liver changes and prevented steatosis in mice. Alwayn et al. [26] also demonstrated that fish oil supplementation in mice with preexisting macrovesicular hepatic steatosis resulted in marked reversal of steatosis and reduction of serum liver enzyme levels. Other animal models have shown that parenteral fish oil does not impair biliary flow, yet may prevent hepatic steatosis and PN-associated cholestasis [19,27–29]. In humans, omega-3 fatty acids have been shown to accelerate clearance of chylomicron triglycerides

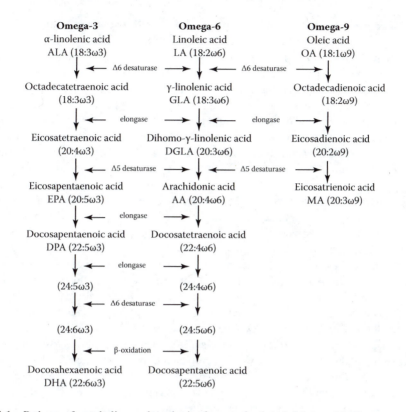

**FIGURE 21.1** Pathway of metabolism and synthesis of omega-3, -6, and -9 fatty acids. Upstream omega-3, -6, and -9 fatty acids, such as α-linolenic acid (ALA), linoleic acid (LA), and oleic acid (OA) are converted into longer chain downstream products, such as eicosapentaenoic acid (EPA), arachidonic acid (AA), and mead acid (MA) by the same set of enzymes in the preference omega-3 > omega-6 > omega-9.

and reduce triacylglycerol concentrations in serum [30]. Other studies have shown a reduction in lipogenesis through suppression of sterol response element binding protein-1 (SREBP-1), hypothesized to be involved in the protection against PNALD [31,32].

## 21.3 CLINICAL EXPERIENCE WITH FISH OIL IN THE MANAGEMENT OF PNALD

Fish oil has been introduced either as a supplement to soybean oil-based ILEs or as an ingredient in a combination emulsion [33]. Fish-oil-based ILE as monotherapy has recently been used in patients with IF, with promising results [33–41]. In 2005, Gura et al. described the first case in which Omegaven, the only commercially available fish-oil-based lipid emulsion, was used as the sole intravenous (IV) lipid source in one patient with a severe soy allergy who was previously unable to tolerate any parenteral fat emulsion [38]. Since that case report, Omegaven monotherapy has been used at the authors' institution under a compassionate use protocol for PN-dependent patients with cholestasis. In 2006, Gura et al. reported the reversal of PNALD and normalization of serum bilirubin levels within 60 days through substitution of a fish-oil-based versus soybean oil-based lipid emulsion in two pediatric patients [35,37].

Following these results, more than 140 children with PNALD have subsequently been treated with the fish-oil-based emulsion at the authors' institution. Inclusion criteria for treatment consideration include PN dependence and risk for significant hepatic injury due to prolonged use of PN (>30 days), significant hepatic dysfunction (direct bilirubin of ≥2 mg/dL) due to PN despite utilization of all conventional therapies, and signed patient/parental informed consent. Patients are excluded if pregnant, have chronic liver disease unrelated to PN (e.g., hepatitis C, biliary atresia, α-1 antitrypsin deficiency), and/or if already enrolled in another clinical trial involving an investigational agent. Treatment with Omegaven, as monotherapy, is initiated at the goal dose of 1 g/kg/day and infused over −10–24 h, without allowing the infusion rate to exceed 0.15 g/kg/h. Omegaven is infused in the same manner as conventional fat emulsions through a central or peripheral line. It is compatible with PN solutions and may be coinfused with PN; it should not be compounded as a total nutrient admixture due to a lack of stability information. Patients may continue Omegaven as an additional source of calories after the dextrose/protein portion of PN is discontinued. Patients treated with Omegaven are monitored for appropriate growth, spontaneous bleeding (e.g., unexplained bruising, oozing), maximum triene/tetraene ratio, trends in prealbumin (age standardized levels), triglyceride levels, and liver function tests. Fatty acid profiles (e.g., triene/tetraene ratios, omega-6 and omega-3 FA, total saturated, total monounsaturated, and total polysaturated fatty acids) and specific FA (e.g., arachidonic, stearic, oleic, and linoleic) are evaluated before treatment with Omegaven and then weekly after treatment initiation until direct bilirubin <2 mg/dL, followed by monthly blood draws until discontinuation of Omegaven.

An analysis of the initial 18 patients undergoing treatment for PNALD on Omegaven monotherapy demonstrated reversal of cholestasis, compared to 21 historical controls who received the conventional soybean oil-based lipid emulsion [36]. In both studies, patients tolerated the therapy well with no report of any adverse reactions. Recent findings of an open-label trial of Omegaven at the authors' institution showed patients receiving the fish-oil-based lipid emulsion experienced reversal of cholestasis approximately six times faster (95% CI: 2.0–37.3) than those receiving the soybean oil-based lipid emulsion [35]. The reversal of cholestasis permitted PN independence and development of enteral tolerance. Two infants receiving the soybean oil-based lipid emulsion underwent liver transplantation compared to none of the infants receiving the fish-oil-based lipid emulsion. The provision of the fish-oil-based lipid emulsion was not associated with hypertriglyceridemia, EFAD, coagulopathies, growth impairment, or an increased number of central venous catheter infections [40]. Furthermore, recent evidence has shown that the frequency of hypertriglyceridemic events were more common among control patients [35,39].

Similar results have been reported by other centers [41,42]. One study reported combination therapy using Omegaven 0.5 g/kg + Intralipid 1.5 g/kg for 1 week to ensuretolerance (of Omegaven) followed by 1 g/kg of each lipid emulsion; however, if PNALD failed to improve or worsened despite Omegaven therapy, the Intralipid was reduced or discontinued and Omegaven was continued alone [34]. Of the 12 subjects in the study, nine had complete resolution of hyperbilirubinemia (serum conjugated bilirubin = 0 μmol/L) within a median of 24 weeks (range 7–37 weeks); however, in 5/9 patients, resolution occurred only after transition to Omegaven monotherapy [34]. Other studies have shown that administration of a fish-oil-based lipid emulsion lowered substrates derived from AA and plasma concentrations of TNF-α and IL-6, while improving liver and pancreas function [43–45].

## 21.4   CONCERNS WITH FISH OIL AS A LIPID SOURCE

Despite its success, fish oil administration has been questioned regarding potential risk of coagulopathy, EFAD, and increased infection rate although clinical experience does not support these concerns. Incidence of coagulopathy and/or EFAD has not been demonstrated clinically, including patients completely dependent on PN [33,35,36,38,46,47]. At the authors' institution, children receiving the fish-oil-based emulsion had lower mean INR and overall rate of bloodstream infections than children who received the conventional soybean oil-based emulsion [35]. In addition, fish-oil-based lipid emulsion used as monotherapy has been questioned by critics for its lack of the traditionally defined essential fatty acids (i.e., ALA and LA) and the potential to restrict growth [18]. While recent evidence from murine models suggest AA and DHA provision alone is sufficient to prevent biochemical and physiologic evidence of EFAD [48], an ongoing double-blind randomized controlled clinical trial comparing the soybean oil-based lipid emulsion Intralipid to the fish-oil-based lipid emulsion Omegaven is imperative in the current debate regarding the efficacy and safety of parenteral fish-oil-based lipid emulsions [49].

In Boston, MA, one such randomized controlled trial (NCT00512629) was initiated in 2007 to evaluate the current standard of care in the management of PNALD in infants and children. Inclusion criteria include a need for full or partial PN with assignment to the conventional soybean oil-based Intralipid or fish-oil-based Omegaven, as the only source of IV lipid [50]. The primary outcome will be the number of PN-associated cholestatic events, defined as serum direct bilirubin levels >2 mg/dL for 2 consecutive weeks, in neonates and infants (<3 months old) diagnosed with a congenital or acquired gastrointestinal disease which requires PN for greater than 3 weeks. Secondary clinical and developmental outcomes include markers of hepatic function, fatty acid profiles, PN duration, neurodevelopment, and mortality. Safety and tolerability outcomes include frequency of central venous catheter infections, bronchopulmonary dysplasia, and coagulopathy. These findings are anticipated to enhance the current understanding of parenteral fish-oil-based lipid emulsions and determine its role as monotherapy in PN-dependent patients.

Fish oil has additional benefits and involvement in retinal disease (e.g., retinopathy of prematurity), bone health, and neurodevelopment. Studies have demonstrated reduced pathological retinal angiogenesis with increased dietary intake of omega-3 PUFA; in particular, EPA and DHA have been shown to reduce pathologic neovascularization through enhanced vessel regrowth after vascular loss/injury, suggesting supplementation of omega-3 FAs may help prevent proliferative retinopathy [51]. Studies evaluating bone health and the effect of fish oil have shown increased bone mineral density, decreased bone turnover, and increased calcium absorption following fish oil supplementation. Further studies suggest omega-3 FA beneficially impact neurodevelopment in infants [52–54]. Neurodevelopmental outcomes following Omegaven administration are currently under review at the authors' institution.

## 21.5 CONCLUSION

The composition of an ILE administered in combination with PN to provide dense calories and prevent EFAD, can significantly contribute to the development of PNALD. The aforementioned experimental murine studies have demonstrated that fish oil prevented and reversed steatosis. Utilization of a fish-oil-based lipid emulsion in PN-dependent neonates and infants appears to reverse cholestasis and prevent further progression of liver disease and development of EFAD. These benefits may result from the absence of soybean oil, the pharmacologic effects of fish oil, the ability to introduce enteral nutrition, or a combination of the aforementioned factors. A randomized clinical trial to determine the role for fish-oil-based emulsions in the prevention of PNALD in PN-dependent pediatric patients is currently underway. At present, however, its use is restricted to experienced pediatric centers for compassionate use only.

Refer to The Oley Foundation (http://www.oley.org) for further information on obtaining Omegaven.

## REFERENCES

1. Wretlind A. Development of fat emulsions. *JPEN* 1981;5:230–5.
2. Edgren B, Wretlind A. The theoretical background of the intravenous nutrition with fat emulsions. *Nutr Dieta Eur Rev Nutr Diet* 1963;13:364–86.
3. Clayton PT, Whitfield P, Iyer K. The role of phytosterols in the pathogenesis of liver complications of pediatric parenteral nutrition. *Nutrition* 1998;14:158–64.
4. Dichtl W, Ares MP, Jonson AN et al. Linoleic acid-stimulated vascular adhesion molecule-1 expression in endothelial cells depends on nuclear factor-kappaB activation. *Metabolism* 2002;51:327–33.
5. Park HJ, Lee YW, Hennig B, Toborek M. Linoleic acid-induced VCAM-1 expression in human microvascular endothelial cells is mediated by the NF-kappa B-dependent pathway. *Nutr Cancer* 2001; 41:126–34.

6. Tilley SL, Coffman TM, Koller BH. Mixed messages: Modulation of inflammation and immune responses by prostaglandins and thromboxanes. *J Clin Invest* 2001;108:15–23.

7. Aksnes J, Eide TJ, Nordstrand K. Lipid entrapment and cellular changes in the rat myocard, lung and liver after long-term parenteral nutrition with lipid emulsion. A light microscopic and ultrastructural study. *APMIS* 1996;104:515–22.

8. Chen WJ, Yeh SL, Huang PC. Effects of fat emulsions with different fatty acid composition on plasma and hepatic lipids in rats receiving total parenteral nutrition. *Clin Nutr* 1996;15:24–8.

9. Calder PC, Sherrington EJ, Askanazi J, Newsholme EA. Inhibition of lymphocyte proliferation *in vitro* by two lipid emulsions with different fatty acid compositions. *Clin Nutr* 1994;13:69–74.

10. Monson JR, Sedman PC, Ramsden CW, Brennan TG, Guillou PJ. Total parenteral nutrition adversely influences tumour-directed cellular cytotoxic responses in patients with gastrointestinal cancer. *Eur J Surg Oncol* 1988;14:935–43.

11. Grimminger F, Mayser P, Papavassilis C et al. A double-blind, randomized, placebo-controlled trial of n-3 fatty acid based lipid infusion in acute, extended guttate psoriasis. Rapid improvement of clinical manifestations and changes in neutrophil leukotriene profile. *Clin Investig* 1993;71:634–43.

12. Waitzberg DL, Torrinhas RS, Jacintho TM. New parenteral lipid emulsions for clinical use. *JPEN* 2006;30:351–67.

13. Lee S, Gura KM, Puder M. Omega-3 fatty acids and liver disease. Hepatology 2007;45:841–5.

14. Prescott SM. The effect of eicosapentaenoic acid on leukotriene B production by human neutrophils. *J Biol Chem* 1984;259:7615–21.

15. Camandola S, Leonarduzzi G, Musso T et al. Nuclear factor kB is activated by arachidonic acid but not by eicosapentaenoic acid. *Biochem Biophys Res Commun* 1996;229:643–7.

16. Chen MF, Lee YT, Hsu HC, Yeh PC, Liau CS, Huang PC. Effects of dietary supplementation with fish oil on prostanoid metabolism during acute coronary occlusion with or without reperfusion in diet-induced hypercholesterolemic rabbits. *Int J Cardiol* 1992;36:297–304.

17. Lee S, Gura KM, Kim S, Arsenault DA, Bistrian BR, Puder M. Current clinical applications of omega-6 and omega-3 fatty acids. *Nutr Clin Pract* 2006;21:323–41.

18. Carlson SE, Cooke RJ, Werkman SH, Tolley EA. First year growth of preterm infants fed standard compared to marine oil n-3 supplemented formula. *Lipids* 1992;27:901–7.

19. Yeh SL, Chang KY, Huang PC, Chen WJ. Effects of n-3 and n-6 fatty acids on plasma eicosanoids and liver antioxidant enzymes in rats receiving total parenteral nutrition. *Nutrition* 1997;13:32–6.

20. Mayer K, Meyer S, Reinholz-Muhly M et al. Short-time infusion of fish oil-based lipid emulsions, approved for parenteral nutrition, reduces monocyte proinflammatory cytokine generation and adhesive interaction with endothelium in humans. *J Immunol* 2003;171:4837–43.

21. Rallidis LS, Paschos G, Liakos GK. Velissaridou AH, Anastasiadis G, Zampelas A. Dietary alpha-linolenic acid decreases C-reactive protein, serum amyloid A and interleukin-6 in dyslipidaemic patients. *Atherosclerosis* 2003;167:237–42.

22. Novak TE, Babcock TA, Jho DH, Helton WS, Espat NJ. NF-kappa B inhibition by omega-3 fatty acids modulates LPS-stimulated macrophage TNF-alpha transcription. *Am J Physiol Lung Cell Mol Physiol* 2003;284:L84–9.

23. Babcock TA, Novak T, Ong E, Jho DH, Helton WS, Espat NJ. Modulation of lipopolysaccharide-stimulated macrophage tumor necrosis factor-alpha production by omega-3 fatty acid is associated with differential cyclooxygenase-2 protein expression and is independent of interleukin-10. *J Surg Res* 2002;107:135–9.

24. Alwayn IP, Gura K, Nose V et al. Omega-3 fatty acid supplementation prevents hepatic steatosis in a murine model of nonalcoholic fatty liver disease. *Pediatr Res* 2005;57:445–52.

25. Alwayn IP, Javid PJ, Gura KM, Nose V, Ollero M, Puder M. Do polyunsaturated fatty acids ameliorate hepatic steatosis in obese mice by SREPB-1 suppression or by correcting essential fatty acid deficiency. *Hepatology* 2004;39:1176–7; author reply 1177–8.

26. Alwayn IP, Andersson C, Zauscher B, Gura K, Nose V, Puder M. Omega-3 fatty acids improve hepatic steatosis in a murine model: Potential implications for the marginal steatotic liver donor. *Transplantation* 2005;79:606–8.

27. Araya J, Rodrigo R, Videla LA et al. Increase in long-chain polyunsaturated fatty acid n-6/n-3 ratio in relation to hepatic steatosis in patients with non-alcoholic fatty liver disease. *Clin Sci (Lond)* 2004;106:635–43.

28. Van Aerde JE, Duerksen DR, Gramlich L et al. Intravenous fish oil emulsion attenuates total parenteral nutrition-induced cholestasis in newborn piglets. *Pediatr Res* 1999;45:202–8.

29. Chen WJ, Yeh SL. Effects of fish oil in parenteral nutrition. *Nutrition* 2003;19:275–9.

30. Putadechakum S, Tanphaichitr V, Leelahagul P, Pakpeankitvatana V, Surapisitchart T, Komindr S. Long-term treatment of N-3 PUFAS on plasma lipoprotein levels and fatty acid composition of total serum and erythrocyte lipids in hypertriglyceridemic patients. *J Med Assoc Thai* 2005;88:181–6.
31. Park Y, Harris WS. Omega-3 fatty acid supplementation accelerates chylomicron triglyceride clearance. *J Lipid Res* 2003;44:455–63.
32. Sekiya M, Yahagi N, Matsuzaka T et al. Polyunsaturated fatty acids ameliorate hepatic steatosis in obese mice by SREBP-1 suppression. *Hepatology* 2003;38:1529–39.
33. de Meijer VE, Gura KM, Le HD, Meisel JA, Puder M. Fish oil-based lipid emulsions prevent and reverse parenteral nutrition-associated liver disease: The Boston experience. *JPEN* 2009;33:541–7.
34. Diamond IR, Sterescu A, Pencharz PB, Kim JH, Wales PW. Changing the paradigm: Omegaven for the treatment of liver failure in pediatric short bowel syndrome. *J Pediatr Gastroenterol Nutr* 2009;48:209–15.
35. Puder M, Valim C, Meisel JA et al. Parenteral fish oil improves outcomes in patients with parenteral nutrition-associated liver injury. *Ann Surg* 2009;250:395–402.
36. Gura KM, Lee S, Valim C et al. Safety and efficacy of a fish-oil-based fat emulsion in the treatment of parenteral nutrition-associated liver disease. *Pediatrics* 2008;121:e678–86.
37. Gura KM, Duggan CP, Collier SB et al. Reversal of parenteral nutrition-associated liver disease in two infants with short bowel syndrome using parenteral fish oil: Implications for future management. *Pediatrics* 2006;118:e197–201.
38. Gura KM, Parsons SK, Bechard LJ et al. Use of a fish oil-based lipid emulsion to treat essential fatty acid deficiency in a soy allergic patient receiving parenteral nutrition. *Clin Nutr* 2005;24:839–47.
39. Lee SI, Valim C, Johnston P et al. Title: The Impact of fish oil-based lipid emulsion on serum triglyceride, bilirubin, albumin levels in children with parenteral nutrition-associated liver disease. *Pediatr Res* 2009;66(6):698–703.
40. de Meijer VE, Gura KM, Meisel JA, Le HD, Puder M. Parenteral fish oil as monotherapy for patients with parenteral nutrition-associated liver disease. *Pediatr Surg Int* 2009;25:123–4.
41. Calhoun AW, Sullivan JE. Omegaven for the treatment of parenteral nutrition associated liver disease: A case study. *J Ky Med Assoc* 2009;107:55–7.
42. Cheung HM, Lam HS, Tam YH, Lee KH, Ng PC. Rescue treatment of infants with intestinal failure and parenteral nutrition-associated cholestasis (PNAC) using a parenteral fish-oil-based lipid. *Clin Nutr* 2009;28:209–12.
43. Heller AR, Rossel T, Gottschlich B et al. Omega-3 fatty acids improve liver and pancreas function in postoperative cancer patients. *Int J Cancer* 2004;111:611–6.
44. Wachtler P, Konig W, Senkal M, Kemen M, Koller M. Influence of a total parenteral nutrition enriched with omega-3 fatty acids on leukotriene synthesis of peripheral leukocytes and systemic cytokine levels in patients with major surgery. *J Trauma* 1997;42:191–8.
45. Weiss G, Meyer F, Matthies B, Pross M, Koenig W, Lippert H. Immunomodulation by perioperative administration of n-3 fatty acids. *Br J Nutr* 2002;87 Suppl 1:S89–94.
46. Strijbosch RA, Lee S, Arsenault DA et al. Fish oil prevents essential fatty acid deficiency and enhances growth: Clinical and biochemical implications. *Metabolism* 2008;57:698–707.
47. de Meijer VE, Le HD, Meisel JA, Gura KM, Puder M. Parenteral fish oil as monotherapy prevents essential fatty acid deficiency in parenteral nutrition-dependent patients. *J Pediatr Gastroenterol Nutr* 2010;50:212–8.
48. Le HD, Meisel JA, de Meijer VE, Gura KM, Puder M. The essentiality of arachidonic acid and docosahexaenoic acid. *Prostaglandins Leukot Essent Fatty Acids* 2009;81:165–70.
49. Morgado N, Rigotti A, Valenzuela A. Comparative effect of fish oil feeding and other dietary fatty acids on plasma lipoproteins, biliary lipids, and hepatic expression of proteins involved in reverse cholesterol transport in the rat. *Ann Nutr Metab* 2005;49:397–406.
50. U.S. National Institutes of Health. Efficacy of an omega-3 enriched intravenous fat emulsion in the prevention of parenteral nutrition induced injury in infants. http://www.clinicaltrials.gov/ct2/show/NCT00512629.
51. Connor KM, SanGiovanni JP, Lofqvist C et al. Increased dietary intake of omega-3-polyunsaturated fatty acids reduces pathological retinal angiogenesis. *Nat Med* 2007;13:868–73.
52. Makrides M, Gibson RA, McPhee AJ et al. Neurodevelopmental outcomes of preterm infants fed high-dose docosahexaenoic acid: A randomized controlled trial. *JAMA* 2009;301:175–82.
53. Bouwstra H, Dijck-Brouwer J, Decsi T et al. Neurologic condition of healthy term infants at 18 months: Positive association with venous umbilical DHA status and negative association with umbilical *trans*-fatty acids. *Pediatr Res* 2006;60:334–9.
54. Crawford MA, Costeloe K, Ghebremeskel K, Phylactos A, Skirvin L, Stacey F. Are deficits of arachidonic and docosahexaenoic acids responsible for the neural and vascular complications of preterm babies? *Am J Clin Nutr* 1997;66:1032S–41S.

# 22 Osteopenia and Bone Health in Patients with Intestinal Failure

*Steven A. Abrams*

## CONTENTS

## 22.1  INTRODUCTION

This chapter discusses potential etiologies and approaches to the diagnosis and management of bone mineral deficiency in patients with intestinal failure (IF). Unfortunately, data, either from controlled trials or metabolic studies, are extremely limited related to this condition. The focus of this discussion will be on infants and small children, and in particular those who do not have other major comorbidities (e.g., renal failure).

Few data have assessed bone outcomes in this group of patients [1,2]. To evaluate bone outcomes it is helpful to consider the components of the diet and environment that lead to bone mineralization and how they may be affected by IF. These include deficiency of dietary or absorbed vitamin D, calcium (Ca), phosphorus (P), and other bone mineral components, as well as the possibility of less sunshine exposure and physical activity. Of these, it is likely that, especially in children, vitamin D deficiency and low amounts of retained Ca and P are the primary factors involved in causing low bone mineralization.

## 22.2   NUTRIENT DEFICIENCY

Numerous causes for bone mineral insufficiency exist in patients with IF. Some of the key ones are identified in Table 22.1 and will be considered below.

### 22.2.1   VITAMIN D

Vitamin D deficiency can affect bone health in numerous ways. Severe vitamin D deficiency and rickets in IF was described in the late 1970s and early 1980s in infants requiring long-term parenteral nutrition (PN) [3,4]. Additional reports related to IF and osteoporosis in adults also exist from that era [5,6]. In addition to its classic effects on Ca absorption, severe vitamin D deficiency will lead to increased parathyroid hormone (PTH) levels and bone turnover associated with hyperparathyroidism [7]. It is likely that vitamin D deficiency is largely related to loss of bowel needed for vitamin D absorption and to steatorrhea leading to increased fecal losses of Ca and vitamin D. In adults with Crohn's disease, osteoporosis is best predicted by ileal resection [8]. Decreased enterohepatic circulation of vitamin D may also be involved in low vitamin D levels in children with short bowel syndrome [9]. Of note is a case report of a premature infant with abnormal vitamin D absorption associated with a limited jejunal resection [10].

Other factors may also be involved in vitamin D deficiency. Infants with IF and long-term hospitalization may not have as much sunlight exposure as other infants. Feeding intolerance may limit oral vitamin D intake. In adults, micronutrient and vitamin intakes are often decreased in those with IF [11].

Vitamin D is a component of vitamin-supplemented total PN. The optimal level of vitamin D in PN is unresolved, although excluding low-birthweight infants it is common to provide 400 IU/day. Low-birthweight infants more commonly are given 160–200 IU/day in PN. Especially in children, vitamin D deficiency increases in PTH and bone turnover are more likely to be harmful to bone growth than PTH suppression due to excessive vitamin D. Excess vitamin D may however be problematic in some patients [12]. A study in France [13] suggested that daily average vitamin D intakes

---

**TABLE 22.1**

**Causes of Bone Demineralization in Intestinal Failure Patients**

#### Enteral Nutrition

Inadequate feeding volume

Specialized formulas with poorer mineral bioavailability

Decreased vitamin D intake

Decreased vitamin D absorption due to fat malabsorption

Insolubility of mineral supplements

Decreased Ca absorption due both to insolubility and vitamin D deficiency

#### Parenteral Nutrition

Lower concentration of Ca and P

Decreased fluid volume in sick infants

Increased renal losses due to acidosis, diuretics

#### Other Factors

Decrease exercise/mobility

Lower sun exposure

---

of 1200 IU/day were associated with nephrocalcinosis and bone pain that did not occur when vitamin D was removed from the PN. There are few recent data however to address the issue of optimal vitamin D content of PN.

## 22.2.2 CALCIUM AND PHOSPHORUS DEFICIENCY

The intakes of Ca and P are key variables in determining bone health in children with IF. This is especially the case for premature infants who have a very high incidence of osteopenia and rickets. This risk is much greater when they also have IF, such as that caused by necrotizing enterocolitis (NEC). In this case, premature infants often cannot tolerate a full volume of enteral nutrition or even PN with enough Ca and P to meet bone growth needs.

### 22.2.2.1 Parenteral Nutrition

Calcium and phosphorus are likely to be inadequate in infants who receive PN as their primary nutritional source for more than 2 weeks. This is related to the need to limit mineral concentrations because of their solubility in PN solutions and to the need to limit the volume of PN given. However, increased administration of Ca and P improves mineral retention. As an example, in a study of 24 VLBW infants receiving total PN, administration of 17 mmol/L (680 mg/L) Ca and 20 mmol/L (660 mg/L) P resulted in net retention of 70–80 mg/kg per day Ca and P [14]. This is close to the *in utero* Ca retention rate of about 100–120 mg/kg/day.

In considering PN, neonatal PN can be provided which should meet about 80% of the rapidly growing infant's needs. However, in practice, infants may not tolerate the volume of PN needed for this over a long period of time. Intermittent episodes of sepsis or significant pulmonary disease may require decreases in fluid volume or use of peripheral PN with lower Ca concentrations.

The use of diuretics, especially furosemide and similar medications which act via affecting mineral transport in the loop of Henle will lead to an increase in urinary Ca excretion. This increase also places the infant at risk for nephrolithiasis. Usually, urinary Ca will increase by approximately 3–5 mg/kg/day with daily furosemide therapy. This is substantial, but is <10% of the daily Ca retention. In comparison, fluid restriction of 20–40% below usual intake (e.g., to 100 mL/kg/day of PN) as might be needed with severe lung disease would likely have a larger net effect on decreasing retained Ca than the use of furosemide. Nonetheless, in the presence of bone demineralization, limiting the use of loop diuretics or adding a thiazide diuretic may be helpful. Controlled trials evaluating different strategies for limiting urinary Ca excretion in children are not available.

### 22.2.2.2 Enteral Nutrition

The content of Ca and P in unfortified human milk is insufficient for infants <1800–2000 g birthweight to achieve intrauterine bone mineral accretion rates or normal bone mineralization. It may also be inadequate for larger infants who have IF. Of note is that in low-birthweight infants the deficiency of P in unfortified milk exceeds that of Ca. Very premature infants fed unfortified human milk will have high levels of urinary Ca reflecting a P deficiency in excess of the Ca deficiency. However, both minerals are deficient and supplementation of human milk with both Ca and P improves growth; increases bone mineralization; and normalizes serum Ca, P, and alkaline phosphatase activity [15,16]. Net mineral retention and bone mineral content are also improved. The absorption of Ca from human milk is approximately 60% of intake. Absorption of Ca from infant formulas is more variable but can range generally for 30–60% of intake [16]. There are no data specific to the absorption of Ca in IF patients.

With regard to IF and mineral absorption, numerous factors will lead to a lower amount of bioavailable Ca being absorbed and available for bone mineralization. In seeking to minimize the use of PN, clinicians caring for infants with IF will often increase feeding volume to the maximum tolerated and then increase concentration. This approach may lead to adequate fluid so that less or no PN is needed, and, with the use of modular macronutrient supplements, adequate energy for growth without PN. However, the provision of adequate minerals, especially Ca, in this approach can be difficult.

For premature infants, the use of specialized elemental formulas (partially or completely hydrolyzed whey proteins) is associated both with lower mineral intake than use of formulas designed for premature infants and the possibility of lower Ca absorption. The concentration of these formulas may not overcome this effect. There are no data at all related to the bioavailability of minerals in IF patients receiving hydrolyzed formulas with or without the concentration of minerals.

A crucial unanswered question is whether it is better to provide more minerals enterally at a fixed volume intake by increasing concentration of formula or by adding bone minerals individually. Adding Ca and P individually is problematic in small infants and would not add other minerals such as magnesium and zinc that are needed to optimize bone mineralization. Furthermore, the individual sources of Ca and P are hyperosmolar leading to poorer enteral tolerance in this population and potentially an increased risk of NEC.

## 22.3  OTHER FACTORS

### 22.3.1  ALUMINUM TOXICITY

There has been persistent concern related to the possible role of aluminum or other heavy metal toxicity and bone disease in both parenterally and enterally fed infants [6,17]. Case reports and larger series of patients have documented this problem and although have shown improvement in recent years, have not been completely resolved [18]. Ongoing problems with providing extremely low aluminum-containing PN solutions persist [19]. This problem is under active evaluation [20].

Bone pain and abnormalities of bone metabolism have been reported related to aluminum in PN for approximately 30 years. A detailed review of the likely pathophysiology of this condition by Klein et al. [17] concluded that multiple mechanisms are likely including suppression both of PTH and of 1-α hydroxylation of 25-OHD. The current degree to which bone mineral abnormalities in IF patients is related to aluminum toxicity is uncertain, although it is not likely a primary etiology at this time.

Nonetheless, a recent study from Fewtrell et al. [21] suggests that long-term consequence of decreased bone mass may be associated with early childhood exposure to increased levels of aluminum in PN.

### 22.3.2  EXERCISE AND SUNSHINE EXPOSURE

An effect of lack of physical activity cannot be entirely excluded as part of the etiology of bone loss in children with IF. It is clear, even in small children, that a combination of adequate substrate (minerals) and physical activity is needed for optimal bone growth. Children with IF receiving PN are unlikely to be spending as much time outdoors as other children, especially during the summer months. Furthermore, although exercise may not be directly limited by IF, this is likely to be problematic in such infants and children. There are no specific studies of this topic in children.

### 22.3.3  OTHER DIETARY FACTORS: ZINC AND MAGNESIUM DEFICIENCY

Development and mineralization of bones require multiple micronutrients as well as adequate protein. Efforts to focus only on Ca and P may lead to omission of these other critical factors. Among the key micronutrients that may not be provided adequately are zinc and magnesium. Zinc losses may be excessive in PN-dependent patients with IF, especially those who have an ileostomy. This problem has been lessened in recent years due to supplementation of zinc in PN. Nonetheless, zinc is a critical component of bone and zinc status may need to be assured to prevent osteoporosis [22].

Vitamin deficiencies, especially vitamins C and K may also occur in children with IF and lead to abnormal bone mineralization. These also are likely less common at present with supplementation practices that are in place.

## 22.4 EVALUATION OF BONE MINERAL INSUFFICIENCY IN INTESTINAL FAILURE

Biochemical, densitometric, and radiological approaches are all used in evaluating bone mineral insufficiency in IF patients. A generalized approach related to infants, in whom bone densitometry is not usually performed for clinical purposes is provided in Table 22.2. Aspects of the evaluative process are discussed below.

### 22.4.1 RADIOGRAPH

Although numerous techniques exist to evaluate bone mineral status, in infants, the clinical standard remains a standard radiograph of the bones. In general, radiographs are obtained of either the knee or the radius. These should be interpreted by an experienced radiologist who can comment both on bone appearance and on classical findings of rickets or metabolic bone disease. Films should be evaluated for the presence of healing fractures and review of available chest radiographs also done to ensure that no fractures are present. Caution needs to be applied however to prevent overinterpreting the results of radiographs. It is difficult to clearly identify osteopenia on radiographs and this is a poorly defined term. It is generally accepted that at least 20% of bone mineral must be deficient before a routine radiograph is able to identify bone mineral loss, making radiographs a low sensitivity test of bone mineralization defects.

Radiographs are likely to be particularly beneficial in premature infants or other infants who are on prolonged PN. Radiographic findings of overt rickets resemble those seen in classic vitamin D-deficient rickets in infants and toddlers. When rickets or fractures that are believed to be related to osteopenia are identified, it is necessary to aggressively pursue potential interventions to improve Ca, P, and vitamin D status. In infants with rickets or severe osteopenia, it is usually not necessary to monitor radiographs more often than once every 6–8 weeks as changes occur slowly. The course

---

**TABLE 22.2**

**Approach to Evaluation of Possible Bone Demineralization in Infants with Intestinal Failure**

**Serum Alkaline Phosphatase Activity**

If 400–600 IU/L, then monitor biweekly until <400 IU/L

If 600–800 IU/L, monitor weekly

If >800 IU/L, then obtain serum P and radiograph of wrist or knee

If radiograph shows osteopenia without rickets, continue weekly monitoring of APA

If x-ray shows rickets, consider intervention with high-dose vitamin D, calcitriol, or additional mineral supplements

Repeat radiograph 6 weeks after initial radiograph if it shows osteopenia or rickets

In presence of significant cholestasis, may consider bone-specific alkaline phosphatase activity

**Serum 25-OHD**

Unless history consistent with severe maternal vitamin D deficiency, does not need routine monitoring before 6 weeks of age

Assess at 6 weeks of age

Values < 20 ng/mL usually require intervention

Values 20–32 ng/mL should be followed but may not require specific therapeutic changes

Generally need to follow every 3–6 months

May be helpful to obtain intact PTH

of serum alkaline phosphatase activity, serum 25-hydroxyvitamin D concentration (25-OHD), and possibly the serum P (see below) can be followed more often to assess the effects of any intervention. In the setting of severe osteopenia, care should be taken in handling of these infants at the bedside and during procedures to avoid fractures.

## 22.4.2 DUAL ENERGY X-RAY ABSORPTIOMETRY

An increasing published database is available to evaluate dual energy x-ray absorptiometry (DXA) values for bone mineral content and bone mineral density in infants and small children. Standard databases separated by gender exist for the most commonly available equipment [23]. Problems remain in standardizing software for interpreting scans. Most commonly, whole body scans to measure total body bone mineral content and bone mineral density (excluding the head region) are obtained in children, although regional scans are of value in some cases.

Recent guidelines from an International working group related to the use of DXA are of importance in guiding the use of DXA. Key recommendations include the use of scans of the total body without the head, the spine, and areal bone mineral density. The diagnosis of osteoporosis should not be made entirely based on DXA scan results but include evidence of a history of fracture. An important issue is that the young adult normalized data (referred to as the T-score) should not be used in children, but that appropriate age, race, and gender-normalized data should be used for the standard of comparison (the Z score) [24]. Although guidelines vary, following DXA scans annually in very high-risk patients is reasonable. If scans on a stable diet show little change in total body bone mineral content, these can be less common.

## 22.4.3 OTHER TECHNIQUES

The use of bone ultrasound and quantitative CT scanning are currently being investigated in adults and in children. At present, ultrasound does not appear to be sufficiently sensitive for use in children to identify early or moderate bone mineral deficiency and there are few normal data for quantitative CT. At present these alternatives are not useful outside of a research context for patient evaluation.

## 22.4.4 BONE TURNOVER MARKERS

In adults, the use of turnover markers of bone formation and resorption is well established and widely used clinically. The situation in pediatrics however, is more complex. Total serum alkaline phosphatase activity is a highly sensitive and specific marker for bone mineral status in premature infants [25]. On the other hand, the use of other bone turnover markers, especially serum osteocalcin and N-telopeptide has had a variable course in the pediatric literature. In general, bone-formation markers, like osteocalcin are indicative of some aspects of bone mineral status [26,27]. However, the sensitivity of these and their clinical use to follow bone mineral loss in IF is uncertain. Outside of the research setting, using serum osteocalcin or N-telopeptide to guide therapy is not currently supported by adequate literature.

An important potential additional marker is the bone-specific alkaline phosphatase activity (BS-ALP). As some children with IF have liver dysfunction as well, the total ALP may not be as sensitive as the BS-ALP [28]. When followed in a longitudinal fashion, the BS-ALP may therefore be of some value in chronic illnesses, although clear normal standards are not readily available in children [29].

In infants without liver failure, it is common to monitor serum total alkaline phosphatase activity and serum P. Serum Ca may also be followed although this is not usually clinically useful except to ensure that significant hypercalcemia does not develop. In infants, radiological rickets is associated with an ALP >800 IU/L and often with a low serum P [25]. When used as a screening tool, we carefully follow infants with a serum alkaline phosphatase >600 IU/L and consider obtaining a radiographic study when the value is over 800 IU/L (see Table 22.2).

## 22.4.5 VITAMIN D AND PTH LEVELS

In many cases, it can be helpful to assess vitamin D status in children with IF. There are no obvious clinical markers of vitamin D deficiency so it is necessary to routinely evaluate vitamin D status. For most children, the diagnostic evaluation is optimally performed by measuring a serum 25-OHD level and a serum intact PTH level. Although several methodologies exist for these measurements, it is most important to utilize a laboratory measuring 25-OHD that participates in a national quality assurance program. Recently, reference standards have been released for 25-OHD leading to the ability to ensure high quality and accurate measurements [30].

Use of appropriate methods and standards ensures that both 25-OHD$_2$ and 25-OHD$_3$ are measured, that longitudinal data on an individual is useful and that research can be based on high-quality evidence.

A common question is whether 1,25-OHD should also be measured. Although it is the active form of vitamin D, it is generally agreed that in the absence of renal disease, or the clinical use of calcitriol or an analog in a patient, assessment of serum 1,25-OHD is not clinically useful and is expensive. The reasons that serum 1,25-OHD is not a clinically useful measurement are only partly understood. It appears that it is a relatively acute phase marker and is commonly increased even in the presence of vitamin D deficiency, probably related to PTH elevation. In infants, the blood volume needed for measuring 1,25-OHD may be of concern (usually 2–3 mL of blood is obtained).

Although it is generally of value to assess serum intact PTH, the results are often difficult to clinically interpret. An elevated value may be of concern related to vitamin D deficiency. In the presence of renal disease or uncertainty, consultation with an expert in pediatric nephrology or pediatric endocrinology is helpful.

With regard to serum 25-OHD, a challenging, and as yet unresolved issue is to identify a normal value and more specifically to identify the value that requires intervention. How best to provide that intervention is a further challenge. In adults, some experts recommend a minimum value of approximately 80 nmol/L (32 ng/mL) [31]. This value has not been accepted however by other experts or by governmental panels in the United States. It is however, common for clinical laboratories to report values of serum 25-OHD <32 ng/mL in adults and children as vitamin D "insufficiency."

The data are even less clear about optimal serum 25-OHD levels in children. Guidelines from the Lawson Wilkins Pediatric Endocrine Society [32] describe a value of 50 nmol/L or less (20 ng/mL) as being insufficient or deficient. Almost all would agree that values below 50 nmol/L are of concern, especially in the setting of IF.

Whether it is advantageous to target higher serum 25-OHD levels, such as a value >80 nmol/L specifically in children with IF is unclear. No trials have addressed this issue and it would be very difficult to isolate the effects of higher serum 25-OHD levels on bone health in this population. Furthermore, achieving levels this high can be extremely difficult. With regard to excess vitamin D, Misra et al. [32] define this as a value >250 nmol/L (100 ng/mL). This is probably a reasonable level, although some would be concerned with values >80 ng/mL. It would be extremely hard for a child with IF to achieve levels this high unless they were being supplemented with massive doses of vitamin D on a very regular (almost daily) basis.

Children with IF who have been weaned from PN are at special risk of micronutrient deficiencies, including vitamin D. As a result, it makes most sense to screen these patients after PN has been discontinued for 4–6 weeks as well as periodically thereafter as clinically indicated.

## 22.5 INTERVENTIONS

It is certainly important for bone health that those with IF be encouraged to exercise as much as is possible. Judicious sunshine exposure, in keeping with guidelines for the use of sun-block agents may also be recommended. However, for most children with IF, emphasis will need to be provided on optimizing nutrient intake to enhance bone health.

## 22.5.1 MAXIMIZATION OF MINERAL INTAKE

In infants, especially premature infants or other small infants with IF requiring PN, the single most important key to therapy is to maximize the intake of Ca and P. This can be a tremendous challenge and requires close cooperation between physicians, dietitians, and pharmacists. For those requiring PN, maximizing the intake of Ca and P in PN requires use of available nomograms, forms of these minerals that are most soluble in solution and adjustments of PN (e.g., use of cysteine), and maintenance of room temperature so as to promote maximal solubility. A considerable amount of pharmaceutical literature exists related to this and should be consulted [33].

For those who are able to tolerate some oral feedings, the amount and form of Ca and P that should be provided and are tolerated need to be considered. For preterm infants, especially those <2 kg bodyweight, the use of either preterm formulas or human milk fortifiers is optimal as these are very high in Ca and P. However, many babies who have ostomies or otherwise poorly functioning intestines may not tolerate these products well or may not tolerate an adequate volume of them to provide enough mineral intake.

Many infants with IF are fed using elemental or semielemental formulas. The quantity of Ca and P in some widely used formulas is shown in Table 22.3. There are very few data related to the bioavailability of Ca in these formulas and none specific to IF patients. It is likely that the lack of lactose has a small effect in decreasing Ca absorption. Nonetheless, it is also probably the case that bioavailability related to the formula itself (or human milk fortifier) is less of a problem than is the underlying low mineral intake and intestinal malabsorption due to limited bowel and low vitamin D status.

The use of human milk has many potential benefits in virtually all infants and should be provided whenever possible in IF patients. However, as noted previously, from a mineral perspective, human milk is relatively low in Ca and P. The high bioavailability of these minerals in healthy infants may not apply in IF and the mineral content may be inadequate to prevent a cumulative deficit in those who have had a prolonged period on PN or were premature. Furthermore, in human milk, but less so in formula, Ca binds to fat and when fed continuously, may be lost in the tubing and not reach the patient.

## Table 22.3
## Mineral and Vitamin D Intake of Feedings Commonly Provided to Infants with Intestinal Failure

| Feeding | Elecare (180 mL/kg) | Nutramigen AA (180 mL/kg) | Pregestimil 20 (180 mL/kg) | Neocate (180 mL/kg) | Neosure (165 mL/kg) | Enfacare (165 mL/kg) | Human Milk Unfortifed (180 mL/kg) |
|---|---|---|---|---|---|---|---|
| Calcium intake at 120 kcal/kg/d (mg) | 140 | 115 | 113 | 149 | 129 | 147 | 50 |
| Phosphorus intake at 120 kcal/kg/d (mg) | 103 | 65 | 63 | 112 | 76 | 81 | 27 |
| Vitamin D intake at 120 kcal/kg/d (IU) | 50 | 61 | 59 | 72 | 86 | 97 | <40 |
| % fat as MCT | 33% | 0% | 55% | 5% | 25% | 20% | <1% |

*Notes:* Elecare, Neosure = Abbott Nutrition, Columbus, OH; Nutramigen AA, Pregestemil 20, Enfacare = Mead-Johnson, Nutrition, Evansville, IN; Neocate = Nutricia North America, Gaithersburg, MD; Vitamin D content of unfortified human milk is variable, but unless high dose maternal supplements given, is generally <50 IU/liter.

The use of Ca and P as individual supplements is widely done in this patient population. Concern exists about this practice however, for several reasons. First, in very small infants, the liquid preparations commercially available and widely used for Ca and P supplementation are hyperosmolar and likely to be poorly tolerated or even increase the risk of NEC. Second, even in the presence of adequate vitamin D, the absorption of these supplements may be poor due to poor solubility. This can be a particular problem with calcium carbonate, which, in a less acidic environment (e.g., in a newborn), may be poorly solubilized and absorbed.

In summary, providing adequate Ca and P intake in patients with IF is a tremendous challenge. Communication among caregivers related to forms of the minerals, their delivery system and tolerance are needed to provide optimal intakes. Failure to provide adequate intake is at least as substantial a problem in many cases as poor bioavailability or increased excretion.

### 22.5.2 Vitamin D

Vitamin D can be provided via several possible sources to patients with IF. In general, it is best to provide it to patients with IF as part of a day multivitamin supplement. However, some patients will not absorb the vitamin adequately to maintain desired 25-OHD levels. High-dose supplementation can be considered, using one of the strategies recently outlined [32]. Parenteral therapy may also be provided, although details of the forms and availability of these vary by country. For some patients, it may be necessary to provide 1,25 dihydroxy vitamin D (calcitriol) or an analog. This should usually be done with the consultation of the appropriate expert in the use of these medications. Of note is that currently there is no source of 25-hydroxyvitamin D (calcidiol) marketed in the United States.

There remains uncertainty about the relative advantages of providing vitamin D2 compared to vitamin D3 [34,35]. In general, either may be used, although there remains a general consensus to some advantage for vitamin D3 when possible [36].

### 22.5.3 Anti-Bone Resorptive Therapy

Bisphosphonates and other anti-bone resorptive therapy can be considered in any patient with significant bone mineral deficiency. Specific data related to their use are very minimal in this population, but have been described [37]. Benefits appear to be modest, although identifiable [38].

## 22.6 SUMMARY AND CONCLUSIONS

Nutritional management of patients, especially children with IF is a tremendous challenge. Bone demineralization and rickets/osteomalacia are well-known in this population. During early infancy, evaluation using standard radiographs is usually needed. Later in childhood, DXA may be used and standards that are age, gender, and race match applied.

The etiology of bone demineralization in these patients is primarily related to deficient availability of absorbed Ca and P, although other factors, including immobility are also involved. Increasing intake and absorption of Ca is a challenge as well as providing Ca and P via parenteral routes. However, availability of relatively high mineral-containing PN, use of high-dose vitamin D supplements and other approaches can be used with appropriate monitoring.

## REFERENCES

1. Dellert, S. F., Farrellm, M. K., Specker, B. L., and Heubi, J. E. Bone mineral content in children with short bowel syndrome after discontinuation of parental nutrition. *J Pediatr* 1998;132:516–9.
2. Hurley, D. L. and McMahon, M. M. Long-term parenteral nutrition and metabolic bone disease. *Endocrinol Metab Clin North Am* 1990;19:113–31.

3. Compston, J. E. and Horton, L. W. Oral 25-hydroxyvitain D3 in treatment of osteomalacia associated with ileal resection and cholestyramine therapy. *Gastroenterology* 1978;74:900–2.
4. Klein, G. L., Cannon, R. A., Diament, M. et al. Infantile vitamin D-resistant rickets associated with total parenteral nutrition. *Arch Pediatr Adol Med* 1982;136:74–6.
5. Shike, M., Harrison, J. E., Sturtridge, W. C. et al. Metabolic bone disease in patients receiving long-term total parenteral nutrition. *Ann Intern Med* 1980;92:343–50.
6. de Vernejoul, M. C., Messing, B., Modrowski, D., Bielakoff, J., Buisine, A., and Miravet, L. Multifactorial low remodeling bone disease during cyclic total parenteral nutrition. *J Clin Endocrinol Metab* 1985;60:109–13.
7. Touloukian, R. J. and Gertner, J. M. Vitamin D deficiency rickets as a late complication of the short gut syndrome during infancy. *J Pediatr Surg* 1981;16:230–5.
8. van Hogezand, R. A., Bänffer, D., Zwinderman, A. H., McCloskey, E. V., Griffioen, G., and Hamdy, N. A. Ileum resection is the most predictive factor for osteoporosis in patients with Crohn's disease. *Osteoporos Int* 2006;17:535–42.
9. Ryzko, J., Lorenc, R. S., Socha, J., Lukaszkiewicz, J., and Preiss, U. Changes in vitamin D metabolism in children following partial intestinal resection. *Monatsschr Kinderheilkd* 1989;137:447–50.
10. Markstead, T., Akses, L., Finne, P. H., and Aarskog, D. Decreased vitamin D absorption after limited jejunal resection in a premature infant. *J Pediatr* 1982;101:1001–3.
11. Estívariz, C. F., Luo, M., Umeakunne, K. et al. Nutrient intake from habitual oral diet in patients with severe short bowel syndrome living in the southeastern United States. *Nutrition* 2008;24:330–9.
12. Verhage, A. H., Cheong, W. K., Allard, J. P., and Jeejeebhoy, K. N. Increase in lumbar spine bone mineral content in patients on long-term parenteral nutrition without vitamin D supplementation. *JPEN* 1995;19:431–6.
13. Larchet, M., Barabedian, M., Bourdeau, A., Gorski, A., Goulet, O., and Ricour, C. Calcium metabolism in children during long-term total parenteral nutrition: The influence of calcium, phosphorus, and vitamin D intakes. *J Pediat Gastroent Nutr* 1991;13:367–75.
14. Prestridge, L. L., Schanler, R. J., Shulman, R. J. et al. Effect of parenteral calcium and phosphorus therapy on mineral retention and bone mineral content in very low birth weight infants. *J Pediatr* 1993;22:761–8.
15. Schanler, R. J., Abrams, S. A., and Garza, C. Mineral balance studies in very low birth weight infants fed human milk. *J Pediatr* 1988;113:230–8.
16. Abrams, S. A., Esteban, N. V., Vieira, N. E., and Yergey, A. L. Dual tracer stable isotopic assessment of calcium absorption and endogenous fecal excretion in low birth weight infants. *Pediatr Res* 1991;29:615–8.
17. Klein, G. L. and Coburn, J. W. Total parenteral nutrition and its effects on bone metabolism. *Crit Rev Clin Lab Sci* 1994;31:135–67.
18. Advenier, E., Landry, C., Colomb, V. et al. Aluminum contamination of parenteral nutrition and aluminum loading in children on long-term parenteral nutrition. *J Pediatr Gastroenterol Nutr* 2003;36:448–53.
19. Poole, R. L., Hintz, S. R., Mackenzie, N. I., and Kerner, J. A. Aluminum exposure from pediatric parenteral nutrition: Meeting the new FDA regulation. *JPEN* 2008;32:242–6.
20. Charney, P. J. American Society for Parenteral and Enteral Nutrition Aluminum Task Force. A.S.P.E.N. Statement on aluminum in parenteral nutrition solutions. *Nutr Clin Pract* 2004;19:416–7.
21. Fewtrell, M. S., Bishop, N. J., Edmonds, C. J., Isaacs, E. B., and Lucas, A. Aluminum exposure from parenteral nutrition in preterm infants: Bone health at 15 year follow-up. *Pediatrics* 2009;124:1372–9.
22. Lowe, N. M., Fraser, W. D., and Jackson, M. J. Is there a potential therapeutic value of copper and zinc for osteoporosis? *Proc Nutr Soc* 2002;61:181–5.
23. Kalkwarf, H. J., Zemel, B. S., Gilsanz, V. et al. The bone mineral density in childhood study: Bone mineral content and density according to age, sex, and race. *J Clin Endocrinol Metab* 2007;92:2087–99.
24. Bianchi, M. L., Baim, S., Bishop, N. J. et al. Official positions of the International Society for Clinical Densitometry (ISCD) on DXA evaluation in children and adolescents. *Pediatr Nephrol* 2010;25(1):37–47.
25. Mitchell, S. M., Rogers, S. P., Hicks, P. D., Hawthorne, K. M., Parker, B. R., and Abrams, S. A. High frequencies of elevated alkaline phosphatase activity and rickets exist in extremely low birth weight infants despite current nutritional support. *BMJ Pediatr* 2009;9:47.
26. O'Connor, E., Mølgaard, C., Michaelsen, K. F., Jakobsen, J., Lamberg-Allardt, C. J., and Cashman K. D. Serum percentage undercarboxylated osteocalcin, a sensitive measure of vitamin K status, and its relationship to bone health indices in Danish girls. *Br J Nutr* 2007;97:661–6.

27. Kalkwarf, H. J., Khoury, J. C., Bean, J., and Elliot, J. G. Vitamin K, bone turnover, and bone mass in girls. *Am J Clin Nutr* 2004;80:1075–80.

28. Rauch, F., Middelmann, B., Cagnoli, M., Keller, K. M., and Schönau, E. Comparison of total alkaline phosphatase and three assays for bone-specific alkaline phosphatase in childhood and adolescence. *Acta Paediatr* 1997;86:583–7.

29. Barera, G., Beccio, S., Proverbio, M., and Mora, S. Longitudinal changes in bone metabolism and bone mineral content in children with celiac disease during consumption of a gluten-free diet. *Am J Clin Nutr* 2004;79:148–54.

30. Phinney, K. W. Development of a standard reference material for vitamin D in serum. *Am J Clin Nutr* 2008;88:511S–2S.

31. Holick, M. F. and Chen, T. C. Vitamin D deficiency: A worldwide problem with health consequences. *Am J Clin Nutr* 2008;87:1080S–6S.

32. Misra, M., Pacaud, D., Petryk, A., Collett-Solberg, P. F., Kappy, M., and on behalf of the Drug and Therapeutics Committee of the Lawson Wilkins Pediatric Endocrine Society. Vitamin D deficiency in children and its management: Review of current knowledge and recommendations. *Pediatrics* 2008;122:398–417.

33. Wong, J. C., McDougal, A. R., Tofan, M., Aulakh, J., Pineault, M., and Chessex, P. J. Doubling calcium and phosphate concentrations in neonatal parenteral nutrition solutions using monobasic potassium phosphate. *J Am Coll Nutr* 2006;25:70–7.

34. Thacher, T. D., Obadofin, M. O., O'Brien, K. O., and Abrams, S. A. The effect of vitamin D2 and vitamin D3 on intestinal calcium absorption in Nigerian children with rickets. *J Clin Endocrinol Metab* 2009;94:3314–21.

35. Pietras, S. M., Obayan, B. K., Cai, M. H., and Holick, M. F. Vitamin D2 treatment for vitamin D deficiency and insufficiency for up to 6 years. *Arch Intern Med* 2009;169:1806–8.

36. Leventis, P. and Kiely P. D. The tolerability and biochemical effects of high-dose bolus vitamin D2 and D3 supplementation in patients with vitamin D insufficiency. *Scand J Rheumatol* 2009;38:149–53.

37. Haderslev, K. V., Tjellesen, L., Sorensen, H. A., and Staun, M. Effect of cyclical intravenous clodronate therapy on bone mineral density and markers of bone turnover in patients receiving home parenteral nutrition. *Am J Clin Nutr* 2002;76:482–8.

38. Raman, M., Aghdassi, E., Baun, M. et al. Metabolic bone disease in patients receiving home parenteral nutrition: A Canadian study and review. *JPEN* 2006;30:492–6.

# 23 Micronutrient Deficiencies in Intestinal Failure

*Gil Hardy*

## CONTENTS

## 23.1 INTRODUCTION

Intestinal failure (IF) occurs when there is reduced intestinal absorption so that nutrients and/or water and electrolyte supplements are needed to maintain health and/or growth [1]. Conditions leading to IF include short bowel syndrome (SBS), non-short bowel diarrhea/malabsorption, active disease, or obstruction [2].

Most patients with insufficient gastrointestinal (GI) function are unable to maintain adequate nutrition or hydration without oral and/or parenteral supplementation and invariably will also be depleted in micronutrients. Many will have high demands caused by inadequate GI absorption, excessive losses, or abnormalities in storage or metabolism. These may be as a result of poor long-term diet for medical or cultural reasons or insufficient recent intake by the elderly, especially those in long-term care facilities, who often eat little food. Consequently, they are at risk of deficiencies, especially of the water-soluble micronutrients, at the time of hospital admission [3]. Patients with a history of drug abuse or excessive intake of alcohol are particularly likely to be depleted. While folate and vitamin C are the most commonly altered, the most clinically important is thiamine because of the danger of refeeding syndrome in such patient groups. Deficiencies may also occur during nutrition support therapy because of increased requirements or increased bodily losses [4]. Loss of bile results in fat malabsorption and eventually, loss of fat-soluble vitamins. Limited absorption of fat-soluble vitamins may also be associated with low protein intakes. Chylous leaks and fistulas, conditions for which parenteral nutrition (PN) is often required, result in additional losses, due to the large volumes of protein-rich fluid lost each day. These deficiencies can deleteriously affect enzyme functions and other biochemical processes, leading to organ dysfunction, muscle weakness, poor wound healing, and altered immune status [5]. Micronutrient depletion can lead to clinical compromise; therefore, the Nutrition Support Team (NST) and other health care providers need to appreciate their importance and ensure that there is adequate provision of micronutrients in PN regimens [6].

The remarkable achievements of pediatric NST in sustaining infants for longer periods on PN have created a clinical setting in which micronutrient deficiencies have often only been manifested and unmasked during prolonged courses of PN, demonstrating the importance of prophylactic addition of adequate vitamins and trace elements. Neonates have special dietary requirements. Premature and full-term infants on prolonged PN, after GI surgery, with large intestinal fluid losses are at special risk of deficiencies without supplementation. Their micronutrient requirements therefore need to be separately considered.

## 23.2   GUIDELINES

The most recent Dietary Guideline Recommendations for Americans [7] incorporate a significant change, which has considerable practical implications for artificial nutritional therapy. A new paradigm expands the original basis of the RDA or Adequate Intake (AI), beyond simple prevention of deficiency states and decreasing the risk of various chronic diseases. The AI recommendations now include figures with upper levels for avoiding the possibility of adverse effects when micronutrients are consumed in excess through consumption of fortified foods and/or dietary supplements.

The US Food & Drug Administration, in 2000, increased the recommended doses for certain multivitamin products and included vitamin K for the first time [8]. However, a similar updated recommendation for trace elements has not been made. Likewise, the Australasian (AuSPEN) trace element guidelines for PN have not been updated since 1998 [9]. Recently published guidelines for PN supplementation and monitoring may seem somewhat contradictory but are qualitatively similar. The combined ASPEN–society of critical care medicine (SCCM) guidelines for the critically ill make no mention of micronutrient supplementation [10], whereas the UK National Institute for Clinical Excellence (NICE) guidance document, published in 2006, states that "provision of PN without adequate micronutrient content must be avoided" [6, p. 137]. The 2009 European Society for Clinical Nutrition and Metabolism (ESPEN) Guidelines on PN make a Grade C recommendation that: "in those patients after surgery who are unable to be fed via the enteral route, and in whom total or near-total parenteral nutrition is required, a full range of vitamins and trace elements should be supplemented on a daily basis" [11, p. 383]. For adult home parenteral nutrition (HPN), Staun et al. [12] for ESPEN, emphasize that care should be taken to provide AIs and not to provide excess in patients with cholestasis or renal failure and recommend monitoring of micronutrients at 12 monthly intervals. On the other hand, routine monitoring of most micronutrients is recommended every 3–6 months by NICE [6] and ESPEN [13] and every 6 months for long-term (HPN) patients by AuSPEN [14]. Serum levels of 25-OH vitamin D, vitamin B12, and folate are readily available in most countries for routine use in clinical practice. The status of other micronutrients may be obtained on request from specialized reference laboratories.

The main focus of this chapter is to review the causes of deficiencies and address the needs for micronutrition therapy in IF patients who require long-term hospital or home nutrition support. It is drawn extensively from two recently published literature reviews [5,15].

## 23.3 TRACE ELEMENTS

In IF patients, trace element requirements have been estimated from the proportion of the element absorbed from a normal oral diet, but the information available is limited. Absorption of trace elements is difficult to study, and can range from 1% for chromium (Cr) to 75% for selenium (Se). When used at recommended doses, toxicity due to trace elements is unlikely, but the chemical form of the element, antagonistic or facilitatory ligands and competitive interactions between trace elements, can affect absorption via the GI tract and hence bioavailability [5].

### 23.3.1 Chromium

Cr is important in protein, carbohydrate, and lipid metabolism. It is absorbed in the ileum and potentiates the action of insulin, which is crucial in the synthesis of glucose tolerance factor, a cofactor in insulin action. Cr deficiency has been observed during long-term PN and reports of decreased levels in the blood and urine of elderly diabetics with impaired glucose tolerance, unexplained weight loss, and peripheral neuropathy indicate a potential need for correction [15]. Over 30 years ago, the depleted Cr status and glucose intolerance of patients who developed insulin-resistant hyperglycemia on long-term PN were rapidly corrected by Cr chloride supplementation [16]. Assessing and monitoring Cr levels is difficult with few accurate indicators of Cr status. Demonstrating insulin resistance, or abnormal glucose clearance that improves after Cr supplementation, still seems to be the best monitoring option [17].

The PN guidelines for Cr supplementation from ASPEN in 2002 [18] and ESPEN in 2004 [13] suggested 10–15 µg/day (0.2–0.3 µmol/day). However, the optimum daily supplement may be higher for many patients in postsurgical states where increased urinary excretion of Cr is evident. For pediatric patients, the recommended doses of 0.14–0.2 µg/kg/day (0.003–0.004 µmol/kg/day) were designed to meet maintenance and growth needs, but can elevate serum levels above normal and need careful monitoring [19].

Enterally, the organic form of Cr is better absorbed but for parenteral use Cr should be administered in the Cr (III) oxidation state, for example, chromic chloride, because the Cr (VI) form is toxic. Care should be taken if any metal chelating agents such as EDTA have been used as stabilizing agents for the other PN components, as these may bind or precipitate [20]. Cr contamination in PN solutions may be sufficient to exceed current recommendations for supplementation and requirements for long-term PN may need to be reduced.

### 23.3.2 Copper

Copper (Cu) is a component of several metalloenzymes, mainly oxidases, hydroxylases, and superoxide dismutases. Cu is absorbed in the ileum and largely excreted in the bile, so biliary obstruction can result in high levels leading to hepatic necrosis, renal failure, and death. Conversely, excessive losses through biliary drains or high output stomas may quickly lead to a deficiency characterized by a microcytic, hypochromic anemia unresponsive to iron therapy, neutropenia, poor wound healing, and osteoporosis [21]. Other less common complications include skin depigmentation and hair loss. Serum ceruloplasmin and serum Cu decline progressively, with clinical symptoms becoming apparent within 5–8 months [22]. It is advisable to check Cu levels in patients with severe liver disease and in long-term PN to avoid overdosing. Cu status can be assessed from hemoglobin, hematocrit, circulating plasma, serum, or erythrocyte concentration. Low ceruloplasmin can reflect Cu status but as an acute phase reactant it may be elevated during inflammation. Other nutrients can interact with Cu and affect bioavailability. Under suitable anaerobic conditions and pH, vitamin C can reduce Cu from the cupric (II) to the cuprous (I) form with concomitant oxidation of the ascorbic acid, thus compromising the prescribed dose of both nutrients. Interactions between Cu and zinc (Zn) have also to be considered.

Current practices suggest that 0.3–0.5 mg/day (5–8 µmol/day) is sufficient for most PN patients but in the presence of burns, diarrhea, or increased fluid loss through GI stomas or fistulas, the Cu requirements may increase. Intravenous recommendations for infants are similar to those for adults at 20 µg/kg/day (0.3 µmol/kg/day) [7]. Doses should be halved for patients with liver disease [22].

### 23.3.3  IRON

Iron (Fe) is a component of a number of metalloenzymes, mainly dehydrogenases in the brain and skeletal muscle, and is thought to be involved in cognitive function and T-cell immunity. Fe is absorbed in the duodenum and proximal jejunum, but enteral absorption can be decreased by phytates and/or fiber in the formulas [5]. Deficiency symptoms include fatigue, lowered resistance to infection, dry skin, and microcytic, hypochromic anemia. Hyperferremia is an important cause of oxidative stress and may enhance bacterial growth and virulence by impairing the chemotactic and phagocytic properties of neutrophils to cause infections [23]. However, Swoboda et al. [24] showed that surgical ICU patients who received intravenous Fe did not have significantly higher rates of bloodstream infections. Monitoring Fe status from the relative levels of hemoglobin, transferrin saturation, and free erythrocyte protoporphyrin is extremely important. However, anemia can be caused by other nutritional factors, not specific to Fe deficiency. Serum ferritin is also a useful tool but in patients with systemic inflammation, ferritin levels may *rise* in the presence of Fe deficiency [25].

The majority of IF patients who need PN or EN have adequate Fe stores to meet daily requirements. Routine supplementation is therefore not necessary and may result in Fe overload with an increased risk of adverse effects such as infections and cardiovascular disease. When supplementation is deemed necessary, usually for long-term patients, a level of 1.0–1.2 mg/day (18–20 µmol/day) is recommended (Table 23.1). Similarly, HPN patients are at risk of Fe deficiency anemia and a dose of 25–50 mg once per month or 10 mg per week may be necessary [26], but with careful monitoring to avoid Fe overload [27]. Term infants usually have sufficient Fe stores for 3–6 months' growth and red cell mass expansion, but premature or low-birth-weight (LBW) infants have not had the chance to accumulate Fe. In such cases, supplementation is warranted at 200 µg/kg/day with doses of up to 3–4 mg/kg/day (54–71 µmol/kg/day) in infants weighing <1 kg.

Ferric (Fe III) iron is stable, and compatible with most aqueous solutions at physiological concentrations, but in the presence of oxygen and light, ferrous (Fe II) is oxidized to ferric, forming insoluble polymers and free radicals that cause peroxidative damage to vital cell structures. Fe dextran is not compatible with lipid-containing PN formulations because $Fe^{3+}$ can destabilize the negative surface charge on lipid particles and result in coalescence of the emulsion [20]. For supplemented Fe to be incorporated into new erythrocytes, adequate supplies of the other hematinic nutrients (i.e., vitamin $B_{12}$, folic acid, Cu and pyridoxine) must also be provided.

### 23.3.4  ZINC

Zn is essential to the structural integrity of proteins. It is a component of metalloenzymes, such as pyruvate dehydrogenases, alkaline phosphatase, DNA, and RNA polymerases. Zn is absorbed mainly in the duodenum and jejunum, so many common diseases and clinical situations predispose to Zn deficiency. Patients with GI and biliary fistulas are vulnerable and perioral or perineal rashes are common in severe Crohn's disease. Zn absorption is decreased by the presence of phytates or fiber but absorption is aided by citric acid. Fe depresses the absorption of Zn; Zn depresses Cu absorption and vice versa, resulting in deficiencies of both elements [28]. Moreover, Zn binds to albumin and to certain amino acids (i.e., histidine, lysine, and threonine in PN admixtures) whose excretion may contribute to an increase in urinary Zn losses. Clinical manifestations of Zn deficiency, especially in LBW infants include growth retardation, depressed immune function, anorexia, dermatitis, skeletal abnormalities, diarrhea, alopecia, and altered taste acuity. Delayed pubertal development can occur in older children. Decreased serum alkaline phosphatase levels can also be indicative of Zn deficiency. Its principal toxic effect results from interference with normal Cu metabolism, leading to Cu-deficiency anemia, or depressed immune function [15].

Current ASPEN guidelines [18] for parenteral Zn supplementation suggest 2.5–5 mg/day (38–76 µmol/day). This may be suboptimal but should probably not exceed 30 mg/day. Increased intake of Zn is recommended during high GI fluid losses, where an additional 12–17 mg (185–260 µmol) is required for each liter of intestinal fluid lost. Zn is very important in neonates due to their rapid rate of growth. This gives rise to a recommendation for term infants, less than 3 months old, of 250 µg/kg/day (3.8 µmol/kg/day), decreasing to 100 µg/kg/day (1.5 µmol/kg/day) for children over 3 months of age (Table 23.1). Premature infants are at an even higher risk of developing a deficiency as about two-thirds of Zn stores are accumulated in the last 10–12 weeks of gestation. Hence much higher supplementation levels of 400 µg/kg/day (6.2 µmol/kg/day) are required for the premature infant [13].

There is still no reliable indicator of Zn nutritional status, which must be undertaken using a battery of tests. There is a Zn redistribution related to the patients' different pathologies and to the inflammatory process, contributing to the difficulty of interpretation of Zn values. Nevertheless, plasma and 24 h-urinary Zn levels, are the most common indicators due to the feasibility of sample collection. Both indicators are maintained by homeostatic mechanisms and respond quickly to changes in the dietary Zn content. Zn supplements appear to be quite stable in PN mixtures at physiological concentrations and there are no known reports of incompatibilities. PN product quality has improved but may vary from country to country and a number of components used for admixtures can be contaminated with Zn.

### 23.3.5 Selenium

Se, as the amino acid selenocysteine, occupies an essential part of more than 30 selenoenzymes [29] including glutathione peroxidase (GPx), iodothyronine deiodinases, and thioredoxin reductase; GPx can inhibit the activation triggered by proinflammatory cytokines of the nuclear factor (NF) κB which regulates genes that encode inflammatory cytokines [30]. The most common parenteral form of Se (IV) is selenite (selenious acid or the sodium salt). Sodium selenite has a biphasic action: first as a transient pro-oxidant compound and second as an antioxidant when converted into the selenoenzymes. Common presentations of Se deficiency in PN patients are Keshan cardiomyopathy and myositis. Loss of skin and hair pigmentation, as well as whitening of the nail beds, can also occur. Clinical states that are associated with Se deficiencies and can contribute to the onset of symptoms in unsupplemented PN regimens are, most notably: cystic fibrosis, some cancers, AIDS, and burns [15].

Normal serum Se levels are generally in the range 46–143 µg/L (0.61–1.9 µmol/L). Requirements range from 10–15 µg/day for infants to 100 µg/day for adults if GPx activity in platelets is used as the measure of Se repletion [31]. Supplementation of at least 30–70 µg/day (0.4–0.84 µmol/day) is recommended to maintain Se balance in adults (Table 23.1) [32] and 3 µg/kg/day (0.04 µmol/kg/day) is sufficient to maintain normal plasma levels in infants. Preterm and term infants may need up to 30 µg/day if receiving PN for longer than 4 weeks.

Se toxicosis has only been observed from long-term oral ingestion. Se is absorbed mainly in the duodenum and jejunum but there are no reports of Se toxicity from Se-supplemented PN, where patients are already Se depleted and supplementation has not been for more than 2–3 weeks. In cases of severe depletion, doses of 250 μg/day (3.2 μmol/day) can be administered in IF before normalization occurs. Up to 400 μg/day of parenteral Se is safe, although higher amounts have been administered with no apparent short-term adverse effects. The optimal dose of parenteral Se to improve outcome for critically ill systemic inflammatory response syndrome (SIRS) patients with no adverse effect is 800–1000 μg/day [33]. Se status is commonly assessed by measuring blood levels with atomic absorption spectrophotometry. For short-term PN plasma Se appears to respond quickest to changes in intake and disease state but reflects acute fluxes between compartments rather than recent dietary intake. Routine monitoring of renal failure and long-term IF patients is recommended.

The inorganic selenite additives are compatible at physiological concentrations with most constituents of a PN mixture. However, when mixed directly with vitamin C in unbuffered intravenous solutions at low pH, the selenite is reduced to elemental Se, which is not biologically available. Fortunately, this reaction proceeds slowly in All-in-One PN mixtures around neutral pH and is inhibited by the presence of amino acids and other buffering agents [34].

### 23.3.6 MANGANESE

Manganese (Mn) is a component of the metalloenzymes: superoxide dismutase and pyruvate carboxylase, which play a significant role in antioxidant protection and energy metabolism. Mn deficiency in humans is rare and there have been no cases of deficiency in PN patients. Although Mn is relatively nontoxic, excess intake can lead to accumulation of Mn in the brain, especially in pediatrics [35], and postmortem data on long-term HPN patients confirm the accumulation effect of Mn supplementation over time [36]. Routine measurement of Mn in whole blood in combination with regular MRI is recommended to monitor potential accumulation in the brain for long-term pediatric and adult PN patients and those with renal or hepatic dysfunction [37].

Interactions or incompatibilities in PN mixtures have not been reported at physiological concentrations but ubiquitous Mn contamination of PN products makes it difficult to assure consistent intake so that doses may often be excessive. In PN-dependent patients, the intestinal regulatory mechanism is bypassed and intravenously delivered micronutrients are completely bioavailable. As Mn is secreted almost entirely in the bile, parenteral Mn supplementation may contribute to cholestasis [38], thus patients with cholestatic disease should normally be administered Mn-free PN regimens. ASPEN [18] and ESPEN [13] recommend 60–100 μg/day or 1 μg/kg/day for adults with a maximum of 50 μg/day for children receiving long-term PN. However, the optimal supplementation for adult HPN is likely to be no more than 1 μmol/day (55 μg/day) [39]. A lower recommendation of 1–1.5 μg/kg/day (0.02–0.03 μmol/day) has also been made for Mn supplementation in LBW infants on PN. The growing evidence for Mn toxicity suggests supplementation for long-term pediatric and for adult HPN patients remains too high and is usually unnecessary. There is thus a persuasive argument for not routinely adding Mn for short-term PN [37].

### 23.3.7 IODINE

The major role of iodine (I) is in thyroid function, where it is incorporated mainly into the hormones thyroxine ($T_4$) and triiodothyronine ($T_3$). Tests for free T3, T4, and TSH, total thyroxine, or triiodothyronine levels are used to observe thyroid function. Iodine deficiency affects growth, development, and mental impairment if these thyroid hormones are not produced [40].

The recommended adult daily dose is 70 μg/day (0.6 μmol/day), but intakes up to 1 mg/day are well tolerated. Parenteral iodine supplementation for premature infants should range from 4–5 μg/kg/day (0.03–0.04 μmol/kg/day), and for full-term infants 5–15 μg/kg/day (0.04–0.12 μmol/kg/day). There have been few reports of iodine deficiency symptoms and no incompatibility problems during PN [20]. Despite low parenteral intakes in a recent study of children with SBS or intestinal diseases, there were no signs of thyroid dysfunction [41].

### 23.3.8 MOLYBDENUM

Molybdenum (Mo) is incorporated into xanthine oxidase, which takes part in the metabolism of purines, and sulfite oxidase which oxidizes the sulfite formed from the metabolism of the sulfur-containing amino acids; methionine and cysteine [42]. Mo deficiency is rare but has been reported in a long-term severely malnourished PN patient with Crohn's disease [43]. Mo appears physically compatible in PN mixtures at physiological concentrations. An excess of either Cu or Mo in the presence of sulfate can give rise to a Cu–Mo–S complex which will result in a deficit of the metals. Care should therefore be taken to monitor Cu levels as well. Mo can be measured using either neutron activation analysis or electron-emission spectroscopy, but neither of these techniques is widely available. Alternatively, levels of xanthine oxidase and sulfite oxidase can be measured.

Addition of 100–200 µg/day (1.0–2.1 µmol/day) as ammonium molybdate has been recommended for adults [13,18] but other PN constituents can contain Mo as a contaminant. The recommended parenteral supplement for both premature and full-term pediatric patients is 0.25 µg/kg/day (0.003 µmol/kg/day) [13].

## 23.4 OTHER TRACE ELEMENTS

There are various other elements, which may play a role in human nutrition. The most significant is cobalt (Co), which is known to be essential as a constituent of vitamin $B_{12}$ which is reviewed later. The only recognized role for fluoride (F) in humans is its presence in bone and tooth enamel. Fluoride status of PN patients is rarely monitored. The bone content would probably provide the best evaluation but is impractical for routine use. Normal requirements are 1.5–4.0 mg/day (50–200 µmol/day). If fluoride is to be administered as a supplement to PN solutions, there are no reported stability problems and the recommended dosage for adults is 0.95 mg/day (50 µmol/day). For the pediatric patient 1 µg/mL PN solution (0.05 µmol/mL) is recommended. Alternatively, for infants on long-term PN a daily dose of 500 µg (26 µmol) has been suggested (Table 23.1) [15].

## 23.5 VITAMINS

The requirement for vitamins in IF may be higher than for healthy individuals (Table 23.2). Serum levels of some vitamins decrease with the inflammatory response [44], but vitamins B1, B2, B12, and folate are not affected by inflammation, and decreased levels may represent a true deficiency. Deficiencies can occur in patients with inflammatory bowel disease from losses through high output GI fistulas or with diarrhea. Refeeding of upper GI secretions into the jejunum, either via a nasojejunal tube or jejunostomy [45], will facilitate absorption of fat-soluble vitamins that require bile and pancreatic secretions for optimal absorption [5]. Most water-soluble vitamins are absorbed easily from the proximal GI tract and may occur in relatively short lengths of jejunum or residual ileum. Fat-soluble vitamins are absorbed in the mid- and distal ileum as digestion of fat by bile and pancreatic lipase is required. If the terminal ileum is missing, then these vitamins plus B12 become depleted. In conditions where fat malabsorption can occur, such as pancreatic insufficiency and bile loss, deficiency of fat-soluble vitamins is common.

Complex interactions between vitamins, trace elements, and drug–nutrient interactions during compounding, storage, and administration of PN admixtures can all substantially reduce the amount of individual micronutrients delivered to the IF patient. Protection from air and sunlight can minimize many chemical losses [15] but it may also be necessary to compensate for vitamin losses by increased dosage. Toxicity from water-soluble vitamins is unlikely, and up to 100 times the RDA can be safely administered. Fat-soluble vitamin toxicity can occur, and it is generally recommended that a safe limit is 10 times the RDA [46].

**TABLE 23.1**

**Summary Recommendations for Trace Elements in PN**

| Trace Element | DRI for Oral Intake | Daily Parenteral Dose | | Status Assessment |
|---|---|---|---|---|
| | | **Adults** | **Children** | |
| Chromium | 35 µg | 10–15 µg (0.2–0.3 µmol) 20 µg (0.4 µmol) in ICU 5–10 µg/day for long-term PN | 0.14–0.2 µg/kg (0.003–0.004 µmol/kg) 0.05 µg/kg for long-term PN | Plasma Cr |
| Copper | 0.9 mg | 0.3–0.5 mg (5–8 µmol) 1.3 mg (20 µmol) in major burns and GI losses | 20 µg/kg (0.3 µmol/kg) | Plasma Cu or ceruloplasmin with CRP |
| Iron | 8 mg | 0–1.0–1.2 mg (18–20 µmol) | 200 µg/kg 3–4 mg/kg (54–71 µmol/kg) in LBW infants | Serum ferritin |
| Zinc | 11 mg | 2.5–5 mg (38–76 µmol) plus 2.5–4 mg (38–62 µmol) in catabolic states but not more than 30 mg in ICU 12–17 mg (185–260 µmol) with GI losses | Prematures: 400 µg/kg (6.2 µmol/kg) <3 months old: 250 µg/kg (3.8 µmol/kg) >3 months old: 100 µg/kg (1.5 µmol/kg) | Plasma and serum Zn with albumin and CRP |
| Selenium | 55 µg | 30–70 µg (0.4–0.84 µmol) 250–400 µg (3.2–5.1 µmol) in ICU 2000 µg as a bolus plus 1000 µg (12.8 µmol) over 14 days in severe sepsis | 3 µg/kg (0.04 µmol/kg) 30 µg for long-term PN | Plasma or serum Se Whole blood Se RBC GPx |
| Manganese | 2.3 mg | 0–55 µg (1 µmol max) | 1–1.5 µg/kg (0.02– 0.03 µmol) with max 50 µg for long-term | Whole blood Mn MRI |
| Iodine | 150 µg | 70 µg (0.6 µmol) | Prematures: 4–5 µg/kg (0.03–0.04 µmol/kg) Full term: 5–15 µg/kg (0.04–0.12 µmol/kg) Long-term PN 1 µg/kg (0.01 mmol/kg) | Serum $T_3$, $T_4$, TSH |
| Molybdenum | 45 µg | 100–200 µg (1.0–2.1 µmol) | 0.25 µg/kg (0.003 µmol/ kg) | Urinary hypoxanthine and xanthine sulfite oxidase |
| Fluorine | 4.0 mg | 0.95 mg (50 µmol) | 1 µg/mL (0.05 µmol/mL) PN 500 µg (26 µmol) for long-term PN | Blood levels and urine excretion |

*Source:* Adapted from Hardy G, Menendez AM, Manzanares W. *Nutrition* 2009;25:1073–1084. With permission.

*Note:* CRP: C-reactive protein; DRI: dietary reference intakes; GI: gastrointestinal; GPx: glutathione peroxidase; ICU: intensive care unit; LBW: low birth weight; MRI: magnetic resonance imaging; PN: parenteral nutrition; RBC: red blood cell; TSH: thyroid-stimulating hormone.

**TABLE 23.2**

**Summary Recommendations for Vitamins in PN**

| Vitamins | DRI for Oral Intake[a] | Daily Parenteral Dose | |
|---|---|---|---|
| | | Adult | Pediatric |
| Vitamin A | Infants and young children: 400–500 RAE[b] Adults: M[c]: 900 RAE F[d]: 700 RAE | 1000 μg | Infants: 150–300 μg/kg/day Children: 15 μg/day |
| Vitamin D | Infants and young children: 5 μg Adults: M: 5–15 μg F: 5–15 μg | 5 μg | Infants: 0.8 μg/kg/day Children: 10 μg/day |
| Vitamin E | Infants: 4–5 α-TE[c] (mg)/day Young children: 6–7 α-TE (mg)/day Adults: M: 15 α-TE F: 15 α-TE | 10 mg | Infants: 2.8–3.5 mg/kg/day Children: 7 mg/day |
| Vitamin K | Infants: 2.0–2.5 μg Young children: 30–55 μg Adults: M: 120 μg F: 90 μg | 150 μg | Infants: 10 μg/kg/day Children: 200 μg/day |
| Vitamin B1 (Thiamine) | Infants: 0.2–0.3 mg Young children: 0.5–0.6 mg Adults: M: 1.2 mg F: 1.1 mg | 3.0–3.5 mg | Infants: 0.35–0.5 mg/kg/day Children: 1.2 mg/day |
| Vitamin B2 (Riboflavin) | Infants: 0.3–0.4 mg Young children: 0.5–0.6 mg Adults: M: 1.3 mg F: 1.1 mg | 3.6–4.9 mg | Infants: 0.15–0.2 mg/kg/day Children: 1.45 mg/day |
| Vitamin B3 (Niacin) | Infants: 2–4 mg Young children: 6–8 mg Adults: M: 16 mg F: 14 mg | 40–46 mg | Infants: 4.0–6.8 mg/kg/day Children: 17 mg/day |
| Vitamin B5 (Pantothenic Acid) | Infants: 1.7–1.8 mg Young children: 3–5 mg Adults: 2–3 mg M:5 mg F: 5 mg | 15 mg | Infants: 1.0–2.0 mg/kg/day Children: 5 mg/day |
| Vitamin B6 (Pyridoxine) | Infants: 0.1–0.3 mg Young children: 0.5–0.6 mg Adults: M: 1.3–1.7 mg F: 1.3–1.5 mg | 4.0–4.5 mg | Infants: 0.15–0.2 mg/kg/day Children: 1.0 mg/day |
| Folic acid | Infants: 65–80 μg Young children: 150–200 μg Adults: M:400 μg F: 400 μg | 400 μg | Infants: 56 μg/kg/day Children: 140 μg/day |

*continued*

**TABLE 23.2    (continued)**
**Summary Recommendations for Vitamins in PN**

| Vitamins | DRI for Oral Intake[a] | Daily Parenteral Dose | |
|---|---|---|---|
| | | Adult | Pediatric |
| Vitamin B12 (Cyanocobalamin) | Infants: 0.4–0.5 µg<br>Young children: 0.9–1.2 µg<br>Adults:<br>  M: 2.4 µg<br>  F: 2.4 µg | 5.0–6.0 µg | Infants: 0.3 µg/kg/day<br>Children: 1.0 µg/day |
| Vitamin H (Biotin) | Infants: 5 µg/day<br>Young Children: 8–12 µg/day<br>Adults:<br>  M: 30 µg<br>  F: 30 µg | 60–69 µg | Infants: 5.0–8.0 µg/kg/day<br>Children: 20 µg/day |
| Vitamin C | Infants: 40–50 mg<br>Young children: 15–25 mg<br>Adults:<br>  M:90 mg<br>  F: 75 mg | 100–125 mg | Infants: 15–25 mg/kg/day<br>Children: 80 mg/day |

[a] From U.S. Department of Agriculture, Agricultural Research Service: Nutrient Database for Standard Reference, in *Krause'S Food & Nutrition Therapy*, International Edition, 12e ISBN: 978–0–8089-.

[b] RAE, Retinol activity equivalents, I RAE = 1 µg of retinol; RAEs from plant sources are calculated based on 12 µg β-carotene: 1 RAE.

[c] Male.

[d] Female.

[e] α-TE, α-Tocopherol equivalents (1 IU = 1 mg).

### 23.5.1    FAT-SOLUBLE VITAMINS

#### 23.5.1.1    Vitamin A

Vitamin A (retinol) comprises a number of β-ionone derivatives of β-carotene, the most biologically active of which is all-*trans*-retinol. It is required for vision, bone development, and immune function but may be poorly absorbed due to the steatorrhea of SBS. Postoperative patients exhibit decreased levels of vitamin A and septic patients excrete high levels in the urine. Supplementation of excess vitamin E may antagonize vitamin A function in IF patients. Vitamin A is usually employed in PN multivitamin additives as the acetate or palmitate ester. Retinol acetate is relatively more lipophilic and migrates to the inner surfaces of plasticized containers and PVC giving sets, accounting for up to 30% loss during administration [47]. In contrast, retinol palmitate does not absorb and no losses to plastic surfaces are observed during storage [48]. Retinol is also highly sensitive to daylight, undergoing rapid degradation by a photolytic reaction induced by ultraviolet (UV) radiation. Losses can amount to more than 90% during infusion if no precautions are taken [49]. It is therefore essential to cover the PN container with a light-protecting overwrap when infusing in daylight.

#### 23.5.1.2    Vitamin D

Ergocalciferol (vitamin D2) and cholecalciferol (D3) have similar sterol-like structures. They are considered to be biologically equivalent in humans but 25-hydroxyvitamin D3 (25-OH-D) is the form measured to determine vitamin D status. Serum levels should be monitored in IF patients, and maintained at 30–100 ng/mL [50]. Vitamin D is required for bone synthesis, immunomodulation, and cardiovascular function. Autoimmune and inflammatory bowel diseases such as Crohn's disease or any malabsorption syndrome will interfere with vitamin D absorption in the GI tract [51]. Small bowel absorption of calcium is dependent on an adequate supply of vitamin D. It regulates induction of proteins that enable the gut enterocytes to transport calcium into plasma. Calcium losses combined with insufficient vitamin D can lead to hypocalcemia, osteomalacia, and increased risk of fractures. Hypovitaminosis D is associated with alterations in glucose and lipid metabolism and increases the risk of osteoporosis and heart disease. In contrast, correction of hypercalcemia and hypercalciuria observed in some long-term PN patients, by withdrawal of vitamin D from the PN regimen, has led to the suggestion that metabolic bone disease could be vitamin D related. However, other factors such as the calcium and phosphorus intake could also be responsible and removing vitamin D completely from PN regimens would be detrimental to bone repair and other important metabolic functions [50]. Since the capacity to synthesize vitamin D from sunlight is reduced in the elderly some supplementation or UV radiation is invariably necessary, but bioavailability studies in children have suggested that vitamin D status is maintained during long-term HPN [52]. However, losses may be incurred in PN admixtures. Gillis et al. [53] reported significant cholecalciferol depletion from non-fat-containing PN bags, during simulated administration, speculating that binding to the plastic bag and administration set occurs. In contrast, Dahl et al. [54] reported no losses during infusion in a fat emulsion, which may have a protective effect. Light protection is therefore advisable.

### 23.5.1.3   Vitamin E

Vitamin E activity can be identified in eight naturally occurring antioxidants, all comprising a six-chromanol ring structure. Deficiencies are rare but absorption of vitamin E requires adequate biliary and pancreatic function. A serum $\alpha$-tocopheral:cholesterol ratio <2.47 mg/g is consistent with deficiency [55]. Malabsorption conditions such as Crohn's disease may be at risk. Moreover, vitamins E and C are synergistic so that vitamin C deficiency in postoperative patients also decreases vitamin E function [56,57]. The four tocopherol isomers, the usual artificial sources of vitamin E, have variable biological activity, but are relatively stable after addition to PN mixtures, at least when light protected [58] If exposed to daylight then degradation occurs by a photooxidative reaction in the presence of oxygen. This can account for losses amounting to 30–50% during administration [53]. Some fat emulsions also contain $\alpha$-tocopherol and may be light protective.

### 23.5.1.4   Vitamin K

Vitamin K has an important role in bone health, blood clotting, and regulation of several enzymatic reactions. The revised AI for adults is 120 $\mu$g/day for men and 90 $\mu$g/day for women [59]. However, ingested vitamin K in the form of phylloquinone is poorly absorbed due to the disorders of bile acid secretion, or other metabolic derangements of SBS. Antimicrobial drugs that alter the intestinal flora, responsible for synthesis of vitamin K, may also cause depletion. Hypoprothrombinaemia with prolonged blood clotting time can result from the vitamin K deficiencies occasionally reported in SBS. Measurement of phylloquinone in serum is a useful indicator of vitamin K status, whereas International Normalized Ratio (INR) is an insensitive method [59]. The natural form of the vitamin is also present in lipid emulsions with relatively high levels in soybean oil, while the synthetic derivative used in some additives is a mixture of *cis*- and *trans*-isomers, but contains more than 80% of the natural *trans*-isomer. The US FDA recommends that parenteral multivitamin products should provide 150 $\mu$g/day [8] but NST need to be aware that this could be almost doubled from the lipid content when considering supplementation [60]. Vitamin K is stable in PN mixtures during storage for at least 20 days at 4°C, but losses may occur from daylight exposure.

### 23.5.2   WATER-SOLUBLE VITAMINS

### 23.5.2.1   Biotin (Vitamin H)

Biotin is important for carboxylase enzymes involved with carbohydrate and fat metabolism. There is insufficient information to make firm recommendations for extra dosages of biotin. Deficiencies are rare, but symptoms include dermatitis, conjunctivitis, alopecia, and paresthesias, with hallucinations and may be seen in long-term PN patients without supplementation. A scaly red rash, oftentimes confused with that seen with Zn deficiency or essential fatty acid deficiency can develop around the eyes, nose, mouth, or genital area. Indirect evidence from vitamin status studies provide the evidence that blood biotin levels are maintained during long-term PN administration [61]. Information on the stability of biotin in PN mixtures is sparse. Only Dahl et al. [54] reported data, which indicates that biotin is stable for at least 4 days at 2–8°C in an all-in-one mixture.

### 23.5.2.2   Thiamine (Vitamin B1)

Thiamine diphosphate (cocarboxylase), employed in many parenteral multivitamin products, is the coenzyme form of vitamin B1. Thiamine is relatively unstable in aqueous solution, and is particularly prone to reaction with strong reducing agents, for example, bisulfite, which is used as a stabilizer in some amino acid products. Degradation rates are such that losses will reduce the shelf life to only 1–3 days, depending on the final volume and concentration of bisulfite after compounding [62]. Most malnourished patients are thiamine deficient and require supplementation. Without supplementation, large carbohydrate loads will trigger thiamine deficiency. Thiamine is rapidly consumed in glycolysis and can cause lactic acidosis with impaired glucose metabolism when levels become depleted as pyruvate cannot be decarboxylated and thus cannot enter the Krebs cycle. This leads to failed synthesis of adenosine triphosphate and an energy deficit resulting in beriberi, with patients experiencing hypotension, tachycardia, and severe metabolic acidosis that does not respond well to bicarbonate therapy [63]. Other symptoms include altered mental status, diplopia, vomiting, and abdominal pain. Although alcoholics frequently exhibit low folate and vitamin C levels, the most clinically important deficiency is thiamine because of the dangers of Wernicke–Korsakoff syndrome in which neurological damage can ensue from aggressive refeeding [64]. An increased erythrocyte transketolase activity from baseline after the addition of thiamine pyrophosphate confirms diagnosis, although clinical suspicion is often sufficient to warrant immediate administration of parenteral thiamine, 10–25 mg intramuscularly or intravenously [65].

### 23.5.2.3   Riboflavin (Vitamin B2)

Riboflavin comprises an isoalloxazine ring attached to a butyl side chain. It has numerous roles as coenzyme in critical oxidation–reduction reactions. Deficiency symptoms are nonspecific and include nausea, vomiting, abdominal pain, weight loss, and fatigue, but can be easily reversed by supplementation, through its beneficial effect on mitochondrial function [5]. Riboflavin is stable in acid conditions, but less stable at higher pH. It also shows some sensitivity to light. More than 80% riboflavin remained after 8 weeks' refrigerated storage in a range of PN mixtures, but, like most vitamins, significant losses occurred during administration in daylight [66].

### 23.5.2.4   Nicotinamide (Nicotinic Acid, Niacin, Vitamin B3)

Nicotinic acid is a pyridine-3-carboxylic acid. Nicotinamide, or niacin, the physiologically active compound, is the amide derivative. It can also be generated from tryptophan by biotransformation in the liver. Requirements for niacin are increased in pyridoxine (vitamin B6) and riboflavin (vitamin B2) deficiencies [5]. Nicotinamide is one of the most stable vitamins and is insensitive to light, oxidizing or reducing agents. This vitamin would therefore be expected to be stable after addition to PN mixtures.

### 23.5.2.5   Pyridoxine (Vitamin B6)

Pyridoxine is the generic name for 3-hydroxy-2-methylpyridine derivatives with biological activity. It serves as an essential coenzyme in a variety of reactions involving fat, amino acid, and carbohydrate metabolism. Although deficiency is rare, it can occur as a result of chronic drug therapy and malabsorption. Isoniazid can increase urinary pyridoxine excretion. Moreover, pyridoxine requirements are increased in the presence of malignancy. Deficiency is characterized by neurologic changes including irritability and depression in adults, while convulsions have been seen in neonates receiving a pyridoxine-free diet. Supplementation is also not without risk. Pyridoxine can antagonize levodopa's therapeutic activity by stimulating the decarboxylation of dopa to dopamine in peripheral tissues. Pyridoxine is formulated as the hydrochloride salt and is a relatively stable compound but is sensitive to direct daylight. It should not be given as an undiluted injection as it may predispose patients to dizziness, syncope, and tissue irritation.

### 23.5.2.6  Cyanocobalamin (Vitamin B12)

Cyanocobalamin is a complex molecule, comprising four pyrrole groups joined in a large ring with a Co atom attached to a cyanide group. The vitamin is relatively stable in PN but may be sensitive to strong light. The requirement for B12 is similar for older and younger adults but the former may have consumed less meat, the principal source of the vitamin, because of poor dentition, dysphagia, and signs of deficiency may take years to develop. Pancreatic enzymes are needed for optimal vitamin B12 absorption, and therefore deficiency may occur with pancreatitis. Malabsorption, gastrectomy, or terminal ileum resection may also lead to vitamin B12 deficiency. Loss of the ileum (>100 cm) is metabolically much more significant than loss of the jejunum, since it is the site of absorption of intrinsic factor-bound B12. Nitrous oxide administration during anesthesia and use of PPI or H2 receptor antagonists can also interfere with B12 metabolism [67,68]. Typically, patients at greatest risk for B12 deficiency include those with a history of surgical resection >15–45 cm of ileum as infants, chronic acid suppression, and those with bacterial overgrowth. Vitamin B12 deficiency alters intestinal mucosal cell morphology and intestinal cell-wall transport function. B12 deficiency is associated with megaloblastic anemia and potentially irreversible neurocognitive complications. Diagnosis of deficiency states is often done by detecting increased levels of methylmalonic acid as serum assays are less precise. Patients with B12 deficiency secondary to ileal resection will not respond to oral supplementation and should be treated with either intramuscular injections on a monthly basis or daily intranasal administration of the vitamin. Since the hematological changes of B12 deficiency may be masked by high folate intake, careful monitoring is imperative so as to avoid neurologic complications.

### 23.5.2.7  Ascorbic Acid (Vitamin C)

The biologically active form of vitamin C is L (+) ascorbic acid. Scurvy is the best-known manifestation of severe vitamin C deficiency but in IF and postoperative patients, vitamin C depletion is often associated with poor wound healing and decreased vitamin A function. Ascorbate is an important antioxidant, a cofactor for several enzymes which is involved in the synthesis of carnitine, dopamine, serotonin, and the metabolism of cholesterol. Nevertheless, there is no clear indicator of inadequate vitamin C status. A serum level <20 µmol/L has been advocated, but plasma concentrations will be altered by inflammation [69]. The new US dietary reference intakes (DRI) recommends 75 mg/day for females and 90 mg/day for males increasing to 200 mg/day for parenteral use [8]. A dosage of 100–150 mg/day has been the European practice in PN and is probably sufficient for stable HPN patients [13]. However, PN supplementation requires care. Ascorbic acid is the least stable vitamin in solution. The compound reacts directly with oxygen, to form dehydroascorbic acid, which in turn is rapidly hydrolyzed to 2,3-diketogluconic acid. This reaction is catalyzed by heavy metals, in particular Cu and Fe. The final stage of the degradation pathway leads to oxalate formation, which is toxic. Both the rate and extent of losses of ascorbic acid in PN mixtures depend on the quantity of oxygen present during storage and administration. Losses due to this process can be prevented by multilayered plastic bags, which are largely impermeable to oxygen, and mixtures prepared in such containers may be assigned extended shelf lives [70]. Some initial loss of ascorbic acid after addition to a PN mixture is inevitable, but the reaction with dissolved oxygen will be complete within a few hours and can be compensated for by increasing the dose.

### 23.5.2.8 Pantothenic Acid (Vitamin B5)

Pantothenic acid is an essential component of the biologically active coenzyme A, and is essential for many acetylation reactions, especially the tricarboxylic acid cycle. Deficiencies are rare in humans, and diarrhea is the only reported evidence of any toxicity [5]. Only the D (+) enantiomer of this vitamin has biological activity and it is usually provided as the alcohol, D-pantothenyl alcohol (dexpenthanol), which is expected to be relatively stable for at least 4 days when stored at 2–8°C in PN mixtures with neutral pH . It is the form incorporated into the various multivitamin preparations used for routine PN supplementation at DRI daily doses ranging from 2 mg for infants, 10 mg for older children up to 15 mg for adults.

### 23.5.2.9 Folic Acid

Folic acid is a B-complex vitamin consisting of a pteridine molecule linked through a methylene bridge to *p*-aminobenzamide, which is bonded to glutamic acid. This structure enables folate to function as a coenzyme in single carbon (methylene) transfers for the metabolism of amino acids and nucleic acids. Folate intake may have been limited by special diets or its uptake reduced by interference from certain medications. Given that folate is absorbed throughout the small bowel, with the majority primarily in the proximal third, deficiency is uncommon in SBS. Folic acid can be degraded by reducing agents (e.g., ascorbic acid), by hydrolysis and light. Riboflavin also has adverse effects on folate stability. It is therefore not surprising that the stability of folic acid in PN mixtures remains poorly defined. Conflicting reports have been published, indicating, the possibility of absorption to the container which may effect chemical stability during storage [71,72].

## 23.6  SUMMARY AND CONCLUSIONS

With the increased use of PN over the past few decades, it has become clear that supplementation with micronutrients is vital in order to prevent clinical symptoms associated with a deficiency of one or more vitamins or trace elements. Supplementation of PN regimens with micronutrients should be mandatory whenever PN is instituted [6,73]. Whether a patient has depleted stores due to cachexia, or has suffered severe long-term losses, the micronutrient levels must be restored and any remaining reserves maintained by supplementation on the first day of nutrition therapy. Routine supplementation of PN regimens, with the readily available multitrace element or vitamin combination products, is essential, but more individual additives should now be made available. Manufacturers of amino acid solutions and additives for PN also need to carefully monitor, and reduce trace element contamination in their products.

Routine measurement of most micronutrients is not essential in short-term PN. Nevertheless, careful observation and monitoring of blood levels and reassessment of clinical symptoms is important in patients with renal, hepatic, or intestinal dysfunction and those on long-term PN to determine any additional micronutrient requirements. More research is required to understand true trace element and vitamin requirements for malnourished and IF patients. As more is learned about deficiency syndromes and monitoring techniques, so too must practitioners become more aware of the physicochemical interactions between individual nutrients that could ultimately affect their bioavailability and patient outcomes.

## REFERENCES

1. Nightingale J. Definition and classification of intestinal failure. In: Nightingale J, editor. *Intestinal Failure.*. London: Greenwich Medical Media; 2001.
2. Chatriwalla EG, Parekh NR, Steiger E, Siedner DL, Su L-C, Lopez R. Factors associated with micronutrient deficiency in intestinal failure. *JPEN* 2008;32:323–324.
3. Johnson KA, Bernard MA, Funderburg K. Vitamin nutrition in older adults. *Clin Geriatr Med* 2002;18:773–799.

4. Sriram K, Cue J. Micronutrients in critical care. In: Cresci G, editor. *Nutrition Support in the Critically Ill*. Boca Raton FL: Taylor & Francis, CRC Press; 2005. pp. 109–123.
5. Sriram K, Lonchyna VA. Micronutrient supplementation in adult nutrition therapy: Practical considerations. *JPEN* 2009;33:548–562.
6. National Institute for Clinical Excellence. Nutrition support in adults: Oral nutrition support, enteral tube feeding and parenteral nutrition. 2006. pp. 137 (cited from www.rcseng.ac.uk).
7. Dietary Reference Intakes for vitamin A, vitamin K, arsenic, boron, chromium, copper, iodine, iron, molybdenum, nickel, silicon, vanadium and zinc. Standing Committee on the Scientific Evaluation of Dietary References Intakes, Food and Nutrition Board & Institute of Medicine, National Academy of Sciences, Washington, DC, 2001.
8. Food and Drug Administration (FDA). Parenteral multivitamin products; Drugs for human use; Drug efficacy study implementation; Amendment. *Fed Regist* 2000;65:21200–21201.
9. Russell D. AuSPEN guidelines for intravenous trace elements and vitamins. *AuSPEN* 1998;1–32. Available at www.auspen.org.au.
10. McClave SA, Martindale RG, Vanek VW, McCarthy M, Roberts P, Taylor B, Ochoa J, Napolitano L, Gresci G. Guidelines for the provision of nutrition support therapy in the adult critically ill patient *JPEN* 2009;33:277–316.
11. Braga M, Ljungqvist O, Soeters P et al. ESPEN guidelines on parenteral nutrition: Surgery. *Clin Nutr* 2009;28:378–386.
12. Staun M, Pironi L, Bozzetti F et al. ESPEN guidelines on parenteral nutrition: Home parenteral nutrition in adult patients. *Clin Nutr* 2009;28:467–479.
13. Shenkin A. Trace elements and vitamins in enteral and parenteral nutrition. In: Sobotka L, Allison S, Furst P, Meier R, Soeters P, editors. *Basics in Clinical Nutrition. ESPEN*. 3rd ed. Prague: Galen; 2004. pp. 169–175.
14. Gillanders L, Angstmann K, Ball P et al. AuSPEN HPN AuSPEN clinical practice guideline for home parenteral nutrition adult patients in Australia & New Zealand. *Nutrition* 2008;24:998–1012.
15. Hardy G, Menendez AM, Manzanares W. Trace element supplementation in parenteral nutrition: Pharmacy, posology and monitoring guidance. *Nutrition* 2009;25:1073–1084.
16. Jeejeebhoy KN, Chu RC, Marliss E et al. Chromium deficiency, glucose intolerance and neuropathy reversed by chromium supplementation in a patient receiving long-term PN. *Am J Clin Nutr* 1977;30:531–538.
17. Vincent JB. Quest for the molecular mechanism of chromium action and its relationship to diabetes. *Nutr Rev* 2000;58:67–72.
18. ASPEN. Board of Directors and the Clinical Task Force. Guidelines for the use of parenteral and enteral nutrition in adult and pediatric patients. *JPEN J Paren Enteral Nutr* 2002;26 (Suppl):23SA.
19. Mouser JF, Hak EB, Helms RA et al. Chromium and zinc concentrations in pediatric patients receiving long-term parenteral nutrition. *Am J Health Syst Pharm* 1999;56:1950–1956.
20. Hardy G, Reilly C. Technical aspects of trace element supplementation. *Curr Opin Clin Nutr Metab Care* 1999;2:277–285.
21. Spiegel J, Willenbucher R. Development of severe copper deficiency in a patient with Crohn's Disease receiving parenteral nutrition. *JPEN* 1999;23:169–172.
22. Shike M, Roulet M, Kurian R et al. Copper metabolism and requirements in total parenteral nutrition. *Gastroenterology* 1981;81:290–297.
23. Tielemans CL, Lenclud CM, Wens R et al. Critical role of iron overload in the increased susceptibility of haemodialysis patients to bacterial infections. Beneficial effects of desferrioxamine. *Nephrol Dial Transplant* 1989;4:883–887.
24. Swoboda SM, Lipsett PA. Intravenous iron as a risk factor for bacteremia in the surgical intensive care unit patient. *Surg Infect* 2005;6:158.
25. WHO/UNICEF/ICCIDD. Iron deficiency anemia: Assessment, prevention and control. WHO 2001, Geneva, WHO/NHD/013.
26. Lapointe M. Iron supplementation in the intensive care unit: When, how much, and by what route? *Crit Care* 2004;8(Suppl 2):S37–S41.
27. Kumpf VJ. Update on parenteral iron therapy. *Nutr Clin Pract* 2003;18:318–326.
28. Kenny F, Sriram K, Hammond J. Clinical zinc deficiency during adequate enteral nutrition. *J Am Coll Nutr* 1989;8:83–85.
29. Kohrle J, Brigelius-Flohe R, Bock A et al. Selenium in Biology: Facts and medical perspectives. *Biol Chem* 2000;381:849–864.
30. Rayman MP. The importance of selenium to human health. *The Lancet* 2000;356:233–241.

31. Thomson CD, Robinson MF, Butler JA et al. Long term supplementation with selenate and selenome-thionine: Selenium and glutathione peroxidase in blood components of New Zealand women. *Br J Nutr* 1993;69:577–588.

32. Berger MM, Shenkin A. Vitamins and trace elements: Practical aspects of supplementation. *Nutrition* 2006;22:952–955.

33. Manzanares W, Hardy G. Selenium supplementation in the critically ill. *Curr Opin Clin Nutr Metab Care* 2009;12:273–280.

34. Hardy IJ, Martin H, Hardy G. Selenium stability in vitamin and glutamine mixtures. *Clin Nutr* 2005;24:596.

35. Reynolds N, Blumsohn A, Baxter JP. Manganese requirement and toxicity in patients on HPN. *Clin Nutr* 1998;17:227–230.

36. Howard L, Ashley C, Lyon D et al. Autopsy tissue trace elements in 8 long-term parenteral nutrition patients who received the current US FDA formulation. *JPEN* 2007;31:388–396.

37. Hardy IJ, Gillanders L, Hardy G. Is Manganese an essential supplement for parenteral nutrition? *Curr Opin Clin Nutr Metab Care* 2008;11:289–296.

38. Dickerson RN. Manganese intoxication and parenteral nutrition. *Nutrition* 2001;17:689–693.

39. Takagi Y, Okada A, Sando K et al. Evaluation of indexes of *in vivo* manganese status and the optimal intra-venous dose for adult patients undergoing home parenteral nutrition. *Am J Clin Nutr* 2002;75:112–118.

40. Zimmermann MB. Iodine in clinical nutrition and public health: A review. *Gastroenterology* 2009; 137:S36–S46.

41. Cicalese MP, Assante L, Vicinanza A et al. Asking for iodine supplementation in children on parenteral nutrition. *Dig Liver Dis* 2008;40:A115.

42. Johnson JL, Rajagopalan KV, Cohen HJ. Molecular basis of the biologic function of molybdenum. *J Biol Chem* 1874;249:859–866.

43. Abumrad NN, Schneider AJ, Steel D, Rogers LS. Amino acid intolerance during prolonged total paren-teral nutrition reversed by molybdate therapy. *Am J Clin Nutr* 1981;34:2551–2559.

44. Galloway P, McMillan DC, Sattar N. Effect of the inflammatory response on trace element and vitamin status. *Ann Clin Biochem* 2000;37:289–297.

45. Sriram K, Sridhar R. Gastroduodenal decompression and simultaneous nasoenteral nutrition: "Extracorporeal gastrojejunostomy." *Nutrition.* 1996;12:440–441.

46. Demling RH, De Biasse MA. Micronutrients in critical illness. *Crit Care Clin* 1995;11:651–673.

47. Howard L, Ohu R, Feman S, Mintz H, Ovesen L, Wolf B. Vitamin A deficiency from long-term parenteral nutrition. *Ann Int Med* 1980;93:576–577.

48. Billion-Rey F, Guillaumont M, Frederich A, Aulanger G. Stability of fat-soluble vitamins A(retinol pal-mitate), E(tocopherol acetate) and K1(phylloquinone) in total parenteral nutrition at home. *JPEN* 1993;17:56–60.

49. Allwood MC, Plane JH. The wavelength-dependent degradation of vitamin A exposed to ultraviolet light. *Inter J Pharmaceutics* 1986;31:1–7.

50. DeLuca HF. Vitamin D. *Gastroenterology* 2009;137:S79–S91.

51. Cantorna MT. Vitamin D and its role in immunology: Multiple sclerosis, and inflammatory bowel dis-ease. *Prog Biophys Mol Biol* 2006;92:60–64.

52. Davis AT, Franz FP., Coutney DA, Ullrey DE, Scholten DJ, Dean RE. Plasma vitamin and mineral status in home parenteral nutrition patients. *JPEN* 1987;11:480–485.

53. Gillis J, Jones G, Penchardz P. Delivery of vitamins A, D and E in total parenteral nutrition solutions. *JPEN* 1983;7:11–14.

54. Dahl GB, Jeppson RI, Tengborn HJ. Vitamin stability in a TPN mixture stored in an EVA plastic bag. *J Clin Hosp Pharm* 1986;11:271–279.

55. Louw JA, Werbeck A, Louw MEJ. Blood vitamin concentrations during the acute phase response. *Crit Care Med.* 1992;20:934–941.

56. Thurnham DJ, Davies JA, Crump BJ et al. The use of different lipids to express serum tocopherol lipid ratios for the measurement of vitamin E status. *Ann Clin Biochem* 1986;23(Pt5):514–520

57. Agarwal N, Norkus E, Garcia C. Effect of surgery on serum antioxidant vitamins. *JPEN* 1996;20(Suppl):32S.

58. McGee CD, Mascarwnhas MG, Ostro MJ, Rasallas G, Jeejeebhoy K. Selenium and vitamin E stability on parenteral solutions. *JPEN* 1985;5:568–570.

59. Shearer MJ. Vitamin K in parenteral nutrition. *Gastroenterology* 2009;137:S105–S118.

60. Singh H, Duerksen DR. Vitamin K and nutrition support. *Nutr Clin Pract* 2003;18:359–365.

61. Hariz MB, De Potter S, Corriol O, Goulet O, Chaumont P, Forget D, Ricour C. Home parenteral nutrition in children: Bioavailability of vitamins in binary mixtures for 8 days. *Clin Nutr* 1993;12:147–152.
62. Kearney MCJ, Allwood MC, Hardy G. The stability of thiamine in TPN mixtures stored in EVA and multilayered bags. *Clin Nutr* 1995;14:295–301.
63. Champ P, Harvey P, editors. *Lippincott's Illustrated Reviews: Biochemistry* 2nd ed. Philadelphia, USA: J.B. Lippincott Company; 1994. Chapter 28. pp. 319–342.
64. Austin P, Stroud M, editors. *Prescribing Adult Intravenous Nutrition*. London: Pharm Press; 2007.
65. Doolman R, Dinbar A, Sela BA. Improved measurement of transkeolase activity in the assessment of "TPP" effect. *Eur J Chem Clin Biochem* 1995;33(7):445–446.
66. Chen MF, Boyce W, Triplett L. Stability of B vitamins in mixed parenteral nutrition solution. *JPEN* 1983;7:462–464.
67. Schilling RF. Is nitrous oxide a dangerous anesthetic for vitamin B12-deficient subjects? *JAMA* 1986;255:1605–1606.
68. Marian R, Sacks G. Micronutrients and older adults. *Nutr Clin Prac* 2009;24:179–195.
69. Berger MM. Vitamin C requirements in parenteral nutrition and other conditions. *Gastroenterology* 2009;137:S70–S78.
70. Allwood MC, Brown PE, Ghedini C, Hardy G. The stability of ascorbic acid in TPN mixtures stored in a multilayered bag. *Clin Nutr* 1992;11:284–288.
71. Barker A, Hebron BS, Beck PR, Ellis B. Folic acid and total parenteral nutrition. *JPEN* 1984;8:3–13.
72. Halsed CH. Intestinal absorption and malabsorption of folates. *Annu Rev Med* 1980;31:79–87
73. ASPEN Board of Directors. Safe practices in parenteral nutrition. *JPEN* 2004;28:S39–S70.

# 24 Bacterial Overgrowth of the Small Intestine

*Esi S. N. Lamousé-Smith and Samuel Kocoshis*

## CONTENTS

## 24.1 DEFINITION

Any definition of small intestinal bacterial overgrowth (SIBO) must differentiate between SIBO itself and the SIBO syndrome. Essential to the definition of SIBO is the concept that under conditions of health, the small intestine, via a number of mechanisms, keeps the number of bacteria populating it very low. An increased number of bacteria within the small intestinal lumen is the *sine qua non* of SIBO. By convention, $>10^5$ colony forming units per milliliter of small intestinal fluid (CFU/mL) are the accepted minimum number of bacteria that define bacterial overgrowth [1]. However, as described in detail later in this chapter, pitfalls exist in accepting this number too strictly.

The SIBO syndrome is operationally defined as an increased number of a colonic type of bacteria (coliforms, *Enterococci*, and Gram-positive anaerobes) associated with nutrient malabsorption caused by those bacteria or toxicity to the host due to bacterial metabolites such as D-lactate, ammonia, or ethanol.

A historical perspective of the SIBO syndrome is enlightening, and can help to explain how these operational definitions were derived. SIBO syndrome was first recognized in the era during which the Billroth 2 operation was employed as a treatment for chronic ulcer disease. That procedure requires the surgical creation of a blind loop which, if it does not empty effectively, becomes populated with excessive quantities of a "colonic" type of flora. Those patients who developed steatorrhea following a Billroth 2 procedure were likely to have excessive numbers of colonic bacteria populating their proximal small intestine. When bacterial counts were quantitated, it was shown that those patients consistently had $>10^5$ CFU/mL of luminal fluid. The presence of steatorrhea in the face of $>10^5$ CFU/mL in all patients who had naturally occurring blind loops or surgical blind loops was defined as "blind loop syndrome," "stagnant loop syndrome," or "intestinal stasis" syndrome. When similar symptoms, signs, biochemical findings, and/or microbiologic findings were observed in entities such as short bowel syndrome unassociated with anatomic blind loops, the term small intestinal bacterial overgrowth syndrome (SIBO) or small bowel bacterial overgrowth syndrome came into popular usage.

The fact that some patients have signs and symptoms of bacterial overgrowth syndrome with fewer than $10^5$ CFU/mL and conversely, some patients are asymptomatic with >$10^5$ CFU/mL, mandates that simple bacterial overgrowth be differentiated from SIBO syndrome which is present when the small intestinal flora are exerting deleterious effects upon the host.

## 24.2  SYMPTOMS

Patients suffering from SIBO are likely to experience bloating, early satiety, crampy postprandial abdominal pain, and steatorrhea or diarrhea. Among patients who have SIBO associated with short bowel syndrome, the symptoms cannot often be differentiated from the typical symptoms engendered by rapid small intestinal transit and colonic fermentation. In those patients, the syndrome can go unrecognized until some toxic metabolic product of small intestinal bacterial metabolism exerts its deleterious effect. The fact that the symptoms produced by the SIBO syndrome and short bowel syndrome itself are identical should prompt circumspection when the decision to treat the SIBO syndrome is contemplated.

Many of the products produced by the enteric flora that populate the small intestine during SIBO are neurotoxic. For example, D-lactic acidosis is quite commonplace among patients with SIBO [2]. Hyperammonemia [3] and "autointoxication" from ethanol [4] are extremely rare complications. However, any of the above substances can produce somnolence, dementia, ataxia, seizures, or coma. Patients who have SIBO with excessive production of the above substances may also experience more subtle neurodevelopmental findings. Therefore, among patients with neurologic symptoms and underlying gastrointestinal (GI) disease putting them at risk for SIBO, D-lactate, ethanol, and ammonia levels should be obtained in blood.

## 24.3  PATHOGENESIS OF SIBO

SIBO is typically prevented by normal physiologic functions of the GI tract that can be perturbed by infection, autoimmune inflammation, or surgical alteration. Inhibition of gastric acid secretion, pancreatic exocrine enzyme production, or intestinal motility are important contributing factors in the development of SIBO and can occur in a variety of intestinal and systemic conditions. SIBO has been well described in patients with many forms of intestinal failure including: in short gut syndrome (congenital or postsurgical) [5]; following any surgery that creates a blind intestinal loop [6,7]; intestinal pseudo-obstruction [8]; in radiation-induced enteropathy [9]; scleroderma [10]; and in Crohn's disease, including following ileocecal resection [11]. In addition, SIBO is also implicated in the pathogenesis of acute pancreatitis [12]; liver cirrhosis [13,14]; non-alcoholic steatohepatitis (NASH) [15]; and irritable bowel syndrome [16–18].

Normal intestinal motility is required to prevent intestinal stasis, which, when it occurs, leads to bacterial proliferation and overgrowth of populations in segments of the small intestine resulting in the symptoms of SIBO (bloating, cramping, diarrhea, malabsorption). Normal intestinal motility is probably the most important regulator of bacterial population growth. The requirements for normal intestinal motility has been examined in animal models and in humans where it has been shown that disruption of phase III of the intestinal migrating motor complex (MMC) is associated with the development of SIBO [19–21].

Normal gastric and pancreatic secretions help to maintain normal intestinal pH and prevent the integration of pathogenic bacteria into the otherwise well-balanced bacterial niches inhabiting the upper and lower intestine. Gastric acid prevents the outgrowth of ingested bacteria and thus limits bacterial burden in the upper intestinal tract [22]. The prevalent use of proton pump inhibitors may

## TABLE 24.1
## Distribution of Bacterial Populations in the Gastrointestinal Tract

| | | |
|---|---|---|
| Mouth | $10^{7-8}$/mL | Aerobes and anaerobes: *Streptococcus* (*mitis, salvarius, viridans*), *Veillonella* sp., *Peptostreptococcus* sp., HACEK |
| Stomach | $0-10^3$/g | *Helicobacter pylori, Lactobacillus* sp. |
| Duodenum | $10-10^3$/g | Facultative anaerobes or aerobes: Streptococci, Lactobacilli, Gammaproteobacteria, *Enterococcus* and *Bacteroides* |
| Jejunum | $10^{3-5}$/g | Facultative anaerobes or aerobes: Streptococci, Lactobacilli, Gammaproteobacteria, *Enterococcus* and *Bacteroides* |
| Ileum | $10^{7-9}$/g | Aerobes Lactobacillus and facultative anaerobes: *Lactobacillus* sp., *Enterococcus faecalis*, Bacteroides, Coliforms, Bifidobacteria |
| Cecum and colon | $10^{10-12}$/g | Anaerobes: *Bifidobacterium, Lactobacillus, Clostridium, Bacteroides, Eubacterium, Peptostreptococcus*<br>Facultative aerobes: *Enterococcus, Enterobacteria* sp. (incl *E. coli*), *Staphylococcus* |

*Source:* Hayashi H et al. *J Med Microbiol*. 2005;54:1093–101; Eckburg PB et al. *Science*. 2005;308:1635–8.

be a potential contributor to SIBO [23]. It is important to take note of the potential effects that acid suppression may have on the integrity of the normal bacterial flora in the population of patients with intestinal failure, where H-2 and proton pump inhibitor therapy is commonly used to treat postresection hypergastrinemia.

Typically, the upper intestinal tract is home to $10^3–10^5$ CFU/g of bacteria, while the lower tract (TI, cecum, colon) is home to up to $10^{12}$ CFU/g of predominantly anaerobic bacteria (*Clostridia, Bacteroides*) (Table 24.1). Culture-based techniques have identified Gram-positive aerobes and facultative anaerobes in normal jejunal aspirates [24] and molecular approaches have determined that colonic-type bacteria (specifically, *Clostridium* sp) are not typically found in the jejunum [25]. Intestinal bacterial communities (niches) are established in close approximation to the epithelial mucosa of the intestine. This close approximation of intestinal bacteria with GI epithelial cells is instrumental for the regulation of a large number of important and synergistic metabolic functions critical to host survival and function. These include: degradation and absorption of otherwise indigestible nutrients (e.g., amino acids, complex carbohydrates, plant cell wall polysaccharides, and fats), bile acid conjugation, metabolism of essential vitamins (e.g., vitamins K and B12), maintenance of gut epithelial integrity, and mucosal (and systemic) immune homeostasis [26]. Therefore, the presence of unusual bacterial species or abnormal function of the intestinal flora within the small intestine can be interrogated by analyzing the products or by-products of bacterial metabolism: hydrogen, carbon dioxide, or methane gases (the basis for the application of breath tests), or short-chain fatty acids (SCFA; end products of bacterial metabolism within the large intestine) [27], which are unlikely to be present in the absence of small intestinal overgrowth.

Intestinal bacteria utilize ingested nutrients to remain viable themselves. Thus, expansion of one or more populations as occurs in the small intestine during SIBO results in competition with the host for nutrients in addition to the overall upregulation of the normal metabolic capacities of specific bacterial species. Elevated concentrations of unabsorbed substances within the intestinal lumen results in the symptoms associated with SIBO: bloating, diarrhea, steatorrhea (due to increased bile salt deconjugation and secondary fat malabsorption), malabsorption (secondary to mucosal damage associated with SIBO), and vitamin deficiencies (specifically vitamins B12, A, D, E, and K). Therefore, the major complicating morbidities in patients with SIBO are anorexia and malnutrition, inability to wean from transparenteral nutrition (TPN) [28], weight loss, and poor growth (Table 24.2).

**TABLE 24.2**

**Complications Associated with SIBO**

Gastrointestinal symptoms (bloating, diarrhea, anorexia, poor growth)

Malabsorption (fat, carbohydrate, vitamin B12, fat-soluble vitamins)

Failure to wean from total parenteral nutrition

Bowel inflammation (gross and histologic)

Bacterial translocation (endotoxemia, bacteremia, central line sepsis)

D-Lactic acidosis, hyperammonemia, ethanol "autointoxication"

D-Lactic acidosis is a unique form of acidosis well described in patients with short bowel syndrome or jejunoileal bypass who are thereby predisposed to develop overgrowth of anaerobes in the small intestine, or have relatively increased delivery of glucose and starches typically absorbed in the small intestine to the colon for fermentation by colonic anaerobic bacteria [2]. The by-product of carbohydrate fermentation by anaerobic bacteria in the intestine is D-lactate. In humans, the lack of specific metabolizing enzymes and slow renal clearance of D-lactate may result in abnormal serum accumulation when excess production or intake occurs. High levels of serum D-lactate cause metabolic acidosis and may also result in recurrent episodes of encephalopathy, although the exact mechanisms by which neurologic symptoms develop are not well understood. The neurologic presentation of D-lactic acidosis in patients is varied, but typical symptoms include: slurred speech, confusion, inability to concentrate, somnolence, hallucinations, clumsiness, weakness, ataxia, unsteady gait, nystagmus, irritability, and abusive behavior [29].

An imbalance of bacterial species within the small intestine may also trigger activation and upregulation of inflammatory cytokines both in the intestinal mucosa and systemically [30–32]. This may occur when alterations in bacterial populations within compartments of the intestinal tract trigger innate and adaptive immune responses that lead to damage of intestinal epithelial integrity. Enhanced penetration of bacteria and bacterial products into submucosal intestinal immune compartments that are typically exposed to limited or very small bacterial antigenic loads may thus ensue [33,34]. Thus, the altered immune regulation that is sometimes associated with SIBO may not simply be attributable to general malnutrition and stress.

## 24.4 DIAGNOSIS OF SIBO

One of three approaches is typically used to diagnose SIBO in patients: culture of jejunal aspirates, breath tests, and presumptive, based upon symptom response to therapy (Table 24.3). One or more may be applied and general consensus regarding which test is the best for diagnosis is still lacking.

The "gold standard" definition for the diagnosis of SIBO is the culture of $>10^5$ CFU/mL of organisms from small intestinal aspirates and the identification of colonic-type flora. The acceptance of

**TABLE 24.3**

**Diagnostic Approaches for SIBO**

Small bowel aspirates (and/or biopsies) and culture

    Aerobic and anaerobic cultures

Breath testing

    Glucose—fasting >20 ppm or rise >12 ppm from baseline in the first 2 h

    D-Xylose—dose: 1 g; catabolized by Gram-negative bacteria

    Lactulose—early $H_2$ peak; not reliable if slow or fast intestinal transit

Presumptive treatment (treat presumed symptoms or recurrence)

    Antibiotics

this quantity of bacteria as abnormal originated from early studies of patients who had undergone Billroth II gastro-jejunostomies. Those who experienced malabsorption following this procedure were most likely to have $>10^5$ CFU/mL of duodenal fluid. However, the relationship between the number of cultivatable species within the duodenum and the presence of steatorrhea was not uniform. Such difficulties emphasize the limitations of duodenal culture as a reliable test to diagnose SIBO. In practice, the location of small bowel fluid recovery is highly variable among practitioners and for practical ease, the duodenum is often sampled applying the standard definition of $>10^5$ CFU/mL to diagnose SIBO. Obtaining samples for culture relies upon upper endoscopy and while this is a fairly straightforward and safe procedure, there are multiple potential technical problems that can reduce the reliability of the aspiration and culture-based approach. These include: contamination of the endoscope and aspiration catheter by upper GI tract and oropharyngeal organisms, location of sampling, and difficulty of aspirating samples through the catheter. Further, reproducibility of the sampling procedures (reported to be as low as 38%), reproducibility and yield of bacterial cultures, and lack of definition regarding *which* bacterial organisms correlate with specific symptoms and complications of SIBO are additional major limitations and criticisms of this approach. A recent review of diagnostic tests used to diagnose SIBO found that the utilization of culture-based approaches varied widely and many studies did not specify a gold standard (i.e., culture of $>10^5$ organisms from small bowel aspirates) in their diagnosis of SIBO [35]. Finally, a major issue in applying the culture-based approach is the lack of validation with normal controls—what truly describes normal?

Alternative and less invasive techniques are therefore commonly applied and breath testing has become a favored approach to diagnose SIBO. Breath tests are performed based upon the production of hydrogen gas from bacteria following carbohydrate fermentation. Theoretically, an increase in lumenal bacteria can be directly correlated with their increased capacity to digest and ferment ingested dietary carbohydrates resulting in increased hydrogen gas ($H_2$) production within the intestinal lumen. Exhaled $H_2$, the by-product of bacterial metabolism, is safely and easily recovered and measured from individuals at baseline or following ingestion of a defined amount of carbohydrate (glucose, lactose, lactulose, xylose).

There are drawbacks with the application of breath tests in the diagnosis of SIBO. Slow or rapid intestinal transit (often a problem in patients with short gut syndrome, diabetes, and intestinal pseudo-obstruction) may impede test result accuracy. In addition, 15–25% of the general population harbor bacteria that preferentially produce methane and thus the application of breath tests that rely on the production of hydrogen and not methane gas (lactulose) will underestimate the activity of bacteria in a subset of patients. There are wide variations in the sensitivity and specificity of these tests when compared to the gold standard of aspirate and culture and validation against this standard has not been confirmed with most breath tests [36,37]. Nonetheless, the ease and inexpensive nature of breath tests has led to their common and widespread use to diagnose and monitor the response therapy of SIBO.

The glucose breath test has been most widely used and has been applied in most situations of SIBO. Glucose is mostly absorbed in the proximal intestine and the test is simple and inexpensive. Fasting breath hydrogen levels of $>20$ ppm or an increase from the baseline fasting hydrogen level to values $\geq 12$ ppm following ingestion of 50 g of glucose is considered abnormal [38]. This test may be less accurate in patients with liver cirrhosis [39] and false positives occur due to rapid intestinal transit when substrate is delivered to the colon where it is metabolized by colonic flora.

The xylose breath test is another favored test. Unlike the glucose breath test, which measures hydrogen produced by bacteria, this test measures radio-labeled carbon dioxide ($^{14}$C-D-xylose) or the stable compound ($^{13}$C-D-xylose). $^{14}CO_2/^{13}CO_2$ is released following fermentation of the substrate xylose by Gram-negative bacteria in the small intestine and exhaled. Initial reports using this technique seemed to indicate improved sensitivity and specificity when compared to the glucose hydrogen breath test although reported sensitivity and specificity have ranged from 42% to 100% and 40% to 100%, respectively [37]. This $^{14}$C-D-xylose test is not advocated for use in pregnant women or children due to the use of a radioactive substrate and instead the $^{13}$C-D-xylose can be utilized [40].

Application of other noninvasive tests with high sensitivity would be attractive for the diagnosis of SIBO. The urine indican test was one such initially promising test. Indican is a by-product of tryptophan metabolism by bacteria and therefore could be used as a surrogate marker for bacterial colonization of the intestine [41,42]. Unfortunately, the test suffers from the same drawbacks as all tests measuring bacterial by-products in patients with rapid GI tract transit. The synthesis of indican from tryptophan may occur within the colon after rapid transit of unabsorbed substrate through the small intestine. Hence, the indican test has been relatively unreliable in its ability to diagnose SIBO and it has not been properly validated against the gold standard, and therefore it is not widely used.

In the absence of aspirate culture or breath tests, many clinicians diagnose SIBO clinically and thus choose to treat the condition empirically using a therapeutic trial of antibiotics shown to effectively treat the condition. If symptoms diminish and/or diagnostic tests normalize, then the diagnosis is made. This approach has become increasingly common for the treatment of irritable bowel syndrome (IBS) and in conditions where SIBO is known to occur with increased prevalence.

A final comment on the correlation between tissue biopsy specimens and SIBO also deserves mention. Intestinal inflammation has been noted in children with intestinal failure and is associated with failure to wean from TPN [28] and a few studies have demonstrated increased intra-epithelial lymphocytes (IEL) in patients with SIBO [31,43]. However this latter finding is neither sensitive nor specific for SIBO. There have been no rigorous studies performed to date to demonstrate that specific histologic changes in the intestinal mucosa are directly caused by the dysbiosis associated with SIBO.

## 24.5    TREATMENT OF SIBO

### 24.5.1    ANTIBIOTICS

#### 24.5.1.1    Indications

Antibiotic therapy for SIBO should be predicated upon eradicating a specific symptom or undesirable consequence of bacterial overgrowth. It is virtually impossible to differentiate the symptoms caused by the SIBO syndrome from those caused by intestinal failure itself, but several clues can prompt the astute clinician to initiate therapy aimed as SIBO. In the early phase following a resection, small intestinal transit is rapid, and the bowel caliber remains normal. Therefore, it is unlikely that excessive numbers of bacteria are either contaminating the proximal bowel or contributing to symptoms. However, months to years after a resection, when the small intestine is dilated and transit has slowed or other risk factors for SIBO exist, an antibiotic course may be warranted. A therapeutic trial is therefore appropriate, and if symptoms improve, SIBO syndrome may be inferred. If symptoms do not improve, the underlying intestinal failure symptoms may be at play.

Treatment of SIBO syndrome is warranted for reasons beyond treating malabsorption, flatulence, and diarrhea. If a patient has neurological symptoms and evidence of a D-lactate-induced metabolic acidosis with an anion gap, or if the patient experiences an elevated serum ammonia level or elevated blood ethanol level, antibiotics can be given until these toxic metabolites disappear from the serum.

It is virtually impossible to permanently eradicate the organisms responsible for SIBO, so the goal of therapy should be to reduce the small intestinal load of offending bacteria and/or to reduce the circulating levels of toxins produced by those bacteria.

Finally, treatment of SIBO is justified in the absence of SIBO syndrome if the patient has evidence of bacterial translocation and repeated blood stream infections with enteric organisms. The concept of bacterial translocation from intestinal lumen to blood stream is somewhat controversial in humans, but it has been shown in animal models of short bowel syndrome [44]. Indirect evidence of the occurrence of translocation in humans is derived from the fact that blood stream infections in patients with intestinal failure frequently arise from organisms present in their intestinal lumen. It is possible that direct contamination of central line hubs can occur following contact with feces, but

**TABLE 24.4**

**Treatment of SIBO**

Antibiotics

    Amoxicillin/clavulanic acid

    Metronidazole

    Nitazoxanide

    Tobramycin

    Colistimethate

    Ciprofloxacin

    Tetracycline

    Rifaximin

Surgical (correction of anatomic defect; intestinal tapering or lengthening; transplantation)

Correction of nutritional deficiencies (TPN, parenteral nutrition (PN), fat-soluble vitamins, vitamin B12, zinc)

Prokinetics (erythromycin, metaclopramide, cisapride, amoxicillin/clavulanic acid, octreotide)

Probiotics

Prebiotics

the presence of infections with enteric organisms despite meticulous line care suggests that translocation from lumen to blood does occur in humans.

Complete eradication of the enteric flora is an unattainable goal. Instead, the goal should be eradication of symptoms while concomitantly reducing the absolute number of offending organisms populating the upper GI tract (Table 24.4).

### 24.5.1.2 Types of Antibiotics

When the goal is to improve energy balance or to rid the patient of a toxic bacterial metabolite, the ideal antibiotic should target anaerobes. In order to minimize selection of resistant bacterial species, an antibiotic with a limited aerobic spectrum is probably preferable to a broad-spectrum antibiotic. Therefore, metronidazole is chosen by many clinicians treating the SIBO syndrome. This agent can be quite effective, but can produce unwanted side effects. It may alter the metabolism of other drugs such as calcineurin inhibitors or anticonvulsants. It may produce both central nervous system abnormalities such as headaches or seizures and peripheral neuropathy resulting in paresthesias. It may also produce a disulfiram-like effect if taken with ethanol. For some of the above reasons, prescribing it in 7–14-day cycles followed by 14–21-day off periods may be preferable to giving it continuously.

For those patients unable to take metronidazole, nitazoxanide has a similar *in vitro* antimicrobial spectrum. No large studies of efficacy for SIBO have been conducted, but it theoretically should be just as effective as is metronidazole. The safety profile is excellent as well.

Adults with SIBO and irritable bowel symptoms have been successfully treated with rifaximin [16]. A nonabsorbable analog of rifampin, rifaximin possesses several theoretical advantages. As a nonabsorbable antibiotic, it affects only the flora of the GI tract without affecting the flora of the nasopharynx, urogenital tract, or skin. Hence, patients are less likely to suffer from fungal infections and other side effects. In addition, while it possesses a broad aerobic and anaerobic spectrum, it is bacteriostatic rather than bacteriocidal. Therefore, it probably does not affect bacterial sensitivities—even if given continuously for a long period of time.

Another broad-spectrum antibiotic which possesses two theoretical advantages is amoxicillin/clavulanic acid [45]. This agent is cidal for about 90% of aerobic and anaerobic species that populate the GI tract. It also has prokinetic properties that might theoretically enhance intestinal motility. Its disadvantage is that with continuous, long-term use, it could theoretically select multidrug-resistant bacterial strains. Furthermore, many individuals on amoxicillin/clavulanic acids experience dyspepsia and/or diarrhea as significant side effects.

Tetracycline should be mentioned primarily for historic interest. When the SIBO syndrome was first described during the middle of the twentieth century, the antibacterial spectrum of tetracycline lent itself satisfactorily for the treatment of this disorder. However, more recent trials suggest that it is relatively ineffective because of the changing bacterial-resistance patterns [46].

The strategy of "selective decontamination" to minimize blood stream infections is far from universal acceptance. Indeed, there are no published studies of efficacy for patients with short bowel syndrome. However, the literature does suggest that it reduces the frequency of bloodstream infections among patients who have undergone liver transplantation [47]. If it is chosen as a therapy, the goal should be to reduce the numbers of Gram-negative aerobic bacteria and *Enterococci* which translocate readily in animal models while preserving Gram-positive anaerobic bacteria which seldom if ever translocate. Therefore, antibiotics with broad anticoliform and anti-Enterococcal profiles are ideal. Ciprofloxacin would appear to be better suited for selective decontamination than for treatment of SIBO syndrome because it is excellent for coliform and for *Enterococcus* coverage while possessing a relatively limited anaerobic spectrum with significant activity only against *Clostridium perfringens* and *Propionibacterium acnes*. However, ciprofloxacin has been associated with headache, irritability, somnolence, or dizziness. In addition, significant drug interactions may occur. Rhabdomyolysis and spontaneous tendon rupture are uncommon but have adverse events.

In order to minimize disruption of the systemic ecology while altering the GI ecology, a nonabsorbable antibiotic cocktail is frequently utilized for decontamination. A typical cocktail would include colistimethate, tobramycin, and either mycostatin or amphotericin B [48].

Another strategy designed to minimize the risk of selecting multidrug-resistant organisms is the cycling of 7–14-day courses of antibiotics with 14–21-day off periods as opposed to continuous treatment with antibiotics.

### 24.5.2   Probiotics and Prebiotics

Current evidence from studies performed in normal hosts suggests that the antibiotic-induced alterations of the GI flora is temporary and the composition of flora eventually returns to baseline. As discussed, antibiotics can effectively manage SIBO. An alternative strategy to utilizing antibiotics would alter the overall composition of the flora by introducing specific nonpathogenic bacteria that counteract the effects of imbalance in the GI microbial flora. Selecting specific species of bacteria with beneficial properties may thus result in a similar treatment effect without the inherent side effects of antibiotics, which with repeated use, enhance the risk for selecting antibiotic-resistant bacteria.

Probiotics are defined as "live organisms when ingested in adequate amounts confer health benefit to the host." These are nonpathogenic bacterial species cultivated from the normal human intestinal tract and have been used for centuries in food production and as food supplements. Common and commercially used probiotics include the *Lactobacillus*, *Bifidobacteria*, and *Saccharomyces* (a nonpathogenic yeast) species. To date, the selective use of probiotics to treat SIBO has not been adequately studied or established and very limited data exist. Vanderhoof et al. [49] demonstrated that *Lactobacillus plantarum299v* may delay or prevent symptom recurrence in children with short bowel syndrome and recurrent difficult to manage SIBO following antibiotic therapy. Other strains that have been tried and with variable results include: *L. casei, L. acidophilus, Bifidobacterium breve*, and *S. boulardii* [50–52]. Probiotics may also confer specific benefit on certain symptoms and complications of SIBO as they have been shown to enhance intestinal motility and may also help to improve vitamin and mineral absorption [53].

An alternative to ingesting live nonpathogenic bacteria is to enhance the growth of these desirable species within the host's natural flora. Prebiotics are defined as nondigestible fermentable foodstuffs that are beneficial to the host by selectively stimulating the growth of bacteria in the intestine, especially the growth of beneficial bacteria. Prebiotics have been shown to stimulate the growth of probiotic species of *Bifidobacteria* and *Lactobacillus* [54] and are not absorbed in the small intestine but are fermented by bacteria in the colon. Examples of prebiotics include oligosaccharides found in human breast milk, inulin-type fructans, and fructo-oligosaccharides. The use of prebiotics in the treatment of SIBO, while theoretically feasible to stimulate the growth of desirable bacteria in the intestine, is not at all established and has not been evaluated in clinical trials.

The topic of probiotics and prebiotics in intestinal failure is more fully considered in Chapter 28.

### 24.5.3 MOTILITY MEDICATIONS

One of the physiologic responses to the human small intestine is the phenomenon of "adaptation" following a significant resection. One mechanism of improving the absorptive capacity of the GI tract is by an increase in surface area. Two means by which the surface area increases are by the elongation of villi and increase in bowel diameter. Because the bowel diameter study follows La Place's law, as its diameter increases, the peristaltic contractile force decreases, thereby increasing small intestinal transit time. If transit is so disrupted that motility is impaired SIBO will be fostered. For this reason, prokinetic agents are utilized in an attempt to restore satisfactory motility and housekeeping.

Few data are available favoring the use of prokinetic agents in short bowel syndrome associated with abnormally slow motility. In one study, octreotide seemed to provide benefit to patients with bacterial overgrowth associated with scleroderma [55]. However, subsequent studies have failed to duplicate these results, and while octreotide induces migrating myoelectric complexes, it appears to lengthen small bowel transit rather than shortening it [56]. Hence, it may be more effective in the treatment of rapid transit than the treatment of slow transit.

Other agents commonly in use include amoxicillin/clavulanic acid, metoclopramide, and erythromycin. Cisapride and tegaserod have also been utilized by some clinicians for this off label indication, but both of these agents have been removed from the market and are only available for compassionate use by the food and drug administration following investigational review board approval.

Amoxicillin/clavulanic acid has not only antibacterial but also prokinetic properties. It appears to increase that amplitude and duration of propagated small intestinal contractions during the fasting state. Its mechanism is unknown, but it may have a motilin-like effect or it may competitively inhibit gamma aminobutyric acid in either the central nervous system or the myenteric plexus [45].

Erythromycin clearly has a motilin-like effect, and it enhances small intestinal motility in both the fed and fasting state [57]. At low dose (1–2 mg/kg/dose), it enhances gastric emptying as well as small bowel motility, but when the dose is increased, the amplitude of antral contraction may be enhanced enough to paradoxically produce antral spasm and vomiting. Tachyphylaxis occurs quite commonly necessitating frequent drug "holidays" for the drug to regain effectiveness [58].

Metoclopramide functions by both a central nervous system effect and an enteric nervous system effect. In the central nervous system, it antagonizes dopamine by binding to dopaminergic receptors. Peripherally, it augments acetylcholine release by presynaptic neurons and inhibits 5-hydroxytryptamine release, thereby accelerating esophageal clearance, gastric emptying, and small bowel motility [59]. Dystonic reactions occur quite frequently. Indeed, the occasional association of tardive dyskinesia (characterized by involuntary repetitive movements) with the use of metoclopramide, has mandated a "black box" warning on the package insert highlighting the risk of this complication which may persist indefinitely, even after withdrawal of the drug. Additionally, metoclopramide can be associated with excessive somnolence in older individuals or excessive irritability in infants. As with erythromycin, tachyphylaxis may also limit long-term usage and may require periodic drug holidays.

## 24.6   NEW DIRECTIONS IN THE DIAGNOSIS OF SIBO

Interest in analyzing the microbial community of the human intestine has increased significantly in the last decade. Sequencing of bacterial 16srRNA genes has determined that >500 different species of bacteria exist in the human intestine with densities reaching $10^{12}$–$10^{14}$ CFU/mL in the colon of a normal host [26]. Since >85% of *all* of the bacteria in the intestine are not cultivated by traditional culture techniques [60] research of the complex microbial community in the human intestine utilizes sensitive metagenomic techniques of sequence analysis to describe this dense intestinal community. These techniques have discovered bacterial and yeast species in the intestine that were previously unknown, and have yet to be characterized, due to reliance on culture-based techniques [61,62].

Sequencing of the 16S rRNA genes from human fecal samples has demonstrated that populations of bacteria differ between normal individuals and among groups of individuals diagnosed with various diseases. Thus, patients with Crohn's disease harbor bacterial populations distinct from those of patients with another form of IBD, ulcerative colitis, *and* from normal individuals without known GI disease [63,64]. Infants born by cesarean section also harbor a distinct colonizing flora that contains more pathogenic bacteria as compared to infants born vaginally [65]. Finally, short-term use of antibiotics was shown to significantly and temporarily alter the intestinal microbial community in adults and in infants [66].

These exciting advances utilizing rapid high-throughput analysis of the complex intestinal flora may lead to the development and application of microarray or chip-based diagnostic tests that can be routinely applied in the clinical setting to diagnose specific disease entities in which bacterial dysbiosis is known to contribute to pathogenesis. As one example, Flanagan et al. [67] applied the Phylochip to monitor the endotracheal secretions of ICU patients. The Phylochip is a microarray that contains sequence tags for hundreds of bacteria and can identify a heterogeneous microbial community to the species level. The chip was used to demonstrate that the normally sterile lung, is rapidly colonized following intubation, and that antibiotics cause a marked reduction in the microbial diversity of the colonizing community that facilitates the outgrowth of pathogenic bacterial species. Interestingly, in all patients, *Pseudomonas aeruginosa* was isolated as the dominant bacterial species in the lung environment following antibiotic treatment. This highly sensitive yet broadly selective approach of microarray analysis could also be applied to better define the specific microbial imbalances that occur in SIBO, to correlate the presence of bacterial species with symptoms, and to refine and monitor response to therapy.

## REFERENCES

1. Donaldson RM, Jr. Normal bacterial populations of the intestine and their relation to intestinal function. *N Engl J Med.* 1964;270:1050–6 CONCL.
2. Petersen C. D-lactic acidosis. *Nutr Clin Pract.* 2005;20:634–45.
3. Shah SM, Roberts PJ, Watson CJ et al. Relapsing encephalopathy following small bowel transplantation. *Transplant Proc.* 2003;35:1565–6.
4. Spinucci G, Guidetti M, Lanzoni E, Pironi L. Endogenous ethanol production in a patient with chronic intestinal pseudo-obstruction and small intestinal bacterial overgrowth. *Eur J Gastroenterol Hepatol.* 2006;18:799–802.
5. Dibaise JK, Young RJ, Vanderhoof JA. Enteric microbial flora, bacterial overgrowth, and short-bowel syndrome. *Clin Gastroenterol Hepatol.* 2006;4:11–20.
6. Di Stefano M, Miceli E, Missanelli A, Mazzocchi S, Corazza, G.R. Absorbable vs. non-absorbable antibiotics in the treatment of small intestine bacterial overgrowth in patients with blind-loop syndrome. *Aliment Pharmacol Ther.* 2005;21:985–92.
7. Farivar S, Fromm H, Schindler D, Schmidt FW. Sensitivity of bile acid breath test in the diagnosis of bacterial overgrowth in the small intestine with and without the stagnant (blind) loop syndrome. *Dig Dis Sci.* 1979;24:33–40.
8. Swan RW. Stagnant loop syndrome resulting from small-bowel irradiation injury and intestinal by-pass. *Gynecol Oncol.* 1974;2:441–5.

9. Husebye E. Gastrointestinal motility disorders and bacterial overgrowth. *J Intern Med.* 1995;237:419–27.

10. Parodi A, Sessarego M, Greco A et al. Small intestinal bacterial overgrowth in patients suffering from scleroderma: Clinical effectiveness of its eradication. *Am J Gastroenterol.* 2008;103:1257–62.

11. Castiglione F, Del Vecchio Blanco G, Rispo A et al. Orocecal transit time and bacterial overgrowth in patients with Crohn's disease. *J Clin Gastroenterol.* 2000;31:63–6.

12. Van Felius ID, Akkermans LM, Bosscha K et al. Interdigestive small bowel motility and duodenal bacterial overgrowth in experimental acute pancreatitis. *Neurogastroenterol Motil.* 2003;15:267–76.

13. Morencos FC, de las Heras Castano G, Martin Ramos L, Lopez Arias MJ, Ledesma F, Pons Romero F. Small bowel bacterial overgrowth in patients with alcoholic cirrhosis. *Dig Dis Sci.* 1995;40:1252–6.

14. Bauer TM, Steinbruckner B, Brinkmann FE et al. Small intestinal bacterial overgrowth in patients with cirrhosis: Prevalence and relation with spontaneous bacterial peritonitis. *Am J Gastroenterol.* 2001;96:2962–7.

15. Wigg AJ, Roberts-Thomson IC, Dymock RB, McCarthy PJ, Grose RH, Cummins AG. The role of small intestinal bacterial overgrowth, intestinal permeability, endotoxaemia, and tumour necrosis factor alpha in the pathogenesis of non-alcoholic steatohepatitis. *Gut.* 2001;48:206–11.

16. Pimentel M, Chow EJ, Lin HC. Eradication of small intestinal bacterial overgrowth reduces symptoms of irritable bowel syndrome. *Am J Gastroenterol.* 2000;95:3503–6.

17. Pimentel M, Soffer EE, Chow EJ, Kong Y, Lin HC. Lower frequency of MMC is found in IBS subjects with abnormal lactulose breath test, suggesting bacterial overgrowth. *Dig Dis Sci.* 2002;47:2639–43.

18. Kurtovic J, Segal I, Riordan SM. Culture-proven small intestinal bacterial overgrowth as a cause of irritable bowel syndrome: Response to lactulose but not broad spectrum antibiotics. *J Gastroenterol.* 2005;40:767–8.

19. Vantrappen G, Janssens J, Hellemans J, Ghoos Y. The interdigestive motor complex of normal subjects and patients with bacterial overgrowth of the small intestine. *J Clin Invest.* 1977;59:1158–66.

20. Husebye E, Hellstrom PM, Sundler F, Chen J, Midtvedt T. Influence of microbial species on small intestinal myoelectric activity and transit in germ-free rats. *Am J Physiol Gastrointest Liver Physiol.* 2001;280:G368–80.

21. Nieuwenhuijs VB, Verheem A, van Duijvenbode-Beumer H et al. The role of interdigestive small bowel motility in the regulation of gut microflora, bacterial overgrowth, and bacterial translocation in rats. *Ann Surg.* 1998;228:188–93.

22. Gray JD, Shiner M. Influence of gastric pH on gastric and jejunal flora. *Gut.* 1967;8:574–81.

23. Spiegel BM, Chey WD, Chang L. Bacterial overgrowth and irritable bowel syndrome: Unifying hypothesis or a spurious consequence of proton pump inhibitors?. *Am J Gastroenterol.* 2008;103:2972–6.

24. Bhat P, Albert MJ, Rajan D, Ponniah J, Mathan VI, Baker SJ. Bacterial flora of the jejunum: A comparison of luminal aspirate and mucosal biopsy. *J Med Microbiol.* 1980;13:247–56.

25. Hayashi H, Takahashi R, Nishi T, Sakamoto M, Benno Y. Molecular analysis of jejunal, ileal, caecal and recto-sigmoidal human colonic microbiota using 16S rRNA gene libraries and terminal restriction fragment length polymorphism. *J Med Microbiol.* 2005;54:1093–101.

26. O'Hara AM, Shanahan F. The gut flora as a forgotten organ. *EMBO Rep.* 2006;7:688–93.

27. Hoverstad T, Bjorneklett A, Fausa O, Midtvedt T. Short-chain fatty acids in the small-bowel bacterial overgrowth syndrome. *Scand J Gastroenterol.* 1985;20:492–9.

28. Kaufman SS, Loseke CA, Lupo JV et al. Influence of bacterial overgrowth and intestinal inflammation on duration of parenteral nutrition in children with short bowel syndrome. *J Pediatr.* 1997;131:356–61.

29. Uribarri J, Oh MS, Carroll HJ. D-Lactic acidosis. A review of clinical presentation, biochemical features, and pathophysiologic mechanisms. *Medicine (Baltimore).* 1998;77:73–82.

30. Deitch EA, Xu DZ, Qi L, Berg RD. Bacterial translocation from the gut impairs systemic immunity. *Surgery.* 1991;109:269–76.

31. Riordan SM, McIver CJ, Wakefield D, Duncombe VM, Thomas MC, Bolin TD. Small intestinal mucosal immunity and morphometry in luminal overgrowth of indigenous gut flora. *Am J Gastroenterol.* 2001;96:494–500.

32. Riordan SM, McIver CJ, Wakefield D, Thomas MC, Duncombe VM, Bolin TD. Serum immunoglobulin and soluble IL-2 receptor levels in small intestinal overgrowth with indigenous gut flora. *Dig Dis Sci.* 1999;44:939–44.

33. Berg RD, Garlington AW. Translocation of certain indigenous bacteria from the gastrointestinal tract to the mesenteric lymph nodes and other organs in a gnotobiotic mouse model. *Infect Immun.* 1979;23:403–11.

34. Berg RD, Wommack E, Deitch EA. Immunosuppression and intestinal bacterial overgrowth synergistically promote bacterial translocation. *Arch Surg.* 1988;123:1359–64.

35. Khoshini R, Dai SC, Lezcano S, Pimentel M. A systematic review of diagnostic tests for small intestinal bacterial overgrowth. *Dig Dis Sci.* 2008;53:1443–54.
36. Corazza GR, Menozzi MG, Strocchi A et al. The diagnosis of small bowel bacterial overgrowth. Reliability of jejunal culture and inadequacy of breath hydrogen testing. *Gastroenterology.* 1990;98:302–9.
37. Rana SV, Bhardwaj SB. Small intestinal bacterial overgrowth. *Scand J Gastroenterol.* 2008;43:1030–7.
38. Kerlin P, Wong L. Breath hydrogen testing in bacterial overgrowth of the small intestine. *Gastroenterology.* 1988;95:982–8.
39. Bauer TM, Schwacha H, Steinbruckner B et al. Diagnosis of small intestinal bacterial overgrowth in patients with cirrhosis of the liver: Poor performance of the glucose breath hydrogen test. *J Hepatol.* 2000;33:382–6.
40. Dellert SF, Nowicki MJ, Farrell MK, Delente J, Heubi JE. The $^{13}$C-xylose breath test for the diagnosis of small bowel bacterial overgrowth in children. *J Pediatr Gastroenterol Nutr.* 1997;25:153–8.
41. Mayer PJ, Beeken WL. The role of urinary indican as a predictor of bacterial colonization in the human jejunum. *Am J Dig Dis.* 1975;20:1003–9.
42. Tohyama K, Kobayashi Y, Kan T, Yazawa K, Terashima T, Mutai M. Effect of lactobacilli on urinary indican excretion in gnotobiotic rats and in man. *Microbiol Immunol.* 1981;25:101–12.
43. Kakar S, Nehra V, Murray JA, Dayharsh GA, Burgart LJ. Significance of intraepithelial lymphocytosis in small bowel biopsy samples with normal mucosal architecture. *Am J Gastroenterol.* 2003;98:2027–33.
44. Ford HR, Avanoglu A, Boechat PR et al. The microenvironment influences the pattern of bacterial translocation in formula-fed neonates. *J Pediatr Surg.* 1996;31:486–9.
45. Caron F, Ducrotte P, Lerebours E, Colin R, Humbert G, Denis P. Effects of amoxicillin-clavulanate combination on the motility of the small intestine in human beings. *Antimicrob Agents Chemother.* 1991;35:1085–8.
46. Di Stefano M, Strocchi A, Malservisi S, Veneto G, Ferrieri A, Corazza GR. Non-absorbable antibiotics for managing intestinal gas production and gas-related symptoms. *Aliment Pharmacol Ther.* 2000;14:1001–8.
47. Safdar N, Said A, Lucey MR. The role of selective digestive decontamination for reducing infection in patients undergoing liver transplantation: A systematic review and meta-analysis. *Liver Transpl.* 2004;10:817–27.
48. Schultz MJ, de Jonge E, Kesecioglu J. Selective decontamination of the digestive tract reduces mortality in critically ill patients. *Crit Care.* 2003;7:107–10.
49. Vanderhoof JA, Young RJ, Murray N, Kaufman SS. Treatment strategies for small bowel bacterial overgrowth in short bowel syndrome. *J Pediatr Gastroenterol Nutr.* 1998;27:155–60.
50. Gaon D, Garmendia C, Murrielo NO et al. Effect of *Lactobacillus* strains (*L. casei* and *L. acidophillus* strains *cerela*) on bacterial overgrowth-related chronic diarrhea. *Medicina (B Aires).* 2002;62:159–63.
51. Kanamori Y, Hashizume K, Sugiyama M, Morotomi M, Yuki N. Combination therapy with *Bifidobacterium breve, Lactobacillus casei,* and galactooligosaccharides dramatically improved the intestinal function in a girl with short bowel syndrome: A novel synbiotics therapy for intestinal failure. *Dig Dis Sci.* 2001;46:2010–6.
52. Uchida H, Yamamoto H, Kisaki Y, Fujino J, Ishimaru Y, Ikeda H. D-Lactic acidosis in short-bowel syndrome managed with antibiotics and probiotics. *J Pediatr Surg.* 2004;39:634–6.
53. Verdu EF. Probiotics effects on gastrointestinal function: Beyond the gut? *Neurogastroenterol Motil.* 2009;21:477–80.
54. Macfarlane S, Macfarlane GT, Cummings JH. Review article: Prebiotics in the gastrointestinal tract. *Aliment Pharmacol Ther.* 2006;24:701–14.
55. Soudah HC, Hasler WL, Owyang C. Effect of octreotide on intestinal motility and bacterial overgrowth in scleroderma. *N Engl J Med.* 1991;325:1461–7.
56. von der Ohe MR, Camilleri M, Thomforde GM, Klee GG. Differential regional effects of octreotide on human gastrointestinal motor function. *Gut.* 1995;36:743–8.
57. Peeters T, Matthijs G, Depoortere I, Cachet T, Hoogmartens J, Vantrappen G. Erythromycin is a motilin receptor agonist. *Am J Physiol.* 1989;257:G470–4.
58. Catnach SM, Fairclough PD. Erythromycin and the gut. *Gut.* 1992;33:397–401.
59. Kowalewski K, Kolodej A. Effect of metoclopramide on myoelectrical and mechanical activity of the isolated canine stomach perfused extracorporeally. *Pharmacology.* 1975;13:549–62.
60. Hugenholtz P, Goebel BM, Pace NR. Impact of culture-independent studies on the emerging phylogenetic view of bacterial diversity. *J Bacteriol.* 1998;180:4765–74.
61. Eisen JA. Environmental shotgun sequencing: Its potential and challenges for studying the hidden world of microbes. *PLoS Biol.* 2007;5:e82.

62. Eckburg PB, Bik EM, Bernstein CN et al. Diversity of the human intestinal microbial flora. *Science*. 2005;308:1635–8.

63. Frank DN, St Amand AL, Feldman RA, Boedeker EC, Harpaz N, Pace NR. Molecular-phylogenetic characterization of microbial community imbalances in human inflammatory bowel diseases. *Proc Natl Acad Sci U S A*. 2007;104:13780–5.

64. Bibiloni R, Mangold M, Madsen KL, Fedorak RN, Tannock GW. The bacteriology of biopsies differs between newly diagnosed, untreated, Crohn's disease and ulcerative colitis patients. *J Med Microbiol*. 2006;55:1141–9.

65. Palmer C, Bik EM, DiGiulio DB, Relman DA, Brown PO. Development of the human infant intestinal microbiota. *PLoS Biol*. 2007;5:e177.

66. Dethlefsen L, Huse S, Sogin ML, Relman DA. The pervasive effects of an antibiotic on the human gut microbiota, as revealed by deep 16S rRNA sequencing. *PLoS Biol*. 2008;6:e280.

67. Flanagan JL, Brodie EL, Weng L et al. Loss of bacterial diversity during antibiotic treatment of intubated patients colonized with Pseudomonas aeruginosa. *J Clin Microbiol*. 2007;45:1954–62.

# Part IV

Nursing Management

# 25 Ostomy Management

*Sandy Quigley and Ellen A. O'Donnell*

## CONTENTS

## 25.1 OVERVIEW

Short bowel syndrome (SBS) is a consequence of intestinal loss or resection [1] that frequently necessitates a surgically placed opening in the intestine for the drainage of luminal contents to the skin that is called an ostomy or stoma. A proximal intestinal ostomy may be present along with a distal portion of "defunctionalized" bowel that is not in continuity. If the defunctioned portion of the intestine is brought out to the skin it is termed a mucous fistula. The amount of time a patient has a stoma or stomas is dependent upon a series of factors including the underlying disease process, general physical condition, and extent of bowel adaptation. Intestinal function is generally improved by reanastomosis (reconnection) of the bowel [2].

Advances in stoma care have contributed to more rational use of ostomies and a wider acceptance of them by the medical and lay communities. Nonetheless treating a patient with an ostomy can be a daunting task, especially if there is a large amount of stomal output. Fluid loss may sometimes be ameliorated by "refeeding" ostomy effluent into a mucous fistula. This promotes nutrient absorption, electrolyte balance, adaptation of the distal bowel [3], and the enterohepatic circulation [4].

Patients who are school age or older, often have psychosocial concerns related to living with an ostomy. For example, the daily containment of 1–2 L of stomal output in a traditionally sized ostomy pouch requires constant emptying, odor management, peristomal skin protection, and vigilance regarding nighttime leaks. Families obtain information regarding ostomies from a multitude of internet sites that are at times confusing and may even be misleading, so providing accurate information and long-term guidance to patients with stomas is imperative. The encouragement of parents to treat their child with stomas as normally as possible and reinforcing the concept that the presence of an ostomy does not delay cognitive development is also important. Networking with other patients with similar disease processes, including patient support groups (see Chapters 36 and 38) may also facilitate a positive adjustment to living with an ostomy.

### 25.1.1  PRINCIPLES OF GASTROINTESTINAL OSTOMY MANAGEMENT

Successful adjustment to ostomy surgery begins during the preoperative phase and continues until changes in body image and function have been fully integrated. The first step is selection of a appropriate stoma site on the abdominal surface. With emergent surgery, the surgeon's priority is to bring out the ostomy in an area away from skin folds or incision lines. Ideally, the stoma should be placed away from the umbilical cord in newborns, and below the belt line in older patients. The underlying principle is to allow adequate surface area for the ostomy appliance to adhere. A poorly placed stoma can make ostomy pouching more difficult due to hip movement or an uneven peristomal skin surface. It should be noted that growth and change in body habitus may adversely affect even a well-positioned stoma.

### 25.1.2  GASTROINTESTINAL STOMA ASSESSMENT

Postoperative assessment of the stoma or stomas should include the following: anatomic level (i.e., small bowel vs. colon), mucosal appearance, degree of protrusion, position on the abdominal wall, and diameter. Clinicians should always review the operative report to determine the specific type of stoma constructed. Healthy stomas are normally moist, well perfused, and described as "beefy" red. Although the height of the stoma can range from flush with skin level to protruding, the ideal stoma should be at least slightly above skin level. A flush stoma or stoma that is below skin level can make it difficult to obtain a secure seal with the ostomy wafer. When the effluent empties at or below skin level, there is a tendency for it to leak underneath the wafer and onto the skin, resulting in skin irritation. Conversely, a stoma that has excessive height and protrudes is more vulnerable to trauma, as well as being aesthetically displeasing.

A transparent pouch allows visualization and assessment of bowel mucosal appearance and is preferred in the early postoperative period. Edema, giving the stoma a somewhat translucent appearance, is a common postoperative finding and may be accentuated by fluid overload. A light pink stoma may indicate anemia. Deep red, purple, or black ostomy tissue reflects ischemia and should prompt assessment by a physician.

Auscultation of bowel sounds and measurement of stool output is also a routine part of every nursing assessment. Return of bowel function after surgery is variable. Ileostomies usually begin to function within 2–5 days. Maintaining pouch adherence to the abdominal skin surface is critical for accurate output measurement. Stoma leakage and the resultant peristomal irritant contact dermatitis are the clinical manifestations the patient most often experiences if there is poor pouch adherence to the abdominal skin surface. Other postoperative complications that may occur include stomal prolapse (the intestine protruding like a proboscis), parastomal hernia, twisting of the stoma under the fascia (manifesting as bowel obstruction) and stomal stenosis that may either cause intermittent watery output or if complete no output whatsoever.

### 25.1.3  PERISTOMAL SKIN

Monitoring peristomal skin integrity is an important aspect of ostomy care. Optimally, it appears healthy and intact, with no difference between the peristomal skin and the adjacent skin surface. Despite meticulous pouch application technique, skin breakdown may still occur. It is often a result of mechanical trauma from improper removal of the pouch, chemical damage due to contact with irritating effluent, contact dermatitis caused by skin products (i.e., adhesive agents such as ostomy paste) or infectious dermatitis (e.g., fungal infection). Peristomal skin damage is evidenced by the presence of erythema, maceration, ulceration, or blister formation. Once the skin is denuded, pouch adhesion is difficult to achieve and this compounds skin breakdown. Appropriate selection of pouches, adhesive removers, skin sealants, and ostomy paste can minimize peristomal skin complications. Table 25.1 summarizes common peristomal skin problems and describes appropriate therapy. Stoma complications tend to occur less frequently than in the past because of improved surgical techniques and stoma care. However, these problems still arise and clinicians must be aware of them to facilitate patient education, formulate effective therapeutic plans, and where possible, initiate preventative measures (see Table 25.2).

### 25.1.4 SPECIAL CONSIDERATIONS: NEONATES

There are some characteristics unique to preterm infants' skin that must be taken into consideration when choosing products for the application of an ostomy pouch. The epidermal barrier is in the outer layer of the skin known as the stratum corneum. It forms *in utero* during the third trimester and increases in maturity rapidly with increasing gestational age. Premature infants have less developed epidermis, and more permeable skin [5]. They also have a higher ratio of body surface area to weight, allowing a relatively increased concentration of chemicals to be absorbed cutaneously. Therefore, it is important to minimize skin sealants, adhesive removers, and other products that contain alcohol in these infants.

Premature neonates also exhibit lower cohesion between the dermal–epidermal junction, leaving the epidermis relatively vulnerable to trauma. Epidermal stripping readily occurs with the removal of adhesives applied to premature skin, because they create a stronger bond with the epidermis than the epidermis has with the underlying dermis [6]. Minimizing the use of tape and adhesives will decrease the disruption of this fragile skin. Additionally, the use of nonalcohol sealants and pectin-backed barriers, as well as moistening wafers prior to their removal are helpful interventions to preserve the skin. All products in contact with the premature infant should be removed slowly while a second hand supports the underlying skin.

Modifying pouching techniques to minimize dislodgement may be necessary in neonates in order to obtain at least 24–48 h of "wear time." Placing cotton balls into the pouch to wick watery effluent helps prevent leakage under the wafer and loss of adhesion. A urology-type "spouted" pouch can be attached to a bedside drainage collection system and has the advantage of minimizing pouch weight. Spouted pouches also have an inner bag that serves as an antireflux mechanism allowing watery effluent to stay in the lower chamber of the pouch, decreasing the risk of leakage under the wafer.

## 25.2  OSTOMY POUCH SELECTION AND APPLICATION

The primary goal of an ostomy pouching system is to provide a means to efficiently collect effluent from a stoma, while protecting the surrounding skin. Furthermore, the pouch offers a means for an odor proof secure seal that will allow the wearer to lead a relatively normal lifestyle. In patients with SBS it is mandatory to have secure adherence of an ostomy pouch in order to facilitate accurate output measurements.

The components of a pouching system include a collection pouch and a skin barrier wafer. Pouches may be one piece, or two piece that attach together similar to a Tupperware seal or the recently introduced "sticky" adhesive mount. Most wafers base plates are manufactured using pectin or similar organic material and are available in a wide variety of sizes to accommodate a person's particular anatomy. The pouch selection will depend upon the patient's size, developmental attainment, activity level, and effluent volume/consistency. In general, fewer product options are available for younger patients.

## TABLE 25.1
## Peristomal Skin Damage and Therapeutic Interventions

**Irritant contact dermatitis:**

Peristomal irritant dermatitis is an inflammation of the skin resulting from contact with a chronic irritant, such as intestinal and urinary effluent, ostomy wafers, deodorants, or solvents. Erythematous and denuded skin may be the result of leakage or adhesive and solvent irritation. A skin level or retracted stoma will increase the risk that effluent will "undermine" an ostomy appliance and expose the skin to damage. Inappropriate technique in appliance care such as cutting the wafer aperture too small or too large and exposing peristomal skin to effluent, or a variety of topical products used in the pouch and on the skin can also lead to irritation.

In older patients, excessive perspiration or activity can also loosen the skin wafer.

**Interventions:**

Check that the aperture cut in ostomy wafer is appropriately sized to leave only minimal amount of skin visible around stoma. If epidermis is denuded, manage with aluminum acetate based astringent soaks (i.e., Domeboro®) that help to constrict blood vessels to promote healing.

Dilute 1 powder packet Domeboro in 8 oz. (240 mL) of tepid water and apply to affected area with gauze as "compress" for 10 min every day with pouch changes until skin heals. Then apply skin barrier powder and sealant as needed.

Finally, if the effluent is of watery consistency and leakage under the wafer persists, consider placing cotton balls in the pouch to "wick" stool away from stoma. Accurate output measurement can be obtained by weighing the cotton balls on a scale similarly used for wet diapers.

**Fungal rash:**

Fungal infection (e.g., *Candida*) may be caused by moisture around or under the stoma appliance or the use of systemic antibiotic therapy that alters the body flora. The clinical features include erythema and maceration of the skin, maculopapular rash with characteristic satellite lesions. However, presentation may be atypical in patients in whom erythema may be to appreciate. Dry skin usually limits the progression of the rash. Patients typically have pruritis in the affected area.

**Interventions:**

In addition to antifungal therapy, the treatment priority is keeping the skin dry. This includes the evaluation and resizing of the appliance opening to fit closely around the base of the stoma, the application of an antifungal powder sparingly to the affected area, and the use of a nonalcohol-based skin sealant such as No-Sting barrier (3M Smith and Nephew, Largo, FL) prior to applying the new ostomy appliance. Changing the pouch every 24–48 h may be indicated to reapply the antifungal powder and reevaluate the skin integrity based upon the severity of the infection.

**Mechanical trauma:**

Damage to the peristomal skin may result from inappropriate skin care (i.e., abrasive cleaning techniques), or incorrect tape removal that occurs if one pulls up on the wafer causing "tenting" of the skin with inadequate counter pressure to support the underlying skin. This is known as epidermal stripping and presents as patchy areas of erythema, or denuded skin under the ostomy wafer resulting in frequent pouch changes and further exacerbation of the problem.

**Interventions:**

Eliminate the cause by appropriate tape removal and proper cleansing techniques. Teach families and patients to limit the amount of adhesives used to secure the pouch and to remove the pouch by pushing down on the skin while gently pulling up the pouch wafer (a "push and pull" technique). Avoid the use of solvents for adhesive removal as much as possible to avoid chemical or irritant dermatitis. If these are used, the patient must completely rinse the area with plain water and small quantities of soap prior to reapplying new pouch.

Denuded areas usually require the use of a skin barrier powder with a skin sealant used over the powder to create an effective adhesive surface until the area is healed.

**Parastomal hernia:**

A parastomal hernia is a protrusion of the bowel or loops of intestine through the fascial opening into the subcutaneous tissue around the stoma. It presents as a bulge around the stoma in the immediate peristomal area. It may be difficult to maintain good pouch adherence to abdominal skin because the peristomal skin alternately stretches and relaxes with changes in positions. Surgical intervention is often required.

**Interventions:**

If a patient is asymptomatic they can be managed conservatively by applying a hernia support belt or binder that offers support for the parastomal hernia, decreases the protrusion. In neonates there are no such products presently available. Clinicians should monitor patients who presents with a hernia for constipation and ensure soft stools by making the appropriate dietary changes, maintaining adequate hydration, and considering a bulk laxative or stool softener.

## TABLE 25.1 (continued)
## Peristomal Skin Damage and Therapeutic Interventions

**Allergic dermatitis:**

An allergic reaction may also occur from product sensitivity. This presents as erythema and pruritis corresponding to an area of skin exposed to allergen. When multiple products are used, there is a chance that the interaction of these ingredients can increase the skin's sensitivity. The cutaneous manifestations can vary in severity from erythema and swelling to ulceration and bleeding that results in significant discomfort to the patient.

**Interventions:**

It may be necessary to do a patch or skin tests of the product(s) to determine the allergen and then avoid its use. Also consider patch testing with an alternative product on an unaffected area of body for at least 24 h. In older children, a topical corticosteroid agent (i.e., spray) may be needed to reduce the inflammation, pain, and itching. Resizing the pouch and changing it as soon as leakage occurs are other effective interventions.

## TABLE 25.2
## Stoma Complications and Therapeutic Interventions

**Stomal bleeding:**

A small amount of stomal bleeding from the capillaries at the mucosal surface is common and should be expected when cleaning the stoma. An improperly sized pouch opening (too small) may injure the mucosa and lead to bleeding. More major bleeding from the stoma can result from inadequate hemostasis during stoma construction, portal hypertension, trauma, underlying disease, and because of some medications, such as prolonged use of antiinflammatory drugs or anticoagulants.

**Interventions:**

If bleeding occurs, treatment is conservative and it is appropriate to apply firm pressure to the stoma with a cool compress. Superficial bleeding that does not stop spontaneously requires cauterization, suture placement, topical hemostatic agents (silver nitrate), or prolonged direct pressure. Frank bleeding presents as blood that runs down the abdominal wall and may come from a "pumping" artery deep to the mucocutaneous junction. Frank bleeding requires prompt surgical notification and maintaining hemodynamic stability.

**Necrosis:**

Stomal necrosis occurs when the blood flow to or from the stoma is impaired or interrupted. Evaluating stomal viability is particularly important during the early postoperative period when necrosis is most likely to occur. Stoma edema begins immediately postoperatively. The stoma looks swollen within 4–6 h, swelling progresses for the first few days, and then often subsides markedly. The stoma continues to decrease in edema (size) for the first 6–8 weeks after surgery. While edematous, the stomal mucosa is pale and translucent but the stomal tissue remains soft. Ischemia and necrosis may occur from excessive tension on the mesentery (or excessive stripping of the mesentery) compromising blood flow, or from interruption of blood supply to the stoma, such as from an embolus or a fascial closure that is too snug around the stoma. Stomal blood supply compromise presents as either ischemia (dark red, to purple), or frank necrosis (brown to black). The stoma may be flaccid or hard and dry. Necrosis may be circumferential or scattered and may be superficial or deep. Necrosis may be scattered or circumferential on the mucosa; the depth may be superficial or deep to the fascia.

**Interventions:**

Ongoing assessment of stoma viability during the edematous phase and sizing the opening of the faceplate are important to prevent stomal constriction and ischemia. The stoma measurement selected for the pouching system should allow for an opening 1/8-inch larger than the stoma size to prevent constriction that could impair stoma blood flow. The postoperative pouching system selected should be transparent or two piece. The two-piece system allows removal of the pouch to assess the stoma without disturbing the wafer.

Necrosis of the stoma should be promptly brought to the attention of the surgeon. Superficial necrosis may be managed expectantly while deep necrosis may require repeat laparotomy and further intestinal resection. Clinically, complications of limited necrosis may include stoma that is flush (skin level, retracted (below skin level)) or stenotic (narrowed). More rarely, a mucocutaneous separation may evolve. This latter problem may heal by secondary intention.

*continued*

**TABLE 25.2 (continued)**
**Stoma Complications and Therapeutic Interventions**

**Prolapse:**

The bowel telescopes out through the stoma. It occurs most frequently in the distal limb of loop stomas than in end stomas. The etiology of prolapse may be secondary to too large a diameter fascial opening during stomal construction, poorly developed fascial support due to weak abdominal musculature, increased abdominal pressure (i.e., coughing, excessive crying). Periodic episodes of abnormal bowel motility as are sometimes seen in children with chronic intestinal pseudo-obstruction and stomal prolapse is sometimes seen. The clinical presentation of a prolapse includes a stoma, that is, increased in size and height, edematous, and bleeds. In severe prolapse, stoma obstruction, and resultant ischemia may result.

**Interventions:**

When a prolapse first occurs, it must be evaluated by a surgeon to determine if there is a component of ischemia or obstruction, either of which requires bedside reduction or operative intervention.

After the initial assessment, the prolapsed stoma should be assessed regularly for perfusion, extent of protrusion (measured from abdominal surface to distal end) and function (i.e., are feedings well tolerated). Clinicians often manage mild to moderate prolapse expectantly as long as there is no ischemia or obstruction. There may be a need to modify the stomal opening in the wafer by cutting extra "snips" at 12, 3, 6, and 9 o'clock to accommodate the larger diameter of the edematous stoma base. Also manually reducing the prolapse and then applying a support binder or hernia support belt with a prolapse flap to hold the stoma in place may be indicated. The clinician reduces the prolapse by having the patient lie down to decrease the intra-abdominal pressure and continuously applies gentle pressure to the distal portion of the stoma returning the stoma to its intra-peritoneal place. If the bowel is edematous, applying a cold compresses or sugar (osmotic therapy) for 10–15 min before stoma reduction may be of benefit.

**Retraction:**

Retraction occurs when the stoma is drawn or pulled back below the skin level. It may also occur when the stoma is in a deep skin fold, resulting in a concave defect in the abdominal wall. It is often preceded by a necrotic stoma and/or mucocutaneous separation. Retraction presents clinically with all or part of the stoma located below skin level or with the surrounding skin pulled in due to the tension. The depth of retraction may increase with sitting. The degree or even presence of retraction can vary with peristalsis. It may cause management problems because of difficulty in obtaining and maintaining a good pouch seal.

**Interventions:**

Maintaining adequate pouch adherence is challenging because stool effluent may undermine the pouching system resulting in persistent leakage, shortened pouch wear time, and peristomal irritant dermatitis. Modifications to the pouching system may be necessary (i.e., use of flexible, one-piece pouches, and barrier pastes to fill any skin folds or indentations).

**Stenosis:**

Stenosis is a narrowing of the lumen of an ostomy and typically occurs at either the fascial or cutaneous (skin) level. Stenosis may present as a bowel obstruction, a decrease in stool output or sometimes an intermittent "explosion" of large quantities of intestinal content. Physician and nursing surveillance for the development of stomal stenosis particularly necessary in patients who have had stomal necrosis, significant weight gain, or a mucocutaneous separation.

**Interventions:**

The initial treatment is gentle digital or soft catheter dilation, but ultimately surgical revision may be indicated. The smallest gloved finger is lubricated and gently inserting into the stoma until the fascial opening is reached. The clinician slides the finger through the fascial opening, holds for 10 s without any twisting motion, removes the finger, and repeats the procedure. Dilators maybe used by a trained clinician or the certified ostomy nurse, although chronic dilations are controversial because they may be associated with further stomal stenosis.

## 25.3 POUCH OPTIONS

There are a wide variety of pouching options available. The two-piece system consists of a separate a wafer with a flange (plastic ring), and a compatible snap-on pouch. One desirable feature of this system is the ability to remove the pouch to examine the stoma without removing the adhesive wafer. Two-piece systems allow patients with high output the option of changing pouches, from an open tailed roll-up bottom to a urinary spouted drainable pouch that can be connected to a gravity drainage bag at night. This reduces pouch weight and minimizes nocturnal leakage. Another advantage of the two-piece pouch is that it can be removed without disturbing the skin barrier wafer. Most two-piece systems are semirigid due to the plastic flange and therefore perform best when there is a flat peristomal skin surface.

In a one-piece pouching system the pouch and the skin barrier wafer are sealed together and cannot be separated. The one-piece pouches have flexibility to mold into skin folds and uneven peristomal surfaces. A one-piece system also requires the fewest number of steps to assemble and apply. Clear or opaque one-piece systems are available. Clear pouches are preferable postoperatively allowing staff to visualize the stoma and pouch contents. They are also of benefit when ostomy care is being initially taught. Opaque pouches are more discreet and conceal the pouch contents. Many people prefer opaque pouches, especially after becoming accustomed to their stoma. Some pouches are manufactured with convexity that is good for flat or retracted stomas and facilitate a better wafer adherence by pressing into the tissue around the stoma, therefore increasing the degree of stomal protrusion. Effluent more readily can project into the pouch and reduces the risk of undermining the wafer adherence. Some pouches are available with integrated filters to vent gas build-up and also deodorize odors. Drainable pouches and pouch clips (many now be integrated into the pouch) are used to facilitate emptying without necessitating pouch removal.

A cut-to-fit wafer can be custom sized for patients who have irregularly shaped stomas, or newly created stomas that are typically edematous and will change contour and size in the first few weeks after surgery. Commercially available precut wafers are more suitable for patients with long-term ostomies where stoma swelling has diminished and stoma size remains constant. Most precut wafers are available with circular apertures and are therefore not conducive to oval, double barrel, or irregularly shaped stomas. This type of wafer provides the family and patient with ease of pouch changes as it eliminates a step in the pouch change process.

### 25.3.1   POUCH APPLICATION

The proper application of the pouch is another consideration that can influence adherence and decrease the risk of skin breakdown. The first few weeks postoperatively, the pouch should be changed at routinely scheduled intervals every 2–3 days to monitor for any leakage under the wafer and to examine the peristomal skin. Waiting to change the appliance only when leakage occurs does not maintain optimal peristomal and incisional skin integrity. Taping a leaking pouch to reinforce the seal only traps stool under the barrier, which leads to skin breakdown.

Pouches should last for several days and occasionally up to 5–7 days with an established stoma. Increased activity of the patient, more watery effluent, a flush or inverted stoma, and poor condition of the peristomal skin are all factors that adversely influence individual "wear" time. A scheduled routine pouch change during periods of reduced stoma activity is ideal. Organizing and keeping all supplies, along with written instructions, at the bedside or in one predetermined place at home will make the process of pouch care more routine.

### 25.3.2   APPLYING AN OSTOMY POUCH

The diameter of the patient's stoma is measured and an appropriate pattern made or selected. This is especially important for an irregularly shaped stoma. The internal diameter of the barrier should be a 16th to an 18th of an inch larger than the stoma [7]. The barrier should fit snugly but not so tightly that it constricts the stoma. Reevaluating pouch equipment as patient gains weight or if clinical condition changes resulting in ostomy edema or prolapse to avoid any trauma that may occur by the stoma rubbing against the wafer borders. This is particularly true for the plastic flange of the two-piece systems. With prolapsed stomas cutting a "notch" 1/8 or 1/4 of an inch at the 12, 3, 6, and 9 o'clock position of the wafer will allow for stoma movement in and out of the abdominal cavity.

Warming the skin barrier between the hands for 1–2 min softens the pectin and allows for better adherence to the skin. A barrier paste can be applied to the peristomal skin to fill in any irregular edges or creases to make a smooth pouching surface. Most preparations contain alcohol and burn when applied directly to irritated skin. The paste is sticky and sometimes difficult to control. Placing a small amount of paste into a syringe allows for a more precise application. If the epidermis is denuded, applying a thin layer of methylcellulose-based powder to nonintact skin then placing the barrier paste, will minimize the irritation and promote healing. Another strategy is to apply a pectin-based seal (Eakin Cohesive Seals, distributed by ConvaTec, Princeton, NJ) to the area where the epidermis is denuded then pouch over the Eakin seal. These pectin seals do not contain alcohol and are malleable. They can thus be molded, or stretched to any shape to accommodate peristomal skin irregularities. A moistened cotton-tipped applicator can help to shape the paste or the pectin seal around the stoma.

When applying the pouching system, the tail of the bag is directed in a downward position to facilitate emptying into the toilet for ambulatory patients. For infants, toddlers, and patients on bed-rest the tail of the pouch should be angled laterally off to the side and emptied into the diaper or a container. The pouch is emptied when it is one-third to one-half full to decrease the amount of weight the appliance must support. Measurement of the fullness of the pouch includes gas because that can pull the skin wafer away from the skin and cause the pouch to leak. Using one-piece tee shirts and outfits will help prevent inadvertent pouch removal by the curious hands of an infant or toddler.

## 25.4   POUCH EMPTYING

For patients on bedrest, empty the pouch into a basin or use a syringe. For ambulatory patients, sitting on the toilet and emptying the pouch between their legs may be the most convenient. Others prefer to stand and face the toilet while emptying. Lift the bottom of the pouch slightly while removing closure to avoid accidental spillage, then empty. Clean the tail end of the pouch with damp tissue or gauze to decrease odor and minimize staining of clothes. It is not recommended to clean the inside of the pouch by squirting water with a syringe because this often decreases adherence of the pectin wafer to the skin and results in leakage. It is more challenging to manage a high-output stoma. For example, daily containment of 2 L or more of fecal output in a traditionally sized ostomy pouch requires repeated emptying, odor management, peristomal skin protection, and drainage of nighttime stool while the patient sleeps [7].

## 25.5   POUCH REMOVAL

Gently remove pouch using both hands to release the adhesive side of wafer while pushing away the skin. Warm water and a soft cloth or gauze can be used to facilitate pouch removal. Adhesive removers are also helpful but are limited to use in full-term infants and patients with intact skin. The peristomal skin is inspected for breakdown and the stoma assessed for physical changes. The skin can be cleansed with mild soap and water and is dried thoroughly before the application of a new appliance. It is normal to have a small amount of bleeding from the stoma when an appliance is manipulated around the vascular stoma tissue. Persistent bleeding requires further evaluation (see Table 25.1).

## 25.6   POUCHING CHALLENGES

### 25.6.1   Poor "Wear Time" (<24 h)

Patients with retracted stomas, irregular peristomal contours, and soft or protuberant abdominal surfaces may require modifications in their pouching system. Careful observation (with the pouch off and in both supine and upright posture) of the stoma and the peristomal contors, as well as, the point and angle that the stoma spout empties will be helpful. Poor pouch wear time often results in skin compromise, but more importantly, inaccurate measurement of output can occur. In patients with short wear times due to frequent leakage clinicians should look for peristomal candidal rashes that may require treatment with an antifungal powder. When using this powder it will be necessary to seal it with a nonalcohol barrier protective wipe. If a barrier sealant is not utilized, the wafer will fail to adhere to the powder layer. One should consider discontinuing ostomy paste during treatment as they contain alcohol. An alternative is to replace the paste with a piece of pectin ring (Eakin Cohesive Seal or Hollister Adapt Barrier Rings) that can be molded around the stoma base and hence facilitates direct application of the pouch. Avoid using tincture of benzoin as it is unacceptably caustic.

### 25.6.2 SCARS, CREASES, AND FOLDS

These may result in leakage or poor adhesion due to an uneven abdominal surface. Fill in these irregularities with a Stomahesive paste to create an adequate seal. If wear time is still <24 h, adjust the amount of paste used.

### 25.6.3 LIFTING EDGES

Urine may undermine the outer borders of the wafer and cause lifting. This is generally more of an issue with boys than girls because the urinary stream is more likely to come in contact with the abdominal surface. Waterproofing the wafer borders with a transparent film dressing may increase wafer integrity.

### 25.6.4 GAS/INCREASED STOOL OUTPUT

The wear time of pouches may be adversely affected if the pouch fills with too much air. Increased gas production in babies and toddlers may be due to ingestion of air during periods of crying or feeding and/or increased stool transit time. In older children, and adults it may be due to chewing gum, air swallowing, or consuming carbonated beverages. Utilizing pouches with integrated air filters may obviate premature detachment from the skin.

Patients with a jejunostomy or ileostomy often have loose, liquid stool output. They are more likely to have issues with pouching related to high volume output that is acidic in nature. Therefore, it is important to monitor output carefully, and empty the pouch when it is 1/3 full to prevent the pouch from becoming too heavy and pulling away from the skin. If the patient is experiencing high output, it is important to monitor for dehydration through strict intake and output records, physical exam, and laboratory assessment. Strongly consider a urinary spouted pouch that can be attached to bedside gravity drainage bag.

## 25.7 PREPARING TO GO HOME

Adjusting to an ostomy is greatly enhanced if patients and/or their families feel confident and have mastered ostomy care. Ostomy teaching is therefore a critical component of nursing care. There is usually ample opportunity to teach patients and families self care because of the prolonged hospitalization that can accompany surgical and medical therapy for intestinal failure. Basic procedures that families and patients must master prior to discharge include pouch emptying and pouch change procedure. The caregivers should provide a list of necessary supplies including manufacturer product numbers and community durable medical equipment supply companies. To ensure a smooth transition to home, hospital case managers should contact local visiting nurse agencies to provide reinforcement and support. They also may wish to place the first supply request order. In some cases a letter of medical necessity and/or prescriptions are required. The older child may need assistance with ostomy care at school. Clinicians should proactively communicate with the school nurse, who is a valuable resource to ensure a smooth transition. Support and teaching can have an incredible impact on a patient's adaptation to life with an ostomy. Sample home care instructions are provided in the Appendix.

## APPENDIX*: HOME CARE INSTRUCTIONS FOR CHANGING AN OSTOMY POUCH (BAG OR APPLIANCE)

An ostomy is a surgically created opening in the intestine (bowel). This opening is also called a stoma. You/your child will be going home wearing an ostomy pouch. A pouch is put over the stoma to collect stool ("poop") or urine. Your nurse will teach you how to change your ostomy pouch, care for your stoma and tell you what supplies you will need. Be prepared and organize supplies before removing old pouch.

### SUPPLIES

**One-Piece System:** Pouch and wafer are made in one piece.
Pouch

OR

**Two-Piece System:** Pouch and wafer are separate. Each one has a plastic ring that "click" together, similar to closing a Tupperware® container.
Pouch

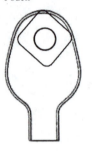

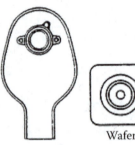

Wafer

**Pouch Clip**
(Not needed for urostomy pouch)

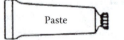

**Scissors**

**Towel or Gauze**

**Measuring Card and Pen**

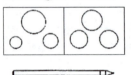

**Stomahesive Powder®:**
Used to dry and protect raw, wet open skin.

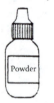

**Skin Barrier Wipes:**
Forms protective film on skin.

Skin barrier wipe

**Stomahesive Paste:**
Used like caulking to prevent leaking, for example: Whenever there is a watery stool ("poop"), to fill in bumpy, uneven skin surfaces so that there is a no gap between the skin and the wafer, or around flat, skin level stomas.

OR

**Eakin Seal:**
Donut shaped, sticky, gum-like material used to mold around the stoma if skin is red or open.

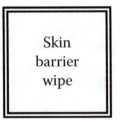

Paste

---

Adapted from teaching materials used at Children's Hospital Boston.

## INSTRUCTIONS

1. With one hand supporting the skin and the other hand lifting the wafer, gently remove the wafer from the skin. **Adhesive remover** pads may be helpful to lift wafer off of skin. **Many contain alcohol** and may be irritating to skin. Make sure to clean skin with soap and water to completely clean off skin.

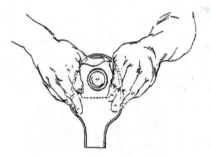

2. **Wash the skin around your stoma with warm water using a washcloth or soft** paper towel. A small amount of bleeding from the stoma is normal when washing the skin.
3. **Look at the stoma**. The color should be pink or red.

*Note:* **If the color is blue, purple, or black this may be considered a medical emergency; contact physician or surgeon.**

4. **Look at your skin around the stoma**.
   - **If there is no irritation,** wipe the skin around the stoma where the wafer will touch the skin with the barrier wipe. It leaves a protective layer on the skin. Skip to step 5.

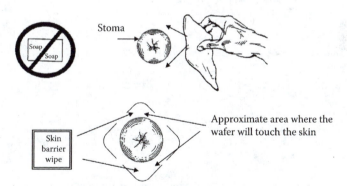

Stoma

Approximate area where the wafer will touch the skin

Skin barrier wipe

   - **If skin is raw, wet or open**, Sprinkle Stomahesive Powder™ only on the wet, open skin. This will help the skin heal.

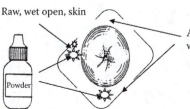

Raw, wet open, skin

Approximate area where the wafer will touch the skin

Powder

- **Then "lightly pat" the barrier wipe** over the powder to form a protective film and "seal" it. Also wipe the skin around the stoma where the wafer will touch the skin. Let the area dry for 1–2 min.

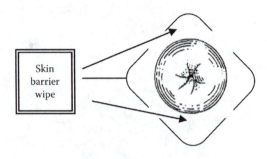

5. **Measure the stoma with the measuring card.** To do this, find the circle size on the card that fits closest to the stoma without touching it. The stoma may change size or shape during the first 3–4 weeks after surgery as the swelling goes down.

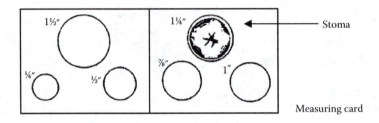

6. Trace the chosen circle onto the back of the paper on the wafer.
7. Cut the wafer to this circle size.

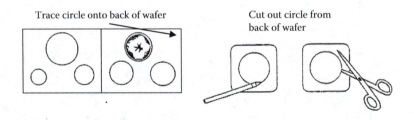

8. **If you have a *two-piece* system, attach the pouch to the plastic ring on the wafer.**

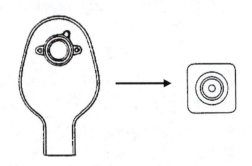

9. **Peel the paper off of the back of the wafer.**

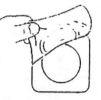

10. **Put stomahesive paste around the opening on the sticky side of the wafer.**
    - Squeeze stomahesive paste around the hole on the wafer, the same thickness that you would squeeze toothpaste onto a toothbrush.

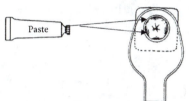

   - **If skin around the stoma becomes red or open**, you may need to stop using Stomahesive Paste and use an Eakin Seal a soft, flexible pectin ring. Mold the Eakin Seal on the skin around the stoma.

11. **Center the pouch around the stoma and place it onto the skin.** Firmly press the wafer to the skin near the stoma and hold for 3–4 min so that the wafer sticks to the skin. A warm facecloth held over stomas may also help wafer to adhere better to the skin.

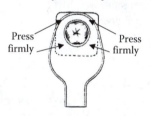

12. Place cotton balls (or absorbent gel packets, i.e., ParSorb at home) if using for watery stool in pouch to avoid it leaking under wafer.
13. Place pouch clip on the end of the pouch. Note: Some pouches have "Velcro-like" closure at bottom of pouch.
14. Wash your hands.

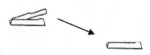

## WHEN SHOULD I EMPTY MY POUCH?

Empty your pouch when it is 1/3 full, at least 3–5 times a day. If a pouch gets too full, it gets heavy and may leak.

## WHEN SHOULD I CHANGE MY OSTOMY POUCH?

- If there is a leak under the wafer, or
- Every 2 to 4 days as instructed by your nurse

## What Supplies Are Needed At Home?

- There are a number of ostomy supply companies. Usually ostomy supplies can be delivered directly to your home.
- A nurse from Children's Hospital will contact one of these supply companies to order what you need. Which company is used usually depends on your health insurance plan.
- After the first delivery, you can contact the company directly for additional orders. Be sure to plan ahead so you do not run out of supplies.
- A nurse from Children's will arrange for a visiting nurse to come to your home. The visiting nurse will help you and answer any questions you may have.
- A follow-up visit with your/your child's doctor is very important. The nurse will help to schedule this before going home.
- Always carry an extra pouch with you in case the pouch needs to be removed during medical exam procedure or the pouch leaks.

## When To Call Your Doctor or Nurse?

Call if:
- any questions or concerns
- a fever higher than 101°F or "feeling very hot"
- vomiting
- sleepiness
- irritability
- bloated belly or abdominal (belly) pain
- very little or no stool from the stoma for more than 4 h,
- a large increase in the amount of stool from the stoma
- diarrhea that is foul-smelling or bloody
- inability to eat or drink
- any questions or concerns
- color of the stoma is blue, purple, or black
- rash, redness, or irritation of the skin around the stoma which does not improve in 2–3 days
- if you have bleeding from the stoma, firmly hold a cool, wet cloth over the area. If it does not stop in 5 min, call your doctor

## REFERENCES

1. Hwang S, Shulman R. Update on management and treatment of short gut. *Clin Perinatol.* 2002;29:181–194.
2. Kamin D, Goulet O. Intestinal failure, short bowel syndrome, and intestinal transplantation. In: Duggan C, Watkins J, Walker WA, editors. *Nutrition in Pediatrics*, 4th ed, pp. 641–662. Ontario: BC Decker, Inc., 2009.
3. Goday PS. Short bowel syndrome: How short is too short? *Clin Perinatol.* 2009;36:101–110.
4. Richardson L, Banerjee S, Rabe H. What is the evidence on the practice of mucous fistula refeeding in neonates with short bowel syndrome? *J Pediatr Gastroenterolo Nutr.* 2006;43(2):267–270.
6. Evans NJ, Rutter N. Development of the epidermis in the newborn. *Biol Neonate.* 1986;49:74–80.
7. Rogers V. Managing preemie stomas: More than just the pouch. *J WOCN.* 2003;30(2):100–110.

# 26 Central Venous Catheter Care

*Sara Gibbons and Denise S. Richardson*

## CONTENTS

## 26.1 OVERVIEW OF CENTRAL VENOUS CATHETERS

Patients diagnosed with short bowel syndrome (SBS) often require parenteral nutrition (PN) and hydration fluids for various periods of time. Often, particularly in the pediatric patient who has not obtained full growth, the shortened length of the gastrointestinal tract is insufficient to absorb enough nutrients to fully support growth and development. Adults with SBS may also require fluids by vein to maintain adequate hydration and/or meet caloric needs.

In order to ensure provision of adequate intravenous (IV) calories in the intestinal failure patient, a central venous catheter (CVC) must be placed such that hyperosmolar parenteral solutions can be administered safely. The catheter is inserted into the central venous system, generally the superior vena cava (SVC), via the external jugular, the internal jugular, or the subclavian vein. Sometimes, the femoral vein approach is used and the CVC is placed into the inferior vena cava (IVC). The SVC is desirable because the high blood flow allows rapid dilution of infusates and thus reduces the risk of phlebitis, thrombosis, and vessel-wall irritation. The different types of catheters and methods of insertion are discussed in greater detail in Chapter 12.

Briefly, three general types of CVCs are used: tunneled, non-tunneled (percutaneous), and totally implanted. The tunneled catheters (e.g., Broviac/Hickman/Leonard [C.R. Bard, Inc., Covington, GA]) and the implanted types are generally placed by a surgeon in the operating room under general anesthesia. The stiffer, short-term, nontunneled catheters (e.g., Arrow [Teleflex Medical, Everett, MA]/Cook [Cook Medical, Bloomington, IN] types) may be placed in the operating room, or at the bedside under local anesthesia. Another type of percutaneous catheter is the peripherally inserted central catheter (PICC), which is an alternative to the non-tunneled CVC for the delivery of PN, medication, and hydration [1]. A PICC may be placed by a nurse certified in placement or by an interventional radiologist.

Upon insertion, the newly placed catheter tip position must be verified prior to use. If the line is placed using fluoroscopy, the position should be noted in the procedure note. Otherwise, placement is confirmed by radiographic exam. Once the catheter tip position is verified, it may then be used for infusion. Placement should be reconfirmed if there are any signs or symptoms of catheter malfunction or if there is any question of migration. It is recommended that placement of long-term catheters also be reconfirmed at least yearly in pediatric patients because children often have significant growth that could change the location of the tip of the catheter [2]. One recommendation is to check the placement of the line annually, using the child's birthday as a guide.

It is recommended that a CVC with the minimum number of lumens essential for the management of the patient be used [2,3]. Regardless of which type of catheter is placed, the principles for care and maintenance are very similar. All require meticulous care, including dressing changes, routine cap changes, flushing with saline, and most often heparin to maintain patency. Once a catheter is inserted, the goal is for it to remain in place throughout the course of treatment with minimal or no complications. In the SBS patient, treatment requiring central venous access may be lifelong. Thus, it is critical to maintain the catheter, paying particular attention to care.

When working effectively, CVCs assist the administration of medication, blood products, nutritional support, and withdrawal of blood samples, thus minimizing the need for venipuncture, easing the trauma of undergoing necessary treatment [4,5]. That being said, every patient should have an established plan of care for each day to include: weaning from IV to enteral medications, introducing and advancing enteral feedings, minimizing the number of catheter manipulations, and continual review of need for the CVC [6,7].

Increased vigilance is needed when caring for patients who have CVCs. Meticulous handwashing, site preparation, and the use of sterile technique during insertion and maintenance are essential to minimize the risk of infection [8]. Catheter care begins at the time of insertion, generally in the hospital by medical personnel, and continues throughout the length of time it is needed. Often, the care may extend into the home setting. Regardless of where the patient is located, it is critical that all those providing care for patients with CVCs are knowledgeable and competent in catheter maintenance.

## 26.2 EXPECTATIONS OF NURSES/NURSING CARE

Staff education has been shown to be the best way to reduce catheter-related complications [9]. Nurses, both in the acute care setting and ambulatory arena, including the home, must be able to identify the type of CVC the patient has and plan nursing interventions to prevent complications. Establishment of protocols for dressing changes, management of connections and IV tubing, as well as flushing to maintain catheter patency must be in place to guide care. When this is done, the risk of complications with CVCs is greatly decreased [10]. An appropriate catheter care regimen must begin with meticulous hand hygiene and aseptic technique.

## 26.3 DRESSING CHANGES

The area where the catheter exits the skin must be routinely cleaned and a dressing applied to the site. The purpose of a dressing is to secure the catheter and prevent dislodgement, as well as provide a barrier to water and bacteria [11]. Kits that contain all the supplies necessary for dressing changes are recommended as they are convenient, cost-effective, and a way to standardize dressing changes [12]. Dressings may be changed on a set schedule (every 2–7 days) and if ever non-occlusive, wet, or soiled. The most common types are either gauze and tape or transparent polyurethane film dressing e.g., SorbaView (Centurion Medical Products, Williamston, MI), Tegaderm (3M, St. Paul, MN), Opsite IV 3000 (Smith & Nephew, St. Petersburg, FL) [4]. There is no difference in the incidence of infectious complications between the types of dressings, including: catheter-related sepsis, exit site, and tunnel infections [4]. The type of dressing selected is dependent on the needs of the patient and there are benefits to both types. Evidence does not support use of one over the other [4,13]. The most important aspect to consider is skin integrity at the site [14].

The CVC site should be visually inspected daily through an intact dressing [10,15]. If there is any evidence of tenderness at the site, fever without obvious source, or symptoms of local or bloodstream infection, the dressing should be removed so that the site can be inspected directly [3,15]. With every dressing change, the site is assessed carefully and palpated for redness, tenderness, or drainage [13]. More frequent dressing changes combined with the use of a topical antibiotic may be necessary if the exit site becomes inflamed or purulent drainage is noted [12,16]. See Table 26.1 for the pros and cons of dressing types.

### 26.3.1 GAUZE DRESSINGS

The advantages of a gauze dressing include its absorptive quality and clean appearance. The disadvantages include: it creates an obscured site, the need to replace once site is viewed, and it requires that it be secured with tape across all surfaces to ensure occlusiveness. The dressing needs to be

**TABLE 26.1**
**The Pros and Cons of Dressing Types**

| Dressing Type | Pros | Cons |
|---|---|---|
| Gauze and tape | Highly absorptive; preferable if site is bleeding or oozing or patient perspires; less costly (per dressing) and readily available | More frequent dressing changes (at least every 48 hours); prevents visualization of catheter insertion site |
| Transparent polyurethane dressing (e.g., Tegaderm, OpSite) | Dressing changes no more than every 7 days; Continuous visualization of catheter insertion site | Not always appropriate for patients who perspire or have a site that is bleeding or oozing |
| Highly moisture permeable transparent polyurethane dressing (e.g., OpSite IV3000) | Dressing changes no more than every 7 days; Continuous visualization of catheter-insertion site | Not always appropriate for patients who perspire or have a site that is bleeding or oozing |

*Source:* Reprinted from *Infusion Nursing—An Evidence-Based Approach*, Gorski, L., Perucca, R., and Hunter, R. Central venous access devices: Care, maintenance, and potential complications. In: Alexander, M., Cotrigan, A., Gorski, L., Gorski, L., Hankins, J., and Perucca R. (eds.), 3rd ed., pp. 495–515. Copyright 2010, with permission from Saunders Elsevier, St. Louis, MO; Reprinted from *Infusion Nursing—An Evidence-Based Approach*, Hadaway, L. C., Infusion therapy equipment. In: Alexander, M., Corrigan, A., Gorski, L., Gorski, L., Hankins, J., and Perucca, R., eds. 3rd ed., pp. 391–436, Copyright 2010, with permission from Saunders Elsevier, St. Louis, MO; Reprinted from *Infusion Nursing—An Evidence-Based Approach*, McGoldrick, M. Infection prevention and control. In: Alexander, M., Corrigan, A., Gorski, L., Gorski, L., Hankins. J. and Perucca, R. (eds.), 3rd ed., pp. 204–228, Copyright 2010, with permission from Saunders Elsevier, St. Louis, MO.

changed at least every 48 hours or more often if it becomes dirty, wet, or non-adherent [14,15]. It can be a good choice for patients who experience site drainage, perspire excessively, or have a sensitivity reaction to the transparent dressings [13,17].

## 26.3.2  TRANSPARENT DRESSINGS

The advantages of a transparent dressing are that it: is occlusive, provides good adherence, and minimizes the need for additional tape. Further advantages include the ability to visualize the site without disturbing the dressing and also the need for less frequent dressing changes [12,13]. A transparent dressing should be changed every 7 days or more often if it becomes wet, dirty, or non-adherent [14,15]. When gauze is used in conjunction with the transparent dressing, the dressing is considered a gauze dressing and should be changed every 48 hours [15].

The CVC site should be visually inspected daily through an intact dressing [10,15]. If there is any evidence of tenderness at the site, fever without obvious source, or symptoms of local or bloodstream infection, the dressing should be removed so that the site can be inspected directly [3,15]. With every dressing change, the site is assessed carefully and palpated for redness, tenderness, or drainage [13]. More frequent dressing changes combined with the use of a topical antibiotic may be necessary if the exit site becomes inflamed or purulent drainage is noted [12,16]. Appendix 1 describes one institution's dressing procedure.

## 26.3.3  CHLORHEXIDINE PATCH

The chlorhexidine gluconate circular patch is another option that may be placed at the catheter site to aid in the reduction of Gram-positive and negative colonization significantly and concurrently, catheter-associated infection. This can be useful in patients with high infection risks [14,18,19]. Like transparent dressing, the patch is changed every 7 days. Silver-impregnated dressings are also an alternative, but studies have shown them to be not as effective as chlorhexidine [13]. See Table 26.2 for more information.

## 26.4  SKIN PREPARATION

The most important aspect, when considering a skin preparation, is whether it is effective at cleaning away microbes, and whether it continues to inhibit pathogen growth between dressing changes [20]. The preferred skin disinfectant for patients older than 2 months of age is 2% chlorhexidine. It has been show to have residual antibacterial activity that remains for several hours after application and has little to no systemic absorption. It is vital to allow the chlorhexidine to dry before applying

---

**TABLE 26.2**
**"Do"s and "Do Not"s of the Chlorhexidine Disk**

| Do | Do Not |
|---|---|
| • Only use the disk for catheters secured at least 1″ (2.5 cm) from insertion site. | • Do not use in neonates who are less than 7 days old or gestational age less than 26 weeks (18). |
| • Ensure skin is completely dry before placing disk. | • Do not place white side up. Antimicrobial white side must face skin. |
| • Place disk around catheter printed side up. | • Do not allow slit edges to straddle catheter. Edges of slit must touch to assure efficacy. |
| • Ensure edges of slit touch completely. | |
| • Align radial slit to the side of the catheter so the pressure of the catheter does not open the edges. | • Do not secure catheter too close to entry point. This will prevent proper placement of disk. |
| • Ensure complete contact between disk and skin. | • Do not place disk on catheter. Disk must have complete contact with skin to assure efficacy. |

*Source:*  Adapted from http://www.ethicon360.com.

any dressing [13]. Chlorhexidine solution has proven six times more effective than alcohol and povi-done–iodine in cleaning the skin [20]. However, although a 2% chlorhexidine-based preparation is preferred, the Center for Disease Control (CDC) and Intravenous Nurses Society (INS) include tincture of iodine or 70% alcohol and iodophor as acceptable prepping alternatives [20] (see Appendix 1, for skin preparation recommendations).

## 26.5 CATHETER STABILIZATION

Catheter stabilization reduces the risk of phlebitis, catheter migration, and dislodgement [13]. Use a method that does not impede vascular circulation or the delivery of the prescribed therapy [15]. Use of a Statlock (C.R. Bard, Inc., Covington, GA) anchoring device has shown some success in reduction of the incidence of catheter migration. In one study, catheter migration fell from 6% to 1.5% after initiation of the use of Statlock on all PICC lines placed [21]. If a stabilization device is used, it should be removed at established intervals, generally every 7 days with dressing change, to allow visual inspection of the site and monitoring of the skin integrity [15].

## 26.6 CVC CAP CHANGES

The benefit of a CVC cap is that it allows venous access without removing the protective covering and maintains a sterile, closed infusion system [13]. CVC caps are attached to the hub of the catheter itself or the end of an implanted port needle tubing set. Whenever accessing the cap, it is cleansed with 70% alcohol, povodine–iodone, or 3.15% chlorhexidine/70% alcohol solution. A vigorous scrubbing motion is done for 15 seconds. The CDC recommends caps not be changed more frequently than every 72 hours, but should be done at the same time a dressing change occurs. In addition, the cap is to be changed whenever it is removed, if residual blood is noted, or contamination occurs [3,22]. At Children's Hospital Boston, we recommend that the cap change be done every 96 hours in addition to the above conditions. (See Appendix 2.)

## 26.7 CVC FLUSHING

CVCs are flushed at established intervals to promote and maintain patency and prevent mixing of incompatible medications and solutions. Indwelling catheters are flushed with an anticoagulant on a routine schedule. The lowest amount and concentration should be used to maintain catheter patency. Heparin solution in low doses (1–10 U/mL of heparin) is used in neonates and pediatric patients because they have tiny veins and a small-gauge catheter is used. A recommended flushing volume is equal to two times the volume capacity of the catheter in extension and needle-free systems [22,23]. Some studies recommend a turbulent manual flush to reduce the intraluminal biofilm but further studies are needed. If resistance is met at any time during the flushing procedure, no further flushing attempts should be made because this could result in catheter rupture or a clot being dislodged into the vascular system [22]. Recommended flushing volumes vary according to patient age, weight, and catheter size. In neonates, 1–3 mL normal saline (NS) with 10 U/mL heparin every 12–24 hours is sufficient. In pediatric patients 2 mL NS with 10 U/mL heparin every 24 hours may be enough [24]. In adults 5–10 mL NS with 2–3 mL of 100 U/heparin may be used. NS with preservatives should not be used in neonates or pediatric patients [13]. It is important to note that flushing is not required during continuous infusions but it is required before and after intermittent infusions [12]. Flushing protocols for tunneled and non-tunneled is a minimum of 5 mL of NS with 10 U/mL heparin intermittently, and pre-PN, pre-blood product administration, and pre-blood draws; some adult centers will use higher concentrations of heparin, typically 5 mL of 100 U/mL. Some catheters, such as the Groshung catheter, only require saline flushes after use as these are closed-ended catheters with internal valve. Post blood product and blood draw requires a minimum of 10 mL flush [13]. The unused CVC is flushed at least once per day for tunneled catheters, monthly for ports, and every 8–12 hours for PICCs [12]. It is important that aseptic technique is used each time a catheter is accessed, with the primary goal being to reduce the introduction of organisms into the lumen [25]. Pre-packaged, single-use-only syringes of NS or NS with heparin should be used because bacterial contamination of multiple-dose vials is reported to be as high as 23% [25]. Additionally, 8% of syringes prepared by nurses were contaminated at the syringe tip, tip cap, or within the fluid. As mentioned above, single-dose containers, including vials of preservative free NS and prefilled syringes are strongly recommended by the Institute for Safe Medication Practices (ISMP) and the Joint Commission to achieve national patient safety goals [25].

Flushing technique is dependent on the type of cap used (negative- and positive-displacement devices), making it imperative that all who flush CVCs understand the type of device being used [25]. In most instances, a syringe is attached and the flush solution is administered using a pulsatile technique. Appendix 3 describes the approach used at Children's Hospital Boston.

## 26.8 BLOOD DRAWING THROUGH A CVC

When drawing blood, it is required that a portion of blood is wasted to remove the solution used to lock the catheter or any fluid that has been infused through the system. One must be wary when frequent blood samples are required because this can lead to nosocomial blood loss and iatrogenic anemia. Additionally, because collecting blood samples from CVCs requires excessive manipulation of the catheter hub, this increases the risk of contamination. An inline blood-sampling system such as the VAMP (Edwards Lifesciences Corporation, Irvine, CA) may be used [14]. This system has a reservoir that conserves blood and enables the collection of undiluted samples while significantly reducing residual-blood buildup.

Withdrawal of blood can also contribute to thrombotic catheter occlusion if the catheter is not adequately flushed after the procedure. The most common method used is the discard method [14]. Before and after blood administration, 1 mL NS for neonates and 3 mL NS for all others is flushed followed by instilling a locking solution or resumption of the infusion. The withdrawal volume for sampling should be three times the volume of the administration tubing and add-on set. Variation in size makes it difficult to recommend a volume for all patients [24]. For example, healthy adults of average size and weight can easily tolerate blood draws as much as 200 mL with minimal risk; however, an ill adult who requires frequent blood draws can tolerate smaller volumes (e.g., 50 mL or 3 mL/kg in an 8-week period). Appendix 3 outlines the blood-draw procedure at Children's Hospital Boston.

## 26.9 ADMINISTRATION OF FLUIDS AND MEDICATIONS VIA A CVC

Care should be taken to avoid contamination during solution or tubing changes [12]. When patients are hospitalized, administration sets used for most IV fluids, medications, and PN should be changed every 96 hours [3,7,17,26]. If lipid-based infusions or medications (i.e., IV fat emulsion, liposomal amphotericin, propofol) are used, then the sets are changed every 24 hours [3,17,26]. In the home setting, all containers and tubing are changed every 24 hours. In the inpatient setting, tubing should be labeled with the patient's name, medical record number, and the start date and time and discard date and time. Any tubing that is not properly labeled should be disposed of [17]. Prior to administration of any medication, fluid, blood product, or PN, the nurse identifies the patient with at least two patient identifiers including, but not limited to, date of birth, patient name, or medical record number. The patient's room number is not considered an identifier [15]. When administering PN, an infusion pump should be used which prevents "free flow" and has reliable, audible alarms [2].

Oftentimes patients requiring PN also receive multiple parenteral medications, and questions arise concerning whether these medications can be co-administered with PN. As discussed in Chapter 10, due to the risks of precipitation and/or infection, the co-administration of medications and PN should be avoided whenever possible. Moreover, medications should not be added directly to the PN bag itself except by pharmacy staff. Medications not directly added to PN should be co-infused via a "y" connection with the IV setup proximal to a filter. Figure 26.1 shows a typical IV

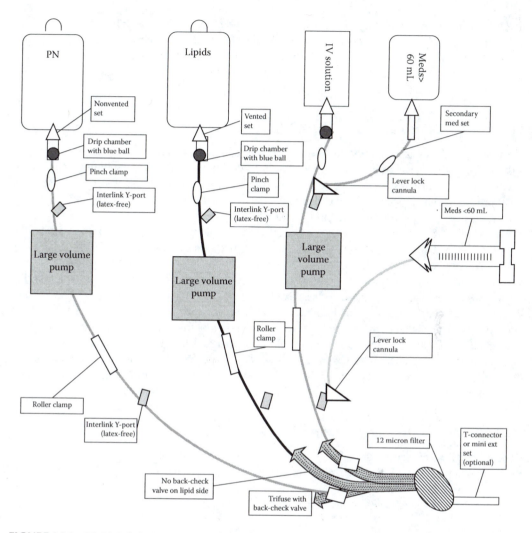

**FIGURE 26.1**    Multiple infusion setup. (Copyright: Children's Hospital Boston.)

setup. Since compatibility is based on a number of factors, whenever the PN formula changes, medications co-administered with the solution should be reviewed.

## 26.10    COMPLICATIONS

Monitoring and meticulous care can increase early detection of and prevention of many complications. The nurse is responsible for catheter care, observing the patient, monitoring how the patient responds to therapy, and providing appropriate nursing interventions [10]. Catheter care includes examination of the insertion site and the surrounding skin for swelling or induration. In addition, the entire arm as well as the neck and clavicle areas should be assessed. Swelling around the neck of the clavicle is an indicator of SVC syndrome [10]. Moreover, the catheter site should be assessed for drainage (color, consistency, amount, and odor). Swabbing the site for culture is necessary as purulent drainage may indicate an infected catheter. Also, if the patient has a fever, blood cultures must be drawn to determine organisms and the source of infection. The most effective way to determine if the infection is related to the catheter is to perform a culture of the catheter tip. This is discussed in detail in Chapter 19. Keeping an infected catheter in place is not recommended as this can result in hematogenous seeding of organisms within the bloodstream. Seeding can also result in catheter-related sepsis if another infection seeds microorganisms on the IV catheter [10]. If the catheter must be removed for any reason, the exit site must be assessed for inflammation, tenderness, erythema, or drainage. The patient should be kept flat and supine for a short time to maintain positive intrathoracic pressure and allow the tract time to seal [10].

### 26.10.1  CVC Occlusions

Obstruction of the IV infusion system is one of the most common complications of PN use. One of the first signs of catheter occlusion is the ability to flush the device but difficulty in aspirating. Initial management consists of ensuring that there are no clamps or kinks present. Using sterile technique, a 3–10 mL flush with NS should then be attempted. Persistent occlusions are often treated with thrombolytic agents. A venogram can be helpful in distinguishing between malpositioned catheters, a fibrin sheath at the CVC tip, or mural thrombi. Complete obstructions, however, cannot be evaluated by contrast studies. Depending on the nature of an intracatheter precipitate, Table 26.3 lists commonly used agents. Appendices 4 and 5 discuss in greater detail the management of CVC occlusions.

In-line filters should always be used to decrease the particulate load of the solution [2]. Microparticulates that are invisible to the naked eye can cause nonthrombotic catheter occlusions. Sources of particulate matter include plastic fibers from the infusion bag, glass particulates from ampoules, and precipitants from incompatible ingredients. Moreover, in-line filters may offer some protection against thombosis by decreasing the amount of particulate matter that can potentially irritate the vasculature endothelium [27]. Dextrose–protein (i.e., 2-in-1 solutions) should be infused through a 0.22 μm in-line filter while 1.2 μm filter should be used for total nutrient admixtures [28,29]. For additional information, please refer to the Appendix 6, for device placement and other considerations.

### 26.10.2  Phlebitis and Extravasation

Phlebitis and extravasation, though less likely, can still occur after placement of a PICC, CVC, or implanted port. Mechanical/sterile phlebitis, irritation of the vein during catheter insertion can lead to loss of the catheter if not assessed and treated promptly. This type of phlebitis is more frequent in a PICC placed in the antecubital fossa rather than the upper arm. Chemical phlebitis rarely occurs

---

**TABLE 26.3**
**Treatment of CVC Occlusion**

| Precipitate Suspected | Clinical Scenario | Pharmacological Agent |
|---|---|---|
| Particulate (e.g., Ca–P) with drugs that are soluble in acidic solution | PN, Ca, and/or P; use of etoposide; or aminoglycosides + heparin | 0.1 N hydrochloric acid |
| Particulate with drugs that are soluble in basic solutions | Phenytoin, imipenem, oxacillin, ticarcillin | Sodium bicarbonate 1 mEq/mL |
| Waxy | PN/IL, propofol | Ethanol 70% in water |
| None (i.e., thrombus suspected) | No precipitate suspected, line sluggish, difficulty drawing bloods off CVC | Alteplase 1 mg/mL or urokinase 5000 U/mL or reteplase 0.4 U/0.4 mL |

*Note:*  Most CVCs require 1 mL of the pharmacological agent chosen, although implantable ports require 2 mL. The agent is allowed to dwell within the lumen of the CVC for 30–60 min before being aspirated with a 10 mL syringe. A NS flush should then be attempted before the infusion is resumed. Occasionally a prolonged infusion of a thrombolytic agent is required. Large thrombi are often unable to be treated successfully, and are generally an indication for catheter removal.

with solutions infused through a PICC because when the solution exits the PICC, adequate hemodilution occurs [30]. However, damage to the catheter inside the vein can lead to chemical phlebitis if the infusion leaks through the damaged catheter into the surrounding vein or tissue. Daily observation of the site and upper arm is vital [31].

Extravasation can occur when a catheter is dislodged or when a venous vessel is perforated. Given that extravasation can cause skin blistering and ulcer formation, it is not considered a benign complication. Central extravasation should be considered when the patient complains of fever, pleuritic pain, upper extremity, and/or neck swelling and can be complicated by severe pain, effusion, dysrhythmia, or mediastinitis. Risk factors include choice of device, type of treatment as well as clinician, and patient-related characteristics. Choice of a large gauge catheter that impedes blood flow can increase the risk of phlebitis and extravasation because it can impede blood flow and slow dilution of infusate. With CVCs, catheter migration, fibrin-sleeve formation, thrombosis, or needle displacement (in the case of an implanted port) can also increase the risk for extravasation. Additionally, the very young and the very old are also at increased risk of extravasation due to fragile veins [31].

## 26.11 POWERPORT™/POWERPICC®

A power-injection port or power-injection PICC is another option for patients and provides access for power-injected contrast-enhanced computed tomography (CECT) scans. Both the PowerPort and PowerPICC are cared for in a manner very similar to a traditional port or PICC. The PowerPort requires a special safety needle set, which enables clinicians to perform power-injected CECT scans. See Table 26.4 for more information about use of a PowerPort or PowerPICC.

## 26.12 HOME CARE EDUCATION

Prior to discharge, patients and caregivers need to be thoroughly educated on the proper handling of a CVC. Nurses help to educate patients and families, encouraging them to promptly notify the primary care provider of any unusual discomfort, erythema, edema, or drainage related to the catheter. Hand hygiene is reviewed and modeled for patients and families. Since patients and families may have a lack of knowledge related to the purpose and function of the catheter, they may also be anxious about the management of the device. Even those with some knowledge may be noncompliant with the administration of medications and the maintenance of the catheter and will require additional training. Because the goal of treatment for all patients is completion of treatment with minimal or no complications, nurses must take adequate time to allay fears, educate patients and families, and provide time for questions and answers.

Because the patient and/or family assumes the responsibility of caring for and maintaining the CVC after discharge from the hospital, nursing staff must take time to provide the necessary education prior to discharge. Ideally, teaching should begin before insertion of the line and should include time for the patient and/or family to practice care and management of the catheter (see Appendix 7). This will allow the nurse to assess technique and identify additional learning needs. Signs and symptoms of infection and whom to contact must be taught. Home-care services must also be coordinated prior to discharge so that the necessary equipment can be ordered and the family can be educated on these products as well. Collaboration between hospital nursing staff and home-care providers is vital to ensure all needs are met at home. Chapter 32, provides additional information on this topic.

### 26.12.1 PEDIATRIC CONSIDERATIONS

For the child on PN, steps should be taken to try to normalize the environment and experience for the child requiring PN. Options include cycled PN to allow time off the pump to allow mobility and development and portable pumps whenever possible [32]. Portable pumps including those using a

**TABLE 26.4**
**Use of a PowerPort or PowerPICC**

| | PowerPort | PowerPICC | Both |
|---|---|---|---|
| Maintenance | It is recommended that a PowerLoc™ safety-infusion set is used to access the PowerPort regardless of use (e.g., IV fluids or CECT) for consistency. The Power Injection Port accessed with a PowerLoc safety infusion set is used the same as the traditional implanted port (e.g., administering medications, IV fluids, and PN/IL). | Can be used for CVP monitoring. A continuous NS infusion is recommended (3 mL/hour) to improve accuracy of CVP results. | The care and maintenance of the power-injection port and PICC are the same as the traditional care outlined in this chapter. Prior to infusions, flush with a minimum of 10 mL NS. Use a pulsatile motion. |
| Flushing | Flush catheter with 10 mL NS before and after each use. Flush port with 5 mL of either 10 U/mL heparin (for infants and children) or 100 U/mL heparin (for adults) per lumen after each use. After blood draw, flush with 20 mL NS and 5 mL heparin. | Flush catheter with 2 mL (infants and children) or 10 mL NS (adults) before each use and with 3 mL NS (infants and children) or 10 mL NS (adults) and heparin after each use. Usually 1 mL of either 10 U/mL heparin (for infants and children) or 100 U/mL heparin (for adults) per lumen is adequate. When infusing TPN and labs are required, flush with 20 mL NS prior to drawing labs. Flush at least weekly when not in use. | Only use syringes 10 mL or larger. |
| CECT studies | Verify the patient has a power-injection port by at least two means and ensure they are accessed with a PowerLoc infusion set prior to use. | When power injecting, use only the lumens marked "Power Injectable" to prevent catheter failure. Use of other lumens for power injection could cause failure of the catheter. | Contrast media is warmed to body temperature prior to power injection. A positive-pressure cap cannot be used with the power injection of contrast. Check for patency, via aspiration and then vigorously flush the PowerPort using 10 mL of sterile NS prior to and immediately following the completion of a power-injection study. Do not flush or inject against resistance. |

| Maximum flow rate/maximum pressure | 19 gauge 5 mL/second and 300 psi<br>20 gauge 5 mL/second and 300 psi<br>22 gauge 2 mL/second and 300 psi | All catheter sizes 5 mL/second 300 psi |
| Identification/ verification | Feel the top of the septum for the three palpation points arranged in a triangle.<br>Palpate the sides of the port for a triangular shape.<br>Request confirmation from the patient or family by asking them to show you the PowerPort patient-identification card, ID bracelet, or keychain they received when the port was implanted.<br>Check for radiographic confirmation. | |

*Source:* Adapted from Bard Access Systems. http://www.bardaccess.com/index.php.

backpack allow mobility for toddlers and older children [32]. Infusion pumps used for children should have the following features:

- Lock-out option
- Capability to do small increment adjustments
- Alarm feature at low psi

Families should be instructed to check catheter site every day and report any changes such as redness, drainage, or pain at the insertion site [3,13]. Families should also be instructed to position the catheter as to prevent infants and small children from scratching or picking at the catheter site, pulling, or biting the catheter and to prevent contamination from the diaper and/or stoma site if applicable [33]. (Special care must be taken with infants who are teething so they do not use the cap to teethe on [32].) Additionally, keeping the dressing intact is one of the most important factors in preventing infection [32]. Families must be educated to look for excessive drooling, stool, or urine output that could soil the dressing [32]. Other lifestyle issues must also be considered. For example, families must be instructed that the child must wait 4 weeks after tunneled-catheter placement before swimming in a chlorinated pool and that the child should not swim in a natural source of water such as a pond, lake, or ocean and should avoid hot tubs and whirlpools [34].

Prior to discharge, other family concerns should also be addressed. Studies show that families express concerns regarding CVC occlusion and these episodes were dominated by fear of venipuncture; other anxieties included the possibility of requiring another line [5]. A third of families expressed feelings of anger and frustration when their child encountered occlusion problems. They also reported feeling disappointed and helpless. Many of the children reported similar feelings with some becoming irritable or visibly upset [5]. Overall the main concerns appeared to surround three main areas: the possibility of needing venipuncture, the fear of total line failure and replacement, and the inconvenience that this can cause to the daily lives of the family. Other concerns included interruptions in treatment, the possibility that occlusion might in some way be painful for the child, and a lack of knowledge regarding the reasons for occlusion [5]. The majority of parents reported that they felt they had received adequate teaching regarding the care of their child's CVC but had difficulty recalling the precise information they had been given [5]. This shows that adequate time for teaching and frequent review is necessary.

Families prefer to be taught how to flush the line sooner to develop their and their child's confidence with the CVC and enhance their feelings of involvement [5]. Families also would have liked to have been aware of this type of complication sooner, so that they could have prepared for the possibility of requiring venipuncture [5]. Families also expressed that the most appropriate time to be taught about this complication would be at the time of insertion. Many families consistently stated that they wanted all the facts from the beginning of treatment and added that this knowledge reduced their anxiety when they encountered the problem for the first time, because they understood that it was not unusual, not their fault and could probably be rectified [5]. The most beneficial factor that enabled the parents to cope with the CVC was actually handing the line themselves, and in particular, being able to undertake the flushing protocol [5]. However, the family's readiness to learn must be assessed as some families may not be ready at the time of insertion because there is a considerable amount of information to absorb under extremely emotional circumstances immediately following diagnosis and the initiation of treatment [5]. Support at home was also vital, including visits by community nurses [5].

The child's own acceptance of the line was the strongest factor enabling families to cope with the CVC at home [5]. Education with children should also occur and be clear and concise. Children often have unrealistic expectations that a CVC will eliminate the need for venipuncture and thus feel betrayed when complications occur. The nurse has a key role in discussing this possibility with the child and family, and by engaging the play specialist may be able to prepare the child for this eventuality [5]. Families should be instructed to store all IV equipment in a designated place within the home so that supplies can be easily located when needed [23]. They should also be instructed that while areas in the home will not be sterile, aseptic technique must still be used for all procedures [11]. A clean, clutter-free area must be identified for CVC care [11]. Additionally arrangements should be made to refer the patient for catheter removal as soon as the CVC is no longer needed [11].

## 26.13 CONCLUSION

Establishing and maintaining central venous access can be very challenging and frustrating for the patient, family, and health-care provider, especially when the patient is dependent on the catheter for long-term nutrition and hydration. Meticulous care and judicious use of a CVC is essential to avoid the need for multiple central catheters and the loss of both peripheral and central veins. Loss of veins can occur when thrombosis occurs. Additionally, once a vessel is accessed via a cut-down technique, it is unlikely to be salvageable for central access. Therefore, over time, it is critical to attempt to reduce the number of CVCs required. Consequently, CVCs should be used as long as possible before removal. Infection is the most common complication leading to removal and patients with SBS have higher rates of infection [12]. Therefore, management of the catheter, especially in young children, by a group of trained healthcare professionals is vital [12]. During inpatient stays, the line should be cared for by the nurse and opportunities for education and re-education should be taken when possible to ensure consistency of care. Manufacturer guidelines and institutional policies should be followed at all times. Needleless systems should be used. All devices should be carefully secured to prevent tugging, irritation to the site, and accidental dislodgement.

It is the hope that once a CVC is inserted, it can remain in for the duration of treatment and barring complications, is not removed until that time. Though complications can be significant, the benefits generally outweigh the risks. Prevention and early detection of catheter-related complications is crucial to reduce patient morbidity and preserve catheter patency.

## APPENDIX 1: DRESSING CHANGE PROCEDURE*

1. Explain procedure to patient and/or parent to promote understanding and cooperation.
2. Open sterile dressing tray and put on mask. Wash hands thoroughly to prevent organisms from contaminating the exit site.
3. Remove old dressing using standard precautions.
4. Assess exit site and surrounding skin for erythema, swelling, tenderness, or drainage. Note if sutures are intact. Document and notify physician of changes.
5. Put on sterile gloves.
6. Do one of the following:
   - *For patients ≥37 weeks gestation:* Use Chloraprep technique: Pinch wings of applicator to crack ampule of Chloraprep. After ampule cracks stop squeezing wings. Press sponge until liquid is visible on skin. Completely wet a 2 in.-wide margin of the skin around line exit site. Apply using *back and forth scrubbing motion.* Apply for 30 seconds on dry sites (chest and antecubital). Apply for 2 min on wet site (groin). Allow to dry.
   - *For patients <37 weeks gestation:* Thoroughly wipe the site with alcohol three times. Allow the alcohol to dry for 1 min. For infants ≤28 weeks gestation, wipe off the alcohol with sterile NS.
7. Minimize catheter manipulation at the catheter site to decrease trauma to tissue, which may increase risk of bacterial colonization and/or infection along subcutaneous tunnel.

---

* Children's Hospital Boston.

8. Cover area with polyurethane adhesive dressing so that the catheter exit site and a surrounding 2 in. margin of skin is covered and intact (see figure). Loop CVC as shown to decrease tension on line.

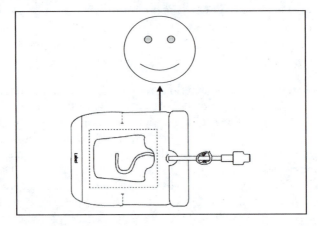

9. Smaller dressing sizes are available for younger children.
10. Ensure that the CVC hub site is *not* allowed to hang down below the patient's waist; near a stoma site; near a GT site; tucked in a diaper; submerged in bath water.
11. Using tape provided, secure CVC to ensure dressing is occlusive (see Figure above).
12. Secure CVC to patient at a second site, by taping or pinning to clothing. Securing at a second site prevents tension on the CVC. If patient safety is an issue, cover safety pin with tape.
13. Place completed CVC label on transparent dressing.
14. Document dressing change.

## APPENDIX 2: CENTRAL VENOUS CATHETER CAP CHANGE PROCEDURE*

1. Explain procedure to patient/parent to promote understanding and cooperation.
2. Mask first, wash hands, and wear protective equipment.
3. Using 10 mL syringe filled with NS solution, prime the positive-pressure cap. Set aside maintaining sterility.
4. Open package of sterile 2 × 2 gauze. Open an alcohol swab. Touching only one corner of the alcohol pad place on gauze. Pick up the gauze with alcohol pad on top. Lay the CVC onto the pad. See figure below.

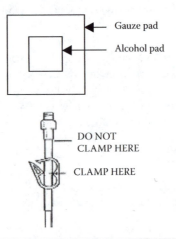

         Gauze pad

         Alcohol pad

         DO NOT CLAMP HERE

         CLAMP HERE

---

* Children's Hospital Boston.

5. Clamp CVC using pinch clamp attached to line. This prevents blood loss and air emboli. All silastic CVCs (e.g., Broviac and Hickman) have reinforced sleeve where clamping is to occur. Clamping close to Luer connection of CVC may perforate silastic.

6. Don sterile gloves. Remove CVC cap and thoroughly scrub the catheter hub site with the alcohol swab for 15 seconds. Be careful not to touch the open CVC hub site or allow CVC to touch skin.

7. Remove protective end cover from new cap and screw onto hub. Do not touch the inner portion that fits into catheter.

8. Unclamp catheter.

9. Scrub positive-pressure cap with alcohol swab for 15 seconds.

10. Using 10 mL syringe filled with heparin solution (10 U/mL) inject 2–3 mLs of solution through the cap into the catheter. Smaller flush volumes are sometimes warranted. Disconnect syringe. Clamp CVC.

11. If necessary for patient safety, secure CVC cap to hub with adhesive tape. Fold a tab over on each end, to facilitate handling tape without touching a sticky surface. Transient hand flora, if heavily inoculated onto sticky side of tape, may wash into system if/when connection loosens.

## APPENDIX 3: BLOOD SAMPLING PROCEDURE*

### BLOOD SAMPLING FROM A CVC WITH A BIFUSE ONE CHECK® VALVE OR MINI-BIFUSE®

1. Calculate the total amount of blood to be drawn. This will help determine the appropriate number of syringes needed.

2. Explain procedure to the patient and/or family to promote understanding and cooperation.

3. Wash hands well and put on gloves to reduce risk of infection or colonization of microorganisms.

4. Open package of sterile $2 \times 2$ gauze. Open an alcohol swab. Touching only one corner of the alcohol pad place on gauze. Pick up the gauze with alcohol pad on top. Lay the CVC onto the pad.

5. Clamp off *IV tubing* as close as possible to the injection site.

6. Turn off the infusion pump.

7. Wait 1 minute before obtaining blood sample.

8. Use the alcohol pad to scrub the Bifuse cap for 15 seconds. The cap must be scrubbed before each entrance into the cap.

9. Connect the prefilled 10 mL NS syringe to the Bifuse cap, unclamp and flush CVC. Draw back 2–3 mL of blood, using same syringe. Drop uncapped syringe into emesis basin. This is the discard sample. Drawing a discard prevents contamination of sample with IV fluid. Smaller flush volumes and blood discard volumes may be warranted.

10. Scrub injection site with alcohol for 10 seconds. Using an empty 10 mL syringe, connect and withdraw the necessary amount of blood for lab tests. Aspirate gently to prevent hemolysis and CVC collapse.

11. Scrub injection site with alcohol for 15 seconds and flush CVC with prefilled 10 mL NS syringe using pulsatile motion. Smaller flush volumes may be warranted.

12. Turn on pump to restart infusion.

13. Fill the blood specimen tubes according to priority.

14. Slightly agitate any tubes containing anticoagulant agents.

15. Label tubes and attach requisitions as per hospital policy and procedure.

16. Send samples to laboratory.

17. Dispose of syringes into an appropriate puncture-proof container.

---

* Children's Hospital Boston.

## BLOOD SAMPLING FROM A HEPARIN-LOCKED CVC

1. Follow blood sampling from a CVC with a Bifuse One Check Valve or Mini-Bifuse steps 1–4 (above).
2. Scrub the positive-pressure cap with alcohol for 15 seconds. The cap needs to be scrubbed before each entry, to prevent the introduction of organisms into the line. For successive entries, the same alcohol pad may be reused if care is taken in handling.
3. Attach the prefilled 10 mL NS syringe to the positive-pressure cap and flush the CVC. Draw back 2–3 mL of blood using same syringe. Disconnect the syringe and drop the discard syringe into the emesis basin. Smaller flush volumes and blood discard volumes may be warranted.
4. Scrub the positive-pressure cap with alcohol for 15 seconds. Attach an empty 10 mL syringe, and withdraw necessary amount of blood for lab tests. Aspirate gently to prevent hemolysis and CVC collapse.
5. Scrub positive-pressure cap with alcohol for 15 seconds. Attach the prefilled 10 mL NS syringe and flush CVC with 3–10 mL prefilled 10 mL syringe of NS solution. Administer 10 mL if no fluid restriction. Smaller flush volumes may be warranted.
6. Scrub the positive-pressure cap with alcohol for 15 seconds. Attach a prefilled 10 mL heparin solution syringe (10 U/mL) and flush CVC. Disconnect syringe and clamp CVC.
7. Continue with blood sampling from a CVC with a Bifuse One Check Valve or Mini-Bifuse steps 13–17 (above).

## APPENDIX 4: CENTRAL VENOUS CATHETER OCCLUSION ALGORITHM*

### DEFINITIONS AND GENERAL INFORMATION

Central venous catheter (CVC) includes all central venous lines, implanted ports, apheresis lines, and PICC lines.

Occlusion is defined as an inability to withdraw 1 mL or more of blood from a line that had a good blood return **or** an inability to flush or infuse through the line. Occlusions may be sudden or gradual with the line becoming increasingly more sluggish or difficult to flush.

CVC-competent nurses are those who have successfully completed CVC competencies.

### REVIEW OF THE LINE HISTORY

(These questions are relevant in determining appropriate treatment of the occlusion.) Complete the line history before activating the algorithm.

1. What happened immediately before the line occluded?
   - Was IV fluid infusing?
   - Was the line used for medication administration?
   - When was the line last accessed/flushed?
   - Was the line flushed with saline and/or heparin?
   - Has the line occluded in the past?
   - Was the line at risk of malposition (e.g., line pulled externally, recent dressing change, change in interthoracic pressure)?
2. If fluids only (no medications) were running:
   - Was TPN infusing? If TPN, check with the Clinical Nutrition Service (CNS) to be certain that the concentrations of calcium and phosphorous are compatible and not prone to precipitation. Review the entire TPN formulation with the CNS to rule out other possible incompatibilities.

---

* Children's Hospital Boston.

- If TPN solution, determine if the bag was allowed to become excessively warm (i.e., placed on top of any infusion pump/under warming lights/inside an isolette).
- Were lipids also being infused? If so, were they:
    - Co-infused into the same IV line as PN or
    - Infused through a different access site?

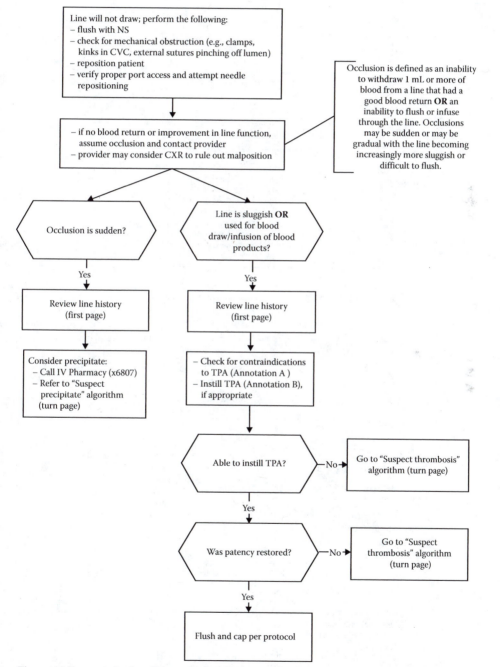

*Note:* These guidelines were developed by a multi-disciplinary group for the management of CVC occlusions. These guidelines are not to established a protocol for all patients with a CVC occlusions, nor are they intended to replace a clinician's clinical judgement.

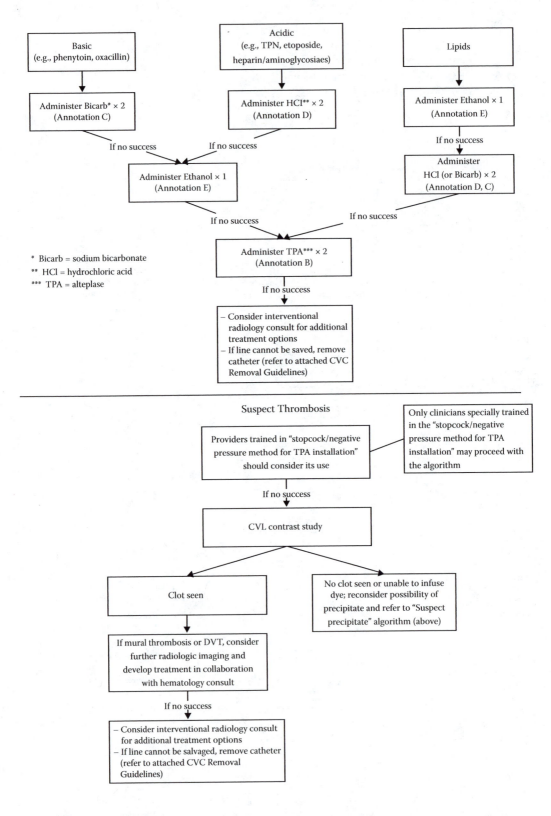

Basic
(e.g., phenytoin, oxacillin)

Acidic
(e.g., TPN, etoposide,
heparin/aminoglycosiaes)

Lipids

Administer Bicarb* × 2
(Annotation C)

Administer HCl** × 2
(Annotation D)

Administer Ethanol × 1
(Annotation E)

If no success        If no success

Administer Ethanol × 1
(Annotation E)

If no success

Administer
HCl (or Bicarb) × 2
(Annotation D, C)

If no success                    If no success

* Bicarb = sodium bicarbonate
** HCl = hydrochloric acid
*** TPA = alteplase

Administer TPA*** × 2
(Annotation B)

If no success

– Consider interventional
radiology consult for additional
treatment options
– If line cannot be saved, remove
catheter (refer to attached CVC
Removal Guidelines)

Suspect Thrombosis

Providers trained in "stopcock/negative
pressure method for TPA installation"
should consider its use

Only clinicians specially trained
in the "stopcock/negative
pressure method for TPA
installation" may proceed with
the algorithm

If no success

CVL contrast study

Clot seen

No clot seen or unable to infuse
dye; reconsider possibility of
precipitate and refer to "Suspect
precipitate" algorithm (above)

If mural thrombosis or DVT, consider
further radiologic imaging and
develop treatment in collaboration
with hematology consult

If no success

– Consider interventional radiology consult
for additional treatment options
– If line cannot be salvaged, remove catheter
(refer to attached CVC Removal
Guidelines)

- Was the solution a TNA solution (e.g., TPN mixed with lipids in one bag) brought in from the patient's home?

3. If medications were given prior to occlusion:
   - Which medications were given?
   - Determine the concentration and length of infusion.
   - How was the medication diluted for administration? (Determine diluent type and volume)
   - Was a filter used?

4. Was there a filter in place?
   - Did the filter occlude? How was it treated? The pharmacist will help to determine what caused the precipitate in the filter and correct the situation.

In some instances, it may be necessary to remove a clogged filter and replace prior to resuming the infusion.

*Never remove a filter and infuse fluids without replacing it with a new one.*

## APPENDIX 5: DECLOTTING A CENTRAL VENOUS CATHETER WITH TISSUE PLASMINOGEN ACTIVATOR INJECTION*

### PURPOSE

To restore patency of a CVC occluded by clotted blood.

### BACKGROUND INFORMATION

Tissue plasminogen activator (tPA) is a thrombolytic agent that activates the endogenous fibrinolytic system by cleaving the arginine–valine bond in plasminogen to produce plasmin, an enzyme that degrades fibrin clots as well as fibrinogen and other plasma proteins including the procoagulant factors V and VIII.

In the premature patient consult with Neonatology and Thrombosis Services. Neonates with small CVC may need a smaller volume of alteplase.

When used for catheter clearance, only small amounts of alteplase could reach the circulation.

The procedure involves slow and gentle injection of alteplase into an occluded CVC. Excessive pressure could result in rupture of the catheter or expulsion of the clot into the circulation.

The concentration strength of alteplase for declotting a CVC is 1 mg/mL. The medication is sent to the unit in 2 mL vials. Use 2 mL for all CVCs except when protocol requires the dose to be consistent with CVC volume.

Alteplase is not an effective treatment for precipitant occlusions. If a precipitant is suspected as the cause of catheter occlusions, notify the physician that Hydrochloric acid (HCl 0.1 m) solution is available in the pharmacy. It is effective in clearing catheters occluded by the precipitation of poorly soluble-fluid components, such as calcium salts or drugs. It acts by increasing the fluid solubility by lowering the pH. A physician administers HCl solution.

### PROCEDURE

1. If unable to flush or aspirate blood, have the patient perform the following:
   a. Raise arms over head
   b. Turn head to opposite side of catheter
   c. Sit upright, take deep breaths
   d. Lie prone or on side
   e. Yawn, cough, sing

---

* Children's Hospital Boston.

2. Verify that there are no external causes for occlusion, such as kinked or clamped tubing.
3. Notify the physician of catheter occlusion. Consider an x-ray to verify catheter tip location.
4. Obtain physician's order for alteplase.
5. Don mask and wash hands. Open package of sterile $2 \times 2$ gauze. Open an alcohol pad. Touching only one corner of the alcohol pad place on gauze. Don clean gloves. Pick up the gauze with alcohol pad on top. Remove CVC cap or disconnect IV tubing. Scrub the connection site with the alcohol pad.
6. Attach alteplase-filled syringe. Gently instill medication and clamp CVC.

   (*Note: NEVER forcefully push on syringe*. Force may cause catheter to rupture or clot to be dislodged. If resistance is excessive, notify physician before proceeding.)

7. Only specially trained practitioners may use a stopcock.
8. Attach positive-pressure cap aseptically and wait for 2 hours.
9. Attach 10 mL syringe, attempt to aspirate alteplase.

---

**Rationale**

A second dose of alteplase is sometimes necessary in resistant cases. If still unsuccessful, consider the possibility of a precipitant occlusion and notify physician. A contrast study may be indicated.

---

10. If a blood return cannot be obtained, wait for two more hours before attempting to aspirate again. If unsuccessful, repeat dose x1.

---

**Rationale**

To remove all medication and residual clot, 2–4 hours is recommended to achieve maximum therapeutic effect.

---

## APPENDIX 6: USE OF IV FILTERS*

### POLICY

- All central venous catheters (CVCs) do not need to be filtered. CVCs are filtered according to solutions infusing, medications being administered, or patient diagnosis.
- All parenteral nutrition (PN) solutions, including lipids, infused via central and peripheral infusions, are administered through a 1.2 µm filter. *Lipids administered without PN do not need to be filtered.*
- *Multiple medications running simultaneously into a single CVC lumen must be filtered at the site closest to the patient.* Single-medication infusions, hydration fluid and peripheral infusions do not require a filter. Contact pharmacy for filter exceptions.
- IV fluids with divalent or trivalent electrolyte additives (e.g., calcium, magnesium, phosphorous) must be filtered. Monovalent electrolyte solutions (e.g., potassium or sodium) do

---

* Children's Hospital Boston.

not need to be filtered unless they are being co-infused with PN or as one of the multiple medication lines being administered simultaneously into a single CVC lumen.

- When infusing medications without IV fluids, an extension set with an in-line 0.22 μm filter may be used.
- Place filter as close to the IV catheter as possible.
- Certain medications containing particulate matter (usually unreconstituted medication) are always filtered. Some other medications may need to be filtered, depending on the concentration and length of infusion. Medications that are formulated as suspension or an emulsion cannot be administered through a 1.2 μm filter.
- Blood products require a filter larger than 1.2 μm.
- Change 1.2 μm filters and tubing every 96 hours unless lipids have been infused through the filter, in which case they are changed every 24 hours.

## PURPOSE

Prevent complications, associated with PN and multiple medication infusions, such as catheter occlusion and air embolism, through effective use of particulate filters.

## PROCEDURE

### Assessment

A 1.2 μm membrane filter removes particulate debris and some microbial contaminants from IV solutions and prevents the passage of air to patients.

Some medication concentrations may decrease dramatically when initially infused through a filter, but will return to normal levels at some point after the start of the infusion. Because the filter's binding site becomes saturated, the remainder of the medication passes through the filter without loss.

### Planning

- Buretteless administration set
- 1.2 μm particulate filter or IV extension-tubing with in-line 0.22 μm filter
- Medication(s) to be infused
- Parenteral nutrition
- Maintenance fluids if indicated
- Bifuse/trifuse set or manifold

### Implementation

*Single Infusion Setup*

1. Using aseptic technique, prepare the buretteless administration set.
2. Spike IV fluid bag with buretteless administration. Prime tubing carefully by gravity to remove air. *Do not use pump to prime tubing.*
3. Insert distal end of administration set into filter inlet with a twisting motion. Secure luer–lock adapter, being careful not to overtighten.

---

**Rationale**

Prevents filter from separating from infusion set. If overtightened, the connector will crack, resulting in patient blood back flow or leakage of solution.

---

4. Prime filter by gravity to remove air following the manufacturer instructions. Hold filter below level of solution container while allowing filter to fill with fluid.

> **Rationale**
> Failure to hold the filter properly when priming may result in entrapped air on the patient side of the filter.

5. Verify that air bubbles are removed from the air filter and tubing. If air bubbles are noted, open clamp and *gently tap* filter and tubing extension to eliminate air. Close clamp.

> **Rationale**
> Medications must be filtered for precipitates after medication mixing has occurred.

6. Remove protective cap from filter and connect male end of filter to T-connector, mini-extension set, or directly to IV catheter.

> **Rationale**
> Prevents filter from separating from infusion set. If overtightened, the connector will crack, resulting in patient blood back flow or leakage of solution.

7. Secure infusion setup to patient. Begin infusion.

> **Rationale**
> Failure to hold the filter properly when priming may result in entrapped air on the patient side of the filter.

*Multiple Infusion Setup*
1. Using aseptic technique, prepare the buretteless administration set.
2. Spike IV fluid bag with buretteless administration. Prime tubing carefully by gravity to remove air. *Do not use pump to prime tubing.*
3. Attach bifuse, trifuse, or manifold set to distal end of administration tubing and prime.
4. Insert male end of bifuse, trifuse, or manifold set into female end of the filter with twisting motion.
5. Attach 1.2 μm filter after the Y-administration set at site closest to the patient.
6. Secure luer–lock adapter, being careful not to overtighten.
7. Prime filter by gravity to remove air following the manufacturer instructions. Hold filter below level of solution container while allowing filter to fill with fluid.
8. Verify that air bubbles are removed from the air filter and tubing. If air bubbles are seen, open clamp and *gently tap* filter and tubing extension-to eliminate air. Close clamp.
9. Remove protective cap from filter and connect male end of filter to T-connector, mini extension-set, or directly to IV catheter.
10. Secure infusion setup to patient. Begin infusion.

## Evaluation

Observe patency of filter, IV tubing, and catheter. Report any problems with precipitate or catheter occlusion to the physician or nurse practitioner and pharmacist. Evaluate effectiveness of the procedure and patient outcomes.

## Documentation

Complete *patient care documentation* per policy.

## APPENDIX 7: EXAMPLE OF FAMILY EDUCATION SHEETS (PEDIATRIC)*

Your child is going home with a CVC. The CVC is an IV IV line that is placed by a doctor or nurse into a large vein close to the heart. Children usually have a CVC placed when there is a long-term need for IV medication, fluids, nutrition, or for obtaining blood tests.

There are three kinds of CVCs used in children.

- Some are used for short periods of time. These are called Arrow, PICC, or deep venous long lines (see Figure).

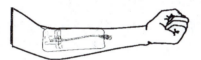

- Others are used for longer periods of time. These are called Broviac, Hickman, or Leonard lines (see Figure). These lines have a cuff that is placed under your child's skin. The cuff helps to hold the CVC in place.

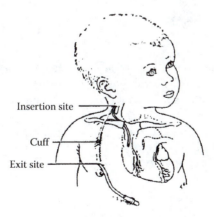

- The third kind is completely under the child's skin. These lines are called implanted ports (see Figure).

---

* Children's Hospital Boston.

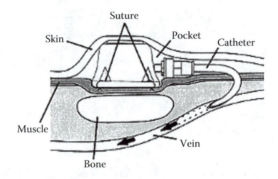

There is a clamp and a cap on the end of every CVC or the attached tubing. These prevent blood loss and air entry into the vein. Care of your child's CVC involves:

- Changing the dressing
- Changing the cap
- Flushing the line

## WHEN TO CALL YOUR CHILD'S DOCTOR OR NURSE

There are some problems that can occur with CVCs. It is important that you understand what these problems might be and how to take care of them. Most can be corrected if noticed early enough.

### Infection
Sometimes the line or site can become infected. Call immediately if you notice:

- Redness, swelling, drainage, or pain at the catheter site
- Increased tiredness or irritability
- Fever >100°F
- Shaking chills

### Breakage
The line is made from a strong rubber kind of material, and it is made to stretch with movement. However, it could break. If you see the line is broken, clamp the line between your child's body and the break. Wrap the broken end with sterile gauze. Call your child's doctor or nurse right away.

### Clotting
The line tip could become blocked with a blood clot. If you are not able to inject the heparin flush easily, the line could be blocked. *Stop* trying to inject the heparin, and call your child's doctor or nurse right away.

### Infiltration
The line could slip out of the vein into the nearby tissue. If this happens, the area near the line will swell during an IV infusion. *Stop the infusion.* Do not give a heparin flush. Call your child's doctor or nurse right away.

### Dislodgement
The line could slip out of the body completely. If this happens, there will be some bleeding at the site. Cover the site with sterile gauze. Apply light pressure with the sterile gauze until the bleeding stops. Call your child's doctor or nurse right away.

### Air Embolism

When removing or replacing the line cap, it is extremely important to clamp the line. This prevents air from entering the vein. This is called an embolism. If a large amount of air gets into the vein, strong chest pains will result. Your child may also have trouble breathing. *Clamp the line right away if you notice these symptoms.* Lay your child on his or her left side to help prevent the air from moving further into the vein. *Call for emergency help right away.*

### IMPORTANT TIPS

- If your child is not able to hold still while you care for the line, have someone help you.
- It is *very important* to keep the line clean to prevent infection. Follow all instructions carefully to help prevent infection.
- Always wash your hands thoroughly before touching the line. It is not only soap but also the *scrubbing* action that cleans your hands well. Proper handwashing is very important in preventing infection. Using sterile technique will also help prevent infection.
- The skin around the line must be cleaned and the sterile dressing changed every 7 days or whenever it becomes wet, soiled, or loose.
- The line cap must be cleaned well with alcohol each time before using it.
- Sponge bathe your child for the first 7–10 days after the CVC is placed. Then baths and showers may continue as usual. Cover the line and dressing with either a larger second layer of transparent dressing, or a plastic wrap (such as Saran Wrap) around the chest. Right after bathing, apply a new line dressing.
- Swimming is not permitted while the line is in place. Swimming could result in an infection because of germs in the water.
- It is important to give the NS and heparin flushes as ordered to help prevent a clot.
- Secure the line so it does not stretch and pull.

## APPENDIX 8: HOME CARE INSTRUCTIONS FOR CHANGING THE CENTRAL VENOUS CATHETER CAP*

Your child's CVC has a cap at the end which protects it from leakage and germ or air entry. It is used to insert medications and fluids your child may need. The cap is also used for routine flushes that keep the CVC from getting blocked. The cap should be changed every 4 days or on Monday and Thursday.

### PREPARATION

1. Prepare a clean work surface by wiping it with rubbing alcohol. For wood surfaces, put down a clean towel.
2. Gather the following items:
   - mask
   - new CVC cap(s)
   - syringe(s) filled with saline
   - two alcohol pads
   - two packages of sterile gauze pads
   - nonsterile gloves (optional)
   - 1 in. wide cloth tape
   - trash bucket

---

* Children's Hospital Boston.

3. Put on mask.
4. Wash your hands with liquid soap and water. Dry your hands with paper towels and turn off the faucet with a paper towel. Proper handwashing is very important in preventing infection. Using sterile technique will also help prevent infection.

## Steps

1. Tell your child what you will be doing. If your child is not able to hold still, have someone help you.
2. Open the new CVC cap package(s). Keep the protective end cover(s) on.
3. Prime (or fill) the cap with saline.
4. Open the packages of sterile gauze pads. Leave the pads on the inside of the package.
5. Open the alcohol pads and place one on each gauze pad (see Figure). Touch only 1 corner of the alcohol pad.
6. Check the CVC clamp(s) to be sure it is closed.

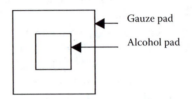

Gauze pad

Alcohol pad

7. If you are using gloves, put them on.
8. Pick up the gauze pad with an alcohol pad on top. Lay the CVC onto the pads.
9. Scrub the connection where the cap meets the CVC hub site with the alcohol pad for at least 15 seconds before removing cap.
10. Remove the old cap and discard. Scrub the CVC hub site with the alcohol pad for at least 15 seconds. Be careful not to touch the CVC hub site or to allow the CVC to rest on your child's body.
11. Remove the protective end cover from the new cap and screw it onto the CVC hub site.
12. If your child has a CVC with two lumens, repeat steps 8 through 12 for the second cap.
13. Discard the old CVC cap(s) in a sharps container. Throw the rest of supplies into a trash bucket.
14. Ask your nurse to show you how to secure the catheter with tape so they do not tug.
15. Wash your hands.

## Important Tips

- Always clamp the CVC whenever you remove the cap.
- Always wash your hands before and after changing the cap.
- If you think you may have touched the end of the new cap, throw it away and get a new one.

## When to Call Your Child's Doctor or Nurse

Call if:
- The CVC hub site is cracked or damaged.
- You cannot remove the old CVC cap.
- Your child has a fever >100° degrees.
- You have any questions or concerns.

## REFERENCES

1. Hertzog, D. R. and Waybill, P. N. Complications and controversies associated with PICCs. *J Infus Nurs* 2008;31:159–163.
2. ASPEN Board of Directors and the Clinical Guidelines Task Force Guidelines for the use of parenteral and enteral nutrition in adult and pediatric patients. *JPEN* 2002;26:1SA–138SA.
3. O'Grady, N. P., Alexander, M., Dellinger, E. P. et al. Guidelines for the prevention of intravascular catheter-related infections. *Infect Control Hosp Epidemiol* 2002;23:759–769.
4. Gilles, D., Carr, D., Frost, J. et al. Gauze and tape and transparent polyurethane dressings for central venous catheters. *The Cochrane Library* 2010;5:1–23.
5. Gordon, K. and Dearmun, A. K. Occlusion problems in central venous catheters: The child and family perspective. *J Child Health Care* 2003;7:55–69.
6. CHCA Clinical Improvement Collaborative: Reducing Central venous Catheter associated Bloodstream Infections–CHANGE PACKAGE. 2006.
7. Marschall, J., Mermel, L. A., Classen, D. et al. Strategies to prevent central line-associated bloodstream infections in acute care hospitals. *Infect Control Hosp Epidemiol* 2008;29:S22–S30.
8. Schmid, M. W. Risks and complications of peripheral and centrally inserted intravenous catheters. *Crit Care Nurs Clin North Am* 2000;12:165–174.
9. East, D. and Jacoby, K. The effect of a nursing staff education program on compliance with central line care policy in the cardiac intensive care unit. *Pediatr Nurs* 2005;31:182–184, 194.
10. Perucca, R. Infusion monitoring and catheter care. In: Hankins, J., Lonsway, R. A., Hedrick, C., and Perdue, M. B. editos. *Infusion Therapy in Clinical Practice*. St. Louis, MO: Saunders, 2001; pp. 389–397.
11. Kelly, L. J. The care of vascular access devices in the community. *Br J Community Nurs* 2008;13:198–205.
12. Othersen, H. B., Glenn, J., and Chessman, K. H. Central lines in parenteral nutrition. In: Baker, S., Baker, R., and Davis, A. editors. *Pediatric Parenteral Nutrition*. 2nd ed. New York, NY: Chapman & Hall, 2007;pp. 331–346.
13. Gorski, L., Perucca, R., and Hunter, R. Central venous access devices: Care, maintenance, and potential complications. In: Alexander, M., Corrigan, A., Gorski, L., Gorski, L., Hankins, J., and Perucca R. (eds.), *Infusion Nursing—An Evidence-Based Approach*, 3rd ed., St. Louis, MO: Saunders Elsevier, 2010; pp. 495–515.
14. Hadaway, L. C. Infusion therapy equipment. In: Alexander, M., Corrigan, A., Gorski, L., Gorski, L., Hankins, J., and Perucca, R., eds. *Infusion Nursing—An Evidence-Based Approach*, 3rd ed., St. Louis, MO: Saunders Elsevier, 2010; pp. 391–436.
15. Infusion Nurses Society. Infusion nurses standards of practice. *J Infus Nurs* 2006;29:S1–S92.
16. Children's Hospital Boston Central Venous Catheters. *Patient Care Manual* 2009.
17. Mermel, L. A. Prevention of intravascular catheter-related infections. *Ann Intern Med* 2000;32:391–402.
18. Timsit, J. F., Schwebel, C., Bouadma, L. et al. Chlorhexidine-impregnated sponges and less frequent dressing changes for prevention of catheter-related infections in critically ill adults: A randomized controlled trial. *JAMA* 2009;301(12):1231–1241.
19. Levy, I., Katz, J., Solter, E., Samra, Z., Vidne, B., Birk, E., Ashkenazi, S. and Dagan, O. Chlorhexidine-impregnated dressing for prevention of colonization of central venous catheters in infants and children: A randomized controlled trial. *Pediatr Infect Dis J* 2005;24:676–679.
20. Moreau, N. L. Are your skin-prep and catheter maintenance techniques up-to-date? *Nursing* 2009;39:15–16.
21. McMahon, D. D. Evaluating new technology to improve patient outcomes. *J Infus Nurs* 2002;25:250–255.
22. McGoldrick, M. Infection prevention and control. In: Alexander, M., Corrigan, A., Gorski, L., Gorski, L., Hankins. J. and Perucca, R. (eds.), *Infusion Nursing—An Evidence-Based Approach*, 3rd ed., St. Louis, MO: Saunders Elsevier, 2010; pp. 204–228.
23. Hamilton, H. Complications associated with venous access devices: Part two. *Nurs Stand* 2006;20:59–65.
24. Frey, A. M. Infusion therapy in children. In: Alexander, M., Corrigan, A., Gorski, L., Gorski, L., Hankins, J. and Perucca, R. (eds.), *Infusion Nursing—An Evidence-Based Approach*, 3rd ed., St. Louis, MO: Saunders Elsevier, 2010; pp. 550–569.
25. Hadaway, L. Technology of flushing vascular access devices. *J Infus Nurs* 2006;29:137–145.
26. Gilles, D., Wallen, M. M., Morrison, A. L. et al. Optimal timing for intravenous administration set replacement. *The Cochrane Library* 2009;2:1–78.
27. Ball, P. A. Intravenous in-line filters: Filtering the evidence. *Curr Opin Clin Nutr Metab Care* 2003;6:319–325.

28. McKinnon, B. T. FDA safety alert: Hazards of precipitation associated with parenteral nutrition. *Nutr Clin Pract* 1996;11:59–65. Erratum in: *Nutr Clin Pract* 1996;11:120.

29. Task Force for the Revision of Safe Practices for Parenteral Nutrition. Safe practices for parenteral nutrition *JPEN* 2004;28:S39–S70.

30. Bowe-Geddes, L. and Nichols, H. A. An overview of peripherally inserted central catheters. *Top Adv Pract Nurs eJ* 2005;5(3). http://currentnursing.com/research/topics_in_advanced_practice_nurs.htm. Accessed August 2, 2010.

31. Sauerland, C., Engelking, C., Wickham, R., and Corbi, C. Vesicant extravasation part 1: Mechanisms, pathogenesis and nursing care to reduce risk. *Oncol Nurs Forum* 2006;33:1134–1141.

32. George, D. E. *Challenges in Pediatric Nutritional Support [PowerPoint Slides]*. Retrieved from http://www.oley.org/documents/Presentations_for_Web/George%20TPN%20PEDs%2009.pdf. Accessed June 27, 2010.

33. Sadlier, C. Intestinal failure and long-term parenteral nutrition in children. *Paediatr Nurs* 2008;20:37–48.

34. Kumpf, V. J. *Safe Practices for Sustaining Yourself on Home Parenteral Nutrition (HPN) [PowerPoint Slides]*. Retrieved from http://www.oley.org/documents/Presentations_for_Web/Kumpf%20Safe%20Practices%20for%20HPN_Oley.pdf. Accessed June 27, 2010.

# 27 Medication Administration in the Enterally Fed Patient

*Mark G. Klang*

## CONTENTS

## 27.1 INTRODUCTION

Medication administration through feeding tubes provides a unique challenge to the caregiver. Patients who require nutrition administered through a feeding tube are less likely to tolerate drugs administered orally. Usually, their medications must be administered by the same route as the nutrition support. Often drugs must be compounded to a specific formulation to allow for feeding tube administration. Few drugs have specific guidelines in their package insert. Even fewer have been studied for the success of that formulation administered through a feeding tube. In most cases the administration of drugs via a feeding tube is a not a Food & Drug Administration-approved route of administration.

To prepare and administer an oral drug through a feeding tube requires considerable knowledge of the drug, its oral formulation, solubility, and release kinetics to ensure that the drug will have its intended effect.

## 27.2 OVERVIEW OF FEEDING TUBES

Feeding tubes are inserted to provide nutrition to patients who cannot obtain sufficient nutrients orally. Some feeding tubes are inserted through the nose (nasal) [i.e., nasogastric tube (NGT), nasojejunal tube (NJT)], or the tube is inserted directly through the abdominal wall using either a surgical [i.e., gastric tube (GT), jejunal tube (JT)], or an endoscopic approach [i.e., percutaneous endoscopically placed gastric tube (PEG), or percutaneous endoscopically placed (PEJ) tube]. The distal site is most often in the stomach and to a lesser extent in the jejunum. Some rarer distal sites include the duodenum or the ileum. Chapter 13 discusses the different types of enteral feeding tubes in greater detail.

## 27.3  MINIMIZING FEEDING TUBE OCCLUSIONS

The maintenance of feeding tube flow is crucial to the care of the patient. Strict procedures to avoid clog formation are needed to maintain consistent nutrition. To avoid clog formation, the tube should be rinsed frequently with water since interactions are minimized in diluted environments. Clogs that are formula based are caused by poorly dissolved solids or a reaction of intact protein with stomach acid. A powdered formula requires ample mixing with sufficient fluid to minimize clog formation. Finely crushed medication fragments can also form clogs when insufficiently mixed with water prior to administration.

To minimize clog formation, the feeding tube should be rinsed often with water. The importance of rinsing the feeding tube with water cannot be overemphasized as a preventive measure to minimize the occurrence of clog formation. All powders and medications need to be thoroughly dissolved in water prior to administration. With some medications, making a slurry is insufficient to ensure appropriate drug delivery.

In the adult patient, the rate of administration for gastric nutrition administration should exceed 50 mL/h so as to reduce retrograde clogging of the feeding tube. Slower administration will allow migration of stomach acid along the slower flowing feeding-tube walls. This laminar flow of gastric acid up the tube will eventually lead to clog formation [1]. Clogs can also be caused by the reaction of an acidic medication syrup with the intact proteins contained in the enteral nutrition formula [2]. Liquid medications directly combined with enteral formulas lead to increased thickening of the liquid (Table 27.1) [2].

## 27.4  INTOLERANCE OF MEDICATIONS ADMINISTERED THROUGH FEEDING TUBES

Tube-fed patients are uniquely sensitive to concentrated medications with high osmolarity. Most liquid medications have an osmolarity of >1000 mOsm/L [3]. The tolerable osmolarity of the gastrointestinal (GI) tract is about 285 mOsm/L (Table 27.2). The larger the volume of a dose, the more is the water needed to dilute the dose to a tolerable level [4]. The following formula can be used to determine the amount of water needed for a medication to be diluted:

$$\frac{\text{mOsm of liquid med}}{\text{desired mOsm (285)}} \times \text{volume} = \text{final volume}$$

**TABLE 27.1**

**Examples of Acidic Liquid Medications Prone to Interactions with Enteral Formulas**

| Product Name | Manufacturer | pH Value |
|---|---|---|
| Lomotil liquid | Searle | 3.3 |
| Robitussin expectorant | A.H. Robbins | 2.6 |
| Sudafed syrup | Burroughs-Welcome | 2.5 |
| Feosol elixir | Menley James | 3.3 |
| Neo-calglucon syrup | Dorsey | 4.0 |
| Klorvess syrup | Dorsey | 2.4 |

---

**TABLE 27.2**

**Examples of Osmolalities of Commonly Used Liquid Medications**

| Product Name | mOsm/kg |
|---|---|
| Digoxin concentrate | 3865 |
| Theophylline elixir | 4500 |
| Phenytoin suspension | 1725 |
| Phenytoin injection | 9120 |
| Furosemide liquid | 3375 |

---

For example, theophylline elixir (80 mg/15 mL) has an osmolarity of 4500 mOsm/L. Using the aforementioned formula, to calculate the dilution needed for a single adult dose of 200 mg (12.5 mL of elixir):

$$\frac{4500 \text{ mOsm of liquid med}}{\text{desired mOsm } (285)} \times 12.5 \text{ mL volume} = 197 \text{ mL: final volume}$$

Administration to the stomach allows the residual volume (200–500 mL) to help neutralize the high osmolarity of the liquid medication. Administration to the lower GI tract (jejunum) does not afford this protection. The jejunum has no residual fluid capacity. The administration of concentrated liquids will cause the bowel to react providing adequate dilution with an associative cramping. This action is known clinically as osmotic diarrhea. To determine if a patient is experiencing a concentrate-induced osmotic diarrhea (as opposed to other causes), the stool osmotic gap can be calculated [5]:

$$\text{Stool osmotic gap} = \text{Stool osmolality} - 2 \times (\text{stool Na} + \text{stool K})$$

(Normal fecal fluid values: Osmolality: ~290 mOsm/kg; Na+ : ~30 mmol/L; K+ : ~75 mmol/L.)

A stool osmotic gap >100 mOsm/kg is indicative of the osmotic laxative effect.

Inert ingredients present in a medication's formulation can often be problematic in the tube-fed patient. Sorbitol is a sweetener added to many liquid medications. Sorbitol is effective in dissolving many poorly water-soluble drugs. It is of the class referred to as Generally Recognized as Safe group of excipients. Sorbitol is also active as a cathartic, being more potent than lactulose, which is used specifically for that indication. As an excipient, manufacturers are not required to note the amount of sorbitol present on the labeling or in the package insert. To get this information, the manufacturer must be contacted with a specific lot number. To further complicate matters, generic products can contain sorbitol, while the original trade name product may not. In one case, a generic form of the antidiarrheal agent, Lomotil (diphenoxylate) actually caused diarrhea due to its high sorbitol content [6]. Despite this, the generic product's manufacturer (Roxanne) continued to use sorbitol as a vehicle for its formulation of diphenoxylate liquid. Manufacturers may also change the amount of sorbitol present in their products between different lots without noting it on the product label. Table 27.3 describes the key points associated with the sorbitol content in liquid medications.

## 27.5 DRUGS THAT SHOULD NOT BE CRUSHED

Solid medications (tablets and capsules) cannot be administered directly through a feeding tube. It is important to be familiar with which tablets can be crushed and which capsules can be opened.

**TABLE 27.3**

**Sorbitol Memory Tool**

**Characteristics Commonly Associated with Sorbitol-Containing Medications**

Sticky—it is a sugar

Osmolarity—causes diarrhea

Reproducible—NOT, content changes often

Bloated feeling—causes gas

Ignites—cauterizes diabetic bowel

Theophylline—contains the most sorbital

Obscure—amount not on label

Liquids—present in most liquid medications

Dosage formulations that should not be crushed include enteric-coated and extended-release medications [7]. These products, when crushed, will release the entire dose quickly, possibly producing toxic effects (Table 27.4). Table 27.5 lists common examples of medications that should not be crushed.

Enteric coating on a tablet medication provides a film protection from the stomach acid and reduces hydrolysis in water-sensitive solid medications. Combining the coated medication with water will activate the surface to become sticky and adhere to other tablets. These coated tablets require additional fluid to ensure that they are fully dissolved prior to administration. Some coatings

**TABLE 27.4**

**Guidelines to Recognizing Medications That Should Not Be Crushed**

There are many tables available in the literature that provide lists of drugs that should not
be crushed. The following summarizes key points to determine whether or not a solid
dosage form should be crushed.

1. Extended, delayed, or controlled-release drugs can release the entire long-acting dose
   in a short time period. This release can cause more side effects since the immediate
   absorption can reach toxic levels. Drugs designed for immediate release are usually the
   best choice for feeding-tube administration.

2. Enteric-coated medications are generally considered inappropriate for feeding-tube
   administration since crushing the medication will expose the drug to degradation by the
   acid of the stomach. Another reason is that the enteric coating shards will form clogs,
   or react with water to form a paste. In some cases, there is no alternative route for the
   drug administration. For those setting concomitant sodium bicarbonate, administration
   can neutralize stomach acid, dissolve enteric coating, and reduce clog formation.

"Do not crush" tables are a good guide, but not always appropriate as a guide for
feeding-tube administration. Some important exceptions of drugs found on do not crush
lists, but can be administered through a feeding tube:

1. Drugs that have a bitter taste when crushed. (This does not apply to drugs that have
   irritant properties.)

2. Capsules that contain enteric-coated PPI-type medications (lansoprazole and
   omeprazole). These medications can be mixed with an acidic juice to be administered
   directly through a feeding tube.

3. Sublingual drugs. If the drug is absorbed under the tongue, (e.g., nitroglycerin), then
   the drug should not be administered through a feeding tube. Orally disintegrating
   tablets (ODTs) are also administered under the tongue, but is actually absorbed in the
   lower GI tract. These sublingual ODTs can be mixed with water and administered
   through a feeding tube into the stomach.

**TABLE 27.5**

**Examples of Medications That Should Not Be Crushed**

| Rationale for Not Crushing | Example |
|---|---|
| Anesthetizes local mucosa | Benzonatate (Tessalon Perles) |
| Bitter taste | Cefuroxime (Ceftin) |
| Enteric-coated | Bisacodyl (Dulcolax) |
| | Divalproex sodium (Depakote) |
| | Enteric-coated aspirin (Ecotrin) |
| | Lansoprazole (Prevacid) |
| | Omeprazole (Prilosec) |
| | Pancreatic enzymes (Pancrease) |
| Extended-release | Diltiazem controlled-dissolution (Cardizem CD) |
| | Divalproex sodium extended-release (Depakote ER) |
| | Fexofenadine/pseudoephedrine (Allegra-D) |
| | Mesalamine (Asacol, Pentasa) |
| | Oxybutynin extended-release (Ditropan XL) |
| | Propranolol long-acting (Inderal LA) |
| | Tamsulosin (Flomax) |
| | Verapamil sustained-release (Calan SR, Isoptin SR) |
| | Alendronate (Fosamax) |
| Irritating to mucosa | Atomoxetine (Strattera) |
| | Diflunisal (Dolobid) |
| | Isotretinoin (Accutane) |
| | Valproic acid (Depakene) |
| Safety | Finasteride (Proscar) |
| | Mycophenolate (Cellcept) |

are intended to protect the medication from the acidic degradation effects of stomach acid. The crushing of enteric-coated medications will allow exposure of acid-labile drug to stomach contents, resulting in drug degradation. In other cases (e.g., aspirin and bisacodyl) the coating acts to protect the gastric mucosa from the irritant effects of the drug. Removal of the coating will expose the GI tract to the direct irritating effects of the medication.

Generally, enteric-coated medications should not be administered through a feeding tube. A notable exception is proton-pump inhibitors (PPIs). These are all enteric coated to avoid stomach acid degradation. Sufficient literature that documents the safety and efficacy of exposing the coating to sodium bicarbonate solution to erode the coatings off [8] exists. This will result in some degradation, but sufficient PPI is delivered to the site of action to ensure that a clinical effect is achieved. Further, the continual administration of the PPI allows for a reduced stomach acid production and subsequent reduced acidic degradation.

## 27.6   FEEDING TUBE DYNAMICS

Long feeding tubes (NGT/NJT) have more bends and allow more potential for clog formation. These tubes generally have a smaller diameter than surgically placed tubes. The smaller diameter tubes (8–12 French) are better tolerated, but they clog easier when undissolved solids are administered. Surgically placed tubes (i.e., percutaneous, endoscopically placed gastrostomy and jejunostomy—PEG/PEJ) have a larger internal bore and are relatively short. These tubes generally clog less frequently than the small-bore NGT/NJT.

Aqueous liquid medication formulations can be grouped as solutions, suspensions, or slurries. Solutions are visually clear and the ingredients are fully dissolved in the aqueous phase. A drug in a solution will have a faster onset than a drug which must dissolve first in endogenous fluids such as simple syrups. A suspension is used when a drug exhibits low solubility in aqueous environment. A significant amount of liquid is usually needed to bring the solids in a suspension to become fully dissolved. This type of formulation has a suspending agent to increase viscosity and reduce precipitate formation. Suspending agents react with acids and/or nutrients to form clogs and sometimes limit dissolution. This is one theory why the phenytoin suspension has an interaction with an enteral formula.

A slurry is an extemporaneously mixed compound of a drug and water. There is no suspending agent involved, and the solids precipitate out readily upon standing.

Ideally, the solution formulation of a medication should be used when administering medications through a tube <8 French. Suspensions and slurries have a tendency to form clogs when administered with feeding tubes <10 French. To minimize this risk, suspensions and slurries should be diluted with additional water until all the particles are dissolved to reduce clog formation.

Not all liquid medications are suitable for administration via feeding tubes. Clarithromycin and ciprofloxacin suspensions have specialized liquid formulations that have produced clogs when administered through a feeding tube. These microcapsule formulations form obstructions within small-bore bending tubes. The tablet formulations of these two medications must be used; however, they do not crush easily. In order to safely administer these products through a tube, the crushed tablet fragments must first be dissolved in water.

Most feeding tubes are placed with distal site in the stomach. Medication administration via a GT has unique challenges. The acidic content reacts with the intact protein in the formula and congeals. This protein–acid complex will clog feeding tubes. Medications formulated as acidic liquids further contribute to an increased risk of clog formation. If the distal site of the tube is in the stomach, the principle issue is a reaction within the acid milieu. In some cases, the tube is placed past the pyloric sphincter and into the jejunum. The jejunum is acutely sensitive to osmolarity (as discussed above). The jejunum also has an increased pH value of ~7.0. Thus, drugs that are weak bases (e.g., diphenhydramine) will have poor absorption as they will not ionize in the basic environment.

Very few drugs are absorbed only in the stomach (e.g., itraconazole and $n$-acetylcysteine). To allow jejunal absorption, itraconazole can be dissolved in a weak acid (i.e., 0.1 N HCl) to enhance delivery. Other drugs will have reduced acidic degradation if administered directly into jejunum. Drugs that have a narrow therapeutic window (e.g., phenytoin, warfarin, and digoxin) should be monitored closely as there will be a change in extent of absorption when these drugs are administered directly into jejunum.

## 27.7  EXCIPIENTS

For any orally administered medication to be absorbed, the drug must first dissolve. Many excipients are added to enhance the dissolution process. For drugs that are highly water-soluble, the excipient content is minimal, but for the majority of physiologically active drugs, there is a degree of lipid solubility, making the use of these additives necessary. Excipients are added to oral formulations to enhance solubility, improve dissolution, reduce hydration, lubricate process machinery, add compression factors, fill space, neutralize acid release, reduce ultraviolet exposure, protect against acid or enzymatic degradation, provide timed release, improve taste/appearance, impart color, resist crushing, or enhance absorption.

Many products are not designed for administration via feeding tubes. There are significant differences between oral administration and administration of a medication through a feeding tube. Solid dosage formulations have coatings to reduce shelf degradation from moisture and to improve enteral passage through the alimentary tract. These coatings reduce surface tension to allow the drugs to slide down the throat when given with water. This coating, however, act as an adhesive with other tablets when mixed with a small amount of water. For example, adding a small amount of water to a bottle of coated aspirin will cause the tablets clump. Similarly, this phenomenon will happen when multiple drugs are crushed together for enteral administration. Medication administration through feeding tubes is a primary cause for clogged feeding tubes, often resulting in increased trauma to the patient due to replacement of the tube, as declogging enzymes are ineffective at restoring flow to drug-occluded feeding tubes [9]. Management of clogs produced by precipitated drugs requires continual flushing with water to restore patency. Stylets and mechanical cleaning devices have been used with some success; but pose a risk of perforation of both the tube and the patient. A shift in pH (acidic juice) may dislodge an accumulation of drug coatings, or the use of ethanol can disrupt a soap formation caused by salts reacting with oils, but these types of remedies require knowledge of the composition of the clog that resides generally near the distal tip of the catheter.

Tablets are formed by the compression of excipients combined with the active pharmaceutical ingredient. Various excipients are used in each tablet formulation to enhance the release, dissolution, and absorbance of the drug. Poorly water-soluble drugs are sometimes formulated with coprecipitates. Coprecipitates can include sugars, (e.g., mannitol, xylitol, and sorbitol) or proteins (e.g., albumin and povidone) [10]. These coprecipitates dissolve rapidly and stimulate the flux of the dissolved drug on the surface of poorly dissolving drug particles. The proximity of the drug and coprecipitate is crucial for dissolution. If the drug does not completely dissolve *in vitro*, it will have less opportunity to dissolve once administered. In some cases, crushing the medications will separate the dissolution enhancer from the active drug and thereby, reduce the amount of medication released.

Various forms of cellulose are added to attract water and cause the solid tablet to swell when exposed to acidic milieu of the stomach. The goal of the swelling is to disperse the API fragments into many smaller pieces. The rate dissolution is dependent on the size of the initial particle size. This is especially important in the case of poorly water-soluble drugs where the surface area exposure is proportional to the rate of dissolution. A minimum of 15 mL is needed for most tablet dissolution, but some tablets that swell may require as much as 60 mL to ensure full dispersion.

In theory, crushing the solid medication in a cup and mixing with water may allow for separation of drugs and excipients, thereby altering the delivery of the drug to the GI tract.

Itraconazole (Sporanox Janssen Pharmaceutica, Titusville, NJ) is available as an oral capsule filled with beads containing sugar and the active drug. Prior to the development of commercially available oral liquid formulation, compounding pharmacies prepared a suspension that was determined not to alter the stability of the active drug [11]. Assays for blood values were conducted on patients receiving this suspension, however, suggested otherwise. Patients had no measurable blood levels of itraconazole, indicating that none had been absorbed. Although the drug was stable in the solution, it could not be absorbed when prepared as a liquid formulation [12]. Janssen Pharmaceutica manufactured the capsule formulation by spraying the sugar granules with a fine coating of itraconazole. When the sugars dissolved, the diffusion would carry the active drug from the matrix and enhance both its dissolution and absorption [8]. Mixing this drug in water allowed the sugar to dissolve and the active drug to settle to the base. Aprepitant (Emend, Merck Research Laboratories, West Point, PA) is another example of a drug formulated as sugar beads. It is not clear if extemporaneous compounding of this medication will result in a similar lack of absorption. One remedy to avoid potential administration concerns is to add the drug to a syringe and then add water to dissolve the contents. The entire contents of the syringe could then be administered through the feeding tube. Problems still can occur even with the technique, however. Patients requiring only a partial dose may not get the exact dose ordered and, due to stability issues, the leftover unused syringe contents cannot be saved for future doses.

Crushing solid dosage forms can be laborious and problematic. The classic mortar and pestle is poorly suited for rigid coated tablets and usually results in much of the drug becoming displaced outside the mortar. These devices must be cleaned between uses to avoid contamination of the next drug with the previous one crushed. Some tablet crushers will keep the drug more contained in packets, but the glassine envelopes can become pierced by shards of poorly crushed tablets. Additional precautions are needed when crushing oral chemotherapy for feeding-tube administration. One method to avoid exposure is to place the antineoplastic tablet in an oral syringe and add water to dissolve the solid. This technique will reduce the possibility of operator exposure to the hazardous powder that is aerosolized whenever an open-container tablet-crushing device is used.

## 27.8 ABSORPTION OF MEDICATIONS ADMINISTERED THROUGH FEEDING TUBES

Some drugs degrade in the acidic contents of the stomach. For example, the antibiotic, ciprofloxacin, is absorbed to a higher degree in the lower GI tract than in the stomach due to extensive degradation in the stomach fluid. The site of the distal port of the feeding tube will alter the degree of drug delivery (Table 27.6). A suspension formulation allows for the delivery of the solid form of a poorly aqueous soluble powder. Suspensions are generally viscous to keep the drug uniformly dispersed such that dosing will be more accurate. Dilution of suspension will allow the maximal release of . drug. Initial dilution, however, will reduce the suspending agent's capacity to keep the drug uniform, so care is needed to dilute until the solid is thoroughly dissolved.

## 27.9 MEDICATION MYTHS: HOLDING NUTRITION FOR 2 H BEFORE AND AFTER A DOSE

To enhance solubility of a poorly soluble drug, the viscosity of the environment must be reduced. If it is a suspension, it must be further diluted so as to remove the interfering agents. For example, phenytoin is a poorly soluble medication in the GI milieu [13]. Moreover, its suspension form is very viscous. Reports involving the original formulation demonstrated that the drug settled over time and required shaking the container before each dose to ensure uniform delivery of all doses in a bottle [14]. The suspension was reformulated to ensure uniformity, although a shaking before use is still recommended.

### 27.9.1 PHENYTOIN–ENTERAL NUTRITION INTERACTION

Reports involving the interaction of enteral nutrition and phenytoin were first reported by Bauer [15] who was monitoring neurology patients who recently had feeding tubes inserted. These patients had been initially stabilized on the oral capsule formulation of phenytoin. Serum values at the time were within the normal range. After feeding tube initiation, they were switched to the suspension form of phenytoin. The patients were also started on continuous enteral feedings given through the same tube as that used for medication administration. Upon reexamination of the phenytoin serum levels, the tests showed a 10-fold decrease for all 12 patients [15].

Bauer et al. [16] recognized that phenytoin is strongly protein bound (about 90%) and that the enteral formula contained intact proteins. The authors speculated that the phenytoin was binding to the nutrition and not getting absorbed. They also noted that patients receiving enteral nutrition were

## TABLE 27.6
## Gastric or Jejunal Medication Administration: Factors for Consideration

| Issue | Gastric | Jejunal |
|---|---|---|
| pH Values | The pH is usually 1–2, but after PPI or antacid use, the pH can be as high as 4 | The pH values are more basic, about 6–7 |
| Residual volume | 500 to <25 mL highly variable, and not always does the higher volume reflect intolerance to tube-feeding | <10 mL |

prone to faster intestinal transit time. With the drug now bound to the nutrition, a patient with active diarrhea would have little opportunity to absorb the slowly absorbing phenytoin. Bauer et al. held nutrition for 2 h before and after drug administration to ensure that the medication would not come into direct contact with the proteins present in the enteral formula that could reduce the amount of drug absorbed. Interestingly, this intervention did not solve the problem. In some patients, the dose had to be increased from the usual dose of 300 mg/day to 1800–1600 mg/day despite the enteral feeding being held. It is not clear from this study why they selected 2 h before and after drug administration, given that phenytoin is typically administered 3–4 times a day. This practice results in 8 h of each day when no nutrition can be administered.

Generally, after 1 h, 65% of a liquid meal has left the stomach. After 2 h, <10% remains. From Kruger's [17] study also evaluating phenytoin absorption, there was no interaction when the drug was separated from the feedings by 1 h. Direct contact of the concentrated drug with the nutrient appears to be the rate limiting factor and not the act of withholding of nutrition for 4 h around each dose. Bauer et al. [18] erroneously assumed the faster transit time occurred in all enterally fed patients. Not all tube-fed patients, however, experience enhanced transit time. In the authors' defense, at the time of the original report, there was an indeed increased incidence of enhanced transit but it was due to the excipients found in liquid medications. These high-osmolarity drugs were responsible for 40% of the cases of diarrhea that had been previously attributed to the enteral nutrition [19].

Since the publication of these papers, Au Yeung and Ensom [20] reviewed all the studies involving phenytoin. There were four single-dose randomized control studies that failed to demonstrate any food interaction with phenytoin. But 23 other studies demonstrated a significant decrease in anticipated serum phenytoin values. These controlled studies allowed for adequate dissolution of the drug prior to administration, unlike the others that did not include any mention of dilution or dissolution of the drug. Possibly prediluting the suspension prior to administration down the feeding tube contributed to the lack of an interaction.

## 27.9.2 CIPROFLOXACIN

There have been reports that it is necessary to hold the enteral feeding when administering fluoroquinolones. Wright et al. showed that when he combined nutrition with the concentrated antibiotic, the loss of drug was about 83% [21]. Nyffeler [22] conducted a review of all the studies that discussed the interaction of ciprofloxacin and enteral nutrition. Interestingly, he discounted the studies that failed to note an interaction occurring [23–26]. A recurrent practice, in each of these studies, was that the drug was dissolved in water before administration. The studies that allowed the drug to be directly mixed with the enteral nutrition showed significant reduction in available ciprofloxacin [27–29]. This concept has since been supported by research conducted at the Sloan-Kettering Institute that demonstrates improved dissolution of the ciprofloxacin when the drug is diluted prior to mixing with enteral nutrition [30].

These aforementioned examples typify a general concept that applies to all drug therapy: a drug medication must be dissolved first in order to be adequately absorbed. When considering an issue with drugs that demonstrate poor aqueous solubility, reduce the viscosity of the mixture and increase the volume with water to improve absorption. This concept becomes especially important when considering the absorption of phenytoin and ciprofloxacin.

## 27.10  PROTEIN BINDING

Another myth initiated by the Bauer reports of phenytoin's lack of absorption is that a medication that is strongly protein bound will adhere to the nutrition and fail to be absorbed. There is no evidence-based literature that supports this concept. If anything, the goal of giving nutrition is the assumption that it will be absorbed. Hence anything that is attached to the protein will follow the same pathway. Further, the attachment of protein to the phenytoin actually enhances the dissolution rate [31].

### 27.10.1 WARFARIN CONSIDERATIONS

Patients receiving warfarin have been documented to experience a reduced anticoagulant response when it is administered via a feeding tube. Efforts have been made to reduce vitamin K content, due to the misconception that was the cause of the interaction [32]. Subsequently, Kuhn et al. [33] conducted an *in vitro* study that showed that warfarin adheres to the protein in the enteral nutrition. The model they used, however, was flawed as it utilized the dissolution bath with a pH value of 8. Nowhere in human GI tract is there a pH value of 8.0 [34]. Nevertheless, the authors advised holding nutrition to avoid this interaction. Dickerson et al. [35] conducted a study on warfarin using the premise that holding nutrition would improve warfarin activity. In this study, the investigators showed improved effect of warfarin in the group that had their nutrition held. But there were several limitations of the study. There were only six patients studied using three different formulas. The amount of vitamin K was significantly different between the two groups. It is not clear that the effect seen in this study was solely due to holding the nutrition to administer the warfarin or due to differences in the composition of the enteral formulas.

There are several factors that may contribute to these conflicting findings. Warfarin is very difficult to work with in a laboratory setting. It adheres to plastic tubing and filters [36]. This binding effect is strongest at acidic pH and weaker as pH values increase. This concept, however, has not been studied clinically. If warfarin is indeed binding to the feeding tube, there is no rationale to support holding the nutrition formula. A consistent method of medication administration is the most important factor.

## 27.11 OTHER CONSIDERATIONS: COMPUTER PHYSICIAN ORDER ENTRY

Physician computer order entry systems are often not geared to specialized routes of medication administration. An internal audit at a major cancer hospital showed that 43% of the medication orders specific for feeding-tube administration were written as "p.o." indicating to be given by mouth [37]. The instructions to give the medications through the feeding tube was either verbally transmitted to the nurse or, since there were no other options, simply understood by the nurse administering the drug. The pharmacists receiving the order would not know of the special administration considerations for a tube-fed patient unless they were actively monitoring the patient. In this scenario, without program enhancements, several drugs that were inappropriate for feeding-tube administration could be given without pharmacist intervention [38]. Computer-generated order entry systems typically block specialized routes of administration that do not appear in the software's list of approved routes of administration. The institution's support staff must create a unique route for each drug and dosage form to ensure that the prescriber and the nurse receive the necessary drug administration alerts.

## 27.12 CONCLUSION

Medication administration via an enteral feeding tube presents a unique set of challenges, especially to the patient with intestinal failure. It should not be confused with the oral route of administration and practices designed for that route should not be automatically extrapolated for the tube-fed patient. Pharmacokinetic properties, dosage formulations, and the site of administration must be taken into consideration. Excipients such as sorbitol should be minimized and therapeutic alternatives or different routes of administration might be necessary. Regardless of the approach used, consistency is key so as to avoid fluctuations in drug response.

## REFERENCES

 1. Hofstetter J, Allen LV, Jr. Causes of non-medication-induced nasogastric tube occlusion. *Am J Hosp Pharm* 1992;49(3):603–607.

2. Cutie AJ, Altman E, Lenkel L. Compatibility of enteral products with commonly employed drug additives. *JPEN* 1983;7(2):186–191.
3. Thompson WG. A strategy for management of the irritable bowel. *Am J Gastroenterol* 1986;81(2):95–100.
4. Estoup M. Approaches and limitations of medication delivery in patients with enteral feeding tubes. *Crit Care Nurse* 1994;14(1):68–72, 77.
5. Duncan A, Robertson C, Russell RI. The fecal osmotic gap: Technical aspects regarding its calculation. *J LabClin Med* 1992;119(4):359–363.
6. Kochevar ME. New York, 2006 [personal communication].
7. Mitchell JF. Oral dosage forms that should not be crushed. (PDF). 2009; http://www.ismp.org/tools/donotcrush.pdf. Accessed September 26, 2009.
8. Woods DJ, McClintock AD. Omeprazole administration. *Ann Pharmacother* 1993;27(5):651.
9. Frankel EH, Enow NB, Jackson KC, II, Kloiber LL. Methods of restoring patency to occluded feeding tubes. *Nutr Clin Pract* June 1, 1998;13(3):129–131.
10. Strickley RG. Solubilizing excipients in oral and injectable formulations. *Pharm Res* 2004;21(2):201–230.
11. Jacobson PA, Johnson CE, Walters JR. Stability of itraconazole in an extemporaneously compounded oral liquid. *Am J Health Syst Pharm* 1995;52(2):189–191.
12. Christensen KJ, Gubbins PO, Gurley BJ, Bowman JL, Buice RG. Relative bioavailability of itraconazole from an extemporaneously prepared suspension and from the marketed capsules. *Am J Health Syst Pharm* 1998;55(3):261–265.
13. Albert KS, Sakmar E, Hallmark MR, Weidler DJ, Wagner JG. Bioavailability of diphenylhydantoin. *Clin Pharmacol Ther* 1974;16(4):727–735.
14. Newton DW, Kluza RB. Prediction of phenytoin solubility in intravenous admixtures: Physicochemical theory. *Am J Hosp Pharm* 1980;37(12):1647–1651.
15. Bauer LA. Interference of oral phenytoin absorption by continuous nasogastric feedings. *Neurology* 1982;32(5):570–572.
16. Bauer LA, Edwards WA, Dellinger EP, Raisys VA, Brennan C. Importance of unbound phenytoin serum levels in head trauma patients. *J Trauma* 1983;23(12):1058–1060.
17. Krueger HA Garnett WR, Comstock TJ, Fitzsimmons WE, Karnes HT, Pellock JM. Effect of two administration schedules of an enteral nutrition formula on phenytoin bioavailability. *Epilepsia* 1987;28(6):706–712.
18. Bauer L. New York, 2005 [personal communication].
19. Edes TE, Walk BE, Austin JL. Diarrhea in tube-fed patients: Feeding formula not necessarily the cause. *Am J Med* 1990;88(2):91–93.
20. Au Yeung SC, Ensom MH. Phenytoin and enteral feedings: Does evidence support an interaction? *Ann Pharmacother* 2000;34(7–8):896–905.
21. Wright DH, Pietz SL, Konstantinides FN, Rotschafer JC. Decreased *in vitro* fluoroquinolone concentrations after admixture with an enteral feeding formulation. *JPEN* 2000;24(1):42–48.
22. Nyffeler MS. Ciprofloxacin use in the enterally fed patient. *Nutr Clin Pract* 1999;14(2):73–77.
23. Yuk JH, Nightingale CH, Quintiliani R et al. Absorption of ciprofloxacin administered through a nasogastric or a nasoduodenal tube in volunteers and patients receiving enteral nutrition. *Diagn Microbiol Infect Dis* 1990;13(2):99–102.
24. Yuk JH, Nightingale CH, Sweeney KR, Quintiliani R, Lettieri JT, Frost RW. Relative bioavailability in healthy volunteers of ciprofloxacin administered through a nasogastric tube with and without enteral feeding. *Antimicrob Agents Chemother* 1989;33(7):1118–1120.
25. de Marie S, VandenBergh MF, Buijk SL et al. Bioavailability of ciprofloxacin after multiple enteral and intravenous doses in ICU patients with severe gram-negative intra-abdominal infections. *Intensive Care Med* 1998;24(4):343–346.
26. Cohn SM, Sawyer MD, Burns GA, Tolomeo C, Milner KA. Enteric absorption of ciprofloxacin during tube feeding in the critically ill. *J Antimicrob Chemother* 1996;38(5):871–876.
27. Piccolo ML, Toossi Z, Goldman M. Effect of coadministration of a nutritional supplement on ciprofloxacin absorption. *Am J Hosp Pharm* 1994;51(21):2697–2699.
28. Healy DP, Brodbeck MC, Clendening CE. Ciprofloxacin absorption is impaired in patients given enteral feedings orally and via gastrostomy and jejunostomy tubes. *Antimicrob Agents Chemother* 1996;40(1):6–10.
29. Mueller BA, Brierton DG, Abel SR, Bowman L. Effect of enteral feeding with ensure on oral bioavailabilities of ofloxacin and ciprofloxacin. *Antimicrob Agents Chemother* 1994;38(9):2101–2105.

30. Klang MG. Influence of enteral formula on ciprofloxacin suspension dissolution. *Nutr Clin Pract* February 2006:21;106–107 P-626-NW.
31. Klang M. Phenytoin binding to enteral formulas in an equilibrium dialysis model as analyzed using HPLC. *J Parenter Enteral Nutr* 2005;29(1):04-P-450-NW.
32. Martin JE, Lutomski DM. Warfarin resistance and enteral feedings. *JPEN J Parenter Enteral Nutr* 1989;13(2):206–208.
33. Kuhn TA, Garnett WR, Wells BK, Karnes HT. Recovery of warfarin from an enteral nutrient formula. *Am J Hosp Pharm* 1989;46(7):1395–1399.
34. Kitagawa K, Nishigori A, Murata, N., Nishimoto, K., Takada, H. Radiotelemetry of the pH of the gastro-intestinal tract by glass electrode. *Gastroenterology* 1966;51(3):368–372.
35. Dickerson RN, Garmon WM, Kuhl DA, Minard G, Brown RO. Vitamin K-independent warfarin resis-tance after concurrent administration of warfarin and continuous enteral nutrition. *Pharmacotherapy* 2008;28(3):308–313.
36. Illum L BH. Sorption of drugs by plastic infusion bags. *Int J Pharm* 1982;10:339–351.
37. Klang M. Issues for the pharmacist monitoring medications administered through a feeding tube. *NY State J Hosp Pharm* 1994;13(4):81–84.
38. Shenderov F, Klang M, Schattner M, Chan A, Lai C, Muller R, Siena G et al. Medication administration in patients with enteral feeding tubes. *Nutr Clin Pract* 2009;24(2):Poster.

# Part V

*Emerging Diagnostic and Therapeutic Methods*

# 28 Intravenous Fat Emulsions

*Vivian M. Zhao and Thomas R. Ziegler*

## CONTENTS

Intravenous lipid emulsions (ILE) have been considered a standard and critical component of parenteral nutrition (PN). ILE consist of triglycerides, egg phospholipids, and glycerin. ILE provide an energy-dense source of calories and essential fatty acids (EFA), linoleic and α-linolenic acid, that are required for the synthesis of the important lipid mediators such as eicosanoids, for the synthesis of lipid rafts involved in cell membrane signaling and other key cellular functions.

## 28.1 SOYBEAN OIL

The first well-tolerated parenteral lipid emulsion for clinical use, Intralipid (Fresenius Kabi AB, Uppsala, Sweden), was introduced in 1961 [1]. It is made of soybean-oil-derived long-chain triglycerides (LCT), which is mainly composed of omega (ω)-6 polyunsaturated fatty acids (PUFA), especially rich in linoleic acid (LA), the precursor of arachidonic acid (AA). This soybean-oil-based ILE has a high amount of ω-6 PUFA and a low amount of ω-3 PUFA, in a ratio of 7:1. The high ratio of ω-6 to ω-3 PUFA has been of concern because of the potential overproduction of proinflammatory lipid mediators in some clinical situations (e.g., sepsis, trauma) that are dominated by an imbalanced inflammatory response [2–7]. ILE with excessive ω-6 fatty acids also may potentially have immunosuppressive properties [2–7]. Available experimental and clinical data have proposed that the most favorable ω-6 to ω-3 ratio is in the approximate range of between 2:1 and 3:1 [5–8]. In addition, ω-6 LA competes with the ω-3 EFA, alpha (α)-linolenic acid, for the elongation and desaturation steps required to produce eicosapentaenoic acid (EPA) and docosahexanoic acid (DHA) [2,9]. High circulating and tissue concentrations of AA might lead to the increased proinflammatory cytokine synthesis and/or activity, while high concentrations of EPA are associated with an increased production of antiinflammatory cytokines [10]. Soybean-oil-based lipid preparation also contains a high content of gamma (γ)-tocopherol but not α-tocopherol, which is the only isoform retained in the liver. The low α-tocopherol content relative to the PUFA of soybean-oil-derived ILE may contribute to oxidative stress [6–7].

According to expert recommendations, newer lipid emulsions should be composed of a reduced content of ω-6 fatty acids, especially LA, and counterbalanced by medium-chain triglycerides (MCT), monounsaturated-fatty acids (MUFA), and long-chain ω-3 fatty acids [11,12]. Furthermore, lipid emulsions should be enriched with an amount of α-tocopherol to maintain an adequate

**TABLE 28.1**

**Compositions of Different Commercially Available Parenteral Lipid Emulsions**

|  | Intralipid® 20%[a] | Lipofundin® 20%[b] | Structolipid® 20%[a] | ClinOleic® 20%[c] | Omegaven® 10%[a] | SMOFlipid® 20%[a] |
|---|---|---|---|---|---|---|
| Lipid source (g/L) |  |  |  |  |  |  |
| Soybean oil | 200 | 100 |  | 40 |  | 60 |
| Coconut oil |  | 100 |  |  |  | 60 |
| Olive oil |  |  |  | 160 |  | 50 |
| Fish oil |  |  |  |  | 100 | 30 |
| Structured triacylglycerol |  |  | 200 |  |  |  |
| Fatty acids per 10 g/100 mL |  |  |  |  |  |  |
| Linoleic | 5 | 2.66 | 3.4 | 0.86 | 0.1–0.7 | 2.85 |
| α-linoleic | 0.9 | 0.1 | 0.49 | 0.115 | <0.2 | 0.275 |
| Oleic | 2.6 | 1.16 | 1.49 | 2.83 | 0.6–1.3 | 2.8 |
| Palmitic | 1 | 0.55 | 0.7 | 0.65 | 0.25–1 | 18.2 |
| Stearic | 0.4 | 0.2 | 0.25 | 0.175 | 0.05–0.2 | 0.33 |
| Arachidonic | – | – | – | 0.025 | 0.1–0.4 | 0.05 |
| EPA | – | – | – | – | 1.28–2.82 | 0.25 |
| DHA | – | – | – | – | 1.44–3.09 | 0.05 |

*Source*: Data provided by the manufacturer:
   [a] Fresenius Kabi, Germany
   [b] B Braun, Germany
   [c] Baxter International, France
DHA: docosahexanoic acid; EPA: eicosapentaenoic acid.

antioxidant status and to avoid lipid peroxidation [13]. Nowadays, there are several ILE commercially available for clinical use in Europe, South America, and Asia that provide differing fatty acid content, lipid sources, and/or additional α-tocopherol to decrease the risk of lipid peroxidation. These ILE include Lipofundin (B. Braun, Melsungen, Germany), Structolipid (Fresenius Kabi AB, Uppsala, Sweden), ClinOleic (Baxter/Clintec Parenteral, Cedex, France), Omegaven (Fresenius Kabi GmH, Bad Homburg v.d.h., Germany), and SMOFLipid (Fresenius Kabi Austria GmbH, Graz, Austria) (Table 28.1).

## 28.2  MCT/LCT

In response to the negative effects observed with the soybean-oil-based ILE, a lipid preparation with reduced ω-6 PUFA content formulated by substituting 50% of the soybean-oil-based LCT with MCT obtained from coconut oil was developed in Europe in the 1980s. This ILE admixture consist of 50% LCT, as soybean oil, and 50% MCT, with the ratio of ω-6 PUFA to ω-3 PUFA of approximately 7:1. MCT are associated with desirable characteristics in that they are not stored in the liver or adipose tissues, are more accessible for metabolic degradation, and are less susceptible to lipid peroxidation [14]. Additionally, MCT neither participate in eicosanoid synthesis nor serve as precursors for oxygen free-radical production, therefore they may proportionally reduce the potential impact on the systemic inflammatory response in relation to ω-6 PUFA [14–16]. MCT represent a rapid source of lipid energy, and exhibit excellent plasma clearance without accumulation in the liver [14]. However, MCT are not a source of EFA; thus, inclusion of LCT remains necessary to prevent EFA depletion in patients requiring PN.

Experimental studies have demonstrated that PN containing MCT/LCT mixtures was associated with less fatty acid deposits in the liver, less interference with the hepatic reticuloendothelial system

(RES), and improved nitrogen balance versus PN containing conventional soybean-oil-based lipid emulsions [2,14]. Available studies performed in both children and adults indicating that MCT/LCT emulsions are clinically safe and well tolerated [14–28], even in patients with liver cirrhosis [17–19] and liver transplant [20].

Some studies have shown that the administration of MCT/LCT may improve hepatic function in patients with PN-induced hepatic dysfunction when compared with soybean-oil-based ILE [7,19,21–25]. Reduction in both total and free bilirubin concentrations has been reported in preterm infants after infusion of PN containing MCT/LCT [21]. In an open label study, 38 postoperative children were randomly assigned to receive PN with either soybean-oil-based ILE or MCT/LCT for 14 days [22]. In the MCT/LCT group, a decrease in total and direct bilirubin concentration, and a normalized serum aspartate transaminase (AST) concentration were observed, whereas these concentrations remained elevated in the LCT group [22].

Similar effects of MCT/LCT infusion on liver function were observed in adults. In a small, randomized, cross-over study, Dennison et al. [23] studied 15 patients, who received 5-day infusions of PN with MCT/LCT or LCT. Plasma bilirubin concentrations were higher in patients receiving LCT than the MCT/LCT group [23]. In patients who required long-term (≥3 months) home PN, infusion of MCT/LCT was associated with normal or progressively improved liver function indices (e.g., bilirubin, AST, and alkaline phosphatase [AP] at 12 and 18 months [24]). Baldermann et al. [25] used ultrasound to examine the liver size and liver fat abundance before and after patients received PN with MCT/LCT or LCT for 7 days. Both the liver size and liver fat values were significantly increased in the LCT group, whereas no changes were observed in patients who received the MCT/LCT infusion. Baldermann et al. [25] concluded that administration of MCT/LCT emulsion in PN could lower the risk of cholestasis and fatty infiltrates in the liver. Another study examined the hematological and biochemical effects of MCT/LCT and LCT in 25 adults [19]. The plasma bilirubin levels were significantly higher in all patients who received LCT, of which over half of these patients had an elevated AST and AP. Although a few patients in the MCT/LCT group had elevated AST and AP, no patient exceeded the upper limit of the reference range for these liver function tests during the study period [19].

In contrast, more recent studies in both infants and adults did not confirm the protective effects of MCT/LCT lipid emulsion [26,27]. Socha et al. [26] compared the effects of LCT versus MCT/LCT on hepatic function in cholestatic infants, who received these ILE in alternating order for 3 days each, separated by a 3-day period without lipid. Both LCT- and MCT/LCT-containing PN were both well-tolerated and improved cholestasis. Although the total bilirubin concentrations were significantly improved after 6 h of infusion of both lipid emulsions, only a significant decrease in direct bilirubin concentrations was observed with the LCT infusion. Interestingly, DHA was also elevated only in the LCT group but not in the MCT/LCT group. Some studies suggested that the availability of DHA during infancy is very important for visual and cognitive development [29,30]; therefore, the use of soybean-oil-derived lipid preparations may be more preferable to the use of MCT/LCT emulsion for infants with severe progressive cholestasis. In a prospective cohort study involving 303 critically ill patients, the use of PN containing an MCT/LCT admixture was associated with elevated liver function tests, particularly in septic patients receiving excessive total PN caloric intakes [27].

## 28.3 STRUCTURED LIPIDS

Structured lipids (SL) were developed with the aim to improve the safety and efficacy of the physical mixture of MCT/LCT lipid emulsion. A commercially available SL, Structolipid, contains triglycerides synthesized from several combinations of LCT from soybean oil and MCT from coconut oil. These structured triglycerides are produced by hydrolysis of LCT and MCT with subsequent random reesterification of long-chain and medium-chain fatty acids to the same glycerol backbone [31]. In animal studies, SL are associated with higher albumin levels, lower infection rate, improved survival, improved nitrogen balance, and growth than conventional MCT/LCT lipid emulsion [31]. The use of SL appeared to be associated with lowered hepatic lipid content [32] and metabolized more efficiently than the LCT/MCT physical mixture in studies in animal models [33].

In human studies involving healthy subjects and in patients studied in various clinical settings, structured MCT/LCT infusion as a component of PN was found to be safe and well tolerated [33–40]. However, the effects of SL on hepatic function are conflicting. Some studies showed no significant difference on liver function tests compared to LCT [28,34–41] and conventional MCT/LCT lipid emulsions [37], whereas others indicated improved liver function parameters [38–41]. In a randomized double-blind study, 40 patients undergoing major elective abdominal surgery were randomly assigned to receive PN with MCT/LCT physical mixture or SL for at least 5 days postoperatively [38]. There was no difference in liver function parameters between groups at baseline; however, patients who received the physical MCT/LCT mixture had a significant increase in AST and alanine transaminase (ALT) on day 6. In the SL group, no liver function abnormalities were observed [38]. In contrast, similarly elevated AST [39], total bilirubin and AP [39,40] concentrations were found in patients who received PN with either structured MCT/LCT or LCT lipid emulsion. However, the elevation of bilirubin and AP was more pronounced in patients receiving LCT infusion in one study in critically ill patients [40]. In another small trial by Rubin et al. [41], 22 patients requiring home PN were studied in a double-blind randomized, cross-over study . Patients were randomly assigned to the treatment sequence of 4-week treatment with LCT emulsion followed by 4-week treatment with SL, or vice versa. No patient developed liver dysfunction during the 4 weeks of SL infusion. However, during the first part of the study, two patients had abnormal liver function tests while receiving LCT infusion. When these patients were crossed over to the SL treatment, all liver function abnormalities returned to normal. The authors concluded that the administration of structured MCT/LCT demonstrated preservation or reversion of liver enzymatic alteration in relation to LCT emulsion [41].

## 28.4  OLIVE OIL

Another ILE with reduced content of ω-6 PUFA by partially replacing ω-6 PUFA with olive oil rich in MUFA was developed in the 1990s [42–43]. This new olive-oil-based lipid emulsion, (ClinOleic), consists of purified olive oil (80%) and soybean oil (20%), which is enough to supply or correct EFA requirement and/or deficiency. The MUFA oleic acid, the main component of olive-oil-based lipid emulsion, may exert modulating effects through competition for incorporation with ω-6 and ω-3 PUFA into membrane phospholipids [42]. The use of olive-oil-based emulsion has been associated with an indirect anti-inflammatory effect and is less prone to peroxidation [43]. Parenteral olive oil is also enriched with α-tocopheral (active form of vitamin E), a major antioxidant, which may prevent oxidative damage and lipid peroxidation [42–43]. Administration of olive-oil-based ILE, either in isolation or combined with glucose and amino acids, has been demonstrated to be clinically safe and well tolerated in a number of settings including animal, healthy subjects, and clinical studies [28,42–53].

In animal models with liver damages, parenteral infusion of olive-oil-based emulsion for a longer period of time has been reported to have protective effects [44,45]. In rats with hepatic resection, the use of olive-oil-based lipid emulsion improved hepatic regeneration rate with minimal hepatosteatosis and liver function tests returned to near normal in comparison with conventional MCT/LCT emulsions [46]. However, no changes in hepatic parameters were observed when parenteral olive oil was used as an alternative to soybean-oil-based emulsion in a rabbit model [47].

In studies involving preterm infants [48] and pediatric patients [49,50], the infusion of lipid emulsion enriched with olive oil led to lower levels of LA with concomitantly higher levels of oleic acid in plasma phospholipids. However, there were no differences in the levels of the long-chain ω-6 and ω-3 fatty acids between the soybean oil and olive oil study groups. The preterm infants who received parenteral olive oil infusion were found to have an increased α-tocopherol, which showed a better indicator of antioxidant activity against lipid peroxidation compared with soybean-oil-based emulsion [48]. Nevertheless, the measures of liver function (AST, ALT, AP, and γ-glutamyl transferase [GGT]) were not significantly different between baseline and end of study in study groups [48–50].

Over the last decade, olive-oil-based lipid emulsions have been studied fairly extensively in patients requiring home PN. Thomas-Gibson et al. [51] investigated the effects of olive-oil-based ILE in home PN patients who had been previously treated with soybean-oil-based emulsion. There were no differences in clinical and nutritional outcome parameters after 6 months of treatment. No significant differences were found for hepatic function parameters in patients receiving home PN containing olive-oil-derived lipid emulsion in relation to soybean-oil-based lipid preparation [4,52] and MCT/LCT [4]. Recently, Puiggròs et al. [28] conducted a prospective randomized double-blind study involved 28 postoperative adults, who were randomly assigned to receive one of four different ILEs: LCT, MCT/LCT, structured lipid, and olive/soybean oil [28]. No significant alterations in liver function tests among the different lipid emulsions administered during the study period were observed.

In a single case report, a patient who underwent extensive small bowel resection for acute peritonitis and septic shock resulting in a short gut in need of home PN showed different results [53]. The patient developed hepatic dysfunction while on home PN with soybean-oil-based lipid emulsion as the source of EFA. After switching the infusion of soybean-oil-based emulsion to the olive-oil-based emulsion, elevated liver enzymes fell significantly and eventually returned to normal values [53]. In a randomized, double-blind trial, García-de-Lorenzo et al. [54] compared PN containing an emulsion enriched in olive oil versus MCT/LCT in patients with severe burn over 6 days. Abnormal liver function tests occurred more frequently in the MCT/LCT group than in the olive oil group [54].

## 28.5 FISH OIL

Another recent development in ILE formulations was the introduction of fish-oil emulsions. Brought to market in Europe in the 1990s, fish-oil ILE is intended to serve as a supplement that is added to conventional soybean-oil ILE. When administered intravenously, the ω-3 fatty acids are rapidly incorporated into the cell membranes without impairing platelet function or coagulation. Due to the anti-inflammatory properties of the ω-3 fatty acids, in particular EPA and DHA, their inclusion is considered beneficial in a variety of clinical conditions such as sepsis, pulmonary disorders, cystic fibrosis, and cancer cachexia. Studies using fish-oil ILE have shown that patients treated with them have shorter ICU stays and decreased morbidity and mortality in comparison to conventionally treated patients [55–58]. In one prospective, randomized, double-blinded clinical trial, 44 patients undergoing elective major abdominal surgery were randomly assigned to receive PN supplemented with either conventional soybean oil (1.0 g/kg body weight daily) for 5 days or a combination of fish oil and soybean oil (fish oil 0.2 + soybean oil 0.8 g/kg body weight daily). Compared to pure soybean-oil patients, subjects treated with fish oil had significantly reduced AST ($0.8 \pm 0.1$ vs. $0.5 \pm 0.1$ mmol/L), ALT ($0.9 \pm 0.1$ vs. $0.6 \pm 0.1$ mmol/L), and bilirubin ($16.1 \pm 5.3$ vs. $6.9 \pm 0.6$ mmol/L) [59]. The authors concluded that fish-oil supplementation improved liver and pancreas function, which might have contributed to the faster recovery of the treated patients. Since that time, other products have been formulated that include fish oil in the finished product.

There are several differences with the type of fish oils used in ILE. Depending upon the product, it may conform to one of two monographs from the European Pharmacopeia. One monograph 2008:1912, titled, "Fish oil, rich in omega-3 fatty acids," describes purified fish oils whereas monograph 2008:1352, "Omega-3 acid triglycerides," describes a synthetic mixture of mono-, di-, and triester of ω-3 acids derived either from the esterification of fatty acids with glycerol or by transesterification of ω-3 acids with ethyl esters. Products, such as Lipoplus (B. Braun, Melsungen, Germany) comply with monograph 2008:1352 whereas both Omegaven and SMOFlipid comply with monograph 2008:1912. Thus, when comparing fatty acid content of the various products, one may consist of entirely purified fish oils (i.e., Omegaven) while another may consist of a combination of fish oils supplemented with additional biosynthesized sources of EPA and DHA (i.e.,

Lipoplus). Despite these differences, all would be in compliance with their respective monographs. It also explains how one product, despite having a lower concentration of fish oil, could have a higher final concentration of EPA and/or DHA.

Recently, the use of fish-oil ILE has garnered interest as a sole source of essential fatty acids in pediatric intestinal failure patients [60]. Using dosing parameters that are significantly different than the manufacturer's recommendations, the role of fish-oil lipid emulsion monotherapy as a treatment in the reversal of PN-associated liver disease is discussed in detail in Chapter 21.

## 28.6  MULTIPLE MIXED LIPID EMULSION

More recently, a lipid emulsion containing a well-balanced fatty acid pattern in accordance with current NIH recommendations have been developed for clinical use. This new lipid preparation combines 30% soybean oil (EFA source), 30% MCT (energy source), 25% olive oil (less immunologic effect and reduced lipid peroxidation), and 15% fish oil (anti-inflammatory effect) into one formulation (SMOF) [7]. The emulsion contains all fatty acids found in the regular human diet ($\omega$-6, MCT, $\omega$-9, and $\omega$-3), therefore it is considered more physiological than other ILE available for clinical use. SMOF has an optimal $\omega$-6 to $\omega$-3 ratio of 2.5:1, which mirrors the nutritional environment for human development [2,42]. Lipid formulations containing $\omega$-6 to $\omega$-3 PUFA ratio of 2:1 have shown immune-neutral characteristics in transplantation models [61]. Furthermore, SMOF lipid has an enhanced content of the antioxidant $\alpha$-tocopherol (200 mg/L). Clinical experience with this new mixed-lipid emulsion, at dosage ranges from 0.85 to 2 g fat per kilogram body weight per day, indicates that the emulsion is safe, well metabolized and well tolerated by healthy volunteers, critically ill, and surgical patients [62–67]. Among currently available studies, SMOF lipid seems to result in a more favorable metabolic profile in relation to triglyceride elimination compared to soybean-oil-based lipid emulsions [61,63,64]. Unblinded observational studies involving 302 surgical patients who received isonitrogenous, isocaloric all-in-one PN with SMOF or soybean-oil-based lipid emulsions postoperatively revealed slightly lower liver enzyme abnormalities (AST, ALT, GGT, and AP) in the SMOF lipid group than in the control group [63,64]. Plasma ALT levels were significantly increased in the control group after 5 days of PN, but not with inclusion of the SMOF lipid in PN [64]. Patients who received SMOF lipid had significantly elevated $\alpha$-tocopherol concentrations, reaching healthy control subject mean values, compared to the emulsion based on soybean oil [63–65]. In addition, length of hospital stay was significantly shorter in SMOF lipid group [63,65]. Of interest, a prospective, double-blind, randomized study of 32 patients who received a maximum daily fat dosage of 2 g/kg body weight for a period of 7–14 days showed no differences in plasma triglycerides, total cholesterol, or liver function test concentrations compared to subjects receiving standard soybean-oil-based lipid emulsion as a component of PN [66].

In 2009, Piper et al. [67] compared the effects of two lipid emulsions (SMOFLipid and ClinOleic) on hepatic integrity in 44 postoperative patients in an ICU. Lipid emulsions were given as 40% nonprotein calories for 5 days. Serial concentrations of a new and more sensitive maker of hepatic dysfunction, $\alpha$-glutathione $S$-transferase ($\alpha$-GST), were obtained in addition to standard hepatic function parameters (AST, ALT, AP, and GGT). There were no significant differences in liver function and triglyceride levels at baseline. However, significantly higher plasma AST, ALT, $\alpha$-GST, and triglyceride levels were found in the control group in relation to the SMOF group on both days 2 and 5. The study results suggested that liver integrity was better preserved with the administration of SMOF lipid versus the olive-oil-based emulsion in PN [67].

## 28.7  CONCLUSION

Lipid emulsions are a crucial component of PN solutions, serving as a source of essential fatty acids and as an alternative to carbohydrates in providing adequate energy. Until recently, lipid emulsions were mainly considered a source of nutrition without pharmacologic benefit. With the development of new products using different oil sources, new findings have emerged to suggest that different formulations may be beneficial in a variety of clinical conditions. Currently, practitioners in the United States are limited to only those products comprised solely of soybean oils. Additional work must be done to allow for importation of these alternative products into the American market.

## REFERENCES

1. Schuberth O, Wretlind A. Intravenous infusion of fat emulsions, phosphatides and emulsifying agents. *Acta Chir Scand.* 1961;278:s1–21.
2. Wanten GJ, Calder PC. Immune modulation by parenteral lipid emulsions. *Am J Clin Nutr.* 2007;85:1171–84.
3. Mayer K, Grimm H, Grimmeringer G, Seeger W. Parenteral nutrition with n-3 lipids in sepsis. *Br J Nutr.* 2002;87:s69–75.
4. Reimund JM, Rahmi G, Escalin G, et al. Efficacy and safety of an olive oil-based intravenous fat emulsion in adult patients on home parenteral nutrition. *Aliment Pharmacol Ther.* 2005;21:445–54.
5. Grimm H, Tibell A, Norrlind B, Blecher C, Wilker S, Schwemmle K. Immunoregulation by parenteral lipids: Impact of the n-3 to n-6 fatty acid ratio. *JPEN.* 1994;18:417–21.
6. Pironi L, Ruggeri E, Zolezzi C, Savarino L, Incasa E, Belluzzi A, Munarini A, Piazzi S, Tolomelli M, Pizzoferrato A, Miglioli M. Lipid peroxidation and antioxidant status in adults receiving lipid-based home parenteral nutrition. *Am J Clin Nutr.* 1998;68:888–93.
7. Waitzberg DL, Torrinhas RS, Jacintho TM. New parenteral lipid emulsions for clinical use. *JPEN.* 2006;30:351–67.
8. Grimm H, Kraus A. Immunonutrition: Supplementary amino acids and fatty acids ameliorate immune deficiency in critically ill patients. *Arch Surg.* 2001;386:369–76.
9. Jensen CL, Chen H, Fraley JK, Anderson RE, Heird WC. Biochemical effects of dietary linoleic/α-linolenic acid ratio in term infants. *Lipids.* 1996;31:107–13.
10. Calder PC, Deckelbaum RJ. Fat as a physiological regulator: The news gets better. *Curr Opin Clin Nutr Metab Care.* 2003;6:127–31.
11. Simopoulos AP, Leaf A, Salem N. Essentiality of and recommended dietary intakes for omega-6 and omega-3 fatty acids. *Ann Nutr Metab.* 1999;43:127–30.
12. Fürst P, Kuhn KS. Fish oil emulsions: What benefits can they bring? *Clin Nutr.* 2000;19:7–14.
13. Carpertier YA, Simoens C, Siderova V, et al. Recent developments in lipid emulsions: Relevance to intensive care. *Nutrition.* 1997;13:s73–8.
14. Ulrich H, Pastores SM, Katz DP, Kvetan V. Parenteral use of medium-chain triglycerides: A reappraisal. *Nutrition.* 1996;12:231–8.
15. Radermacher P, Santak B, Strobach H, Schrör K, Tarnow J. Fat emulsions containing medium chain triglycerides in patients with sepsis syndrome: Effects on pulmonary hemodynamics and gas exchange. *Intensive Care Med.* 1992;18:231–4.
16. Manuel-y-Keenoy B, Nonneman L, De Bosscher H, et al. Effects of intravenous supplementation with α-tocopherol in patients receiving total parenteral nutrition containing medium- and long-chain triglycerides. *Eur J Clin Nutr.* 2002;56:121–8.
17. Fan ST, Wong J. Metabolic clearance of a fat emulsion containing medium-chain triglycerides in cirrhotic patients. *JPEN.* 1992;16:279–83.
18. Druml W, Fischer M, Pidlich J, Lenz K. Fat elimination in chronic hepatic failure: Long vs medium-chain triglycerides. *Am J Clin Nutr.* 1995;61:812–7.
19. Ball MJ. Hematological and biochemical effects of parenteral nutrition with medium-chain triglycerides: Comparison with long-chain triglycerides. *Am J Clin Nutr.* 1991;53:916–22.
20. Kuse ER, Kotzerke J, Müller S, Nashan B, Lück R, Jaeger ST. Hepatic reticuloendothelial function during parenteral nutrition including an MCT/LCT or LCT emulsion after liver transplantation—A double-blind study. *Transplant Int.* 2002;15:272–7.
21. Rubin M, Harell D, Naor N, et al. Lipid infusion with different triglyceride cores (long-chain versus medium-chain triglycerides): Effect on plasma lipids, and bilirubin binding in premature infants. *JPEN.* 1991;15:642–6.
22. Lai H, Chen W. Effects of medium-chain and long-chain triacylglycerides in pediatric surgical patients. *Nutrition.* 2000;16:401–6.

23. Dennison AR, Ball M, Hands LJ, Crowe PJ, Watkins RM, Kettlewell M. Total parenteral nutrition using conventional and medium chain triglycerides: Effect on liver function tests, complement and nitrogen balance. *JPEN*. 1988;12:15–9.
24. Carpentier YA, Siderova V, Bruyns J, Rubin M. Long-term TPN and liver dysfunction. *Clin Nutr.* 1989;8:s31.
25. Baldermann H, Wicklmayr M, Rett K, Banholzer P, Dietze G, Mehnert H. Changes of hepatic morphology during parenteral nutrition with lipid emulsions containing LCT or MCT/LCT quantified by ultrasounds. *JPEN*. 1991;15:601–3.
26. Socha P, Koletzko B, Demmelmair H, et al. Short-term effects of parenteral nutrition of cholestatic infants with lipid emulsions based on medium-chain and long-chain triacylglycerol. *Nutrition*. 2007;23:121–6.
27. Grau T, Bonet A, Rubio M, et al. Liver dysfunction associated with artificial nutrition in critically ill patients. *Crit Care*. 2007;11:R10.
28. Puiggròs C, Sánchez J, Chacón P, et al. Evolution of lipid profile, liver function, and pattern of plasma fatty acid according to the type of lipid emulsion administered in parenteral nutrition in the early postoperative period after digestive surgery. *JPEN*. 2009;33:501–12.
29. Koletzko B, Demmelmair H, Socha P. Nutrition support of infants and children: Supply and metabolism of lipids. *Balliere Clin Gasterenterol*. 1998;12:671–96.
30. Koletzko B, Agostoni C, Carlson SE, et al. Long chain polyunsaturated fatty acids (LC-PUFA) and perinatal development. *Acta Paediatr*. 2001;90:460–4.
31. Fürst P. Old and new substrates in clinical nutrition. *J Nutr.* 1998;128:789–96.
32. Nakagawa M, Hiramatsu Y, Mitsuyoshi K, Yamamura M, Hioki K, Yamamoto M. Effect of various lipid emulsions on total parenteral nutrition-induced hepatosteatosis in rats. *JPEN*. 1991;15:137–43.
33. Simoens C, Deckelbaum RJ, Carpentier YA. Metabolism of defined structure triglyceride particles compared to mixtures of medium and long chain triglycerides intravenously infused in dog. *Clin Nutr.* 2004;23:665–72.
34. Sandström R, Hyltander A, Körner U, Lundholm K. Structured triglycerides to postoperative patients: A safety and tolerance study. *JPEN*. 1993;17:153–7.
35. Sandström R, Hyltander A, Körner U, Lundholm K. Structured triglycerides were well tolerated and induced increased whole body fat oxidation compared with long-cahin triglycerides in postoperative patients. *JPEN*. 1995;19:381–6.
36. Nordenström J, Thörne A, Olivercrona T. Metabolic effects of infusion of a structured-triglyceride emulsion in healthy subjects. *Nutrition*. 1995;11:269–74.
37. Kruimel JW, Naber TH, Van der Vliet JA, Carneheim C, Katan MB, Jansen JB. Parenteral structured triglyceride emulsion improves nitrogen balance and is cleared faster from the blood in moderately catabolic patients. *JPEN*. 2001;25:237–44.
38. Chambrier C, Guiraud M, Gibault JP, Labrosse H, Boulétreau P. Medium- and long-chain triacylglycerols in postoperative patients: Structured lipids versus physical mixture. *Nutrition*. 1999;15:274–7.
39. Bellantone R, Bossola M, Carriero C, et al. Structured versus long-chain triglycerides: A safety, tolerance, and efficacy randomized study in colorectal surgical patients. *JPEN*. 1999;23:123–7.
40. Lindgern BF, Ruokonen E, Magnusson-Borg K, Takala J. Nitrogen sparing effect of structured triglycerides containing both medium- and long-chain fatty acids in critically ill patients: A double blind randomized controlled trial. *Clin Nutr.* 2001;20:43–8.
41. Rubin M, Moser A, Vaserberg N, et al. Structured triacylglycerol emulsion, containing both medium- and long-chain fatty acids, in long-term home parenteral nutrition: A double-blind randomized cross-over study. *Nutrition*. 2000;16:95–100.
42. Grimble R. Fatty acid profile of modern lipid emulsions: Scientific considerations for creating the ideal composition. *Clin Nutr Suppl*. 2005;1:9–15.
43. Sala-Vila A, Barbosa VM, Calder PC. Olive oil in parenteral nutrition. *Curr Opin Clin Nutr Metab Care*. 2007;10:165–74.
44. Nazıroğly M, Çay M, Szende B, Timar F, Hargital B. Olive oil decreases liver damage in rates caused by carbon tetrachloride ($CCl_4$). *Exp Toxicol Pathol*. 1994;46:355–9.
45. Üstündağ B, Aksakal M, Yekeler H. Protective effects of vitamin E on carbon tetrachloride-induced liver damage in rats. *Cell Biochem Funct*. 1999;17:253–9.
46. Ok E, Yilmaz Z, Karaküçük I, Akgün H, Şahin H. Use of olive oil based emulsions as an alternative to soybean oil based emulsions in total parenteral nutrition and their effects on liver regeneration following hepatic resection in rats. *Ann Nutr Meat*. 2003;47:221–7.

47. Kohl M, Wedel T, Entenmann A, et al. Influence of different intravenous lipid emulsions on hepatobiliary dysfunction in a rabbit model. *J Pediatr Gastroenterol Nutr.* 2007;237–44.
48. Göbel Y, Koletzko B, Böhles HJ, et al. Parenteral fat emulsions based on olive and soybean oils: A randomized clinical trial in preterm infants. *J Pediatr Gastroenterol Nutr.* 2003;37:161–7.
49. Goulet O, de Potter S, Antébi H, et al. Long-term efficacy and safety of a new olive oil-based intravenous fat emulsion in pediatric patients: A double-blind randomized study. *Am J Clin Nutr.* 1999;70:337–45.
50. Hartman C, Ben-Artzi E, Berkowitz D, et al. Olive oil-based intravenous lipid emulsion in pediatric patients undergoing bone marrow transplantation: A short-term prospective controlled trial. *Clin Nutr.* 2009;26:631–5.
51. Thomas-Gibson S, Jawhari A, Atlan P, Le Brun A, Farthing M, Forbes A. Safe and efficacious prolonged use of an olive oil-based lipid emulsion (ClinOleic) in chronic intestinal failure. *Clin Nutr.* 2004;23:697–703.
52. Vahedi K, Atlan P, Joly F, et al. A 3-month double-blind randomized study comparing an olive oil-with a soyabean oil-based intravenous lipid emulsion in home parenteral nutrition patients. *Bt J Nutr.* 2005;94:909–16.
53. Reimund JM, Arondel Y, Joly F, Messing B, Duclos B, Baumann R. Potential usefulness of olive oil-based lipid emulsions in selected situations of home parenteral nutrition-associated liver disease. *Clin Nutr.* 2004;23:1418–25.
54. García-de-Lorenzo A, Denia R, Atlan T, et al. Parenteral nutrition providing a restricted amount of linoleic acid in severely burned patients: A randomised double-blind study of an olive oil based lipid emulsion v. medium/long chain triacylglycerols. *Br J Nutr.* 2005;94:221–30.
55. Morlion BJ, Torwesten E, Lessire H, et al. The effect of parenteral fish oil on leukocyte membrane fatty acid composition and leukotriene-synthesizing capacity in patients with postoperative trauma. *Metabolism.* 1996;45:1208–13.
56. Schauder P, Röhn U, Schäfer G, et al. Impact of fish oil enriched total parenteral nutrition on DNA synthesis, cytokine release and receptor expression by lymphocytes in the postoperative period. *Br J Nutr.* 2002;87(Suppl 1):S103–10.
57. Roulet M, Frascarolo P, Pilet M, Chapuis G. Effects of intravenously infused fish oil on platelet fatty acid phospholipid composition and on platelet function in postoperative trauma. *JPEN.* 1997;21:296–301.
58. Tsekos E, Reuter C, Stehle P, Boeden G. Perioperative administration of parenteral fish oil supplements in a routine clinical setting improves patient outcome after major abdominal surgery. *Clin Nutr.* 2004;23:325–30.
59. Heller AR, Rössel T, Gottschlich B, et al. Omega-3 fatty acids improve liver and pancreas function in postoperative cancer patients. *Int J Cancer.* 2004;10:611–6.
60. Le HD, Fallon EM, de Meijer VE, et al. Innovative parenteral and enteral nutrition therapy for intestinal failure. *Semin Pediatr Surg.* 2010;19:27–34.
61. Grimm H, Tibell A, Norrlind B, Schott J, Bohle RM. Nutrition and allorejection impact of lipids. *Transpl Immunol.* 1995;3:62–7.
62. Schlotzer E, Kanning U. Elimination and tolerance of a new parenteral lipid emulsion (SMOF)—A double-blind cross-over study in healthy male volunteers. *Ann Nutr Metab.* 2004;48:263–8.
63. Schulzki C, Mertes N, Wenn A, et al. Effects of a new type of lipid emulsion based on soybean, MCT, olive oil and fish oil (SMOF) in surgical patients. *Clin Nutr.* 1999;18:s7.
64. Antébi H, Mansoor O, Ferrier C, et al. Liver function and plasma antioxidant status in intensive care unit patients requiring total parenteral nutrition: Comparison of 2 fat emulsions. *JPEN.* 2004;28:142–8.
65. Grimm H, Mertes N, Boeters C, et al. Improved fatty acid and leukotriene pattern with a novel lipid emulsion in surgical patients. *Eur J Nutr.* 2006;45:55–60.
66. Genton L, Karsegard VL, Dupertuis YM, et al. Tolerance to a lipid emulsion containing a mixture of soybean, olive, coconut and fish oils compared with a fat emulsion containing only soybean oil. *Clin Nutr.* 2004;23:793.
67. Piper SN, Schafe I, Ceschmann RB, et al. Hepatocellular integrity after parenteral nutrition: Comparision of a fish-oil-containing lipid emulsion with an olive-soybean oil-based lipid emulsion. *Eur J Anaesthesiol.* 2009;26:1076–82.

# 29 Probiotics and Prebiotics

*Sanjiv Harpavat and Robert J. Shulman*

## CONTENTS

Medical management of patients with intestinal failure (IF) is rooted in three well-established principles: maximize enteral feedings, minimize parenteral feedings, and avoid infections. Enteral feedings are maximized according to the simple adage "if the gut works, use it," in an effort to promote weight gain and intestinal adaptation. Parenteral feedings are minimized to prevent central line complications as well as parenteral nutrition-associated (PN) cholestasis. Infections—caused by microbes translocating across the gut wall or colonizing venous catheters—are avoided to give fragile IF patients uninterrupted opportunities to grow [1–3].

Probiotics have been proposed as another management tool in IF. Probiotics are "live organisms that when administered in adequate amounts confer a health benefit to the host" [4]. Probiotics have shown promise in a variety of pediatric gastrointestinal (GI) disorders, from preventing acute infectious diarrhea to treating ulcerative colitis, and are actively being tested in many more digestive illnesses [4]. In IF, probiotic use is still in its infancy. This chapter addresses probiotics in IF, by first summarizing the history of probiotics, then detailing the rationale for using probiotics in IF, and finally discussing the growing collection of studies testing the safety and efficacy of probiotics in IF. As with most of the literature in the field, the majority of data stems from reports in patients with short bowel syndrome (SBS), but we have used the more over-arching term "IF" since the issues we discuss may apply to patients with IF due to other causes as well.

## 29.1 BRIEF HISTORY OF PROBIOTICS

While humans have recognized microbes' culinary benefits for years (in making breads, cheeses, yogurts, and beer), it was not until the twentieth century that the health benefits of microbes were formally recognized. In 1907, Russian scientist Elie Metchnikoff proposed that ingesting "good bacteria" could prolong life by antagonizing "bad bacteria" [5]. Metchnikoff's ideas were controversial, but Metchnikoff had a history of proving skeptics wrong (previously he proved amidst much doubt that macrophages phagocytose bacteria, earning him the 1908 Nobel Prize in Medicine). Metchnikoff so believed in his ideas that he ingested sour milk daily to prove the probiotic effect. However, Metchnikoff's critics won the argument temporarily, when they proved the bacteria Metchnikoff ingested, *Lactobacillus bulgaricus*, did not survive in the small intestine [6].

After Metchnikoff, and through the twentieth century, probiotics and antibiotics became twin opposites with the latter enjoying huge successes. Nevertheless, the idea of "giving bacteria" was never completely silenced by gains in "killing bacteria," and Metchnikoff's theory continued to gain momentum. The term "probiotics" was coined by Kollath in 1953, and was modified to its present meaning by Fuller in 1989 [7,8]. In 1995, the term "prebiotics" was suggested by Gibson and Roberfroid, who recognized the value of poorly digested foods which could stimulate growth of beneficial bacteria in the gut [9]. Soon afterwards, the concept of symbiotics was born: using the combination of taking probiotics and prebiotics to attain maximum benefit. These steps, in the context of new discoveries highlighting the vast and complex gut microbiome, have cemented Metchnikoff's original hypothesis that "good bacteria" may indeed provide tremendous benefit.

If Metchnikoff was alive today, he may be surprised that his original idea has blossomed into a rich, deep, and intensely active field. Scientists study individual probiotic strains to pinpoint the molecular mechanisms behind their effects, while others sequence genomes of hundreds of other bacterial species to create a complete "gut microbiome" map [10]. Industry markets a myriad of probiotic pills and products with broad claims of efficacy, an effort helped in part by probiotics' "dietary supplements" designation which frees them from heavy Food and Drug Administration regulation. Most of these commercially available probiotics are combinations from the genus *Lactobacillus* and *Bifidobacterium*, two Gram-positive lactic-acid fermenting bacilli, though formulations of other microbes such as yeast exist. Clinicians continue to test probiotics in clinical trials spanning a wide variety of diseases. As the probiotic movement gains momentum, one stated future goal is to match beneficial bacterial strains with specific ailments, so that clinicians can prescribe probiotics with the same certainty and confidence they have with antibiotics.

## 29.2 PROBIOTICS IN IF PATIENTS: THEORETICAL MECHANISMS OF BENEFITS

In theory, probiotics could benefit IF children by influencing both neighboring bacteria and underlying mucosal cells (Figure 29.1). With neighboring bacterial cells, probiotics hold promise as agents to prevent or ameliorate bacterial overgrowth. Bacterial overgrowth is a known complication post-bowel resection, likely secondary to multiple factors: proton-pump inhibitors used to treat gastric hypersecretion, reduced bile in the intestinal lumen from PN-associated cholestasis, and/or poor intestinal motility from intestinal dilation associated with the adaptation process after bowel resection [11]. Bacterial overgrowth impairs nutrient absorption by inducing gut mucosal inflammation and deconjugating bile acids, thereby increasing stool losses and prolonging PN dependence. The chronic inflammation and damage at the mucosal surface may also in theory enhance bacterial translocation and promote sepsis [11,12].

Probiotics may address bacterial overgrowth at two levels. The first is by directly producing substances that kill neighboring bacteria. Some probiotic species make natural antibiotics, called bacteriocins, which are secreted and function locally (Figure 29.1, number 6). For example, the probiotic strain *Lactobacillus reuteri* makes reuterin from glycerol through a series of well characterized reactions [13,14]. *In vitro*, reuterin inhibits species such as *Shigella sonnei*, *Salmonella enterica*, *Vibrio cholerae*, enterohemorrhagic *Escherichia coli*, and enterotoxigenic *E. coli* [15]. *L. reuteri*, on the other hand, is resistant to reuterin. Hence, in contrast to broad spectrum antibiotics such as penicillins and cephalosporins, probiotics may create local neighborhoods of antibiotics that selectively remove certain organisms.

The second is by occupying space in the gut lumen and on gut mucosal cells. Ingested probiotic organisms bind mucin and/or intestinal cell surface receptors, and may compete with other bacteria attempting to settle in the same area (Figure 29.1, number 7). In this location the probiotic strains also stimulate host defensin production from neutrophils and lymphocytes, which disrupts microbial membranes and further prevents bacterial overgrowth (Figure 29.1, number 1) [16]. Perhaps the best example demonstrating the importance of the "space occupying" effect is in *Clostridium difficile* colitis. Only when the normal gut microbiome is cleared by antibiotics do pathogenic *Clostridium difficile* appear to colonize. Accordingly, many investigators have tested whether different probiotic regimens can prevent or treat *Clostridium difficile* infections. Some, but not all, studies show benefit, and ongoing studies may help clarify the issue [17–19].

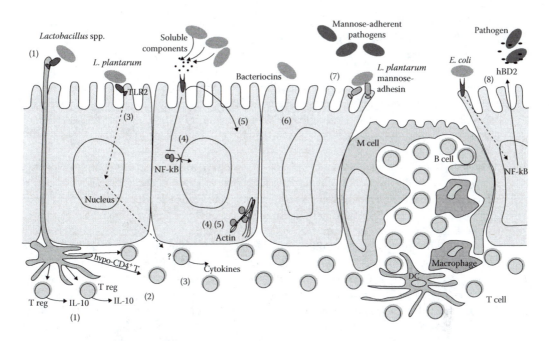

**FIGURE 29.1** Probiotic strains such as *Lactobacillus* spp. can modulate T-cell responses to potential pathogens via interactions with dendritic cells, thereby either upregulating or downregulating (e.g., via IL-10) the immune response (1 and 2). Similarly, via TLR, *L. plantarum* can modulate cytokine production (3). Soluble components of probiotics can, via a number of mechanisms, down regulate the proinflammatory nuclear factor (NF)-κB signaling pathway (4). Probiotics may improve intestinal integrity, decrease permeability, and subsequently reduce systemic infections from bacteria translocating across the gut wall, some acting through activation of actin (5). Some probiotic species make natural antibiotics, called bacteriocins, which are secreted and function locally (6). Ingested probiotic organisms bind mucin and/or intestinal cell surface receptors, and may compete with other bacteria preventing settling in the same area (7). Other probiotics species (e.g., *E. coli* strain Nissle 1917) can induce antimicrobial peptide production [e.g., human β defensin 2 (hBD2)] in intestinal epithelial cells (8). (Adapted from Marco ML et al. *Curr Opin Biotechnol* 2006;17:204–10.)

Equally complex, and very promising therapeutically, is probiotics' influence on underlying mucosal cells. The nature of the probiotic-host relationship is under active investigation, and appears to be one of constant signaling between the two [20]. Microbes stimulate host epithelial and immune cells, either through secreted factors or by direct binding (Figure 29.1, numbers 1, 2, 8). The host, in turn, uses a variety of signaling pathways to respond to microbe signals. The result is a dynamic relationship in which microbe and host collaborate to achieve normal intestinal function. In IF patients, potential probiotic benefits include improving intestinal integrity, modulating immune response, and promoting intestinal adaptation.

Probiotics may improve intestinal integrity, which could impede bacteria translocating across the gut wall and thereby reduce systemic infections (Figure 29.1, number 5). Numerous studies in rodents have shown that probiotics can stimulate epithelial cell tight junction gene expression. For example, Ukena et al. demonstrated that the probiotic strain *E. coli* Nissle 1917 induces zona occludens-1 expression in mice, and can prevent colonic damage in dextran sodium sulfate induced colitis [21]. Similarly, Khailova et al. [22] showed that *Bifidobacterium bifidum* can normalize expression of different tight junction proteins in a rat model of necrotizing enterocolitis. The consequence of improved intestinal integrity may be reduced translocation, as Eizaguirre et al. [23] showed rats given *Bifidobacterium lactis* after massive bowel resection had significantly fewer mesenteric lymph nodes culture positive for bacteria.

Probiotics have well-established roles in modulating the immune system, which may temper chronic inflammation occurring in the intestines of IF patients. Probiotics affect the immune system in a number of ways. Probiotics can stimulate the innate immune system, basally activating toll-like receptors (TLR) which then mediate immune tolerance to the many bacterial antigens present in the gut (Figure 29.1, numbers 1, 2, 3, 4). As a result, host cells allow bacteria in their local environments without mounting an immune attack [24]. Probiotics also affect secreted molecules with powerful immune functions. Probiotics such as *Lactobacillus rhamnosus* are known interleukin-10 (IL-10) stimulators, which in turn promotes immune tolerance [25]. Other probiotics such as *L. reuteri* can reduce monocyte tumor necrosis factor-alpha (TNF-$\alpha$) secretion *in vitro* [26]. Anti-TNF-$\alpha$ therapies dampen inflammation in diseases such as inflammatory bowel disease, raising the possibility that probiotics with TNF-$\alpha$ lowering properties may have similar effects [27].

Probiotics may play a yet undefined role in the holy grail of IF management: inducing adaptation. Gut bacteria are critically important in postnatal intestinal function and development, as seen in germ-free mice which suffer from reduced small bowel mucosal surface area and decreased motility. These mice also have enterocytes with impaired glycan expression and submucosal capillaries that are poorly developed [28,29]. In an analogous way, probiotics may promote redevelopment of lost mucosa following gut resection. While growth factors, rather than probiotics, hold the spotlight in adaptation biology, probiotics may be a critical component that induces epithelial cells to start expressing molecules such as epidermal growth factor and insulin-like growth factor [30,31]. For example, Mogilner et al. administered *L. rhamnosus* GG to rats after bowel resection. After 14 days, the rats showed significant increases in crypt length as well as less apoptosis in the jejunum and ileum [32]. Probiotics may use a variety of molecules in their metabolism which also act as trophic factors for the gut mucosa, including short-chain fatty acids and bile acid metabolites [33].

## 29.3   PROBIOTICS IN IF PATIENTS: CLINICAL EVIDENCE

Given their theoretical benefits, probiotics have been tried in children with IF. These trials vary in the types of bacteria given, duration of treatment, and measured outcomes. A major caveat becomes clear when reviewing the published literature: each probiotic organism may act in different, multiple ways. Thus, to discuss generally "the effects of probiotics" on a disease is overly simplistic at best and misleading at worst. The analogy would be to anticipate that penicillin and ceftriaxone would have the same effect on Gram-negative sepsis. Thus, each probiotic organism or combination must be evaluated in isolation, avoiding the tendency to lump probiotics together as to whether they do or do not "work" for a particular application.

Unfortunately, the majority of published reports are case presentations. Many of these reports are problematic because some improvements in IF, such as adaptation, can take years to occur [34]. In one example, Vanderhoof et al. reported six patients with small bowel bacterial overgrowth refractory to antibiotics [35]. Two patients with a history of volvulus, one as an infant and one as a child, received $1 \times 10^{10}$ colony forming units (cfu) of *Lactobacillus plantarum*. Within "2–3 weeks" and a "few weeks," respectively, the authors reported improved symptoms including more formed stools, less abdominal distension, and less joint pain. When probiotics were stopped, the symptoms returned. Of note, one patient started probiotics while still taking antibiotics. Whether the probiotic regimen improved symptoms before antibiotics were discontinued was unclear.

Candy et al. [36] reported using *Lactobacillus casei* Shirota in a child who underwent intestinal resection for necrotizing enterocolitis. The child had his ileum and colon removed, with 60 cm of jejunum ultimately connecting to rectum. Following the procedure, the child started gastrostomy feedings which caused copious stools and a negative sodium balance (as indicated by low urine sodium). However, after starting $1.5 \times 10^9$ cfu of *L. casei* Shirota 3 times daily, the patient's urine sodium rose to normal within 3 days. His stool frequency also decreased, though it had started improving 3 weeks prior to probiotics treatment when his feedings were switched from a hydrolysate to an elemental formula. Two years later at the time of publication, the patient was still taking *L. casei* Shirota and maintaining normal urine sodium levels. The authors suggested that the probiotic improved mucosal health and sodium absorptive capacity. They also speculated that patients without a colon may benefit more from probiotics, because they have no large reservoir for bacteria to ferment nutrients (i.e., carbohydrates to short-chain fatty acids which subsequently are absorbed).

Kanamori et al. used a symbiotic combination—*L. casei* Shirota, *Bifidobacterium breve* Yakult, and galacto-oligosaccharide (Oligomate, Yakult Honsya, Japan)—and reported their results with seven patients [37]. All patients had some combination of small and/or large bowel resection, including three for Hirschsprung's disease, and each patient had recurrent bouts of "enterocolitis" (defined by the authors as fever, diarrhea, elevated white blood cell count and C-reactive protein). The patients received $1 \times 10^9$ of each bacteria and 1 g galacto-oligosaccharide three times a day for 15–55 months. The authors reported consistent improvements in numerous parameters after treatment was started: frequency of enterocolitis, rate of weight gain, and enteral feeding tolerance. They noted improved serum albumin, prealbumin, and an increase in serum short-chain fatty acids, as well as increased amounts of endogenous *Lactobacillus* and *Bifidobacterium* species in the gut. The children also had reduced hospital admissions while taking the synbiotic preparation. The only patient who did not respond was a child with 20 cm of small bowel (including duodenum) remaining. The authors concluded that this synbiotic regimen may be particularly apt for IF patients, a conclusion seconded later by Uchida et al. [38] who used the same combination in an uncontrolled series of 4 patients with small bowel resection.

To date, only one clinical trial has been performed to evaluate probiotics in SBS. Sentongo et al. [39] hypothesized that *L. rhamnosus* would improve intestinal epithelial cell integrity. They enrolled nine children in an 11-week crossover trial. For the first 4 weeks they received either the probiotic ($1 \times 10^9$ cfu/day) or placebo, followed by a three week wash out period, then 4 weeks of the other treatment (*L. rhamnosus* or placebo). Small intestinal permeability was calculated by measuring the urinary lactose-to-mannitol ratio. The authors first noted that the children had baselines permeabilities similar to healthy controls, a finding suggesting the subjects represented a healthier spectrum of IF patients. After administering *L. rhamnosus*, the authors discovered that permeability did not decrease as would be expected if mucosal integrity improved. The authors conclude that *L. rhamnosus* does not improve small intestinal permeability, though this conclusion is complicated by the normal permeability measurements at the beginning of the study. Other symptoms, such as stool frequency, abdominal distension, and fever were not reported.

These reports highlight the major limitations in the probiotic literature. Some studies use a single strain while others use multiple strains and/or also use prebiotics. Some studies give probiotics indefinitely while others have definitive time points of starting and stopping. In addition, endpoints differ among studies (fever, bowel distention, weight gain, measurements such as intestinal permeability). Finally, the lack of clinical trials (save the study by Sentongo et al.) severely limits interpretation. Thus, it is imperative that well controlled clinical trials using clinically relevant outcomes be carried out.

## 29.4 COMPLICATIONS OF PROBIOTIC USE IN IF PATIENTS

Whereas probiotic species are generally considered safe, they do carry the risk of bacteria entering the bloodstream and causing systemic infection. Boyle et al. reviewed the published cases of probiotic-associated infections and found at least 12 cases (of which five were pediatric) associated with *L. rhamnosus* and *Bacillus subtilis* [40]. Patients in this series ranged from 3 months to 79 years of age, and the majority had bacteremia (two had endocarditis and another had a liver abscess). The bacteria were identified initially by cultures but then compared to the ingested probiotic using DNA fingerprinting, 16S rRNA sequencing, or antibiotic-sensitivity testing. The authors concluded that immune deficient and premature patients are most susceptible to probiotic-associated systemic infections. Other risk factors include presence of a central venous catheter, impaired mucosal barrier, jejunostomy delivery, antibiotic treatments to which the probiotic is resistant, probiotics with increased mucosal adherence, and cardiac valve disease.

Children with IF have many of these risk factors, and hence may be at increased risk of developing bloodstream infections with probiotic treatment. Indeed, 3 of the 12 cases involved IF patients.

Kunz et al. reported the cases of former 36-week and 34-week preterm infants starting $1 \times 10^{10}$ cfu/day of *L. rhamnosus* on day of life 95 and 17, respectively [41]. The first patient developed fever after 23 days whereas the second patient became apneic after 169 days; both grew *L. rhamnosus* in their blood, with the second patient's sample displaying a DNA fingerprint identical to the ingested probiotic. De Groote et al. [42] reported similar findings in a IF patient taking 1/4 the amount of *L. rhamnosus* in the report by Kuntz et al. and confirmed the bacteria identity using 16S rRNA sequencing. While the authors attribute the infection to bacteria crossing a more permeable GI tract, they do report that each patient had a central venous catheter for total parenteral nutrition. Thus, it remains a formal possibility, though less likely, that the infection could be from line contamination rather than bacterial gut translocation.

Finally, note should be made that sepsis from fungal probiotic use with *Saccharomyces boulardii* has been reported in children and adults [40]. An infant with IF and a central venous catheter developed yeast sepsis when the infant in the crib next to her was treated with the *S. boulardii* for chronic diarrhea [43]. Confirmation of the organism's identity was made via mitochondrial DNA analysis and chromosomal profiles.

## 29.5  FUTURE DIRECTIONS

Applying probiotics to children with IF is a practice still in its infancy. There are theoretical benefits but clinical data backing the practice are unclear. As noted above, well designed clinical trials are vitally needed to clarify what organisms, at what dose, and for what duration may provide a benefit in which patients (e.g., with/without a colon) with IF. These studies must be done acknowledging the possibility that probiotics may in rare instances confer more risk than benefit, as seen in the patients who developed probiotic-related sepsis.

In addition, to more clinical trials, "community profiling" of microbes—identifying which microbes are there and which are absent—has yet to be done in IF patients. These experiments involve collecting tissue samples such as stool or intestinal biopsies, extracting bacterial DNA, and identifying microbes based on nucleotide sequence [44]. Such experiments will provide a detailed list of the bacterial members present in the gut, and depending on the techniques used, their amounts relative to other bacteria. From these experiments, clinicians may better understand how the GI microbiome may be altered in patients with IF. Further characterization of the organism/host interaction at the mucosal level will provide vital information to rationally design probiotic preparations that may be of benefit. Such techniques open the treatment possibilities beyond *Lactobacillus* and *Bifidobacterium*, and may be the key in realizing the promising therapeutic potential of giving probiotics to children with IF.

## ACKNOWLEDGMENTS

This research was supported by Grant Number R01 NI NR05337, T32 DK007664, RC2 NR011959, and UH2 DK083990 from the National Institutes of Health, the Daffy's Foundation, the USDA/ARS under Cooperative Agreement No. 6250-51000-043, and P30 DK56338 which funds the Texas Medical Center Digestive Disease Center. The content is solely the responsibility of the authors and does not necessarily represent the official views of the National Institutes of Health. This work is a publication of the USDA/ARS Children's Nutrition Research Center, Department of Pediatrics, Baylor College of Medicine and Texas Children's Hospital, Houston, TX. The contents of this publication do not necessarily reflect the views or policies of the USDA, nor does mention of trade names, commercial products, or organizations imply endorsement by the US Government.

## REFERENCES

1. Carter BA, Shulman RJ. Mechanisms of disease: Update on the molecular etiology and fundamentals of parenteral nutrition associated cholestasis. *Nat Clin Pract Gastroenterol Hepatol.* 2007;4:277–87.

2. Wessel JJ, Kocoshis SA. Nutritional management of infants with short bowel syndrome. *Semin Perinatol.* 2007;31:104–11.
3. Duro D, Kamin D, Duggan C. Overview of pediatric short bowel syndrome. *J Pediatr Gastroenterol Nutr.* 2008;47 Suppl 1:S33–6.
4. Preidis GA, Versalovic J. Targeting the human microbiome with antibiotics, probiotics, and prebiotics: Gastroenterology enters the metagenomics era. *Gastroenterology.* 2009;136:2015–31.
5. Podolsky S. Cultural divergence: Elie Metchnikoff's *Bacillus bulgaricus* therapy and his underlying concept of health. *Bull Hist Med.* 1998;72:1–27.
6. Cheplin HA, Rettger LF. Studies on the transformation of the intestinal flora, with special reference to the implantation of *Bacillus acidophilus*: II. Feeding experiments on man. *Proc Natl Acad Sci USA.* 1920;6:704–5.
7. Hamilton-Miller JM, Gibson GR, Bruck W. Some insights into the derivation and early uses of the word 'probiotic'. *Br J Nutr.* 2003;90:845.
8. Fuller R. Probiotics in man and animals. *J Appl Bacteriol.* 1989;66:365–78.
9. Gibson GR, Roberfroid MB. Dietary modulation of the human colonic microbiota: Introducing the concept of prebiotics. *J Nutr.* 1995;125:1401–12.
10. Turnbaugh PJ, Ley RE, Hamady M, Fraser-Liggett CM, Knight R, Gordon JI. The human microbiome project. *Nature.* 2007;449:804–10.
11. Dibaise JK, Young RJ, Vanderhoof JA. Enteric microbial flora, bacterial overgrowth, and short-bowel syndrome. *Clin Gastroenterol Hepatol.* 2006;4:11–20.
12. Cole CR, Ziegler TR. Small bowel bacterial overgrowth: A negative factor in gut adaptation in pediatric SBS. *Curr Gastroenterol Rep.* 2007;9:456–62.
13. Talarico TL, Casas IA, Chung TC, Dobrogosz WJ. Production and isolation of reuterin, a growth inhibitor produced by *Lactobacillus reuteri. Antimicrob Agents Chemother.* 1988;32:1854–8.
14. Talarico TL, Axelsson LT, Novotny J, Fiuzat M, Dobrogosz WJ. Utilization of glycerol as a hydrogen acceptor by *Lactobacillus reuteri*: Purification of 1,3-propanediol: NAD oxidoreductase. *Appl Environ Microbiol.* 1990;56:943–8.
15. Spinler JK, Taweechotipatr M, Rognerud CL, Ou CN, Tumwasorn S, Versalovic J. Human-derived probiotic *Lactobacillus reuteri* demonstrate antimicrobial activities targeting diverse enteric bacterial pathogens. *Anaerobe.* 2008;14:166–71.
16. Sherman PM, Ossa JC, Johnson-Henry K. Unraveling mechanisms of action of probiotics. *Nutr Clin Pract.* 2009;24:10–4.
17. Graul T, Cain AM, Karpa KD. *Lactobacillus* and bifidobacteria combinations: A strategy to reduce hospital-acquired *Clostridium difficile* diarrhea incidence and mortality. *Med Hypotheses.* 2009;73:194–8.
18. Pillai A, Nelson R. Probiotics for treatment of *Clostridium difficile*-associated colitis in adults. *Cochrane Database Syst Rev.* 2008:CD004611.
19. Miller M. The fascination with probiotics for *Clostridium difficile* infection: Lack of evidence for prophylactic or therapeutic efficacy. *Anaerobe.* 2009;15(6):281–4.
20. Neish AS. Microbes in gastrointestinal health and disease. *Gastroenterology.* 2009;136:65–80.
21. Ukena SN, Singh A, Dringenberg U et al. Probiotic *Escherichia coli* Nissle 1917 inhibits leaky gut by enhancing mucosal integrity. *PLoS One.* 2007;2:e1308.
22. Khailova L, Dvorak K, Arganbright KM et al. *Bifidobacterium bifidum* improves intestinal integrity in a rat model of necrotizing enterocolitis. *Am J Physiol Gastrointest Liver Physiol.* 2009;297(5):G940–9.
23. Eizaguirre I, Urkia NG, Asensio AB et al. Probiotic supplementation reduces the risk of bacterial translocation in experimental short bowel syndrome. *J Pediatr Surg.* 2002;37:699–702.
24. Vanderpool C, Yan F, Polk DB. Mechanisms of probiotic action: Implications for therapeutic applications in inflammatory bowel diseases. *Inflamm Bowel Dis.* 2008;14:1585–96.
25. Pessi T, Sutas Y, Hurme M, Isolauri E. Interleukin-10 generation in atopic children following oral *Lactobacillus rhamnosus* GG. *Clin Exp Allergy.* 2000;30:1804–8.
26. Jones SE, Versalovic J. Probiotic *Lactobacillus reuteri* biofilms produce antimicrobial and anti-inflammatory factors. *BMC Microbiol.* 2009;9:35.
27. Mileti E, Matteoli G, Iliev ID, Rescigno M. Comparison of the immunomodulatory properties of three probiotic strains of *Lactobacilli* using complex culture systems: Prediction for *in vivo* efficacy. *PLoS One.* 2009;4:e7056.
28. Xu J, Gordon JI. Inaugural article: Honor thy symbionts. *Proc Natl Acad Sci U S A.* 2003;100:10452–9.
29. Gordon HA, Pesti L. The gnotobiotic animal as a tool in the study of host microbial relationships. *Bacteriol Rev.* 1971;35:390–429.

30. Chen X, Fruehauf J, Goldsmith JD et al. *Saccharomyces boulardii* inhibits EGF receptor signaling and intestinal tumor growth in Apc(min) mice. *Gastroenterology.* 2009;137:914–23.
31. Drozdowski L, Thomson AB. Intestinal hormones and growth factors: Effects on the small intestine. *World J Gastroenterol.* 2009;15:385–406.
32. Mogilner JG, Srugo I, Lurie M et al. Effect of probiotics on intestinal regrowth and bacterial translocation after massive small bowel resection in a rat. *J Pediatr Surg.* 2007;42:1365–71.
33. Wong JM, de Souza R, Kendall CW, Emam A, Jenkins DJ. Colonic health: Fermentation and short chain fatty acids. *J Clin Gastroenterol.* 2006;40:235–43.
34. Andorsky DJ, Lund DP, Lillehei CW et al. Nutritional and other postoperative management of neonates with short bowel syndrome correlates with clinical outcomes. *J Pediatr.* 2001;139:27–33.
35. Vanderhoof JA, Young RJ, Murray N, Kaufman SS. Treatment strategies for small bowel bacterial overgrowth in short bowel syndrome. *J Pediatr Gastroenterol Nutr.* 1998;27:155–60.
36. Candy DC, Densham L, Lamont LS et al. Effect of administration of *Lactobacillus casei* Shirota on sodium balance in an infant with short bowel syndrome. *J Pediatr Gastroenterol Nutr.* 2001;32:506–8.
37. Kanamori Y, Sugiyama M, Hashizume K, Yuki N, Morotomi M, Tanaka R. Experience of long-term synbiotic therapy in seven short bowel patients with refractory enterocolitis. *J Pediatr Surg.* 2004;39:1686–92.
38. Uchida K, Takahashi T, Inoue M et al. Immunonutritional effects during synbiotics therapy in pediatric patients with short bowel syndrome. *Pediatr Surg Int.* 2007;23:243–8.
39. Sentongo TA, Cohran V, Korff S, Sullivan C, Iyer K, Zheng X. Intestinal permeability and effects of *Lactobacillus rhamnosus* therapy in children with short bowel syndrome. *J Pediatr Gastroenterol Nutr.* 2008;46:41–7.
40. Boyle RJ, Robins-Browne RM, Tang ML. Probiotic use in clinical practice: What are the risks? *Am J Clin Nutr.* 2006;83:1256–64; quiz 1446–7.
41. Kunz AN, Noel JM, Fairchok MP. Two cases of *Lactobacillus* bacteremia during probiotic treatment of short gut syndrome. *J Pediatr Gastroenterol Nutr.* 2004;38:457–8.
42. De Groote MA, Frank DN, Dowell E, Glode MP, Pace NR. *Lactobacillus rhamnosus* GG bacteremia associated with probiotic use in a child with short gut syndrome. *Pediatr Infect Dis J.* 2005;24:278–80.
43. Perapoch J, Planes AM, Querol A et al. Fungemia with *Saccharomyces cerevisiae* in two newborns, only one of whom had been treated with ultra-levura. *Eur J Clin Microbiol Infect Dis.* 2000;19:468–70.
44. Hamady M, Knight R. Microbial community profiling for human microbiome projects: Tools, techniques, and challenges. *Genome Res.* 2009;19:1141–52.
45. Marco ML, Pavan S, Kleerebezem M. Towards understanding molecular modes of probiotic action. *Curr Opin Biotechnol.* 2006;17(2):204–10.

# 30 Tissue-Engineered Intestine

*Tracy C. Grikscheit*

## CONTENTS

## 30.1 INTRODUCTION

To reduce the heavy human and financial costs of intestinal failure, tissue-engineered intestine and other stem-cell-based therapies are attractive research targets. The goal is to increase the available surface area of the gastrointestinal tract and to create reservoir capacity and thereby salvage patients with intestinal failure. Current medical and surgical therapies for short bowel syndrome do not adequately treat all patients, and the morbidity and mortality rates for patients with an inadequate amount of intestine or intestinal function are still unacceptably high. These therapies might replace resected or congenitally absent regions of the gastrointestinal tract.

Dedicated intestinal failure centers, bowel-lengthening surgical procedures, alterations in parenteral nutritional components, and intestinal transplant have all had a measureable effect on the treatment of intestinal failure [1–3]. Intestinal transplantation is gradually improving. A recent review of 141 intestinal transplants in 123 children revealed a 1 year patient survival between 44% and 83% and a 3 year patient survival between 32% and 60%, with graft survival rates presumably lower [4]. However, in a recent review of the past 17 years of experience with pediatric intestinal retransplantation, the physicians reported the mean time of initial graft survival to be 34.2 months, with 71.4% of those patients alive at a mean follow-up time of 55.9 months [5]. Intestinal transplantation is limited by organ supply and matching, the costs and compliance demands of lifelong immunosuppression regimens, overall costs, and complexity. Replacement intestine derived from a patient's own cells might overcome many of these obstacles, and tissue engineering has focused on autologous solutions. Tissue-engineered intestine may also be sourced from different donors, for example, in the case of Crohn's disease the diseased intestine may not be the optimal source for the donor cells. In these cases, the lessons learned in the progress of organ transplantation may also apply to the field of tissue-engineered intestine.

Despite the advances in tissue engineering detailed below, tissue-engineered intestine is not yet clinically available and the timeline to its debut is, at present, unknown. However, these investigations have yielded insights into tissue engineering in general and in engineering the intestine in specific. And this progress has also intersected with and aided investigations into biocompatible materials, the developmental pathways that determine gastrointestinal development, and requirements for the stem-cell niche. In addition, the intestine is an effective model for the study of the stem-cell niche because of rapid and usually faultless cell turnover.

## 30.2   TISSUE ENGINEERING REPLACES OLDER SURGICAL STRATEGIES WITH DISTINCT LIMITATIONS

The goal of tissue engineering and organ fabrication is to create living replacement organs and tissues, with the proposed advantages of more exact replacement with durability related to cellular proliferation and autologous repair [6]. The field of tissue engineering is a new addition to the two essential surgical strategies employed to replace absent tissues.

In the first strategy, multiple procedures evolved that rely on substitution of tissues, as in the transfer of colon, jejunum, or stomach to replace an esophagus. In the second strategy, doctors have relied on the use of a manufactured substitute such as Dacron aortic grafts or mechanical heart valves.

The limitations of the first approach, native substitution, lie in the dilemma of prioritizing the values of various tissues, and the sacrifice of one for the other. In pediatric surgery, there is a fairly limited supply of donor tissue that remains inherently different from the tissue that it replaces. For example, replacement of the native esophagus with colon may result in a tube that has inferior peristalsis and over time may become patulous. The second approach, manufactured substitution, has acknowledged problems: material failure, increased rate of infection, and the destruction by the immune system of the foreign material. In addition, nonliving material does not grow with the patient or adapt to changing circumstances, so pediatric patients may undergo multiple operations with increasing levels of complexity as they outgrow their implanted device. Neither approach can provide a living replacement of composite tissues.

The digestive system is composed of both tubular and solid organs with a variety of distinct physiologic and anatomic functions. In the broadest sense, the gastrointestinal tract may be divided into two functional capacities: transit through hollow viscus organs and secretion of key factors from solid organs such as the pancreas. This chapter addresses progress and problems in regenerating the hollow viscus organs of the digestive system. Generally in bioengineering, complex solid organs have been more difficult to reproduce (e.g., complete liver, complete pancreas). In contrast simple cystic structures or tubular structures as well as hollow viscus organs have been more successful (e.g., bladder, trachea, and intestine). As the radius of perfused tissue increases, the delivery requirements for nutrients and oxygen and the demand for the removal of cellular waste increase exponentially [7]. The distance that oxygen must diffuse between a capillary and a cell membrane is limited to a range of 40–200 μm, and therefore tissues over just 5 mm require comprehensive vascular networks and may not rely on diffusion without central necrosis [7]. In contrast simple cystic structures or tubular structures have a reduced demand because the hollow center of the organ does not have to be supplied with arterial and venous flow.

## 30.3   TISSUE ENGINEERING IS NOT WOUND HEALING OR TISSUE INGROWTH

Because of the wide variety of engineered tissues as well as the variable cell types and approaches to generate these tissues, it is necessary to define what can be considered to be a tissue-engineered portion of the gastrointestinal tract. Some reports of tissue healing and native tissue adaptation or regeneration have been incorrectly classified in the literature as tissue engineering.

A basic example of an approach that does not qualify as tissue engineering would be the body's natural recovery from injury, such as skin components healing a surgical incision or expanding after the placement of an inflatable tissue expander, which is serially enlarged. Other examples that do not qualify as tissue engineering include persistence of implanted cells without formation of a subsequent tissue. Another example is native tissue growth into a foreign material such as silicone tubing or porcine intestinal submucosa. These are more properly termed cell transplantation, tissue expansion, wound healing, adaptation, or tissue ingrowth. In addition, engineering of cells differs from engineering a tissue. While engineered cells may be a precursor to a tissue-engineered organ, most investigators require the multiple layers of the tissue, the epithelium, the mesenchyme, the vasculature, and any other critical components to be present before declaring the result to be an engineered tissue.

True tissue-engineering approaches may make use of organ-specific stem cells or cells resulting from any other strategy including from embryonic stem cells, bone-marrow or amniotic fluid cells, or induced pluripotent stem cells. These cells, often transplanted on a biodegradable construct or scaffold, must grow and result in actual tissues with all necessary components of the organ (intestine) or subpart of the organ (islet) no matter how rudimentary. The tissue that is generated should ideally be expanded from the donor cell population, in order to be clinically useful, as any autologous strategy would be unsuccessful if it returned fewer cells to the patient than were initially collected. Eventually, the goal is to generate tissue identical to native intestine as defined by cellular architecture and function.

For children, generation of engineered intestine from autologous cells would avoid the problems of transplant: immunosuppression and donor supply. In addition to tissue-engineered small intestine emerging as a possible therapy for intestinal failure, other regions of the gastrointestinal tract can be generated by this approach. Engineered large intestine, esophagus, stomach, and specific portions of the gastrointestinal tract such as the gastroesophageal junction [6,8–12], formed by variations of the process of multicellular organoid unit transplantation described below, could aid in future treatments of a great range of problems including trauma, vascular accidents, and gastrointestinal cancer resection.

The autologous multicellular strategies described under the umbrella of transplantation of organoid units are just one approach, described because they have resulted in the most architecturally complete gastrointestinal tissue to date (Figures 30.1 and 30.2) [6,8–12]. As investigators make more progress in the field of intestinal stem cells, the progenitor cells that are necessary and sufficient for the creation of engineered tissues may become better defined.

## 30.4   INTESTINAL PROGENITOR CELLS

In self-renewing tissues, small cadre of stem cells usually participate in the regeneration of the tissue through division, generating transit amplifying cells and through resistance to apoptosis [13]. Gastrointestinal epithelial stem cells are therefore natural candidates for the donor cells of

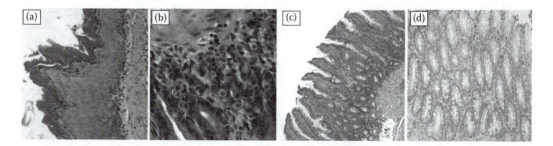

**FIGURE 30.1**   Tissue engineering generates esophagus, stomach, colon, and small intestine in the Lewis rat. (a) Tissue-engineered esophagus, original magnification 20×. Unlike human tissue, the esophagus of the Lewis rat has a squamous epithelium. (b) Tissue-engineered stomach, original magnification 20×. Note large lucent parietal cells and glandular structure. (c) Tissue-engineered small intestine, original magnification 10×. (d) Tissue-engineered colon, original magnification 20×.

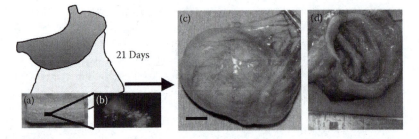

**FIGURE 30.2** Tissue-engineered intestine, in this case, tissue-engineered colon generated in a Lewis rat, is created by implanting organoid units (b) onto a biodegradable polymer (a) into the omentum or other vascular anatomic space. In this case, the organoid units were marked with a fluorescent red membrane dye. After 3 weeks, there is a marked growth of the implant. As seen in (c), a piece of tissue-engineered colon measuring several centimeters has grown from a polymer that initially measured 1 cm long (denoted by black bar). The blood supply is at the top, held by a clamp. The intestine resembles native intestine when opened (d) with a mucosa, serosa, and again the large increase in size from the 1 cm polymer is noted on the included ruler.

tissue-engineered intestine. There is still a healthy debate in the field about definite markers of these progenitor cells, and of course there is some variation throughout the gastrointestinal tract as the esophagus, duodenum, small intestine, and colon vary in their development and therefore the likely stem cells.

Most research has been centered on the stem-cell niche and intestinal epithelial stem cells of the small intestine, which will be discussed here with any important variations noted in the sections for the other regions of the gastrointestinal tract. It is known that the intestinal epithelial stem cells survive in a mesenchymal cell niche toward the base of the intestinal crypt. Intestinal epithelial stem and progenitor cells promote the perpetual regeneration of human small and large intestine. Beyond fetal development, a balanced gut maturation and repair process depends on mesenchyme–epithelial cross talk [14–16]. Wnt, Sonic hedgehog, bone morphogenetic protein, and Notch signaling are known to interact with, regulate, and maintain the rapid self-renewal of the intestinal epithelia. Molecular confirmation of multiple signaling pathways has included a number of soluble signal inhibitors and modulators in the mesenchyme with epithelial effects such as Wnt, Bmp, Fgf, Igf, and Hedgehog among others [15–21].

Early studies before wide availability of transgenic mice and antibodies for immunohistochemistry of specific markers relied on label retention of either [3]H-thymidine or BrdU. Cells that divided rapidly would lose the label, but the label would be retained by longer-cycling cells, presumably therefore stem cells [22,23]. More recently, several putative intestinal epithelium stem-cell markers have been proposed including Bmi1 [24], Lgr5 [25], CD133 [26], DCAMKL1 [27], and Musashi [28]. The Clevers lab has demonstrated growth of "crypt-like structures" *in vitro* from a single Lgr5+ cell with the addition of Wnt agonist R-spondin 1, EGF, and Noggin [29]. Recently, May et al. [27] identified DCAMKL-1, a microtubule associated kinase that is expressed in postmitotic neurons as a putative marker for intestinal stem cells. A follow-up study raises the question if DCAMKL1 is perhaps a marker for tuft cells rather than intestinal epithelial stem cells [30].

Identification of the intestinal epithelial progenitor cell or cells may yield optimized progenitor cell populations for intestinal tissue engineering. Currently, transplantation of these identified populations has not yet resulted in the quantity or function of the tissue-engineered intestine that forms from transplanting multicellular organoid units. This strategy for generating tissue-engineered intestine is distinctive in producing full-thickness tissue that recapitulates native intestine from autologous cells. In order to treat human patients, this is a useful advance: to isolate cells from the patient and return them to the same patient when it is identified that the patient will lose enough intestinal length and thus risk future short bowel syndrome avoids future problems of immunosuppression and rejection.

The sorting processes to purify these single-cell populations are somewhat harsh and time-intensive and it may be difficult to scale up sorted single cells for human therapy unless the purified cells can first expand *in vivo* or *in vitro*. There are encouraging preliminary reports of maintenance and expansion of single-cell populations in cell culture conditions with the addition, as in the Clevers lab, of the Wnt agonist R-spondin 1, with differentiation to goblet and enteroendocrine cells induced by the addition of Notch agonists [31].

Unlike the tissue generated to date by single-cell therapies, tissue-engineered small intestine exactly recapitulates native intestine histology. All differentiated epithelial cell types (enterocytes, enteroendocrine cells, Paneth cells, and goblet cells) are seen in conjunction with a lamina propria comprising intestinal subepithelial myofibroblasts, nerve elements of both Auerbach's and Meissner's plexuses, and a muscularis mucosa [6,8–12,32–34]. However, the multicellular strategy will certainly be altered, improved, and possibly replaced as scientists learn more about the manipulation and preservation of the intestinal stem-cell niche.

## 30.5 TISSUE-ENGINEERED SMALL INTESTINE

The small intestine was the first region of the gastrointestinal tract generated by tissue engineers, and the initial investigators were pediatric surgeons who cared for patients with intestinal failure [35]. The first approach to produce engineered small intestine, transplantation of multicellular organoid units, has subsequently been employed to generate every other region of the alimentary canal from mouth to anus in the Lewis rat [8–12]. This technique has also been adapted to two large animal models, beagle [36] and Yorkshire swine [37].

The generation of a composite tissue resembling small intestine generated from epithelial and mesenchymal intestinal cells which were heterotopically transplanted was first reported in 1998 [35]. Organoid units are multicellular clusters derived from full-thickness biopsies of the intestinal region of interest. These cells are then implanted into a vascularized space such as the omentum, a fatty apron of tissue that is present near the stomach and colon (Figure 30.2). This location has been used because the resulting tissue-engineered small intestine that subsequently grows is then located appropriately inside of the abdomen and can be connected to the shortened small intestine in a later surgery [12]. The scaffolds most commonly used have been constructed of polyglycolic acid and polylactic acid, which are biodegradable (Figure 30.3). As the construct grows into a piece of engineered intestine, the scaffold supporting the cells is degraded through hydrolysis. In most cases, the polymer is essentially absent by the time the engineered intestine is harvested [12]. This process yields tissue-engineered small intestine after 2–4 weeks of growth *in vivo*.

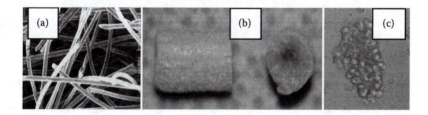

**FIGURE 30.3** Polymer and organoid unit characteristics for the formation of tissue-engineered intestine. (a) Scanning electron micrograph of the scaffold polymer showing the loosely woven biodegradable fibers. Studies have shown that >95% porosity is essential for generating tissue-engineered intestine. (b) The scaffold polymer seen lengthwise and on end. The polymer dimensions for experiments conducted in Lewis rats are a length of 8 mm, an internal diameter of 1 mm, and an outer diameter of 5 mm. The resulting engineered intestine may be several centimeters in length, and the polymer biodegrades during the time of tissue formation, so that it is no longer present when the engineered intestine is fully formed. (c) An organoid unit in culture medium. Organoid units are multicellular, derived from full-thickness biopsies of intestine. Original magnification 10×.

The growth of engineered intestine results in reconstitution of a full thickness piece of intestine, in size several orders of magnitude greater than the original implanted polymer which is hydrolyzed during tissue growth. This regenerated intestine has been used for proof of principle in a replacement model of short bowel syndrome in the Lewis rat. Two groups were compared after greater than 80% resection of their native small bowel. One group also had tissue-engineered small intestine attached to their severely truncated bowel, effectively increasing the intestinal length and surface area. The animals with the additional engineered intestine began to regain weight a week earlier and regained a higher percentage (98.5% vs. 76.8%) of their preoperative weight after 40 days (Figure 30.4) [12].

Animals with the additional engineered small intestine had serum B12 levels in a normal range (439 pg/mL) and animals without were deficient (195.4 pg/mL, $p = 0.0159$). B12 is a vitamin absorbed in the small intestine. The animals with the additional tissue-engineered small intestine also had a longer transit time through the intestine than the animals after massive small bowel resection without any additional engineered segment.

The immune cell population of anastomosed tissue-engineered small intestine at 20 weeks was noted to be similar to native intestine, with no difference in the density or topographical distribution of the mucosal immune system populations of T cells (CD3), B cells (CD32), NK cells (CD56), and macrophages (CD68) [33]. Epithelial mRNA expression topography of SGLT1, a bowel sodium/glucose cotransporter, is also identified in anastomosed engineered small intestine, and increased in animals treated with glucagon-like peptide 2 for 10 days as the engineered intestine grew [34]. Studies of the lymphangiogenesis and angiogenesis of the forming tissue-engineered small intestine found that both processes follow the general pattern of the host animal, rather than that of the donor tissue [32,38]. In tissue-engineered small intestine, as the epithelium and mesenchyme grew, capillary density remained constant, with around 80 capillaries per 1000 nuclei identified [32]. Tissue levels of vascular endothelial growth factor and basic fibroblast growth factor were not as high in the engineered intestine as the source tissue, juvenile intestine [32]. Lymphatic growth also was very similar to the adult host intestine [38].

Investigation in two large animal models shows that tissue-engineered small intestine is not limited to the rodent model. In 2-month-old beagles, one group was unsuccessful in generating

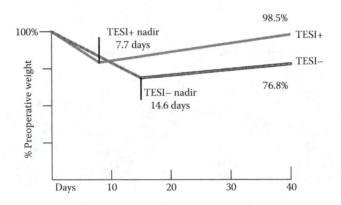

**FIGURE 30.4** Lewis rats with tissue-engineered intestine recover from massive small bowel resection faster than those without. Percentage preoperative weight for TESI+ [rats with a massive small bowel resection rescued with tissue-engineered intestine connected to their shortened intestine (TESI)] and TESI– rats (massive small bowel resection without rescue) over 40 days. TESI+ animals reach their nadir at 7.7 days while animals without TESI lose weight for an additional week. TESI+ animals regain weight to a higher percentage (98.5%) than TESI– animals (76.8%) by day 40. TESI+ animals regained weight more rapidly (0.7% preoperative weight/day regained) than TESI– animals (0.2%/day, $p = 0.004$) after each group reached its nadir.

tissue-engineered intestine from autologous ileum, but allotransplantation of fetal organoid units into 10-month-old canines immunosuppressed with cyclosporine and steroids [36] successfully generated tissue-engineered small intestine.

In 6-week-old Yorkshire swine piglets, similar in size to a newborn human baby, autologous tissue-engineered small intestine and stomach were generated in a model that closely approximates the intended course of human therapy. The animals underwent on-table resection with the organoid units prepared and reimplanted into the same animal during the initial operation. Both tissue-engineered intestine and tissue-engineered stomach formed [37]. This strategy for generating tissue-engineered intestine is distinctive in producing full-thickness tissue that recapitulates native intestine from autologous cells (Figure 30.5).

This is the first description of engineered intestine implanted during a single anesthetic and from autologous tissue [37], presumably arising from organ-specific stem cells, indirectly supported by data identifying some features of an intact stem-cell niche. Success in an autologous large animal model is an important step in a pathway to a human therapy that would avoid the problems of transplantation and subsequent necessary immunosuppression. Further refinements of this technique could allow for options in the human therapy of short bowel syndrome or the replacement of absent intestinal tissue resulting from a wide range of diseases or insults.

All of the successful multicellular organoid unit approaches indicate that at least the epithelial "regenerative unit," presumably containing the stem cells of the intestine, is successfully transplanted, although without distinctly identifying the cell or cells that are sufficient.

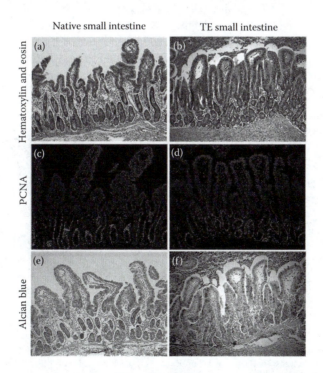

**FIGURE 30.5** Morphological comparison of the differentiated endothelium of the native small intestine and tissue-engineered small intestine generated in Yorkshire swine. (a,b) Hematoxylin and eosin staining of the tissue showing similar architecture of both native and engineered small intestine. (c,d) Immunofluorescence staining of the proliferating cells in the crypt of both engineered and native intestine using an anti-PCNA primary antibody (original magnification 40×). (e,f) Alcian blue staining of the goblet cells (original magnification 10×).

## 30.6  TISSUE-ENGINEERED ESOPHAGUS

Multiple strategies to reconstruct pharyngogastric transit currently exist. Most commonly, the colon or the denervated stomach replace the esophagus [39–42]. Free jejunal grafts can also be used [43]. Esophageal replacements are performed for a variety of conditions including congenital anomalies like long-gap esophageal atresia or tracheoesophageal fistulae in which children are born with an interrupted esophagus, corrosive injury such as ingestion of lye, and resection for injury including long-term exposure to gastroesophageal reflux, or tumor. The most frequent tissues used for surgical replacement of the esophagus include the stomach, jejunum, and large intestine [44,45]. The esophagus is not a vital organ, as feeding through distal tubes into the stomach or jejunum is possible, but loss of the esophagus, and thus oral feeding definitely impacts the quality of life.

In an approach similar to that described in the growth of tissue-engineered small intestine, transplantation of organoid units derived from esophageal tissue results in the growth of tissue-engineered esophagus in Lewis rats [8]. The generated tissue is a complex tissue resembling native esophagus and could be formed from neonatal and adult tissues. Animals with tissue-engineered esophageal replacements were able to eat and gain weight to levels above their preoperative weight over 42 days (Figure 30.6) [8]. Because the engineered esophagus grows orders of magnitude beyond the original implanted construct, this success could lead to an autologous approach to complicated pharyngogastric reconstruction problems when conventional approaches are not useful, perhaps with a laparoscopic implantation of the construct. This technique could possibly be refined aid in cases where native proxy substitution is untenable.

Efforts to refine this approach have been made by changing the polymer supporting the organoid units, using small intestinal submucosa and other variants of the PLGA polymer. One group has also performed an adhesion assay that identified Type-I collagen as binding to rat esophageal epithelial cells better than fibronectin, laminin, or osteopontin [46].

Wound-healing models have shown some promise in decreasing stricture formation after mucosal resection in dogs [47]. An inventive, yet work-intensive process in which human esophageal cells and dermal fibroblasts were cultured in layers with the intent to eventually roll them into a tube anastomosed to the esophagus has also been reported [48].

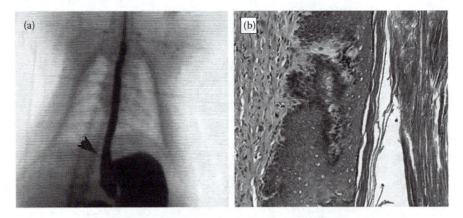

**FIGURE 30.6**  Tissue-engineered esophagus in the Lewis rat is a functional enteral conduit. Lewis rats either underwent patch anastomosis to their native abdominal esophagus or complete interposition graft of the abdominal esophagus, then returned to feeding for 42 days. Animals initially lost weight, but steadily regained weight feeding through the tissue-engineered esophagus until all animals weighed more than their initial preoperative weight at the conclusion of the study. In panel (a), the esophagus below the arrow is tissue-engineered esophagus that has been sutured in place of the animal's native esophagus, and in this upper gastrointestinal x-ray series in which the animal has swallowed radiopaque dye, the contour of the patent esophagus can be evaluated. In panel (b), the histology of the tissue-engineered esophagus shows that the tissue is very similar to the native esophagus of the rat.

## 30.7   TISSUE-ENGINEERED STOMACH

Postgastrectomy morbidity and the rare condition of microgastria both emphasize the difficulties related to inadequate stomach tissue mass and stomach function. More than 70 reconstructive strategies including jejunal interposition (Longmire's procedure) and jejunal pouch formation have been proposed since Schlatter's initial gastrectomy in 1897. Among these strategies, there has been conflicting evidence of improvement of patients' quality of life [49]. Preservation of the duodenal passage for the addition of pancreatic and biliary secretions, and pouch capacity to maximize food intake are important aspects of the stomach or stomach replacements. Congenital microgastria is a very unusual condition with only 26 well-documented accounts. Much less has been demonstrated in the surgical care of this condition [50], but the problems of supplying gastric digestive function and the lack of an appropriate food reservoir remain in cases of resection for tumor or cases where the stomach has been used for esophageal replacement.

Tissue-engineered stomach and esophagus have been published with specific and appropriate full-thickness tissue architecture [8,9]. In the case of tissue-engineered stomach, the central dogma of tissue engineering, exact replacement, has been extended in a series of studies showing that a tissue-engineered gastroesophageal junction can be prepared as well as antrum alone, and either young or old rats can be the syngeneic donor. The tissue stains appropriately for gastrin, has parietal cells, and has the exact architecture of native stomach [9]. These results were confirmed in the same rat model, with the tissue-engineered stomach connected to native intestine [51].

Additionally, tissue-engineered stomach has been generated from an autologous donor and host in 6-week-old Yorkshire swine piglets [37]. The donors and hosts in the previous experiments in Lewis rats were syngeneic, but human therapy could rely on engineered intestine forming from the patient's own cells harvested and implanted during one procedure. Tissue-engineered stomach morphology in the autologous large animal model was similar to the antrum of a native stomach with mucous cells demonstrated by alcian blue and smooth muscle actin immunofluorescence identifying the muscularis mucosae [37].

## 30.8   TISSUE-ENGINEERED LARGE INTESTINE

Removal of the colon is necessary to treat a number of medical problems including most commonly ulcerative colitis, other forms of colitis, and cancer. In pediatric patients with Hirschsprung's disease, a condition in which there is aganglionosis of the intestine leading to functional obstruction, 2–14% of all patients will demonstrate total colonic aganglionosis, with no ganglion cells identified in the entire large intestine, mandating resection [52]. The most common surgical correction after colectomy to replicate storage and absorption properties of the lost native tissue is the formation of an ileal pouch. Although ileal pouch replacement for a resected native large intestine is fairly durable, pouchitis is a common complication after total proctocolectomy, and there are postcolectomy morbidities associated with lack of physiologic large intestinal function. Pouchitis is not trivial, and patients may undergo reoperation, experience greater stool frequency, abdominal cramping, fever, and extraintestinal manifestations [53]. The cumulative frequency of pouchitis at major referral centers approaches 50% over 10 years [54], but earlier problems also occur. A review of 55,934 patients with ulcerative colitis, with a subset of 540 patients who had a colectomy and documented 180 days of postcolectomy follow-up found that 54% of the patients required a second colectomy-related surgery within that timeframe, and mean medical charges for the 180 days following and including the colectomy was $90,445 [55].

In the Lewis rat, tissue-engineered colon grows from neonatal and adult colon as well as from tissue-engineered colon itself, and is very durable [10]. At 4 weeks, tissue-engineered colon histology is very similar to native colon with an appropriate epithelial layer, actin-positive muscularis propria containing S100 positive cells in the distribution of Meissner and Auerbach's plexi (Figure 30.7) as well as lucent adjacent ganglion cells. Transmission electron microscopy of

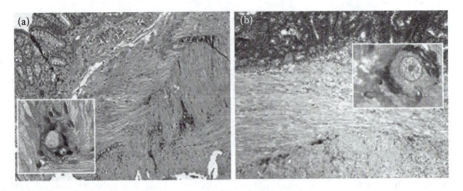

**FIGURE 30.7**  Tissue-engineered intestine has ganglion cells in Meissner's and Auerbach's plexi. In the Lewis rat, immunohistochemical detection of the antigen S100 revealing enteric nerve plexi in native small intestine (a) and tissue-engineered small intestine (b). Ganglion cells are seen surrounded by brown S100 positive nerve (inset). Original magnifications 10× and 20×.

tissue-engineered colon revealed the same ultramicroscopic findings as native colon with abundant mitochondria, apical microvilli, tight junctions, desmosomes with keratin filaments, and goblet cells, indicating successful tube formation with repolarization, re-forming of junctions, and lumen formation (Figure 30.8) [10].

Tissue-engineered colon generated in the Lewis rat was further studied in a replacement model, in which a group of Lewis rats with an end-ileostomy was compared to a group with an anastomosed segment of tissue-engineered colon in lieu of an ileal pouch [11].

In these experiments, animals with a tissue-engineered colon pouch proximal to the ileostomy had a statistically significant physiologic advantage to animals with an end-ileostomy alone, including less weight loss and less relative hyponatremia. There was decreased stool moisture content by 10%. Transit times were more than doubled, and there was observation of more formed stool as well as appropriate short chain fatty acid amounts and types in the animals with tissue-engineered colon. The engineered colon pouch was resilient with no formation of megapouch observed over 41 days, and an overall increase in pouch dimensions of 6% over 41 days. Stool bacteriology was not different between the two groups. The histology was in some cases indistinguishable from native colon. Therefore, the tissue-engineered colon appeared to meet basic physiologic demands in a preliminary demonstration of large intestine replacement.

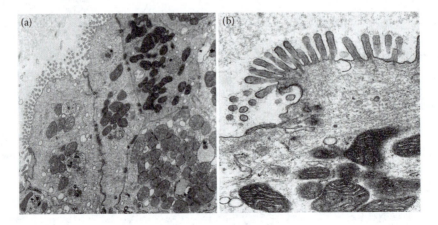

**FIGURE 30.8**  Tissue-engineered colon has the same ultramicroscopic appearance as native colon. In this tissue generated in the Lewis rat, abundant mitochondria, apical microvilli, tight junctions, and desmosomes with keratin filaments are all identified.

## 30.9  IMPEDIMENTS TO TISSUE-ENGINEERED INTESTINE AS A HUMAN THERAPY—POLYMERS, PROGENITORS, AND PROCESSES

Future directions for improving tissue-engineered small intestine in preparation for human therapy may include optimization of polymers [56]. The polymer used in the majority of the studies above is mainly composed of polyglycolic acid, a material that is widely used currently in human applications as absorbable suture material or mesh, and can be stored in moisture-free conditions for long periods of time. Additional approaches include added growth factors such as VEGF or bFGF to implanted polymers, subsequently implanting organoid units [57] or myofibroblasts on the polymers [58].

Other groups have elected to implant the polymer first, adding the organoid units after a delay of weeks in order to "prevascularize" the scaffold, although this entails two procedures and has not yielded superior results [59]. Preliminary reports that small intestinal submucosa, essentially a naturally derived sheet of decellularized collagen, could be surgically interposed in small intestine have been discredited [60], and would be an example of wound healing rather than tissue engineering. Other materials innovations include electrospinning [61] and the incorporation of growth factors and peptides. The obvious choices for factors added to the construct include the Wnt agonist R-spondin 1, as demonstrated in the Clevers and Kuo culture systems or the addition of the other factors needed for culturing Lgr5 cells, EGF, and Noggin [29], or including Notch agonists [31]. These experiments will likely have been completed by several investigators by the publication of this book.

As discussed, there has been recent intensive progress in the field of intestinal epithelial progenitor cell markers, and the necessary and sufficient progenitor cell population will likely be informed by this debate. Optimized progenitor cell populations may be transplanted in the future from autologous or from heterogenous donors, in which cases immunosuppression may be necessary.

Another obstacle to human therapy that will have to be overcome in scaling up any tissue-engineered intestine or stem-cell therapy will be inventing the manufacturing processes including the *in vitro* processing of any donor cells to ensure that regulatory and clinical specifications are met without significant lot to lot variability.

## 30.10  SUMMARY

The focus of tissue engineering as a field is the successful replacement of tissue without resorting to using other tissues by proxy or man-made substitutes that may not be regenerative, an important consideration in pediatric surgery where outgrowing replacement material may lead to numerous operations over a lifetime.

The gross organization of native and tissue-engineered small intestine is homologous. All four types of differentiated intestinal epithelial cells are found in their accustomed locations in engineered and native small intestine. Tissue-engineered small intestine in small and large animal models exactly recapitulates native intestine histology. The crypts in engineered intestine in this model are analogous to those in native intestine with a proliferative zone indicated by PCNA staining. All differentiated epithelial cell types (enterocytes, enteroendocrine cells, and goblet cells) [27] are seen in conjunction with a lamina propria comprising intestinal subepithelial myofibroblasts, nerve elements of both Auerbach's and Meissner's plexuses, and a muscularis mucosa.

Regeneration of the intestine stem-cell niche and full-thickness intestine from autologous cells is a prerequisite to a durable human therapy. Success in an autologous large animal model is an important step in a pathway to a human therapy that would avoid the problems of transplantation and subsequent necessary immunosuppression. Further refinements of this technique could allow for options in the human therapy of short bowel syndrome or the replacement of absent intestinal tissue resulting from a wide range of diseases or insults.

## REFERENCES

1. Reyes J, Bueno J, Kocoshis S, Green M, Abu-Elmagd K, Furukawa H et al. Current status of intestinal transplantation in children. *J Pediatr Surg.* 1998;33(2):243–54.
2. Grant D, Abu-Elmagd K, Reyes J, Tzakis A, Langnas A, Fishbein T et al. 2003 report of the intestine transplant registry: A new era has dawned. *Ann Surg* 2005;241(4):607–13.
3. Sudan D, Thompson J, Botha J, Grant W, Antonson D, Raynor S et al. Comparison of intestinal lengthening procedures for patients with short bowel syndrome. *Ann Surg* 2007;246(4):593–601; discussion -4.
4. Kato T, Tzakis AG, Selvaggi G, Gaynor JJ, David AI, Bussotti A et al. Intestinal and multivisceral transplantation in children. *Ann Surg* 2006;243(6):756–64; discussion 64–6.
5. Mazariegos GV, Machaidze Z. Auxiliary liver transplantation: Location, location, location. *Pediatr Transplant* 2009;13(1):1–2.
6. Grikscheit TC, Vacanti JP. The history and current status of tissue engineering: The future of pediatric surgery. *J Pediatr Surg* 2002;37(3):277–88.
7. Muschler GF, Nakamoto C, Griffith LG. Engineering principles of clinical cell-based tissue engineering. *J Bone Joint Surg Am* 2004;86-A(7):1541–58.
8. Grikscheit T, Ochoa ER, Srinivasan A, Gaissert H, Vacanti JP. Tissue-engineered esophagus: Experimental substitution by onlay patch or interposition. *J Thorac Cardiovasc Surg* 2003;126(2):537–44.
9. Grikscheit T, Srinivasan A, Vacanti JP. Tissue-engineered stomach: A preliminary report of a versatile *in vivo* model with therapeutic potential. *J Pediatr Surg* 2003;38(9):1305–9.
10. Grikscheit TC, Ochoa ER, Ramsanahie A, Alsberg E, Mooney D, Whang EE et al. Tissue-engineered large intestine resembles native colon with appropriate *in vitro* physiology and architecture. *Ann Surg* 2003238(1):35–41.
11. Grikscheit TC, Ogilvie JB, Ochoa ER, Alsberg E, Mooney D, Vacanti JP. Tissue-engineered colon exhibits function *in vivo*. *Surg* 2002;132(2):200–4.
12. Grikscheit TC, Siddique A, Ochoa ER, Srinivasan A, Alsberg E, Hodin RA et al. Tissue-engineered small intestine improves recovery after massive small bowel resection. *Ann Surg* 2004;240(5):748–54.
13. Potten CS, Booth C, Tudor GL, Booth D, Brady G, Hurley P et al. Identification of a putative intestinal stem cell and early lineage marker; Musashi-1. *Differ* 2003;71(1):28–41.
14. Andoh A, Bamba S, Brittan M, Fujiyama Y, Wright NA. Role of intestinal subepithelial myofibroblasts in inflammation and regenerative response in the gut. *Pharmacol Ther* 2007;114(1):94–106.
15. Ramalho-Santos M, Melton DA, McMahon AP. Hedgehog signals regulate multiple aspects of gastrointestinal development. *Dev* 2000;127(12):2763–72.
16. Sancho E, Batlle E, Clevers H. Signaling pathways in intestinal development and cancer. *Annu Rev Cell Dev Biol* 2004;20:695–723.
17. Gregorieff A, Pinto D, Begthel H, Destree O, Kielman M, Clevers H. Expression pattern of Wnt signaling components in the adult intestine. *Gastroenterol* 2005;129(2):626–38.
18. Kaestner KH, Silberg DG, Traber PG, Schutz G. The mesenchymal winged helix transcription factor Fkh6 is required for the control of gastrointestinal proliferation and differentiation. *Genes Dev* 1997;11(12):1583–95.
19. Korinek V, Barker N, Moerer P, van Donselaar E, Huls G, Peters PJ et al. Depletion of epithelial stem-cell compartments in the small intestine of mice lacking Tcf-4. *Nat Genet* 1998;19(4):379–83.
20. Louvard D, Kedinger M, Hauri HP. The differentiating intestinal epithelial cell: Establishment and maintenance of functions through interactions between cellular structures. *Annu Rev Cell Biol* 1992;8:157–95.
21. Ormestad M, Astorga J, Landgren H, Wang T, Johansson BR, Miura N et al. Foxf1 and Foxf2 control murine gut development by limiting mesenchymal Wnt signaling and promoting extracellular matrix production. *Dev* 2006;133(5):833–43.
22. Kalabis J, Oyama K, Okawa T, Nakagawa H, Michaylira CZ, Stairs DB et al. A subpopulation of mouse esophageal basal cells has properties of stem cells with the capacity for self-renewal and lineage specification. *J Clin Invest* 2008;118(12):3860–9.
23. Montgomery RK, Breault DT. Small intestinal stem cell markers. *J Anat* 2008;213(1):52–8.
24. Sangiorgi E, Capecchi MR. Bmi1 is expressed *in vivo* in intestinal stem cells. *Nat Genet* 2008;40(7):915–20.
25. Barker N, van Es JH, Kuipers J, Kujala P, van den Born M, Cozijnsen M et al. Identification of stem cells in small intestine and colon by marker gene Lgr5. *Nat* 2007;449(7165):1003–7.
26. Zhu L, Gibson P, Currle DS, Tong Y, Richardson RJ, Bayazitov IT et al. Prominin 1 marks intestinal stem cells that are susceptible to neoplastic transformation. *Nat* 2009;457(7229):603–7.

27. May R, Riehl TE, Hunt C, Sureban SM, Anant S, Houchen CW. Identification of a novel putative gastrointestinal stem cell and adenoma stem cell marker, doublecortin and CaM kinase-like-1, following radiation injury and in adenomatous polyposis coli/multiple intestinal neoplasia mice. *Stem Cells* 2008; 26(3):630–7.

28. Asai R, Okano H, Yasugi S. Correlation between Musashi-1 and c-hairy-1 expression and cell proliferation activity in the developing intestine and stomach of both chicken and mouse. *Dev Growth Differ* 2005;47(8):501–10.

29. Sato T, Vries RG, Snippert HJ, van de Wetering M, Barker N, Stange DE et al. Single Lgr5 stem cells build crypt-villus structures *in vitro* without a mesenchymal niche. *Nat* 2009;459(7244):262–5.

30. Gerbe F, Brulin B, Makrini L, Legraverend C, Jay P. DCAMKL-1 expression identifies tuft cells rather than stem cells in the adult mouse intestinal epithelium. *Gastroenterol* 2009;137(6):2179–81

31. Ootani A, Li X, Sangiorgi E, Ho QT, Ueno H, Toda S et al. Sustained *in vitro* intestinal epithelial culture within a Wnt-dependent stem cell niche. *Nat Med* 2009;15(6):701–6.

32. Gardner-Thorpe J, Grikscheit TC, Ito H, Perez A, Ashley SW, Vacanti JP et al. Angiogenesis in tissue-engineered small intestine. *Tissue Eng* 2003;9(6):1255–61.

33. Perez A, Grikscheit TC, Blumberg RS, Ashley SW, Vacanti JP, Whang EE. Tissue-engineered small intestine: Ontogeny of the immune system. *Transplantation* 2002;74(5):619–23.

34. Ramsanahie A, Duxbury MS, Grikscheit TC, Perez A, Rhoads DB, Gardner-Thorpe J et al. Effect of GLP-2 on mucosal morphology and SGLT1 expression in tissue-engineered neointestine. *Am J Physiol Gastrointest Liver Physiol* 2003;285(6):G1345–52.

35. Vacanti JP, Morse MA, Saltzman WM, Domb AJ, Perez-Atayde A, Langer R. Selective cell transplantation using bioabsorbable artificial polymers as matrices. *J Pediatr Surg* 1988;23(1 Pt 2):3–9.

36. Agopian VG, Chen DC, Avansino JR, Stelzner M. Intestinal stem cell organoid transplantation generates neomucosa in dogs. *J Gastrointest Surg* 2009;13(5):971–82.

37. Sala FG, Kunisaki SM, Ochoa ER, Vacanti J, Grikscheit TC. Tissue-engineered small intestine and stomach form from autologous tissue in a preclinical large animal model. *J Surg Res* 2009;156(2):205–12.

38. Duxbury MS, Grikscheit TC, Gardner-Thorpe J, Rocha FG, Ito H, Perez A et al. Lymphangiogenesis in tissue-engineered small intestine. *Transplantation* 2004;77(8):1162–6.

39. Samuel M, Burge DM, Moore IE. Gastric tube graft interposition as an oesophageal substitute. *ANZ J Surg* 2001;71(1):56–61.

40. Dreuw B, Fass J, Titkova S, Anurov M, Polivoda M, Ottinger AP et al. Colon interposition for esophageal replacement: Isoperistaltic or antiperistaltic? Experimental results. *Ann Thorac Surg* 2001;71(1):303–8.

41. Gutschow C, Collard JM, Romagnoli R, Salizzoni M, Holscher A. Denervated stomach as an esophageal substitute recovers intraluminal acidity with time. *Ann Surg* 2001;233(4):509–14.

42. Dantas RO, Mamede RC. Motility of the transverse colon used for esophageal replacement. *J Clin Gastroenterol* 2002;34(3):225–8.

43. Pavlovics G, Cseke L, Papp A, Tizedes G, Tabar BA, Horvath PO. Esophagus reconstruction with free jejunal transfer. *Microsurgery* 2006;26(1):73–7.

44. Coopman S, Michaud L, Halna-Tamine M, Bonnevalle M, Bourgois B, Turck D et al. Long-term outcome of colon interposition after esophagectomy in children. *J Pediatr Gastroenterol Nutr* 2008;47(5):458–62.

45. Al-Shanafey S, Harvey J. Long gap esophageal atresia: An Australian experience. *J Pediatr Surg* 2008; 43(4):597–601.

46. Beckstead BL, Pan S, Bhrany AD, Bratt-Leal AM, Ratner BD, Giachelli CM. Esophageal epithelial cell interaction with synthetic and natural scaffolds for tissue engineering. *Biomaterials* 2005;26(31):6217–28.

47. Nieponice A, McGrath K, Qureshi I, Beckman EJ, Luketich JD, Gilbert TW et al. An extracellular matrix scaffold for esophageal stricture prevention after circumferential EMR. *Gastrointest Endosc* 2008; 69(2):289–96.

48. Hayashi K, Ando N, Ozawa S, Kitagawa Y, Miki H, Sato M et al. A neo-esophagus reconstructed by cultured human esophageal epithelial cells, smooth muscle cells, fibroblasts, and collagen. *Asaio J* 2004;50(3):261–6.

49. Parameswaran R, McNair A, Avery KN, Berrisford RG, Wajed SA, Sprangers MA et al. The role of health-related quality of life outcomes in clinical decision making in surgery for esophageal cancer: A systematic review. *Ann Surg Oncol* 2008;15(9):2372–9.

50. Hoehner JC, Kimura K, Soper RT. Congenital microgastria. *J Pediatr Surg* 1994;29(12):1591–3.

51. Maemura T, Shin M, Kinoshita M, Majima T, Ishihara M, Saitoh D et al. A tissue-engineered stomach shows presence of proton pump and G-cells in a rat model, resulting in improved anemia following total gastrectomy. *Artif Organs.* 2008;32(3):234–9.

52. Moore SW Zaahl M. Clinical and genetic differences in total colonic aganglionosis in Hirschsprung's disease. *J Pediatr Surg* 2009;44(10):1899–903.
53. Kirat HT, Remzi FH, Kiran RP, Fazio VW. Comparison of outcomes after hand-sewn versus stapled ileal pouch-anal anastomosis in 3,109 patients. *Surgery* 2009;146(4):723–9; discussion 9–30.
54. Stahlberg D, Gullberg K, Liljeqvist L, Hellers G, Lofberg R. Pouchitis following pelvic pouch operation for ulcerative colitis. Incidence, cumulative risk, and risk factors. *Dis Colon Rectum* 1996; 39(9):1012–8.
55. Loftus EV, Jr., Friedman HS, Delgado DJ, Sandborn WJ. Colectomy subtypes, follow-up surgical proce-dures, postsurgical complications, and medical charges among ulcerative colitis patients with private health insurance in the United States. *Inflamm Bowel Dis* 2009;15(4):566–75.
56. Chen DC, Avansino JR, Agopian VG, Hoagland VD, Woolman JD, Pan S et al. Comparison of polyester scaffolds for bioengineered intestinal mucosa. *Cells Tissues Organs* 2006;184(3–4):154–65.
57. Rocha FG, Sundback CA, Krebs NJ, Leach JK, Mooney DJ, Ashley SW et al. The effect of sustained delivery of vascular endothelial growth factor on angiogenesis in tissue-engineered intestine. *Biomaterials* 2008;29(19):2884–90.
58. Lee M, Wu BM, Stelzner M, Reichardt HM, Dunn JC. Intestinal smooth muscle cell maintenance by basic fibroblast growth factor. *Tissue Eng Part A* 2008 14(8):1395–402.
59. Lloyd DA, Ansari TI, Gundabolu P, Shurey S, Maquet V, Sibbons PD et al. A pilot study investigating a novel subcutaneously implanted pre-cellularised scaffold for tissue engineering of intestinal mucosa. *Eur Cell Mater* 2006;11:27–33; discussion 4.
60. Lee M, Chang PC, Dunn JC. Evaluation of small intestinal submucosa as scaffolds for intestinal tissue engineering. *J Surg Res* 2008;147(2):168–71.
61. Soliman S, Pagliari S, Rinaldi A, Forte G, Fiaccavento R, Pagliari F et al. Multiscale 3d scaffolds for soft tissue engineering via multimodal electrospinning. *Acta Biomater* 2010;6(4):1227–37.

# 31 Assessment of Mucosal Mass and Hormonal Therapy

*David L. Sigalet and Dana Boctor*

## CONTENTS

## 31.1 INTRODUCTION

The care of infants and children with short bowel syndrome (SBS) is primarily focused on meticulous nutritional support, while the remaining intestine undergoes adaptation thereby enhancing nutrient-absorptive capacity (reviewed in Chapter 2). Clinical experience and animal studies have demonstrated that the small intestine adapts through hypertrophy of the mucosa, which increases absorptive abilities [1–4]. Grossly, the bowel dilates, lengthens, and thickens; microscopically villus hyperplasia occurs with increased crypt depth, and muscle thickness [5]. Production of brush-border enzymes is augmented, as well as increases in mucosal weight, protein, RNA, and DNA content [5,6]. Intestinal adaptation begins within 24–48 h of resection, but may continue for several years [7]. Although systematic studies in humans are practically difficult, the data available support similar histological and functional adaptation in infants, which may take several years to complete [8]. Adequate intestinal adaptation is required before a patient with extensive GI resection is able to absorb sufficient enteral nutrients and be weaned from parenteral nutrition (PN) support.

Clinical factors associated with intestinal autonomy include: younger age, limited extent of resection (adults need approximately 50–120 cm and infants about 40 cm + of small intestine to allow successful discontinuation of PN), extent of ileal resection, presence of the ileocecal valve, continuity of colon with small intestine, and adequate general nutritional status [8,9]. It is also important to recall that adaptation, as described here, only occurs if the patient is receiving enteral nutrition, suggesting that nutrients act to stimulate an upregulation of their own absorptive pathways. Further, younger infants and those who have any ileal remnant, however short, have long been appreciated as having an increased ability to adapt. This suggests that different growth and regulatory factors, especially those produced in the ileum, are important in regulating intestinal adaptation. Several hormones and trophic agents have been studied and reviewed including enteroglucagon, growth hormone, insulin-like growth factor, glutamine, glucagon-like peptide 2, epidermal growth factor, cholecystokinin, gastrin, insulin, neurotensin, and peptide YY [10]. This chapter will focus on the major regulatory and growth factors which have been linked to adaptation; these are presented schematically in Figure 31.1.

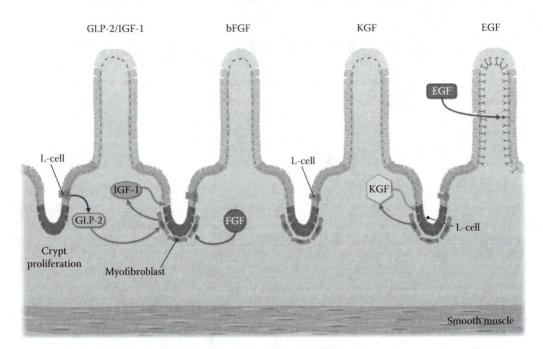

**FIGURE 31.1**  Schematic of growth factors controlling mucosal nutrient-absorptive activity.

## 31.2  GLUCAGON-LIKE PEPTIDE 2

Of these factors, the enteroendocrine hormone glucagon-like peptide 2 (GLP-2) appears to be a key factor in signaling adaptation. GLP-2 is a 33 amino acid peptide produced with GLP-1 from the pro-glucagon gene. This same gene produces pancreatic glucagon, however it undergoes specific post-translational processing in the enteroendocrine L cells of the small intestine to produce the GLP proteins. GLP-2 (with GLP-1) is released by the L-cells primarily in response to direct contact with luminal nutrients, especially long-chain fatty acids in the terminal ileum (Figure 31.2) [7,11–13]. In animal and human subjects after major proximal intestinal resection, GLP-2 levels are significantly elevated [1,14,15]. GLP-2 has a short half-life as an endocrine hormone of 7 min [16]. It acts to stimulate intestinal mucosal crypt-cell proliferation by increasing IGF-1 production by the pericryptal fibroblasts, which increases crypt-cell proliferation, villus height, and surface area, and thus increases nutrient-absorptive capacity [17–19]. There is recent evidence that it acts at the muco-sal level to stimulate elements of the EGF-receptor pathway and chylomicron formation, and at the macroscopic level to slow proximal motility [20,21]. Interestingly, some or all of these effects may be mediated by GLP-2 stimulation of enteric neuronal pathways [22].

In enterally fed animals subjected to massive resection, GLP-2 levels were highly correlated with spontaneous adaptation and ongoing elevated baseline production was noted even after nutrient malabsorption was corrected. This suggests that GLP-2 is important in initiating and maintaining spontaneous adaptation [1]. In animals maintained with enteral nutrition, exogenous GLP-2 increased nutrient absorption by 20%–100%, depending on the length of residual bowel [23–25]. These studies are focused on the "adaptation" of nutrient absorption following intestinal resection; however, it is important to recognize that this is a subtype of the normal physiologic regulation of nutrient absorption which occurs in all mammals. The intestine must respond to such stresses as the wide variations in nutrient availability which occur in the wild, increased nutrient requirements, as seen during pregnancy, or in decreased absorptive capacity as occurs following mucosal damage from disease or toxicity [5,6,26]. In this context, GLP-2 can be viewed as a "master-regulator" of intestinal response to nutrient load (Figure 31.1).

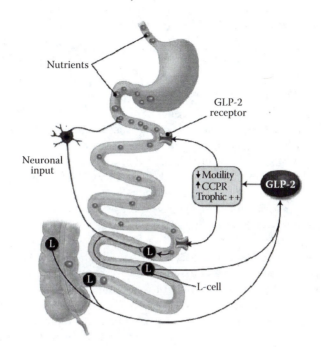

**FIGURE 31.2** GLP-2 release by enteral nutrients and signaling effects.

In adult human studies, GLP-2 or its analogs have been shown to have modest effects on nutrient and fluid absorption [27,28]. A phase-3 trial with teduglutide, a long-acting GLP-2 agonist, has been completed in a population of stable, chronically PN-dependent adult patients with SBS. The preliminary results are positive and suggest that adults achieve a mean 20% reduction in parenteral dependence [29]. This is quite encouraging given the knowledge that the adult bowel is typically not thought to have as great a potential for adaptation in comparison to the infant bowel. At present, studies in pediatric patients are in the planning stages.

It is important to note that this system is constitutively active in premature infants. In fed premature neonates, levels of GLP-2 are very high (up to 450 pM/L), but low in infants not tolerating feeds, showing a regulatory role in this age group [30]. Basal levels are high in these infants without meal stimulation, suggesting a potential role in inducing gut growth in the final weeks of gestation [30–32]. In infants with SBS, serum GLP-2 concentrations were noted to correlate positively with residual small intestinal length and markers of intestinal absorption [15]. Importantly, in these studies, infants without remnant ileum did not produce significant levels of GLP-2, even if the colon was intact. Further, all infants unable to produce GLP-2 levels of >15 pM/L with feeds of >40 kCal/kg died of complications of SBS [15]. In infants with gastroschisis, there is a clear association of GLP-2 production with tolerance of enteral nutrition. Infants with gastroschisis have reduced fasting and stimulated levels of GLP-2 production in the initial weeks of life; when they do begin to tolerate feeds there appears to be a phase of hyper-responsiveness where GLP-2 levels increase significantly [33]. Given that infants with gastroschisis are at increased risk of developing long-term intestinal failure, it is reasonable to plan studies using GLP-2 as a therapy to improve gut function in this population [2,34].

Thus, the mechanism of action of GLP-2 is to stimulate an organ-specific increase in intestinal mucosal crypt-cell proliferation, which in turn increases villus height, intestinal length, and thereby increasing the surface area available for nutrient absorption. An improved understanding of the biology of GLP-2 in controlling adaptation and intestinal growth in human patients should be useful both in planning dietary support for pediatric patients with SBS, and also for planning future studies using GLP-2 ligands as a direct therapy for improving nutrient absorption post-resection.

## 31.3   GROWTH HORMONE AND INSULIN-LIKE GROWTH FACTOR

The model described above also serves to explain the trophic effects of growth hormone (GH) and insulin-like growth factor 1 (IGF-1) (Figures 31.1 and 31.2). IGF-1 has long been known to have trophic effects in most tissues of the body [35,36]; local actions are modulated by a balance between local (paracrine), systemic (endocrine) production, tissue receptor expression, and local expression of avid binding proteins [37]. Although the intestinal mucosa is highly responsive to exogenous IGF-1 production, this is not likely to be a suitable therapy because of the widespread actions of systemic therapy, especially in the growing infant [3,17,38]. There may be instances where a patient is growth restricted because of a primary or secondary reduction in GH or IGF-1 in addition to the nutritional restriction of SBS, so that exogenous supplementation of either GH or IGF-1 would be therapeutic for both problems [39,40]. Systemic GH has been shown to have a modest effect on fluid absorption in adult patient with SBS, and a specific formulation is licensed for use in this population [41,42]. The effects on energy absorption appear to be minimal [43]. The schematic presented in Figure 31.2 explains the likely mechanism of action of GH; acting to increase IGF-1 systemically and thus increase mucosal mass. There are only two small uncontrolled studies of GH in pediatric patients. Socha et al. administered GH for 10 days to children with intestinal resections on PN and showed significant weight gain and increased small bowel concentration of polyamine (thought to mediate intestinal growth) [44]. Goulet et al. report the use of GH in 8 children with SBS on PN for greater than 3 years and receiving greater than 50% of protein-energy requirements from PN. Following 3 months of treatment, all patients were weaned from PN and had increased plasma citrulline levels (a marker of mucosal mass). However, a year later, only 25% remained of PN, 50% decreased their requirements, and 25% did not change in their PN dependency [45]. The side effects reported in adult studies include swelling, fluid retention, myalgias, arthralgias, gynecomastia, carpal tunnel syndrome, nightmares, and insomnia [43]. Thus, given that there is very little data on GH use in pediatrics, and again, because of the number of tissues affected by systemic therapy, GH therapy is not likely to be applicable to the pediatric population. It is possible that localized-delivery systems could be developed which would overcome the unwanted systemic effects of GH or IGF-1 therapy.

## 31.4   EPIDERMAL GROWTH FACTOR

Epidermal growth factor (EGF) is a member of the EGF family of ligands; of these EGF and transforming growth factor-$\alpha$ are the active ligands *in vivo* [46]. EGF is produced by the salivary and Brunner's glands *in vivo*. If the intestinal mucosa is healthy, the ligand is localized in the intestinal lumen. EGF has been shown to be important in both maintaining epithelial tissues, and to induce mucosal trophic actions. The EGF receptor appears to be localized to the basolateral aspect of the epithelial mucosa; thus access (and activity) of the ligand may be increased in states of mucosal damage or increased permeability, which occurs in SBS [46]. A number of elegant knockout studies have shown that EGF is involved in the post-resection adaptive response [47,48]. As noted previously, a recent mechanistic study shows that GLP-2 actually increases the production of some of the important EGF ligands and receptors, thus these two pathways may be complimentary physiologically [21]. There is a limited experience with the use of exogenous enteral EGF clinically in SBS. It appears to have a modest benefit in improving active glucose absorption and possibly reducing the incidence of bacterial translocation in human infants [49]. It is notable that the effect was dependent on continued administration of the hormone. Other studies have focused on the use of parenteral administration of EGF, however the caveats regarding the potential side effects in growing infants noted for GH and IGF-1 are also relevant here.

## 31.5   KERATINOCYTE GROWTH FACTOR

Keratinocyte growth factor (KGF) or basic fibroblast growth factor 7 likely has a mechanistic pathway that is similar to IGF-1. KGF is produced by the peri-cryptal myofibroblast, and acts to stimulate cell division within the crypt "nursery" [50]. KGF may also act to alter the differentiation of dividing cells, and so alter the phenotype of the mucosal cells [51,52]. However, in comparative studies of KGF, GH, and GLP-2, KGF was less potent than GLP-2. KGF was primarily active within the colon, where it specifically increased the production of goblet cells, and mucosal protective factors [51]. Again, there may be overlap with the upstream effects of GLP-2, which stimulates the production of KGF within the colon [53]. Thus, while KGF is useful in protecting the gut, such as in treatment of postchemotherapy mucositis, it does not appear that it will be a useful therapy for SBS patients [54].

## 31.6 ASSESSMENT OF NUTRIENT STATUS AND NUTRIENT-ABSORPTIVE CAPACITY

The day-to-day clinical management of patients with SBS is largely based on empiric observations of well being, weight gain, stool output, and abdominal distension [55–57]. These methods are reasonably adequate for ongoing monitoring within a specific patient, but they do not allow for comparisons between patients or predictive quantification of absorptive capacity. The general parameters that have been used to monitor nutritional status and intestinal functional capacity in SBS are outlined in Table 31.1, and will be reviewed here. Many of these methods are readily available in clinical practice, but are used intermittently, due to a lack of interest and comparative norms for these populations.

## 31.7 NUTRITIONAL STATUS

Anthropometric measurements are a simple, noninvasive, and readily available means to follow the nutritional well-being of patients. It is important to follow multiple measures such as weight, height, and head circumference in children up to 3 years of age. In older children, triceps skinfold, and

**TABLE 31.1**

**Measures of Intestinal Function in Patients with Intestinal Failure**

| Test/Methodology | Ease of Use | Reliability | Utility |
|---|---|---|---|
| Anthropometric measures; height/weight/ Z scores | ++ | ++ | High |
| Radiological measures of body composition: Dexa scanning, MR for lean body mass | - | Not well validated in pediatric populations | Low |
| Blood serum testing Electrolytes, water soluble vitamins, fat soluble vitamins, micronutrients (e.g. Copper, Zn, Selenium) | + + (perhaps overused, contributing to anemia) | + (levels depend as much on PN composition as EN absorption) | High |
| Balance studies | - (difficult to complete, few reliable norms) | + (dependent on institutional expertise) | Low |
| Radiological imaging (contrast studies of intestinal motility, diameter) | + | + (dependent on institutional expertise) | Moderate |
| Hydrogen breath testing | - (difficult, no pediatric norms) | Unknown (in pediatrics) | Low |
| Citrulline levels | + (may require a larger blood draw) | + | + (requires further study) |
| Quantification of nutrient probe absorption | + (may require urinary catheterization) | + (preliminary studies, requires confirmation) | + (requires further study) |

mid-arm circumference become useful measures of fat and protein stores [58]. Other more specific measures of body composition include: isotope-dilution methods to measure body water, dual energy x-ray absorptiometry (DEXA), and magnetic resonance quantification for measurement of fat mass and lean body mass. While they are sensitive and precise measures of body composition, they are however, cumbersome, and not widely used because of a perceived lack of utility for the day-to-day management of patients [59,60]. See Chapters 4 and 5 for detailed discussions of the clinical assessment of IF patients.

The determination of serum levels of electrolytes, vitamin and essential dietary factors, and synthesized proteins is a useful and widely used strategy to monitor nutritional status. The monitoring of water-soluble elements such as electrolytes and the water-soluble vitamins is important in day-to-day management. If electrolytes are abnormal, this may give a gross idea that absorptive capacity is exceeded, however there is limited sensitivity as a measure of absorptive capacity. Fat-soluble vitamins, such as vitamins A, D, E, and K are important indirect but gross methods of assessing fat absorption to monitor, particularly when the full requirements are not being delivered by PN. As well, long-term PN is a risk factor for metabolic bone disease in the infant who may not be receiving adequate amounts of calcium, phosphorus, and vitamin D. Monitoring for vitamin B12 deficiency is important in those with terminal ileal resections. This is more of a long-term concern as depletion occurs over several months. Albumin levels reflect longer term protein synthesis (half-life of 20 days) and prealbumin (half-life of 2–3 days) reflects short-term protein synthesis. However, these are acute-phase proteins and their usefulness is impaired in postoperative or inflammatory states. With intestinal losses, the patient may be at risk for zinc or selenium deficiency; the measurement of these trace elements may not reflect actual stores in the majority of patients [61].

Monitoring of stoma or stool output, and quantification of stool electrolytes, fat, and carbohydrate is useful in the day-to-day management of patients, and may over time reflect nutrient-absorptive capacity. True balance studies are rarely done, but serial assessment of stoma/stool content of neutral fats (by simple microscopy) and quantitative reducing substances are valuable methods of monitoring the adequacy of nutrient absorption when enteral feeds are advanced [4,57].

Radiological imaging plays a role is assessing the functional capacity of the bowel and is used to monitor healing of mucosal lesions and to monitor for the development of strictures or over-adapted, dilated segments of bowel; in addition, a crude assessment of transit time can be done. Such information may help in determining how aggressive the nutrition support plan should be. Short term, in all patients who have undergone a significant resection and in whom there is concern of strictured or dilated segments, a contrast study with small bowel follow-through should be done prior to discharge to establish a baseline. Thereafter, re-imaging can be reconsidered every 6–12 months while the patients are PN dependent, according to symptomatology. See Chapter 7 for details. If unexplained deterioration occurs in a patient who appears to be adapting, then bacterial overgrowth due to a dilated segment should be considered. Bead or dye studies to quantify transit times are interesting, but have not been shown to correlate with any aspect of absorptive capacity. Hydrogen-breath testing is dependent on differential bacterial population between the relatively sterile small intestine versus the high bacterial content of the colon, and has mostly been used to quantify both small intestinal transit and bacterial overgrowth in SBS. However, the interpretation of hydrogen-breath testing may not be reliable for either transit or overgrowth detection in pediatric patients with SBS due to the altered transit time particularly with the loss of the physiologic transition which occurs if the ileocecal valve is resected [62,63].

## 31.8 NUTRIENT-ABSORPTION TESTING

The "gold standard" of nutrient absorption studies is the 48–72 h quantitative stool collection. Bomb calorimetry is a useful reliable tool to measure energy absorption as an indicator of intestinal functional capacity [64]. This is logistically difficult in all cases; in pediatric patients it is further complicated by the necessity of separating stool from urine, and the use of diapers [65,66]. The utility is very dependent on the completeness of the stool collections; this in turn restricts the use to those research centers with the appropriate expertise [65]. True balance studies are rarely done in the management of short bowel patients. However, the absorptive capacity of the intestine is highly correlated with intestinal length, and functional mucosal mass. Thus, measures of the mucosal mass of enterocytes would be theoretically correlated with the nutrient-absorptive capacity of the bowel. As a correlate of mucosal mass, citrulline is a unique amino acid, which is measurable in plasma and is produced almost entirely by the metabolic processing of glutamine and proline by the small bowel enterocyte [67]. Citrulline levels have been shown to be correlated with intestinal length, and nutrient-absorptive capacity in adult and pediatric patients with SBS [68–70]. In pediatric patients, there appears to be a relationship between improving nutrient-absorptive capacity and increased citrulline, which may not be evident in adults [68,71]. Thus, in an appropriate setting, both the initial levels of citrulline, and the changes over time, may be useful in predicting the ability of the remnant intestine to upregulate nutrient-absorptive capacity.

Alternatively as a substitute to the use of balance studies, the quantification of the absorption of specific nutritional probes has much to offer. Theoretically, the absorption of a specific marker molecule would be indicative of the absorption of all nutrients which use the same absorptive pathway. Probes such as radiolabeled Technetium, EDTA, or different forms of polyethylene glycol have been used to monitor the passive uptake of water and electrolytes, while different inert sugars including D-xylose and 3-0 methyl glucose (3-0MG) have been used to quantify both passive and active transport pathways [66,72,73]. The use of a single marker is limited by the variations induced by changes in the speed of transit and contact time on the ultimate absorption. Thus, the use of dual markers, measuring different pathways of uptake, and the expression of the results as a relative ratio, decreases variability, and improves the diagnostic accuracy of the tests [73]. Typically, permeability is assessed by comparing the absorption of a disaccharide sugar such as lactulose or cellobiose to that of a monosaccharide such as mannitol or rhamnose, with quantification by high-performance chromatography. Active transport is likely best assessed by quantification of a marker such as 3-0MG, which is taken up by the SGLT-1 transporter, as opposed to D-xylose, which is passively absorbed [74]. A more precise measure would be the proportional expression of 3-0MG versus a passively absorbed monosaccharide of similar size. To test this hypothesis directly, we have examined the correlation of 3-0MG, mannitol, and lactulose absorption in human infants with SBS, and a small intestinal stoma [66]. There was good correlation with the absolute absorption of 3-0MG and the measured absorption of macronutrients ($r^2 = 0.56$ for carbohydrates, $r^2 = 0.62$ for fats [Figure 31.3]). There was also a significant correlation between 3-0MG absorption and the ability to tolerate enteral feeds (Figure 31.4). In order to validate these methods further, we have repeated these studies in infants with SBS, and the colon in continuity. A total of 11 infants, all with surgical resection of the intestine and defined bowel length, were studied over an 8 month period. The methods for these studies were identical to those reported earlier, except that balance studies were not done; rather enteral absorptive capacity was taken as the percentage of calories tolerated enterally, following a standardized protocol to increase enteral feeds [56,75]. Urinary collection of the absorbed study sugars (3-0MG, mannitol, and lactulose) was done by placement of an indwelling catheter over the study collection period of 8 h. Quantification of marker sugars was done using high-performance liquid chromatography; 3-0MG absorption is presented as a ratio with respect to the absorption of mannitol. We found that the 3-0MG/mannitol absorption was significantly correlated with the tolerance of enteral feeds (Figure 31.5, $r^2 = 0.28$, $p < 0.02$). These results are promising, however, future studies will be required to determine if these findings can be generalized.

The methodology reviewed shows that there are a number of complimentary measures of nutrient absorptive capacity which can and should be used by all centers caring for infants with SBS. The assessment of baseline anthropometric data, and comparison to adjusted norms will provide an ongoing assessment of the adequacy of growth, and thus of nutritional input. Monitoring of clinical

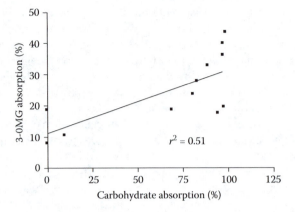

**FIGURE 31.3** Linear correlation analysis of dietary carbohydrate absorption (%) versus 3-0MG absorption (%) in infants with intestinal resection and end stoma. (From Sigalet, D. L., Martin, G. R., and Meddings, J. B. *JPEN J Parenter Enteral Nutr* 2004;28:158–62. With permission.)

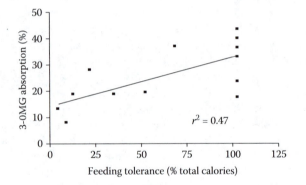

**FIGURE 31.4** Linear correlation analysis of feeding tolerance (% enteral calories) versus 3-0 MG absorption (%) in infants with intestinal resection and end stoma. (From Sigalet, D. L., Martin, G. R., and Meddings, J. B. *JPEN J Parenter Enteral Nutr* 2004;28:158–62. With permission.)

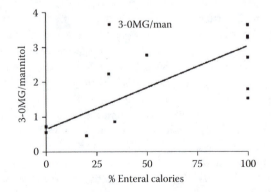

**FIGURE 31.5** Linear correlation analysis of feeding tolerance (% enteral calories) versus 3-0 MG/mannitol ratio in patients with bowel continuity.

input and output, with assessment of fecal fats and reducing substances will aid in the assessment of ongoing nutrient uptake, and facilitate early detection of deteriorations from baseline. Plasma nutrient and fat-soluble vitamin levels will also provide a more long-term measure of nutrient input. The more experimental measures of plasma citrulline and GLP-2 levels appear to be promising both to predict the initial absorptive capacity of the remnant intestine following resection, and the potential for longer term adaptation. Finally, the use of specific nonmetabolized carbohydrate probes should provide a means for quantifying the changes in nutrient uptake as adaptation occurs. Taken together, these measures should provide useful feedback for the care of these patients, beyond the empiric endpoints which are commonly used at present.

# REFERENCES

1. Martin GR, Wallace LE, Hartman B et al. Nutrient-stimulated GLP-2 release and crypt cell proliferation in experimental short bowel syndrome. *Am J Physiol Gastrointest Liver Physiol.* 2005;288:G431–8.
2. Wales PW, de Silva N, Ki JH et al. Neonatal short bowel syndrome: A cohort study. *J Pediatr Surg.* 2005;40:755–62.
3. Sigalet DL, Martin GR. Hormonal therapy for short bowel syndrome. *J Pediatr Surg.* 2000;35:360–3.
4. Sigalet DL. Short bowel syndrome in infants and children: An overview. *Semin Pediatr Surg.* 2001;10:49–55.
5. Williamson RC. Intestinal adaptation (second of two parts). Mechanisms of control. *N Engl J Med.* 1978;298:1444–50.
6. Williamson RC. Intestinal adaptation (first of two parts). Structural, functional and cytokinetic changes. *N Engl J Med.* 1978;298:1393–402.
7. Spence AU, Kovacevic D, Kinney-Barnet M et al. Pediatric short-bowel syndrome: The cost of comprehensive care. *Am J Clin Nutr.* 2008;88:1552–9.
8. Spence AU, Neag A, Wes B et al. Pediatric short bowel syndrome: Redefining predictors of success. *Ann Surg.* 2005;242:403–9.
9. Javid PJ, Collier S, Richardson D et al. The role of enteral nutrition in the reversal of parenteral nutrition-associated liver dysfunction in infants. *J Pediatr Surg.* 2005;40:1015–8.
10. DiBais JK, Youn RJ, Vanderhoof JA. Intestinal rehabilitation and the short bowel syndrome: Part 1. *Am J Gastroenterol.* 2004;99:1386–95.
11. Brubaker PL, Anini Y. Direct and indirect mechanisms regulating secretion of glucagon-like peptide-1 and glucagon-like peptide-2. *Can J Physiol Pharmacol.* 2003;81:1005–12.
12. Roberge JN, Brubaker PL. Secretion of proglucagon-derived peptides in response to intestinal luminal nutrients. *Endocrinol.* 1991;128:3169–74.
13. Xiao Q, Boushey RP, Drucker DJ, Brubaker PL. Secretion of the intestinotropic hormone glucagon-like peptide 2 is differentially regulated by nutrients in humans. *Gastroenterol.* 1999;117:99–105.
14. Jeppesen PB, Hartmann B, Thulesen J et al. Elevated plasma glucagon-like peptide 1 and 2 concentrations in ileum resected short bowel patients with a preserved colon. *Gut.* 2000;47:370–6.
15. Sigalet DL, Martin G, Meddings J, Hartman B, Holst JJ. GLP-2 levels in infants with intestinal dysfunction. *Pediatr Res.* 2004;56:371–6.
16. Hartmann B, Harr MB, Jeppesen PB et al. *In vivo* and *in vitro* degradation of glucagon-like peptide-2 in humans. *J Clin Endocrinol Metab.* 2000;85:2884–8.
17. Dube PE, Forse CL, Bahrami J, Brubaker PL. The essential role of insulin-like growth factor-1 in the intestinal tropic effects of glucagon-like peptide-2 in mice. *Gastroenterol.* 2006;131:589–605.
18. Martin GR, Wallace LE, Sigalet DL. Glucagon-like peptide-2 induces intestinal adaptation in parenterally fed rats with short bowel syndrome. *Am J Physiol Gastrointest Liver Physiol.* 2004;286:G964–72.
19. Sigalet DL, Bawazir O, Martin GR et al. Glucagon-like peptide-2 induces a specific pattern of adaptation in remnant jejunum. *Dig Dis Sci.* 2006;51:1557–66.
20. Hsieh J, Longuet C, Maida A et al. Glucagon-like peptide-2 increases intestinal lipid absorption and chylomicron production via CD36. *Gastroenterol.* 2009;137:997–1005, 1005.
21. Yusta B, Holland D, Koehler JA et al. ErbB signaling is required for the proliferative actions of GLP-2 in the murine gut. *Gastroenterol.* 2009;137:986–96.
22. Sigalet DL, Wallace LE, Holst JJ et al. Enteric neural pathways mediate the anti-inflammatory actions of glucagon-like peptide 2. *Am J Physiol Gastrointest Liver Physiol.* 2007;293:G211–21.

23. Liu X, Nelson DW, Holst JJ, Ney DM. Synergistic effect of supplemental enteral nutrients and exogenous glucagon-like peptide 2 on intestinal adaptation in a rat model of short bowel syndrome. *Am J Clin Nutr.* 2006;84:1142–50.

24. Sangild PT, Tappenden KA, Malo C et al. Glucagon-like peptide 2 stimulates intestinal nutrient absorption in parenterally fed newborn pigs. *J Pediatr Gastroenterol Nutr.* 2006;43:160–7.

25. Scott RB, Kirk D, MacNaughton WK, Meddings JB. GLP-2 augments the adaptive response to massive intestinal resection in rat. *Am J Physiol.* 1998;275:G911–21.

26. Secor SM, Whang EE, Lane JS, Ashley SW, Diamond J. Luminal and systemic signals trigger intestinal adaptation in the juvenile python. *Am J Physiol Gastrointest Liver Physiol.* 2000;279:G1177–87.

27. Jeppesen PB, Hartmann B, Thulesen J et al. Glucagon-like peptide 2 improves nutrient absorption and nutritional status in short-bowel patients with no colon. *Gastroenterol.* 2001;120:806–15.

28. Jeppesen PB, Sanguinetti EL, Buchman A et al. Teduglutide (ALX-0600), a dipeptidyl peptidase IV resistant glucagon-like peptide 2 analogue, improves intestinal function in short bowel syndrome patients. *Gut.* 2005;54:1224–31.

29. Messing B, Bekker P, Jeppesen PB et al. Teduglutide, reduces parenteral nutrition (PN) requirements in PN- dependent short bowel syndrome (SBS) patients: Results of a multi-center, international, placebo-controlled study. *Clin Nutr Suppl.* 2008 2008;3 Suppl 1:12–5.

30. Amin H, Holst JJ, Hartmann B, Wallace L, Sigalet D. Functional ontogeny of the proglucagon derived peptide axis in human neonates. *Pediatrics.* 2008;121:e180–6.

31. Lovshin J, Yusta B, Iliopoulos I et al. Ontogeny of the glucagon-like peptide-2 receptor axis in the developing rat intestine. *Endocrinol.* 2000;141:4194–201.

32. Yoshikawa H, Miyata I, Eto Y. Serum glucagon-like peptide-2 levels in neonates: Comparison between extremely low-birthweight infants and normal-term infants. *Pediatr Int.* 2006;48:464–9.

33. Soon IS, Boctor D, Holst JJ et al. Altered development of the Glucagon Like Peptide 2 response in infants with gastroschisis. *Gastroenterol.* 2009;136 (4 Suppl 1), A716.

34. Wales PW, de Silva N, Kim J et al. Neonatal short bowel syndrome: Population-based estimates of incidence and mortality rates. *J Pediatr Surg.* 2004;39:690–5.

35. Monzavi R, Cohen P. IGFs and IGFBPs: Role in health and disease. *Best Pract Res Clin Endocrinol Metab.* 2002;16:433–47.

36. Lund PK. Molecular basis of intestinal adaptation: The role of the insulin-like growth factor system. *Ann N Y Acad Sci.* 1998;859:18–36.

37. Baxter RC. Insulin-like growth factor (IGF)-binding proteins: Interactions with IGFs and intrinsic bioactivities. *Am J Physiol Endocrinol Metab.* 2000;278:E967–76.

38. Dube PE, Rowland KJ, Brubaker PL. Glucagon-like peptide-2 activates {beta}-catenin signaling in the mouse intestinal crypt: Role of insulin-like growth factor-1. *Endocrinol.* 2008;149(1):291–301.

39. Barksdale E M, Jr., Koehler AN, Yaworski JA, Gardner M, Reyes J. Insulin like growth factor 1 and insulin like growth factor 3: Indices of intestinal failure in children. *J Pediatr Surg.* 1999;34:655–61.

40. Nucci AM, Finegold DN, Yaworski JA, Kowalski L, Barksdale EM, Jr. Results of growth trophic therapy in children with short bowel syndrome. *J Pediatr Surg.* 2004;39:335–9.

41. Byrne TA, Persinger RL, Young LS, Ziegler TR, Wilmore D. W. A new treatment for patients with short-bowel syndrome. Growth hormone, glutamine, and a modified diet. *Ann Surg.* 1995;222:243–54.

42. Messing B, Blethen S, DiBaise JK, Matarese LE, Steiger E. Treatment of adult short bowel syndrome with recombinant human growth hormone: A review of clinical studies. *J Clin Gastroenterol.* 2006;40 Suppl 2:S75–84.

43. Jeppesen PB. Growth factors in short-bowel syndrome patients. *Gastroenterol Clin North Am.* 2007;36:109–21, vii.

44. Socha J, Ksiazyk J, Fogel WA, Kierkus J, Lyszkowska M, Sasiak K. Is growth hormone a feasible adjuvant in the treatment of children after small bowel resection? *Clin Nutr.* 1996;15:185–8.

45. Goulet O, Ruemmele F, Lacaille F, Colomb V. Irreversible intestinal failure. *J Pediatr Gastroenterol Nutr* 2004;38:250–69.

46. Barnar JA, Beaucham D, Russel E, Duboi N, Coffe RJ. Epidermal growth factor-related peptides and their relevance to gastrointestinal pathophysiology. *Gastroenterol.* 1995;108:564–80.

47. Ster LE, Falcon RA, Jr., Huan F, Kem CJ, Erwi CR, Warne BW. Epidermal growth factor alters the bax:bcl-w ratio following massive small bowel resection. *J Surg Res.* 2000;91:38–42.

48. Warne BW, Erwi CR. Critical roles for EGF receptor signaling during resection-induced intestinal adaptation. *J Pediatr Gastroenterol Nutr.* 2006;43 Suppl 1:S68–73.

49. Sigalet DL, Martin GR, Butzner JD, Bure A, Medding JB. A pilot study of the use of epidermal growth factor in pediatric short bowel syndrome. *J Pediatr Surg.* 2005;40:763–8.

50. Finc PW, Rubi JS. Keratinocyte growth factor/fibroblast growth factor 7, a homeostatic factor with therapeutic potential for epithelial protection and repair. *Adv Cancer Res.* 2004;91:69–136.

51. Washizawa N, Gu LH, Gu L, Openo KP, Jones DP, Ziegler TR.. Comparative effects of glucagon-like peptide-2 (GLP-2), growth hormone (GH), and keratinocyte growth factor (KGF) on markers of gut adaptation after massive small bowel resection in rats. *JPEN J Parenter Enteral Nutr.* 2004;28:399–409.

52. Yang H, Antony PA, Wildhaber BE, Teitelbaum DH. Intestinal intraepithelial lymphocyte gamma delta-T cell-derived keratinocyte growth factor modulates epithelial growth in the mouse. *J Immunol.* 2004;172:4151–8.

53. Orskov C, Hartmann B, Poulsen SS, Thulesen J, Hare KJ, Holst JJ. GLP-2 stimulates colonic growth via KGF, released by subepithelial myofibroblasts with GLP-2 receptors. *Regul Pept.* 2005;124:105–12.

54. Finch PW, Rubin JS. Keratinocyte growth factor expression and activity in cancer: Implications for use in patients with solid tumors. *J Natl Cancer Inst.* 2006;98:812–24.

55. DiBaise JK, Young RJ, Vanderhoof JA. Intestinal rehabilitation and the short bowel syndrome: Part 2. *Am J Gastroenterol.* 2004;99:1823–32.

56. Utter S, Duggan C. *Short Bowel Syndrome.* Hamilton: Decker 2000.

57. Vanderhoof JA. Short bowel syndrome in children. *Curr Opin Pediatr.* 1995;7:560–8.

58. Bear MT, Bradford HA. Pediatric nutrition assessment: Identifying children at risk. *J Am Diet Assoc.* 1997; Suppl 2:S107–115..

59. Picaud JC, Lapillonne A, Pieltain C et al. Software and scan acquisition technique-related discrepancies in bone mineral assessment using dual-energy x-ray absorptiometry in neonates. *Acta Paediatr.* 2002; 1991:1189–93.

60. Rigo J. Body composition during the first year of life. *Nestle Nutr Workshop Ser Pediatr Program.* 2006; 58:65–76; discussion 76–8.

61. Forbes GM, Forbes A. Micronutrient status in patients receiving home parenteral nutrition. *Nutr.* 1997;13:941–4.

62. Compher C, Rubesin S, Kinosian B, Madaras J, Metz D. Noninvasive measurement of transit time in short bowel syndrome. *JPEN J Parenter Enteral Nutr.* 2007;31:240–5.

63. Schiller LR. Evaluation of small bowel bacterial overgrowth. *Curr Gastroenterol Rep.* 2007;9:373–7.

64. Jeppesen PB, Mortensen PB. Intestinal failure defined by measurements of intestinal energy and wet weight absorption. *Gut.* 2000;46:701–6.

65. Cooke RJ, Paule C, Ruckman K. Nutrient balance in the preterm infant. 3. Effect of balance duration on outcome measurements. *J Pediatr Gastroenterol Nutr.* 1989;8(3):355–8.

66. Sigalet DL, Martin GR, Meddings JB. 3-0 methylglucose uptake as a marker of nutrient absorption and bowel length in pediatric patients. *JPEN J Parenter Enteral Nutr.* 2004;28:158–62.

67. Rabier D and Kamoun P. Metabolism of citrulline in man. *Amino Acids.* 1995;9:229–316..

68. Bailly-Botuha C, Colomb V, Thioulouse E et al. Plasma citrulline concentration reflects enterocyte mass in children with short bowel syndrome. *Pediatr Res.* 2009;65:559–63.

69. Fitzgibbons S, Ching YA, Valim C et al. Relationship between serum citrulline levels and progression to parenteral nutrition independence in children with short bowel syndrome. *J Pediatr Surg.* 2009;44:928–32.

70. Rhoads JM, Plunkett E, Galanko J et al. Serum citrulline levels correlate with enteral tolerance and bowel length in infants with short bowel syndrome. *J Pediatr.* 2005;146:542–7.

71. Luo M, Fernandez-Estivariz C, Manatunga AK et al. Are plasma citrulline and glutamine biomarkers of intestinal absorptive function in patients with short bowel syndrome? *JPEN J Parenter Enteral Nutr.* 2007;31:1–7.

72. Sigalet DL, Martin GR, Poole A. Differential sugar absorption as a marker for adaptation in short bowel syndrome. *J Pediatr Surg.* 2000;35:661–4.

73. Teshima CW, Meddings JB. The measurement and clinical significance of intestinal permeability. *Curr Gastroenterol Rep.* 2008;10:443–9.

74. Fordtran J, Clodi PH, Soergel KH, Ingelfinger FJ. Sugar absorption tests, with special reference to 3-0-methyl-D-glucose and D-xylose. *Ann Intern Med.* 1962;57:883–91.

75. Sigalet DL, Boctor D, Robertson M, Lam V, Brindle M, Sarkosh K, Dreidger L, Sajedi M. Improved outcomes in paediatric intestinal failure with aggressive prevention of liver disease. *European J of Pediatric Surgery.* 2009;19(6):348–53.

# Part VI

Long-Term Care

# 32 Home Parenteral and Enteral Nutrition

*Darlene G. Kelly, John K. DiBaise, and Megan Brenn*

## CONTENTS

## 32.1 INTRODUCTION

Home parenteral and enteral nutrition (HPEN) have been recognized as critical to the survival of individuals with intestinal failure since the late 1960s. Indeed, some persons have been on these therapies for 35 years or more. The practice of HPN (home parenteral nutrition) and HEN (home enteral nutrition) is typically quite different than when they are used for short-term nutritional support in the hospital.

In the United States, between 1989 and 1992, the estimated annual prevalence of HEN was 415 per 100,000 people compared to 120 per 100,000 for HPN [1]. In most countries, there is approximately five times more HEN than HPN consumers.

For consumers of these home therapies in the United States, financial coverage can be a particularly stressful issue. This is not typically a problem in other parts of the industrialized world where governments cover the majority of the costs of this medical treatment. In the United States, the charges for HPN can be as high as $300–500 daily; the average cost for HEN is about one-tenth that of HPN. In 1981, when these costs were determined to severely limit the availability of HPN for most individuals, Medicare and private insurance reimbursement agreed to cover this expensive therapy and therefore made it possible for virtually anyone who met the clinical criteria set forth by the government and insurance companies to utilize the treatment. Economic evaluations of HPEN have shown that providing nutrition support at home is up to 75% more cost-effective than keeping patients in the hospital [2].

## 32.2   CRITERIA FOR HPEN REIMBURSEMENT

When considering a candidate for HPEN, one of the first issues to be dealt with must be financial coverage, since few persons can afford this therapy without some type of financial assistance. Consequently, either a medical team that is dedicated to HPEN management or a social worker who is experienced with HPEN must address this at the outset of evaluation (see Chapter 34). It is the responsibility of clinicians to supply appropriate documentation to support the need for these therapies [3]. If patients do not fulfill Medicare criteria, a strong supportive letter from the primary clinician may be accepted for reimbursement; however, the clinician should be reminded that these letters must be accurate and not overstate the clinical facts. The indications for HPEN in consumers insured by Medicare include "permanent" oral or intestinal failure, which means that the therapy must be considered to be essential for at least 3 months in the best medical judgment of the responsible clinician.

Private insurance may have criteria that are similar to Medicare for HPEN. The biggest issue in this case is frequently that such insurance has a lifetime maximal allotment. With an expensive therapy such as HPN, this lifetime cap may be met long before consumers are old enough to qualify for Medicare. This can mean that a consumer may need to consider high-risk insurance that is available in some states. The 34 U.S. states having such insurance may be found on the following Web site: http://www.naschip.org/states_pools.html. In states without high-risk insurance, individuals may need to become medically disabled in order to afford the therapy that keeps them alive. In some situations, there may be limitations for preexisting conditions during the initial months of insurance coverage, making foresight important to avoid periods of noncoverage.

### 32.2.1   ACCEPTABLE CRITERIA FOR HPN COVERAGE BY MEDICARE*

For Medicare coverage of HPN, there must be failure of the intestine to absorb or to move the chyme through the small bowel. Isolated failure of gastric emptying, for example, would not be an acceptable indication for HPN, since HEN can be used to deliver the nutrient formula distal to the pylorus. In contrast, chronic intestinal pseudoobstruction may be an acceptable indication because delivery of sufficient nutrients and fluid to the intestine for digestion and absorption, although possible, generally would not be tolerated. In addition, the need for bowel rest for at least 3 months, as might be needed for refractory pancreatitis, enterocutaneous fistulae or extensive Crohn's disease, would also be acceptable criteria for HPN.

Short bowel syndrome (SBS) resulting from intestinal resection or mucosal disease is a major indication for long-term HPN. In this case, Medicare criteria require that the resection has been done within the 3 months prior to starting HPN and that the residual small intestine measures less than 5 ft based on intraoperative or radiological measurement. If either of these is not the case, it becomes important to demonstrate malabsorption that is responsible for weight loss of at least 10% of body weight in the prior 3-month period and an albumin level of less than 3.5 g/dL. Two criteria

---

* https://www.noridianmedicare.com/dme/coverage/docs/trees/tpn_policy_decision_tree.pdf

can be used to demonstrate malabsorption, namely a fecal fat level of at least 50% of an intake of not less than 50 g/day or alternatively, stool losses in excess of 50% of an oral fluid intake of at least 2.5–3 L and a urine output of less than 1000 mL. This must be documented in a 72-h fecal fat test. Because of the need to identify these specific requirements in carefully documented data, the importance of accuracy of records cannot be overemphasized. Occasionally in SBS there may be a benefit from a combination of both HPN and HEN to meet nutritional needs and minimize the dependence on HPN. Typically, however, Medicare will not reimburse for both therapies. Other causes of severe and intractable malabsorption may be covered when weight loss, low albumin, and fat or fluid malabsorption meet the levels described above.

Intestinal dysmotility is another cause of intestinal failure. Acceptable documentation of failure of small bowel motility include x-ray or nuclear transit study showing that oral contrast or radionuclide does not reach the right colon within 6 h after intake. Importantly, these tests must be done at a time when the patient is off all narcotic medications and during use of maximal prokinetic drugs.

In cases of bowel obstruction, a mechanical high-grade obstruction must be present. A partial obstruction or "ileus" does not meet Medicare criteria for HPN. Enterocutaneous fistulae, which originate from a point of the small bowel beyond which a feeding tube can be placed, are also an acceptable indication for HPN. However in both bowel obstruction and fistulae, there must be documentation that surgical intervention is contraindicated at the time of HPN commencement.

In a situation where the precise criteria are not met, a trial of enteral nutrition (EN) is required. Examples include malabsorption with only 25% of ingested fat present in the stool during a 72 h period, slowed small bowel transit but ingested radionuclide appears in the right colon in less than 6 h, or a partial small bowel obstruction. The definition of a failed trial of EN includes the inability to place a feeding tube or intolerance of tube feeding as outlined by Medicare.

### 32.2.2 CRITERIA FOR MEDICARE TO COVER HEN

For Medicare coverage of HEN, reimbursement is generally restricted to those who have impaired delivery of nutrients to the small intestine. Medicare requires that the tip of the feeding tube be placed at or beyond the ligament of Treitz and distal to the site of obstruction or origin of an enterocutaneous fistula. Among underlying conditions that are covered are altered oropharyngeal or esophageal motor function causing dysphagia (e.g., cerebrovascular accident, neuromuscular disease, motor neuron disease, and multiple sclerosis), esophageal obstruction (e.g., malignancy) and gastroparesis [2,4]. Patients in whom there is a reduction in oral intake below the amount needed to maintain nutrition and/or hydration either because they cannot or will not eat (i.e., oral failure) may be treated with HEN, but Medicare coverage is not typical in cases of refusal to eat. HEN is also occasionally used in patients with small bowel malabsorptive conditions to supplement their limited gut function. Complete mechanical obstruction is the only absolute contraindication to HEN. Severe diarrhea or vomiting, enterocutaneous fistulae and intestinal dysmotility, while presenting significant challenges, are not absolute contraindications.

## 32.3 INITIATING HPEN

Successful HPEN administration requires proper patient selection based not only on appropriate diagnostic indication but also on additional considerations such as a clean, safe home environment, physical capability to administer the therapy, a patient and/or caregiver who is willing and able to perform all the procedures safely, availability to competent health professionals and 24 h access to the home care company [4]. Unfortunately, patients are occasionally discharged from the hospital on HPEN without proper indications, education or appropriate follow-up care arrangements, but a designated HPEN team can usually avoid this problem [5,6].

A multidisciplinary nutrition support team consisting of a physician, nurse practitioner or physician assistant, nurse, dietitian, and pharmacist in close collaboration with the patient and primary care provider serves to oversee documentation of criteria needed to assure reimbursement, to help with choosing a quality home infusion agency, to educate and to monitor consumers of HPEN. The team may be assisted by a social worker, hospital case manager, or discharge planner who is experienced with these therapies. While the patient is still in the hospital, a visit by the home infusion nurse can help to familiarize the patient with the HPEN routine and explain the process of HPEN administration. As noted in the Introduction (Multidisciplinary Approach to Intestinal Failure), care from such a multidisciplinary team has been demonstrated to result in improved care, decreased complications and improved cost-effectiveness [7,8].

### 32.3.1  VASCULAR ACCESS FOR HPN

Central venous catheters (CVCs) are essential for patients who require HPN. The permanent catheters that are used most often include tunneled central lines and subcutaneous vascular access catheters. These can be used to access the internal jugular or subclavian vein. The tip of the catheter needs to be at or very near the superior vena cava (SVC)—right atrial junction. Catheter tips placed more superior than this increase the risk of central venous thrombosis [9]. It is important to discuss the advantages and disadvantages of each type of catheter with the patient and to have the patient involved in selecting his/her catheter. While the subcutaneous port is not visible, the catheter requires accessing with a needle. The frequency of accessing varies from daily to weekly, depending on the preferences of the HPN management team and the patient. Although it seems that the subcutaneous port might be less likely to become infected, this is not the case when the catheter is used for HPN [10]. The tunneled catheter offers the advantage of avoiding the accessing step, but the catheter is visible and requires frequent site care. In persons who have had thrombosis, access into the SVC may not be possible, and in this case, an inferior venacaval approach may be necessary. See also Chapter 12.

Peripherally inserted central catheters (PICCs) are occasionally used for HPN; however, they are more prone to thrombosis and possibly to infections and should generally not be used if HPN is planned for greater than a few weeks to months [11]. For many brands of PICCs, there is no cuff or other mode of stabilization so catheter displacement may occur and nursing care may be required to assist with site care. A recent approach in placing these small catheters has been to use them to access the internal jugular vein and then tunnel the catheter down to the chest, similar to placement of a Hickman, Broviac or Groshong catheter. Compared with PICCs, this approach would be expected to decrease the risk of thrombosis since a larger, more rapidly flowing vessel is accessed. In addition, the tunnel likely offers a degree of protection from catheter infection. The risk of displacement remains to be determined, as does optimal care of the catheter to prevent displacement. However, it does have the disadvantage of being a more invasive and expensive placement compared to a traditional PICC. Clearly, the risks and benefits need to be assessed to determine whether they offset the added cost. The ESPEN Home Artificial Nutrition (HAN) Workgroup in the recently published guidelines on parenteral nutrition (PN) states that PICC lines cannot be recommended for HPN [12].

### 32.3.2  ACCESS FOR HEN

The optimal route of administration depends upon the anticipated duration of use, adequacy of intestinal function and risk of aspiration [13]. The stomach is the preferred route of enteral feeding when gastric emptying functions normally. In this case, delivery of nutrients to the small intestine is more analogous to physiological food emptying [14]. However, intragastric feeding should be avoided and the patient fed directly into the jejunum when the stomach is not functioning normally or when there is significant risk for aspiration. In patients whom tube feeding is likely to be required for less than 30 days, the nasoenteric route of enteral nutrition is preferred. Some individuals can be trained to insert and remove a nasogastric tube daily for nocturnal feedings, as is occasionally done in malnourished patients with Crohn's disease for example. Those who will require longer term HEN will require percutaneous gastrostomy, gastrojejunostomy, or jejunostomy tubes (see Chapter 13). Skin-level or low-profile gastrostomy devices (i.e., "buttons") have become popular as replacement catheters in individuals who require long-term enteral nutrition support. The convenience and cosmetic appearance of the skin-level device appear to be the main factors contributing to their greater acceptance by patients [15].

## 32.4 INSTITUTION OF FEEDING

In patients who are severely malnourished, both parenteral and enteral nutrition need to be started slowly and cautiously, preferably in the hospital. These persons are at high risk of development of refeeding syndrome which involves acute decreases of serum potassium, magnesium and phosphorus that may cause respiratory failure, heart failure, cardiac dysrhythmias, and even death [16]. Therefore, close monitoring of laboratory testing and gradual start of the nutrition support is essential. In the case of PN, initially providing a reduced amount of dextrose, decreased volume, increased initial amounts of potassium, magnesium, phosphorus and supplemental thiamine can prevent refeeding issues. In enteral feeding, gradually increasing the infusion rate over several days not only helps improve tolerance to the feeding but also minimizes the risk of refeeding syndrome.

In both HEN and HPN, an estimation of daily energy, nutrient and fluid needs is necessary prior to initiating feeding. For most adult patients, the Harris Benedict equation is helpful in determining caloric needs. This, in conjunction with close observation of weight trends and urine output, will help refine the requirements. In the occasional patient, use of indirect calorimetry or nitrogen balance can provide further optimization of energy needs, particularly in situations where the expected response to therapy is not observed. Although daily caloric and fluid requirements vary, for a normally nourished adult, 20–35 kcal/kg/day and 25–35 mL/kg/day based on ideal body weight is a reasonable starting place.

### 32.4.1 STARTING HPN

The ideal PN formulation for individual patients should contain appropriate calories as well as protein requirements and adequate volume while avoiding excessive dextrose and lipids. Trace elements and vitamins are also required in all PN solutions. The trace element packages (e.g., Multitrace-4, Multitrace-5, American Regent, Shirley, NY) provide fixed amounts of four to five trace elements. The trace elements used in PN were reviewed in a recent National Institutes of Health (NIH)-funded conference [17]. It was concluded that the amounts of some of the trace elements are provided in excessive amounts in the multiple trace element combinations. Notably, manganese appears to be provided in amounts that can be detrimental [17]. Some of the elements are likely provided in adequate amounts as a result of contamination of other components of the PN, and may not need to be added at all. Finally, one of the type of these trace element mixtures (e.g., Multitrace-4) is devoid of selenium, an essential mineral for most species [18]. Vitamin mixtures for parenteral administration are proscribed by the food and drug administration (FDA). Due to stability issues, vitamins are a "patient additive" that must be added to the PN solution within 24 h of starting the infusion. Regular insulin, when needed, is added to maintain blood sugars in a safe range. This, too, must be added to the PN bag by the patient prior to infusion. Provision of excessive calories is associated with development of fatty changes in the liver parenchyma and, in some patients, progressive liver disease. An important study from France identified excessive parenteral lipids as a significant risk factor for this problem [19] (see also Chapters 20 and 21).

Initially, while euvolemia is being established, marked increases in weight may occur. Thereafter, a weight goal needs to be determined and weight monitored to establish gains of 2 lb or less weekly. HPN patients need to have reliable bathroom scales that they use at least weekly, taking care to weigh at the same time of day and should report their weight trends to the HPN management team. Sudden increases in weight may be signs of fluid overload and should be reported immediately.

---

**TABLE 32.1**

**Data Included in Self-Monitoring Worksheet**

Weight (checked weekly)

Temperature

   Before starting infusion

   30–60 min after starting infusion[a]

24-h total urine output

Symptoms (chills, nausea, vomiting, thirst, dizziness, headache)

Blood sugar

   30–60 min after starting infusion[a]

   1 h after stopping infusion

[a] Patients are asked to contact the HPN team with an increase of temperature of >2°F(1°C) over temperature before infusion.

---

Consumers need to be cautioned that shortness of breath occurring during infusion is an emergency that should be assessed promptly as this may be an indication of heart failure. Conversely, rapid weight loss and decreased urine output may be an indication of dehydration.

PN volume requirements can be quite large, particularly in individuals with large stomal or fistula losses. In those with normal renal function, monitoring of urine output is a good indicator of adequate PN volume. A goal urine output in excess of 1 L daily is recommended to prevent kidney failure due to intravascular volume depletion. Excessive urine output can also be very disturbing to the consumer, especially when it is occurs during nocturnal infusion, thereby preventing a restful sleep. It is, therefore, important for the HPN team to evaluate consumer records of urine outputs, as well as weights (Table 32.1).

Typically, HPN is infused overnight, often over a period of 10–14 h. Programmable infusion pumps are used by most consumers. These are usually programmed to infuse the formula with a gradual infusion taper down over the final 1 or 2 h. The taper down period helps to avoid rebound hypoglycemia when the infusion is finished. In adults, a ramp up mode is rarely necessary. Portable pumps that can be carried in a backpack or tote are also available for the HPN patient who needs to infuse PN during the day.

### 32.4.2 FORMULAS AND ADMINISTRATION METHODS FOR HEN

Standard enteral formulae are nutritionally complete emulsions of macro- and micronutrients that consist of intact protein, glucose polymers, and a mixture of long-chain and medium-chain triglycerides. These formulas tend to be isotonic, gluten-free, lactose-free, 1 kcal/mL and meet most nutritional needs depending on the volume given [20]. It is important to consider the individual HEN consumer's food sensitivities and allergies to ensure the most appropriate formula is used. The majority of HEN patients, whether fed into the stomach or jejunum, will tolerate standard formulations.

Specialized formulations are also available and include concentrated formulas (providing 1.5–2 kcal/mL), elemental (containing free amino acids) or semielemental (containing small peptides), fiber-containing, organ-specific (e.g., renal, pulmonary, hepatic), modular products and immune-enhancing (e.g., containing arginine, glutamine, nucleotides, omega-3 fatty acids). Despite the clear theoretical benefits of fiber-containing formulas in the long-term HEN patient, the clinical benefit remains less certain [21,22]. In general, the benefits of most specialized products over standard formulations in the HEN setting remain insufficiently substantiated and they are considerably more expensive. Typically, there must be documentation of the need for specialized formulas for reimbursement by Medicare and some insurance coverage. Therefore, in most circumstances, standard products are recommended and, if not tolerated, a specialty product can be tried.

Methods of formula administration include bolus, gravity, and continuous. In bolus feeding, 200–400 mL is infused with a syringe over 5–10 min several times per day. Bolus feeding is a reliable, easy to comprehend and eliminates the need for an infusion pump; however, it is limited by its propensity to generate high residual volumes and intolerance. Bolus feeding is preferred for intragastric feedings in active, alert patients with low aspiration risk.

Gravity feeding provides an intermittent, continuous drip. Intermittent gravity feeding is sufficient for most patients with a gastrostomy or nasogastric tube and is typically used when the bolus method is not tolerated. This can be accomplished using a closed enteral feeding bag which is a sterile system that allows unused formula to be used at a later time. Alternatively, an open system is clean but not sterile. In this system, cans of formula are poured into a plastic bag that is cleaned at the end of each use. Both the closed and open systems require a pole to hold the container of formula while it is infusing.

Continuous infusion requires a pump and power source but provides accurate, controlled delivery. This is recommended for jejunostomy feeding and for gastrostomy feeding when gastroesophageal reflux and aspiration is a risk or when bolus and/or gravity feeding are not tolerated [23]. For Medicare reimbursement of a pump in gastrostomy feedings, failure of bolus or gravity feedings must be demonstrated. Too rapid delivery, particularly of a hyperosmolar solution, may cause abdominal distension, cramping, and diarrhea because of fluid secretion into the lumen. Compact portable infusion pumps that can be carried around in a backpack or large tote are available for the patient who requires continuous infusion or prefers to infuse during the day.

Similar to HPN, most HEN consumers prefer nocturnal feeding (i.e., cycling over a 10–14-h period overnight) as it allows maximal use of the gut and allows normal activities during the day. Rebound hypoglycemia is uncommonly seen in the HEN setting.

## 32.5 TRAINING THE HPEN CONSUMER

It is important that HPEN patients are carefully trained to ensure safe infusion of the nutrition solution in a sterile manner. Standardized training with well-designed HPEN manuals is critical for successful HPEN administration. Once a consumer has been trained, care should be taken to avoid making suggestions that conflict with the techniques that the consumer has been taught. This can occur at times when a consumer is trained by an HPEN team and a nurse from a different agency is asked to do other cares. A teaching plan should include careful handwashing techniques, storage of HPEN components, maintenance of a clean work area, central venous catheter or feeding tube site care, catheter management, addition of vitamins and other additives to the bag, connection and disconnection of tubing and use of the infusion pump. Consumers need to be taught to recognize signs and symptoms of complications and to respond appropriately. In addition, instructions need to be included for monitoring weight, body temperature, urine output and blood sugars during and after infusion (Table 32.1).

## 32.6 SURVIVAL ON HPEN

In the United States, most information on the outcomes of HPN and HEN comes from the American Society for Parenteral and Enteral Nutrition (ASPEN) and from the Oley Foundation for Home Parenteral and Enteral Nutrition [24]. The underlying diagnosis has the most predictable influence on HPEN outcome, with the highest mortality being seen in AIDS, cancer and those with progressive neurologic illnesses [25,26].

Outcomes of adult consumers on HPN have been published by large HPN programs in France and Minnesota [27–31]. Except for consumers with a primary malignant diagnosis [30], the various published data are comparable; however, it should be noted that all published data are from large, experienced HPN programs. These studies consistently identify that, of those who die while on HPN, most succumb to their underlying disease and not as a consequence of a PN complication.

Indeed, these published survival studies found that only about 10–14% of deaths that occurred while on HPN were directly related to the prolonged HPN therapy. Of those with SBS, survival was 88% at 1 year and 66% at 5 years [29]. In studies of intestinal dysmotility, it was found that younger patients, especially those who could eat, had better survival on HPN [30]. This finding has not been evaluated in older patients in the United States because Medicare criteria do not allow oral intake in beneficiaries who receive HPN because of dysmotility. Mortality while on HPN is also significantly affected by age of the consumer. At the Mayo Clinic, experience over a period representing 1730 catheter years of experience and 942 episodes of care in 887 adult HPN consumers, 56% were tapered off PN primarily because of no further need, 20% died during HPN or within 1 month of discontinuation, 13% remained on PN for up to 32 years while 10% transferred to other programs and were lost to follow-up (Kelly D. G., unpublished data).

In the first 5 years of this decade, the overall median survival of adults on HEN consumers in Italy was 9.1 months in those started on the therapy for all indications [31]. Survival on HEN has been published by French authors indicating that 44% survived 1 year and 29% 2 years [32]. A large retrospective study from the United States found that 1 year after initiating HEN, 48% of those with neuromuscular disorders who had associated dysphagia had died, while 25% remained on HEN and 19% had resumed full oral nutrition. [1]. Of consumers who had suffered a stroke, 14% were able to resume full oral nutrition, emphasizing the need to periodically reassess swallowing in these patients. In cancer patients, data from the ASPEN registry found that after 1 year on HEN, 59% had died, 6% still received HEN and 30% had resumed full oral nutrition [1,25]. These studies also found that HEN consumers with small bowel malabsorptive disease had a 1-year mortality of 18% while 45% had resumed full oral nutrition. Similar to HPN, age also influences survival in HEN consumers—a finding related mainly to the different age-related causes of dysphagia [25]. Only 46% of HEN patients older than 65 years were alive after 1 year compared to 89% of those <25 years of age. Stroke patients older than 75 years of age were shown to be three to four times more likely to die while receiving HEN than those younger than 65 [25].

## 32.7   COMPLICATIONS OF HPN

A chart summarizing HPN complications and associated symptoms is available from the Oley Foundation in their Web site http://www.oley.org/charts/newHEN.pdf. It is advisable to provide copies of this chart to new HPN consumers.

The most common complication of HPN in adults is catheter infection [32]. There are three general types of infection: exit site infection, catheter tract infection and bacteremia or fungemia. Reported frequency of infections includes exit site infection—1 in 10 catheter years; tract infections—1 in 20 catheter years and blood stream infections—1 in 2 catheter years. These data are from a single center with extensive experience with HPN. Rates are variable dependent on experience of HPN management team, consumer training and degree of attentiveness of the consumer (see also Chapter 19).

The importance of salvaging central venous catheters is now well recognized since many HPN consumers will require this therapy for the rest of their lives. Frequent removal of catheters because of infections can result in loss of potential access sites, thus salvage of any possible sites is critical to the HPN-dependent patient. Indeed, some consumers have been referred for transplantation solely because of lack of possible central venous access sites [33]. Catheter infections can be successfully treated in many cases with the catheter *in situ*. In this case, the antibiotic must be given through the central venous catheter and an antibiotic lock left in the catheter when it is not being used for an infusion.

Liver complications are also relatively frequent in consumers of HPN (see Chapters 20 and 21). The exact mechanism of liver disease is uncertain, although recent availability of parenteral lipid formulas in Europe and Asia has provided data suggesting that some lipids may be causative. At present, the only lipid emulsions that are FDA-approved in the United States are manufactured from soybean oil, which contains relatively large amounts of β-sitosterol, a plant sterol that is present in varying amounts in plant-derived lipid (Chapter 28). It has been known for many years that these vegetable sterols are poorly cleared by the human liver [34]. In the Mayo Clinic practice, they have reported that liver enzyme changes can be decreased when soybean-based lipids are infused less frequently than daily [35]. Data in children provide promise that fish-oil emulsions may be helpful in correcting much of the liver disease that is common with HPN [36] (Chapter 21). In patients with liver enzyme abnormalities, hepatic copper has been found to be much higher than in drug-induced cholestasis, with 8 of 28 on HPN and only 1 of 10 with drug-induced cholestasis having levels of copper having levels more than 250 mCg/g of tissue (normal range <35 mCg/g). Liver copper was not correlated with serum copper levels [37]. In addition, manganese is typically elevated in patients with PN-related liver disease (Kelly D.G., unpublished data).

## 32.8  COMPLICATIONS OF HEN

The Oley Foundation also has a chart of complications for HEN. This is available at www.oley.org/charts/newHEN.pdf. A copy of this chart should be provided to HEN consumers.

HEN is relatively safe. The overall complication rate of HEN is about 0.4 per patient per year with little difference between indications for HEN; approximately one-half that of HPN [1]. HEN complications resulting in hospitalization occur an average of once every 3 years.

Complications of enteral feeding include those related to the tube itself and those related to its use with the latter being classified as mechanical, infectious, gastrointestinal, and metabolic [38,39]. Mechanical problems are primarily related to tube size, material, pliability, or location of the tip within the gastrointestinal tract (see also Chapter 13). Infectious complications include those involving the tube exit site, which can be related to contamination at placement of the tube. The use of antibiotics at the time of the tube placement has been shown to decrease skin infections [40]. Careless handling of the formula may cause contamination. In addition, if the feeding formula is left hanging for an extended period spoilage is possible. Common gastrointestinal complications are gastroesophageal reflux, bloating, flatulence, nausea, slowed gastric emptying, and diarrhea. Aspiration of refluxed formula is one of the most common significant problems of tube feeding. Metabolic problems, including excess or deficiency of nutrients, are relatively uncommon when standard enteral formulas are used. However, for patients with preexisting nutrient deficiencies or disorders predisposing to depletion, supplementation with appropriate nutrient(s) may be needed (Chapter 23).

Nutrient–drug interactions may be responsible for decreased absorption of many medications. For example, some medications must be given during a period that the enteral feeding is held. In addition, administration of medications via the feeding tube without adequate water flushes before and after the medication may lead to clogging of the feeding tube. In other situations, the location of the feeding tube needs to be considered before medications are given through the tube. For example, antacids infused into a jejunal tube will only provide an osmotic load, possibly causing diarrhea, while not achieving the desired neutralization of gastric content. Therefore, guidance of medication provision by an experienced pharmacist is ideal (Chapter 27).

## 32.9  LABORATORY MONITORING

Approaches to assessing consumers of HPN have been published on very few occasions [11,41]. The usual Mayo Clinic approach is summarized in Table 32.2. These guidelines are used for consumers who are stable on HPN and based on experience with managing HPN, but have not been subjected to rigorous analysis. During the early part of the HPN course, individuals are typically monitored weekly for the first 3–4 weeks, and then as labs stabilize, the interval between blood tests is lengthened first to every other week, then monthly. Eventually as time progresses and individuals are well, the frequency of monitoring transitioned to the quarterly schedule outlined in the table. An

**TABLE 32.2**
**Adult HPN Monitoring: The Mayo Clinic Routine**

**Quarterly Labs**
**Blood Tests**

| | |
|---|---|
| Sodium | Total protein |
| Potassium | Albumin |
| Chloride | Glucose |
| Bicarbonate, venous | Complete blood count |
| Blood urea nitrogen | Soluble transferrin receptors |
| Creatinine | Magnesium |
| AST | Prothrombin time/ INR |
| Alkaline phosphatase | Copper |
| Bilirubin, total and direct | Selenium |
| Calcium | Zinc |
| Phosphorus | |

**Annual Labs**
**Quarterly Labs Plus:**
**Blood Tests**

| | |
|---|---|
| Vitamin A | Folate |
| Vitamin C | Vitamin B12 |
| Vitamin E | Parathyroid hormone |
| 25 hydroxy vitamin D | Bone alkaline phosphatase |
| Manganese | |

**24-h Urine Tests**

| | | |
|---|---|---|
| Sodium | Creatinine | Calcium |
| Bone mineral density | | |

important NIH—ASPEN research conference on parenteral micronutrients was recently published and provides an intensive discussion by the world experts on trace elements used in PN [16]. However, the guidelines for monitoring the various micronutrients remain largely undefined (see Chapter 23). The ESPEN guidelines for monitoring of the stable patient every 3 month includes: hematology, tests of liver function, creatinine, electrolytes, calcium, phosphate, magnesium, and albumin. Trace elements, vitamins A, E, D, B12, and folic acid as well as bone mineral density are recommended to be measured annually.

Based on clinical experience, it is recommended that blood sugar should be measured early in the infusion and also in the period after the infusion has been completed. In the case of consumers who have very high blood sugar during the early part of the PN, there is often rebound hypoglycemia after stopping the PN because of the high level of endogenous insulin present. In rare cases this can be associated with marked hypoglycemia and even coma. If blood sugars remain stable at less than 150 mg/dL during PN infusion and greater than 70 mg/dL after stopping the infusion, during the initial 2 weeks of PN use, it should not be necessary to continue measuring them unless the PN formula is changed or the patient is ill. If insulin is being added to the PN, measurements of blood sugars should be continued indefinitely.

In general, micronutrient levels should be checked at least annually in HEN patients. However, just as in HPN, there are no prospective or retrospective studies to support specific monitoring recommendations. Enteral formula alone may not provide sufficient water for the patient and water supplementation either orally or via the tube given intermittently by bolus may be required.

## 32.10   QUALITY OF LIFE ON HPEN

Providing enteral and parenteral nutrition support at home may have important psychosocial effects on the patient and their family [42]. Emotions such as fear, anger, and depression are not uncommon and may lead to dysfunctional relationships. In addition, factors such as age greater than 55 years, underlying disease (particularly mesenteric ischemia, malabsorption, scleroderma and pancreatic disease), sleep disturbance, diarrhea, the presence of a stoma and/or use of narcotics can negatively impact the quality of life [11] (see also Chapter 33). Members of the team should be watchful for such issues and address them promptly. Frequently, a visit by an experienced HPEN consumer or caregiver can be very helpful with respect to the psychosocial issues. Introducing the consumer to the Oley Foundation for Home Parenteral and Enteral Nutrition at www//http.www.oley.org (1–800–776–OLEY) will provide important support as well. The Oley Foundation is an organization for consumers, caregivers and clinicians that provides information on practical topics (e.g., body image, travel), regional and national meetings that offer education, an opportunity for networking with other consumers and clinicians and social activities. Involvement by clinicians can strengthen their clinical expertise, as well. Consumer involvement with a support group such as the Oley Foundation has been found to reduce the risk of complications and decrease depression in HPEN consumers [43]. Chapter 38 discusses the importance of organizations such as Oley from the consumer's perspective.

Regarding quality of life on HPN, there have been few studies designed for consumers of HPN [44,45] (see also Chapter 38). A recently validated quality of life tool has been developed specifically for consumers of HPN [46]. Based on this tool, there is an ongoing study originating in Europe under the guidance of members of the Chronic Intestinal Failure (CIF) Work Group of ESPEN. The Oley Foundation is also participating in this study.

The quality of life of HEN consumers has generally been found to be worse compared to the general population; however, this usually relates to their other physical disabilities (e.g., in amyotrophic lateral sclerosis or stroke patients) [47]. Factors that impact on HEN consumers' quality of life include the presence of symptoms such as nausea, vomiting, diarrhea, discomfort while carrying on activities of daily living, fatigue, and issues relating to body image and social isolation [47]. Most consumers and their caregivers rate the feeding tube aspect of their care favorably [48].

Factors that affect successful coping with HEN include having the consumer taking personal responsibility for the enteral nutrition administration, and to seek and accept support, to take charge of their own well-being, to maximize independence and normality and to focus on the positive [49]. In addition, recommendations are found in a self-help manual entitled "Coping Well with HEN" which can be found online at http://www.copingwell.com/copingwell/. Consumers' health care providers and home care companies should also be prepared to improve coping by providing comprehensive HEN education, promoting personal responsibility, encouraging effective coping strategies, allowing flexibility in the HEN regimen, facilitating collaborative decision making, identifying and treating mental health issues and promoting referrals to support groups. Sufficient education will usually allow self-confidence and an improved relationship with their family and the health care team.

## 32.11   PEDIATRIC CONSIDERATIONS

The use of HPEN in pediatrics has long been accepted as an appropriate intervention to optimize quality of life for patients and families and provide an alternative to prolonged hospitalization. Compared to adults, pediatric patients comprise a small percentage of those receiving HPEN in the United States. The lower prevalence is thought to be secondary to the nature of the underlying diseases requiring HPEN in the pediatric population and the increased probability of intestinal adaptation in the first 3 years of life [50]. Estimates suggest that <2.5% of patients receiving HPN are pediatric patients [51]. This may not reflect the true incidence of HPEN given that reporting may be inconsistent. Pediatric HPEN is a rapidly growing field with a new shift toward caring for younger patients [52]. The innate nutritional complexities associated with prematurity, growth and development point toward the importance of pediatric specialists in intestinal failure (IF) management and HPEN provision.

### 32.11.1   BENEFITS

Children with SBS are at increased risk of malnutrition associated with feeding intolerance and malabsorption. Their limited capacity to withstand starvation coupled with high-energy and nutrient requirements necessary for growth and development makes HPEN an invaluable tool in intestinal rehabilitation [53]. One of the primary benefits of HPEN is the ability to provide advanced nutrition support more economically. As previously noted, the cost of HPN as compared to a solution provided in the inpatient setting is roughly 50% less [54]. For the clinically stable child, HPEN allows the clinical team to slowly optimize tolerance of EN utilizing specialized formulae and feeding strategies without compromising fluid and electrolytes status. The combination of PN and EN is crucial in the treatment of children with SBS to prevent the development of micronutrient deficiencies, growth failure, and dehydration.

### 32.11.2   COMPLICATIONS

While the benefits to home nutrition support are obvious, a variety of complications are associated with this therapy. The most common complication is catheter-related blood stream infections (CRBSI). Rates of CRBSI are higher in children than adults secondary to more frequent self dislodgement of CVCs and the propensity of many pediatric patients to manipulate the CVC site [55]. Frequent infections lead to repeated hospitalizations and possible loss of vascular access. Moreover, sepsis may be a risk factor for the onset and progression of parenteral nutrition-associated liver disease (PNALD) (see Chapters 19 and 20).

### 32.11.3   TRANSITION FROM HOSPITAL TO HOME

Children identified for home transfer on HPEN should meet several criteria prior to discharge. These include: the existence of an established and stable nutrition regimen on which the patient has demonstrated growth, tolerance to EN and desired hydration and electrolyte status. Children who are hemodynamically unstable or who require frequent modifications to their nutrition program should not be considered until a stable regimen has been identified. Once a child has been identified for discharge, teaching should begin immediately. Ideally a minimum of two caregivers should be educated on care of feeding tubes and CVCs, use of infusion pumps and medication administration. If a patient is to receive HEN, formula preparation and storage instructions should be provided to the patient or family. As discussed in Chapter 34, Social and Medical Insurance Issues, participation by a case manager is essential when the decision to discharge is made to assist in the selection of the most appropriate home infusion company and medical suppliers. The family's insurance coverage should also be assessed to identify the scope of nutrition coverage. Children on HEN who qualify for the Women Infants and Children (WIC) program should seek out assistance at this time. Careful planning is needed for the WIC-qualified patient as each state varies in the formulas provided. Additional documentation or letters of medical necessity may be needed for a formula not standard to the WIC formulary (http://www.fns.usda.gov/wic/). Once teaching is completed and the homecare agencies are assigned, the child is ready for discharge home. Parents or caregivers should be provided with strict criteria and algorithms to guide the family's decision making, such as when the team should be notified of a problem or when a visit to the emergency department is necessary. This is particularly crucial for the patient being discharged home with a CVC as patients and caregivers need to be educated on signs of CRBSI along with appropriate plans of care. A fever in a child with a CVC should always warrant evaluation even if the cause of elevated temperatures is thought to be related to previously diagnosed infections or noninfectious causes. (e.g., known upper respiratory infection or other clinically apparent infection.)

## 32.11.4   CLINICAL MANAGEMENT OF THE PEDIATRIC HPN PATIENT

A large percentage of children with SBS will be discharged home on PN. In preparation for discharge, the practitioner responsible for prescribing the PN should develop a regimen that is the least disruptive to family life. One example of accomplishing this is the use a cyclical PN infusion schedule. A primary benefit of cyclical PN is that it allows the child time to be disconnected from pumps and tubing. Continual connection to infusion pumps can complicate gross motor skill development in the young child and provide physical and social barriers to such activities as school or work for the older patient. In addition to convenience, cyclical PN is thought to provide physiological benefit as it allows for pauses in substrate utilization more closely mimicking traditional feeding patterns [56]. In one study, infants on cyclical PN did not develop elevations in serum transaminases and showed improved growth velocities in comparison to those receiving continuous PN infusions [57]. While the benefits appear obvious, contraindications exist. A common contraindication to cycling is impairment in hepatic regulation of blood glucose during a fast [56]. This may be true in the very small infant or in those with severe hepatic dysfunction. Prior to discharge, the child's tolerance to cycling should be assessed. Hourly infusion goals can be estimated based on their weight, liver function and age appropriate feeding pattern. For example, a 3-month-old premature infant weighing 3 kg may only tolerate cycling to a 20- or 16-h PN infusion secondary to immature glycolytic pathways and frequent baseline feeding pattern of every 3–4 h [56]. Conversely a 1 year old of average weight who would commonly sleep through the night without requiring a meal to maintain normoglycemia may tolerate a 12–16 h PN infusion, maintaining blood glucose levels via hepatic glycogenolysis. Of note, cycling PN also increases the glucose infusion rate (GIR), another consideration in the child who fails to achieve normoglycemia. A second contraindication to cycling would include unsafe infusion rates of PN components. One example of this is potassium. Guidelines for potassium infusion rates can vary greatly; the HPN practitioner should be well versed in their institutional guidelines as well as those of the home infusion company. For example, at Children's Hospital Boston, potassium infusion rates typically do not exceed 0.25 mEq/kg/h unless a cardiac monitor is used. Because cardiac monitoring is not feasible at home, the risks and benefits of cycling should be carefully weighed against risks of high potassium infusion. Bed wetting is also common for many children on cyclical PN as a majority of the daily fluid volume is provided in a compressed amount of time, typically overnight. This is an especially important consideration in the older child. The benefits of cyclical PN must be carefully weighed against the complications and applied on an individual basis. Not all patients are suitable for cyclic PN administration.

Another HPN consideration is solution compatibility and stability. During a hospital admission, PN solutions are compounded on a daily basis allowing for acute changes and minimal stand time to allow interaction between additives. In the home setting, patients will receive several days' worth of a compounded solution; it is important to assess if the solution is stable for an extended time period to avoid the development of precipitates or disruption of the fat emulsion. One important aspect when assessing compatibility and stability is the method in which intravenous fat emulsions (IFE) will be provided. PN and IFE can be provided in one of two forms, a 2:1 solution in which IFE is separately infused from the PN solution containing dextrose, amino acids and micronutrients, or as a total nutrient admixture (TNA), also commonly referred to as a 3:1 solution, in which the PN and IFE are compounded as a single infusion. There are benefits and drawbacks to each of these systems. TNA eases the process for administration as only one bag is infused at a constant rate thus decreasing the need for multiple infusion pumps. A major limitation for using a TNA is the increased incidence of calcium and phosphorus incompatibility. Due to the higher content of divalent cations (e.g., calcium and magnesium salts) typically present in a pediatric PN, when formulated as a TNA, the risk of reduced particle zeta potential (negative surface charge) can result in coalescence of the lipid emulsion. As noted in the 2004 ASPEN *Safe Practices for Parenteral Nutrition*, TNAs should not be used in the infant receiving PN since calcium and phosphorus solubility is compromised by the addition of the IFE and prohibits desired dosing for bone mineralization [58]. Moreover, the high calcium and phosphate concentration in typical infant PN formulations increases the risk of precipitation, which can go unnoticed due to the opacity of a TNA. Given that many commonly used IV medications are incompatible with lipid emulsions, use of a TNA may require additional PN cycling than the desired number of hours to accommodate medication administration. One major benefit of a 2:1 solution is the ability to modify PN and lipid infusion rates independently thus avoiding the need for interrupting the PN and further cycling. Moreover, 2:1 solutions allow for increased calcium and phosphorus solubility, making them better suited for the infant or patient with existing bone disease. Disadvantages of 2:1 solutions include the need for two pumps at two different infusion rates and the risk of infusion error. Prior to discharge and throughout the HPN management process, solution compatibility should be continually monitored and discussed with the home infusion company for safe and optimal PN provision.

The ultimate goal during the HPN course is to optimize tolerance of EN to allow for decreased support of HPN or supplemental intravenous fluid (IVF). As EN is advanced, growth and tolerance should be closely monitored. The child meeting or exceeding age appropriate growth standards while maintaining desired hydration should be considered for PN weaning (see Chapter 14, Transition to Enteral Nutrition). HPN can be weaned in a variety of ways. One option is for PN volume decrease. This should be considered for the child who has minimal gastrointestinal losses and has demonstrated the ability to maintain hydration enterally. Another option is to wean PN concentration by decreasing the quantities of dextrose, amino acids, and volume of IFE provided. This option may be considered for the child demonstrating excellent growth with enteral advancement and stable GI losses however continuing to require IV hydration and electrolyte administration to maintain homeostasis. Often children with high GI losses and those prone to dehydration may require additional IV hydration from the PN. Every effort should be made to modify solutions so additional hydration fluid is not habitually required. Regardless, families should be educated on signs and symptoms of dehydration and provided algorithms for the use of replacement fluids. Similar infusion guidelines must also be communicated to the home infusion company.

### 32.11.5   Clinical Management of the Pediatric HEN Patient

Most children with intestinal failure (IF) will be sent home on some semblance of EN ranging from complete parenteral independence to small volume trophic feeds to complement the PN regimen. Discharge goals for children on HEN are variable depending on their stage of intestinal rehabilitation. The goal for the child receiving HEN in combination with HPN is to allow for slow enteral feeding advancement and eventual discontinuation of PN. For the child successfully weaned from PN but receiving slow continuous feedings, the goal would include transition to oral or gastric boluses to mimic physiologic feeding. It should be noted that not all patients will proceed through the continuum. While the ultimate goal for children is to demonstrate tolerance to full oral nutrition with desired growth, their anatomy, absorptive capacity, early IF management along with other underlying contributors may prohibit full progression. The overall goal remains to optimize the child's tolerance to EN and to mimic physiologic feeding. Early introduction of enteral feeding is crucial as the likelihood of intestinal adaptation and progression to full enteral independence is most likely in the first 3 years of life [50].

At the time of transition from hospital to home, children with SBS are generally receiving specialized formula to optimizes absorption and feeding tolerance. Formulas such as Neocate and Elecare are commonly used during the early rehabilitation process as the proteins in these products have been completely hydrolyzed to their amino acid constituents. Inflammatory changes associated with bowel resection in the SBS child's intestinal mucosa are thought to increase sensitivity to proteins and peptides introduced in the early stages of life potentially leading to non-IgE-mediated allergic disease and the development of allergic enteropathies [59]. Unlike peptide chains that are capable of creating a bridge between immune receptors leading to a potential allergic response, amino acids fail to create this cross—linking, thus avoiding a reaction. Along with amino acid based products, formulas high in long-chain triglycerides (LCT) have also been shown to be beneficial. Studies have shown subjects fed diets higher in LCT had improved intestinal adaptation and intestinal weight varying in relation to the amount of LCT provided [60,61]. For SBS patients with severe fat malabsorption, medium-chain triglycerides (MCT) may be useful in improving tolerance as micelle formation is not required for absorption into the portal circulation. One study demonstrated that diets high in MCT oil were associated with a decrease in digestive enzyme activity and delayed mucosal hyperplasia [62]. These findings suggest that during the early stages of intestinal intestinal rehabilitation in the young child, use of amino acid-based formulas containing a higher percentage of LCT should be promoted for optimal tolerance and intestinal adaptation. MCT-containing formulas should be reserved for the child who has demonstrated intolerance to a formula containing LCT secondary to suspected fat malabsorption. While some research suggests that the use of these specialized formulas improves intestinal adaptation, they are more expensive and more difficult to obtain. Providers should carefully consider this when prescribing. Insurance coverage varies by patient and state; documentation of medical necessity is commonly required for reimbursement. For the child receiving WIC, state WIC laws and formularies should be carefully reviewed. Table 32.3 contains a full list of commonly used formulas in the management of SBS.

While formula type may play a significant role in intestinal rehabilitation, the method of feeding is also an important consideration. Depending on the degree of adaptation and their anatomy, children may receive feedings via oral bolus, bolus feedings through a gastric feeding tube, or slow continuous feedings provided via gastric or jejunal routes. Continual advancement of enteral feeding volume or concentration is encouraged in the pediatric HPEN patient; however it commonly is done at a slower rate or with longer intervals between changes in comparison to the hospitalized patient. This more cautious approach is implemented as day to day monitoring by skilled IF clinicians is not feasible at home and the risks associated with significant changes in feeding tolerance without appropriate correction can be fatal. Signs of intolerance include: increase in stool output, change in stool consistency from formed to loose or watery and/or abdominal pain or distention. For a child with an ostomy in place, output should be kept <2 mL/kg/h (roughly equal to 50% of the patient's maintenance fluid requirements). For the child in continuity a goal of 10 or less stools daily with desirable consistency may be reasonable [63]. Children with habitually elevated stool losses may require additional intravenous hydration or support from an oral rehydration solution (e.g., Pedialyte) for electrolyte and fluid repletion. Instructions should be provided to patients and families for management of feeding intolerance, mechanisms for rehydration and when clinical status changes may necessitate admission. It is common for many children on their first transition to the outpatient setting to receive continuous enteral feedings for full saturation of brush border enzymes [55]. As the child grows and capacity for EN increases, transition to oral or gastric bolus feedings may be possible. Children with severe gastrointestinal dysmotility who require gastric decompression or those with a history of significant intestinal resection and loss of regulatory valves may not successfully transition to bolus feedings. Furthermore, many infants with SBS present with oral aversions or feeding difficulties associated with lack of oral stimulation at an early age or complications associated with their medical course (see Chapter 35). Feeding therapy is strongly encouraged. Close communication between the feeding therapist and the HEN provider is a critical step in optimizing a patient's enteral regime.

### 32.11.6 MONITORING

Intermittent laboratory assessments are an important part of monitoring for the pediatric patient receiving HPEN. Each patient should have a customized laboratory schedule based upon clinical status. Table 32.4 provides some recommended frequencies for laboratory assessment in the home setting. More frequent lab draws may be required in the setting of acute changes in stool output,

**TABLE 32.3**
**Common Enteral Formulas Used in the Management**

| Formula Type | Infant | | | Child | | |
|---|---|---|---|---|---|---|
| | Product | Calories per Ounce[a] (Osmolality mOsm/kg H₂O) | Notable Characteristics | Product | Calories per Ounce[a] (Osmolality mOsm/kg H₂O) | Notable Characteristics |
| Amino acid-based | Elecare infant | 20 (350) | 33% of fat as MCT oil. Preparation consistent with standard infant formula preparation | Elecare Jr | 30 (590) | Vanilla flavor available for children 1 year and older |
| | Neocate infant / Neocate infant with DHA and ARA | 20 (375) / 20 (375) | 95% of fat as LCT / 33% of fat as MCT | Neocate Junior / Neocate (E028) Splash | 30 (590–700) / 30 (820) | 35% of fat from MCT oil / Ready to feed nutritionally complete hypoallergenic fruit beverage |
| | Nutramigen AA | 20 (350) | 100% LCT fat blend | Pediatric Vivonex | 24 (360) | 68% of fat from MCT oil. Manufactured in the same plant as formulas that contain soy, milk, egg, and wheat |
| Semielemental[b] | Pregestimil lipil[b] | 20 (320) | 55% of fat as MCT oil; used in cases of severe fat malabsorption | Peptamen Jr[b] | 30 (260–400) | 60% of fat from MCT oil; 100% whey protein |
| | Alimentum[b] | 20 (370) | 33% MCT oil; casein hydrolysate blend | Peptamen Jr 1.5[b] | 45 (450) | 60% of fat from MCT oil; unflavored |
| | | | | Pediasure Peptide[b] | 30 (390) | 50% of fat from MCT oil; also available in a 1.5 calorie per mL |
| | | | | Pepdite Junior[b] | 30 (250–390) | Available as unflavored or banana flavored. Not ready to feed |
| Isomeric | Breast milk | 20 (295–300) | First choice for all infants with SBS | Pediasure[b] | 30 (335) | Also comes with fiber. Avilable in a 1.5 calorie: mL |
| | | | | Boost Kids Essential 1.5[b] | 45 (390) | Useful for the patient with fluid restriction or high-energy demand. Also comes with fiber |

a Based on standard preparation/dilution.
b These products should be used only in the patient with known mucosal adaptation and tolerance to milk protein.

**TABLE 32.4**

**Typical Laboratory Monitoring Protocol for Pediatric HPEN Patients[a]**

| | Monthly | Every 6 Months | Annually |
|---|---|---|---|
| Electrolytes | PN[b] | | |
| Liver function tests | PN | | |
| CBC with differential | PN | | EN[c] |
| Lipid panel | PN | | |
| Aluminum | | PN | |
| Selenium | | PN | |
| Zinc | | PN | EN |
| Copper | | PN | |
| Ceruloplasmin | | PN | |
| Carnitine | | PN | |
| 25(OH) vitamin D | | | EN |
| PTH | | | EN |
| Vitamin A | | | EN |
| Vitamin E | | | EN |
| B12 | | | EN |

*Note:* More frequent monitoring may be required in the setting of abnormal values.

[a] Children's Hospital Boston.

[b] PN: patients receiving parenteral nutrition at any level of dependence.

[c] EN: patients weaned completely from PN, sole enteral or oral feeds.

feeding tolerance or changes to the PN formulation. Though laboratory assessment is a critical element in managing HPEN patients, the need for frequent laboratory assessment on a chronic basis may be a contraindication to HPN provision.

Chronic assessment of micronutrient values is an important monitoring tool for the long-term IF patient. See Table 32.4, along with Chapter 10, for additional information on the frequency of micronutrient labs required for the long-term PN patient. For the patient weaned from PN it is important to continue to evaluate micronutrient status. Vitamins A, E, 25(OH) D, zinc, and B12 in particular should be evaluated 4–6 weeks following discontinuation of PN and annually there after. Persistent fat malabsorption and loss of the terminal ileum may predispose patients to malabsorption and need for lifelong micronutrient supplementation (see Chapter 23).

In addition to biochemical parameters, appropriate gains in weight, length and head circumference are the best indicators of adequate nutrient provision in the pediatric population. Children with SBS are at increased risk of growth failure secondary to higher energy and nutrient requirements that accompany malabsorption and growth delays associated with prematurity, a common characteristic amongst pediatric SBS patients. Periodic assessment of anthropometrics in comparison with age appropriate or desired growth velocities is imperative. Acute malnutrition in the pediatric patient is commonly characterized by low weight for height with normal height for age. Chronic malnutrition presents as low to normal weight for height with low height for age, commonly referred to as "stunting." Children with SBS are particularly at risk of delayed linear growth secondary to dependence on PN at an early age and risk of metabolic bone disease, fat malabsorption complicating enteral absorption of calcium and vitamin D, and variations in diurnal calcium absorption due to cyclic PN use [64]. Because of these potential risks, periodic assessment of bone status should be assessed via routine length measurements, serum PTH, bone age, or the gold standard, dual energy x-ray absorptiometry (DEXA) (see Chapter 22). Finally, arm anthropometrics may provide additional benefit in assessing subcutaneous fat stores and lean body mass accretion. Serial measures should be taken and compared to historical data.

## 32.11.7 SURVIVAL

Similar to adults, survival in pediatric patients receiving HPEN is largely dependent upon their underlying diagnosis [52,54]. Survival data for children receiving HEN is not available. For the child receiving HPN, the incidence of therapy associated mortality is higher. Despite this increased risk, children on HPN have higher survival rates than adults on HPN with comparable diagnosis (89% vs. 60% respectively) [52]. One factor that is strongly correlated to patient survival is bowel length [65,66]. It has been theorized that children with <15 cm of small bowel and an intact ileocecal valve (ICV) or >15 cm of small bowel without an ICV have an increased probability of intestinal adaptation [50]. Children with longer small bowel length are more likely to progress to parenteral independence and avoid development of PNALD also closely linked to survival [65]. For both therapies, survival has been linked to the experience and dynamic approach of the team. A study by Modi et al. [67] reported a 19% increase in survival in pediatric IF patients after the establishment of a multidisciplinary team (see Introduction: A Multidisciplinary Approach to Intestinal Failure).

## 32.11.8 TRANSITION FROM THE PEDIATRIC TO ADULT SETTING

As the survival rates for children on HPEN continue to increase, transition of the pediatric patient from a child-centered health care system to one that deals with chronically ill adults is becoming an emerging concern. According to the Society for Adolescent Medicine, transition has been defined as "the purposeful, planned movement of adolescents and young adults with chronic medical and physical conditions to adult-centered health care systems" [68]. In 2003, the Royal College of Paediatrics and Child Care developed guidelines addressing transitional care [69]. Additional recommendations specific to transitioning enterally fed adolescents to adult centers was published by NHS Quality Improvement Scotland (NHS QIS) [70]. Both the young adult and their families may

---

### TABLE 32.5
### Factors That Must Be Considered in Order to Make the Transition Process Successful

#### Prior to Transition

Written and verbal communication between transferring pediatric and receiving adult providers, which has the young person's long-term goals considered

Creation of an individualized transition plan that includes educational and other health-care-related goals to be reached by specific dates

Identification of a dedicated healthcare worker, often a nurse or social worker, to work with the young individual in the planning process

Independent health care visits with the patient, without the parents. This is an opportunity for building self-confidence to navigating and negotiating services

The patient should have an opportunity to meet the adult physician before transfer

#### Key Features of Transition

Discussions regarding transition should begin early, around age 12

Transfer to adult health care facility should be determined by the readiness of the young person and usually occurs after they have finished growth, puberty, and school

Transfer should include a comprehensive transfer of health information

Transfer should be an active process that continues even after the young adult has been accepted into an adult program

The transition process should be flexible and adapted to the young person's needs and views

*Source:* Adapted from Protheroe S. *Proc Nutr Soc* 2009;68:441–445.

---

---

**TABLE 32.6**

**Issues Faced by Adolescents in Transition**

**Self-Care**

Making and getting to medical appointments

Establishing contacts with homecare companies, pharmacies

Central venous catheter care

Stoma care

Connecting PN to administration tubing/CVC

Setting infusion pump rates

Storing/preparing enteral formula

**Lifestyle Issues**

Maintaining appropriate sleep patterns

Sexual health

Exercise habits

Substance abuse

Self-esteem/body image concerns

**Social Issues**

Knowledge of health benefits/support groups

Self advocacy

Work/educational goals

*Source:* Adapted from Protheroe S. *Proc Nutr Soc* 2009; 68:441–445.

---

be concerned about the reduction or loss of services following transfer to an adult center. A key factor in making a successful transition was to have dedicated dietetic and nursing support [68]. Poorly planned transition can result in problems when young adults attempt to access adult services. Given that in many instances transitional care is based on clinical experience, having dedicated professionals was reported to be essential for providing advice and support to families with the goal to develop hospital outreach services, cooperation with schools, and liaison with social services [68]. Table 32.5 discusses factors that must be considered in order to make the transition process successful. Failure to plan for the transition period can result in an increased risk of noncompliance or lack of follow-up, and may increase the risk of morbidity and mortality [71]. Given the multitude of issues that young adults encounter during this period (Table 32.6), age and developmentally appropriate educational, vocational, and psychosocial services must be included in this process. Young adults may have inadequate organizational skills. If they have not achieved the appropriate level of cognitive maturity and autonomy, skills such as setting up their HPN may be delayed [72]. As part of their desire to separate from parenteral controls, medical care may become ignored. Risk-taking behaviors may become more common. Young adults on HPN may be prone to anxiety and depression due to a lack of freedom which can also impact their economic independence [73]. The HPEN team should be familiar with these issues and assist the patient in obtaining the necessary psychosocial support or life skills training. Also during this period, parents may be fearful of transferring care to their child on HPEN to an adult program and their concerns must also be addressed. Support groups can be helpful in this helping patients and families through this often stressful process.

## 32.12  CONCLUSION

Home parenteral and enteral nutrition (HPEN) has resulted in substantially improved survival of patients who have had devastating disease causing oral and intestinal failure. These therapies are associated with complications and detriments to quality of life. Nevertheless, with appropriate care, education and counseling of the HPEN patient, many of these problems can be avoided or reduced in frequency and/or severity. Only a small proportion of deaths involving HPEN consumers are directly related to the nutrition support. One of the most important interventions for those on HPEN is involvement in the Oley Foundation for Parenteral and Enteral Nutrition, which provides access to expert clinicians, education, networking and social activities for consumers.

## REFERENCES

1. Howard L, Ament M, Fleming CR et al. Current use and clinical outcome of home parenteral and enteral nutrition therapies in the United States. *Gastroenterology* 1995;109:355–365.
2. Howard L, Heaphey LL, Timchalk M. A review of the current national status of home parenteral and enteral nutrition from the provider and consumer perspectives. *JPEN* 1986;10:416–424.
3. Kelly DG. The clinician's responsibility for the consumer's financial well-being. *Nutr Clin Pract* 2006;21:539–541.
4. ASPEN Board of Directors and Kovacevich DS, Frederick A, Kelly D, Nishikawa R, Young L. ASPEN standards for specialized nutrition support: Home care patients. *Nutr Clin Pract* 2005;20:579–590.
5. Howard L, Malone M. Current status of home parenteral nutrition in the United States. *Transplantation Proc* 1996;28:2691–2695.
6. Howard L, Malone M, Wolf BM. Home enteral nutrition in adults. In: Rombeau JL, Rolandelli RH, editors. *Clinical Nutrition: Enteral and Tube Feeding*. 3rd ed. Philadelphia: WB Saunders; 1997. pp. 510–522.
7. Powers DA, Brown RO, Cowan GSM et al. Nutrition support team vs. non-team management of enteral nutrition support in a veteran's administration medical center teaching hospital. *JPEN* 1986;10:635–638.
8. Hamaoui E. Assessing the nutrition support team. *JPEN* 1987;11:412–421.
9. Verso M, Agnelli G., Kamphulsen PW et al. Risk factors for upper limb deep vein thrombosis associated with use of central vein catheter in cancer patients. *Intern Emerg Med* 2008; 3:117–122.
10. Howard L. Claunch. C. McDowell R, Timchalk M. Five years of experience in patients receiving home nutrition support with the implanted reservoir: A comparison with the external catheter. *JPEN* 1989;13:478–483.
11. Cowl CT, Weinstock JV, Al-Jurf A et al. Complications and cost associated with parenteral nutrition delivered to hospitalized patients through either subclavian or peripherally-inserted central catheters. *Clin Nutrition* 2000;19: 237–243.
12. Staun M, Pironi L, Bozzetti F et al. ESPEN guidelines on parenteral nutrition: Home parenteral nutrition (HPN) in adult patients. *Clin Nutrition* 2009;30:1–13.
13. Kirby DF, Delegge MH, Fleming CR. American gastroenterological association medical position statement: Guidelines for the use of enteral nutrition. *Gastroenterology* 1995;108:1280–1301.
14. Taylor CA, Larson DE, Ballard DJ et al. Predictors of outcome after percutaneous endoscopic gastrostomy: A community-based study. *Mayo Clin Proc* 1992;67:1042–1049.
15. Gauderer MWL, Picha GJ, Izant RJ. The gastrostomy "button"—a simple, skin-level, non-refluxing device for long-term enteral feedings. *J Pediatr Surg* 1984;19:803–805.
16. Solomon SM, Kirby, DF. The refeeding syndrome: A review. *JPEN* 1990;14:90–97.
17. Buchman AL, Howard LJ, Guenter P et al. Micronutrients in parenteral nutrition: Too little or too much?. The past, present, and recommendations for the future. *Gastroenterology*. 2009;137(5 Suppl):S1–S6.
18. Hardy G. Manganese in parenteral nutrition: Who, when and why should we supplement? *Gastroenterol* 2009;137:S29–S35.
19. Shenkin A. Selenium in intravenous nutrition. *Gastroenterology* 2009;137:S61–S69.
20. Cavicchi M, Beau P, Crenn P et al. Prevalence of liver disease and contributing factors in patients receiving home parenteral nutrition. *Ann Intern Med* 2000;132:525–532.
21. Chen Y, Peterson SJ. Enteral nutrition formulas: Which formula is right or your adult patient? *Nutr Clin Pract* 2009; 24:344–355.
22. Yang G, Wu XT, Zhou Y, Wang YL. Application of dietary fiber in clinical enteral nutrition: A meta-analysis of randomized controlled trials. *World J Gastroenterol*. 2005;11:3935–3938.
23. Barrett JS, Shepherd SJ, Gibson PR. Strategies to manage gastrointestinal symptoms complicating enteral feeding. *JPEN* 2009;33:21–26.
24. Ciocon JO, Galindo-Ciocon DJ, Tiessen C, Galindo D. Continuous compared with intermittent tube feeding in the elderly. *JPEN* 1992;16:525–528.
25. North American Home Parenteral and Enteral Nutrition Patient Registry, Annual Reports 1985–1992, Albany, NY: Oley Foundation, 1987–1994. Enteral feeding. *Gastrointest Endosc Clin N Am* 1998; 8:705–722.

26. Howard L, Patton L, Scheib-Dahl R. Outcomes in long-term enteral feeding. *Gastrointestinal Endoscopy Clin N Amer*. 8(3):705–22, 1998.
27. Van Gossum A, Bakker H, Bozzetti F et al. Home parenteral nutrition in adults: A European multicenter survey in 1997. *Clin Nutr* 1999;18:135–140
28. Messing B, Lemann M, Landais P et al. Prognosis of patients with nonmalignant chronic intestinal failure receiving long-term home parenteral nutrition. *Gastroenterology* 1995; 109:355–365.
29. Scolapio JS, Fleming CR, Kelly DG et al. Survival of home parenteral nutrition-treated patients: 20 years of experience at the Mayo Clinic. *Mayo Clin Proc* 1999;74:217–222.
30. Nehra V, Pedersen RA, Kim WR, Kelly DG. Survival in patients with short bowel syndrome on home parenteral nutrition: Mayo Clinic experience. *Clin Nutr* 2008;3(Suppl 1):76.
31. Amiot A, Joly F, Alves A, Panis Y, Bouhnik Y, Messing B. Long-term outcome of chronic intestinal pseudo-obstruction adult patients requiring home parenteral nutrition. *Amer J Gastroent* 2009;104(5):1262–70..
32. Nehra V, Pedersen RA, Kim WR, Kelly DG. Survival in patients with intestinal dysmotility on home parenteral nutrition: Mayo Clinic experience. *Clin Nutr* 2009;(Suppl 2):59–60.
33. Rodrigues AF, van Mojurik IDM, Sharif K et al. Management of end-stage central venous access in children referred for possible small bowel transplantation. *J Pediatr Gastroenterol Nutr* 2006; 42:427–433.
34. Clayton PT, Whitfield P, Iyer K. The role of phytosterols in the pathogenesis of liver complications of pediatric parenteral nutrition. *Nutrition* 1998;14:158–164.
35. Hwa YL, Nadeau JM, Kelly DG. Long-term parenteral nutrition (PN)-related liver disease: Soybean-based lipids (SBL) as a potential causative factor. 2009 XIth International Small Bowel Transplant Symposium Proceedings. p. 147.
36. Puder M, Valim C, Meisel JA et al. Parenteral fish oil improves outcomes in patients with parenteral nutrition-associated liver injury. *Ann Surg* 2009;250:395–402.
37. Blaszyk H, Wild PJ, Oliveira A et al. Hepatic copper in patients receiving long-term total parenteral nutrition. *J Clin Gastroenterol* 2005;39:318–320.
38. McClave SA, Chang W-K. Complications of enteral access. *Gastrointest Endosc* 2003;58:739–751.
39. DiBaise JK, Decker GA. Enteral access options and management in the patient with intestinal failure. *J Clin Gastroenterol* 2007;41:647–656.
40. Jain NK, Larson DE, Schroeder KW et al. Antibiotic prophylaxis for percutaneous endoscopic gastrostomy. A prospective randomized, double-blind clinical trial. *Ann Intern Med* 1987;107:824–828.
41. Kelly DG. Guidelines and available products for parenteral vitamins and trace elements *JPEN* 2002;26(5 Suppl):S34–S36.
42. Tucker E, Kelly DG. Specialized Nutrition: The patient perspective. In: Matarese LE, Steiger E, Seidner DL, editors. *Intestinal Failure and Rehabilitation: A Clinical Guide*. 1st ed.. Boca Raton, FL: CRC Press; 2004. vol. 1. pp. 353–366.
43. Smith CE, Curtas S, Werkowitch M et al. Home parenteral nutrition: Does affiliation with a national support and educational organization improve patient outcome. *JPEN* 2002;26:159–163.
44. Howard LJ. Length of life and quality of life on home parenteral nutrition. *JPEN* 2002;26:S55–S59.
45. Winkler MF. Quality of life in adult home parenteral nutrition patients. *JPEN* 2005;29:162–170.
46. Baxter JP, Fayers PM, McKinlay AW. The clinical and psychometric validation of a questionnaire to assess the quality of life of adult patients treated with long-term parenteral nutrition. *JPEN* 2010;34:131–142.
47. Bannerman E, Pendlebury J, Phillips F, Ghosh S. A cross-sectional and longitudinal study of health-related quality of life after percutaneous endoscopic gastrostomy. *Eur J Gastroenterol Hepaol* 2000;12:1101–1109.
48. Brotherton AM, Judd PA. Quality of life in adult enteral tube feeding patients. *J Hum Nutr Diet* 2007; 20:513–522.
49. Thompson CW, Durrant L, Barusch A, Olson L. Fostering coping skills and resilience in home enteral nutrition (HEN) consumers. *Nutr Clin Pract* 2006;21:557–565.
50. Quirós-Tejeira RE, Ament ME, Reyen L et al. Long-term parenteral nutrition support and intestinal adaptation in children with short bowel syndrome a 25 year experience. *J Pediatr* 2004;145:157–163.
51. Spencer AU, Kovacevich D, McKinney-Barnett M et al. Pediatric short-bowel syndrome: The cost of comprehensive care. *Am J Clin Nutr* 2008;88:1552–1559.
52. Colomb, V. Long-Term outcome of children receiving home parenteral Nutrition: A 20 year single-center experience in 302 patients. *J Pediat Gastroent and Nutr* 2007;44:347–353.
53. Howard, L. Home parenteral nutrition: Survival, cost and quality of life. *Gastroenterology* 2006;130(2 Suppl 1):S52– S59.

54. Torres C, Sudan D, Vanderhoof J et al. Role of an intestinal rehabilitation program in the treatment of advanced intestinal failure. *J Pediatr Gastroenterol Nutr* 2007;45:204–212.
55. Spencer AU, Neaga A, West B et al. Pediatric short bowel syndrome: Redefining predictors of success. *Ann Surg*. 2005;242:403–409.
56. Modi BP, Langer M, Ching YA et al. Improved survival in a multidisciplinary short bowel syndrome program. *J Pediatr Surg*. 2008;43:20–24.
57. Duggan C, Rizzo C, Cooper A et al. Effectiveness of a clinical practice guideline for parenteral nutrition: A 5 year follow-up study in a pediatric teaching hospital. *JPEN* 2002;26:377–381.
58. Johnson T, Sexton E. Managing children and adolescents on parenteral nutrition: Challenges for the nutrition support team. *Proc Nutr Soc* 2006;65:217–221.
59. Jensen AR, Goldin AB, Koopmeiners JS et al. The association of cyclic parenteral nutrition and decreased incidence of cholestatic liver disease in patients with gastroschisis. *J Pediatr Surg* 2009; 44:183–189.
60. Takehara H, Hino M, Kameoka K, Komi N. A new method of total parenteral nutrition for neonates: Is it possible that cyclic tpn prevents intrahepatic cholestasis? *Tokushima J Exp Med* 1990; 37:97–102.
61. Mirtallo J, Canada T, Johnson D. Safe practices for parenteral nutrition: Taskforce for the revision of safe practices for parenteral nutrition. *JPEN* 2004;28:S39–S70.
62. Vanderhoof, JA Young RJ. Hydrolyzed versus nonhydrolyzed protein diet in short bowel syndrome in children. *Pediatr Gastroenterol Nutr* 2004;38:107.
63. Andorsky DJ, Lund DP, Lillehei CW et al. Nutritional and other postoperative management of neonates with short bowel syndrome correlates with clinical outcomes. *J Pediatr* 2001;139:27–33.
64. Kollman KA, Lien EL, Vanderhoof JA. Dietary lipids influence intestinal adaptation after massive bowel resection. *J Pediatr Gastroenterol Nutr* 1999;28:41–45.
65. Vanderhoof JA, Grandjean CJ, Kaufman SS et al. Effect of high percentage medium chain triglyceride diet on mucosal adaptation following massive bowel resection in rats. *JPEN* 1984;8:685–689.
66. Utter S, Duggan C. Short Bowel Syndrome. In: Hendricks KM, Duggan C, editors. *Manual of Pediatric Nutrition*. 4th ed. Hamilton, Ontario: BC Decker Inc.; 2005. pp. 718–732.
67. Goodman WG, Misra S, Veldhuis JD et al. Altered diurnal regulation of blood ionized calcium and serum parathyroid concentration during parenteral nutrition. *Am J Clin Nutr* 2000;71:560–568.
68. Johnson T, Sexton E. Managing children and adolescents on parenteral nutrition: Challenges for the nutritional support team. *Proc Nutr Soc* 2006;65:217–221.
69. Royal College of Paediatrics and Child Health. Bridging the gaps: Health care for adolescents. 2003; www.rcphch.ac.uk (accessed May 2010)
70. NHS Quality Improvement Scotland Best Practice Statement ~ September 2007: Caring for children and young people in the community receiving enteral tube feeding; http://www.nhshealthquality.org/nhsqis/files/ChildrensHealth_Enteraltubefeeding_Sept2007.pdf (accessed May 2010).
71. Protheroe S. Symposium 6: Young people, artificial nutrition and transitional care. Transition in young people on home parenteral nutrition. *Proc Nutr Soc* 2009;68:441–445.
72. Sawyer S, Drew S, Yeo M et al. Adolescents with a chronic condition: Challenges living, challenges treating. *Lancet* 2007;369:1481–1489.
73. Huisman-de Waal G, Schoonhoven L, Janeen J et al. The impact of home parenteral nutrition on daily life—A review. *Clin Nutr* 2007;26:275–288.

# 33 Quality of Life

*Robert S. Venick and Khiet D. Ngo*

## CONTENTS

## 33.1 BACKGROUND

Over the past 30 years, home parenteral nutrition (HPN) and intestinal transplantation (ITx) have become clinically feasible treatments for children and adults with intestinal failure (IF) [1,2]. Medical and surgical advancements have significantly improved the outcomes in this field, and have enabled clinicians to devote attention not only to the quantity of their patients' lives, but also to their health-related quality of life (HRQOL). Relative to other more mature areas of medicine, there is a paucity of HRQOL data and even validated tools for IF and ITx patients. As multidisciplinary teams gain additional experience, there are increasing opportunities to develop a better understanding of the issues and challenges facing these patients and their families. In this chapter, we aim to review the components and measurements of HRQOL, explain what constitutes a good HRQOL instrument, highlight important practical points and unique challenges faced when implementing HRQOL assessment, and identify future research needs.

## 33.2 HEALTH-RELATED QUALITY OF LIFE

The five aspects of health that make up the multidimensional construct of HRQOL defined by the World Health Organization and other experts in this field include physical health, mental health, social functioning, role functioning, and general health perceptions [3–5]. HRQOL is a fundamental aspect of medical treatment and refers to those aspects of quality of life (QOL) directly related to health and potentially affected by the health care system [6]. A new emphasis on HRQOL is a reflection of the awareness of the critical link between physical and psychological health regarding disease and treatment-related morbidity [7].

Examples of QOL definitions offered by various authors and reviewed by Pais [8] include the following: (a) QOL is a state of complete physical, mental, and social well-being and not merely the absence of disease [9]; (b) QOL is the subjective perception of satisfaction or happiness with life in domains of importance to the individual [10]; (c) QOL is a person's sense of well-being that stems from satisfaction or dissatisfaction with the areas of life that are important to him or her [11]; (d) QOL is the difference between a person's expectations and actual experience [12]; and (e) QOL is an individual's perception of their position in life in the context of the culture and value system in which they live and in relation to their goals, expectations, standards, and concerns [13]. Based on the chosen definition of QOL, specific instruments can be selected to measure HRQOL.

## 33.3   SELECTING THE RIGHT HRQOL INSTRUMENTS: RELIABILITY AND VALIDITY

Psychometrics is the field of survey analysis that enables researchers to determine the quality of an instrument being considered. The two main principles involved in selecting a useful instrument to measure HRQOL are knowing that the instrument is both reliable and valid [14,15]. Reliability refers to the extent to which a measure consistently yields the same score each time it is administered to an individual patient assuming that all other things are equal. It is a statistical measure of reproducibility or stability of the data gathered by the survey, and it is typically assessed in four forms: test–retest, alternate form, interobserver variability, and internal consistency. Reliability is often measured using correlation coefficients ($r$ values). Instruments that have correlation coefficients $\geq 0.70$ are, generally speaking, considered clinically acceptable. Validity is the degree to which an instrument accurately reflects that which it is intended to measure. It is possible that an instrument consistently measures a construct other than the intended one, making it reliable yet not valid. Validity must be documented when developing a new instrument or when applying an existing generic instrument to a new population. In assessing an instrument, one can measure several types of validity, including content, construct, and criterion, as well as responsiveness. Content validity relates to issues of patient population and item sufficiency and refers to the degree to which an instrument samples a representative range of the content under study. Construct validity refers to whether an instrument correlates with the theorized psychological construct that it purports to measure. Criterion validity involves assessing an instrument against the gold standard measurement, while responsiveness refers to the ability of a measure to reflect underlying change.

## 33.4   SIGNIFICANCE OF STUDYING HRQOL IN IF AND ITx PATIENTS

Physiological parameters, medical testing, and survival rates have traditionally been the benchmark by which the health of IF and ITx patients have been measured and currently there are no large studies of HRQOL in IF patients followed longitudinally on HPN and/or after ITx. As the medical field evolves toward patient- and family-centered health care, HRQOL plays an increasingly central role in redefining the standards of care. Gaining a thorough understanding of the way in which disease and health care interventions affect HRQOL clearly has significant clinical implications. For one, this will help practitioners and families anticipate the changes in daily life that can be expected with a particular disease process or treatment course, so that the best decisions possible can be made for the patient. Detecting patient-perceived HRQOL problems may also enable medical teams to identify and advocate for interventional services that many of these patients may qualify for. HRQOL data may potentially be helpful in identifying behaviors or issues that interfere with adherence to admittedly complicated medical and nutritional regimens.

Additionally, HRQOL studies can help guide decision making for IF patients. While we currently have absolute indications for ITx such as loss of central vascular access, irreversible intestinal failure-associated liver disease, and severe fluid and electrolyte abnormalities [16], there are many patients for whom the optimal timing of ITx is not clear-cut. The ability to obtain a better handle on patients' and families' perceptions on HPN and following ITx will be invaluable in addressing these complex decisions. Finally, the extensive and close follow-up that many of these patients receive, and the fact that they are cared for by comprehensive multidisciplinary teams of, gastroenterologists, surgeons, nutritionists, social workers, pharmacists, and nurse coordinators makes this patient population well positioned to valuably participate in and obtain meaningful data from HRQOL studies.

## 33.5 EXISTING INSTRUMENTS AND STUDIES FOR HRQOL IN IF AND ITx PATIENTS

### 33.5.1 PEDIATRIC HRQOL INSTRUMENTS

Measurement of HRQOL in children in the past has been complicated by the need to account for changes in expected role functioning with growth and age [17]. Furthermore, the use of parental proxy instruments that accurately assess children's HRQOL has taken time to properly develop [18]. Validated instruments that measure functional outcomes and HRQOL in pediatric patients have only become available within the last 15 years [19–22]. These new surveys include domains of vital importance to pediatric populations, including cognitive and academic performance, self-esteem, social role function, and family function.

A summary of available pediatric HRQOL instruments is shown in Table 33.1. Currently, there are no disease-specific, age-appropriate HRQOL questionnaires that have been validated for pediatric IF or ITx patients. Nonetheless, the two most widely used instruments to assess HRQOL in pediatrics are (1) the Child Health Questionnaire (CHQ), and (2) the Pediatric Quality of Life Inventory (PedsQL). Both questionnaires address the five domains of HRQOL and both have a child/adolescent self-reporting form as well as a parent proxy form. These instruments are available in both English and Spanish, and have been tested in normative populations and children with various chronic diseases including attention deficit hyperactivity disorder, asthma, cystic fibrosis, renal failure, juvenile rheumatoid arthritis, epilepsy, and solid organ transplant recipients [20,23].

The CHQ is designed to assess 14 subscales of function: physical functioning, role/social function owing to emotional status, role/social function owing to behavioral status, role/social function owing to physical status, bodily pain, general behavior, mental health, self-esteem, general health perceptions, parental impact in terms of time and emotion, family activities, family cohesion, and change in health status. The PedsQL is a more recently developed, shorter, generic instrument that aims to examine physical, emotional, and social function [24].

Items on each survey are initially assigned a raw score that is then converted to a 100-point scale with higher scores suggestive of better HRQOL. The PedsQL has the advantage of being shorter (21–23 items) compared to the CHQ (50–87 items), therefore, making it potentially easier to administer and complete. However, the PedsQL, unlike the CHQ, does not have domains for assessing parental and family impact. Developers of the PedsQL have subsequently published the PedsQL™ Family Impact Module designed to measure the impact of pediatric chronic health conditions on parents and the family; this can be administered at the same time as the main survey [25]. The PedsQL also has patient self-administered surveys for children as young as 5 years old. Currently, the self-administered CHQ survey is only available for children aged 10–18 years old. Parent proxy surveys for the PedsQL are available from 2 years of age, while the CHQ parent proxy survey (CHQ-PF50) is designed for parents of children aged 5–18 years. More recently, developers of the CHQ released the 97-item Infant Toddler Quality of Life (ITQOL) survey designed for parents of patients' aged 2 months to 5 years. Although the ITQL is validated, large normative data are not widely available [26]. For the CHQ and PedsQL, depending on the patient or parent familiarity with the survey, it may be completed in 10–15 min, a duration that has been suggested as the optimal time for completion of a survey [8]. Despite its brevity, the PedsQL has been found in prior studies with pediatric liver transplant (LTx) recipients to explain more of the variance in physical function than the CHQ [27].

**TABLE 33.1**
**Features of Selected Pediatric Generic HRQL Instruments**

| Instrument | Population | Administration | No. of Items | Original Language/ Translations (Y/N) | Domains |
|---|---|---|---|---|---|
| Pictured Child's Quality of Life Self-Questionnaire (AUQUEI) (www.mapi-trust.org) | Pediatrics | Self | 3–5-year-old children: 26 6–11 year-old children: 33 | French/Y | Family life, social life, children's activities (school and leisure), health |
| Child Health and Illness Profile (CHIP) Child Edition (CHIP-CE); CHIP-Adolescent Edition (CHIP-AE) (www.chip.jhu.edu) | Pediatrics Adolescents | Self Proxy | CHIP-CE: Child Report: 45; Standard Parent Report: 45; Comprehensive Parent Report: 76; CHIP-AE: 153; Additional disorders module: 41 | English for the United States/Y | Activities, comfort, satisfaction with health, disorders, achievement of developmental expectations, resilience |
| Child Health Questionnaire (CHQ) (www.healthactchq.com) | Pediatrics Adolescents | Self (10–18 years) Proxy (5–18 years) | Parent Form: 50 items (PF50) and 28 items (PF28/Youth Form: 87 items (CF87) | English for the United States | Global health, physical functioning, limitations to the role or social functions (owing to emotional, behavioral, or physical reasons), bodily pain, behavior, mental health, self-esteem, parental impact in terms of time and emotions, family activities, family cohesion, and change in health status |

| Instrument | Population | Respondent | Items | Language | Concepts |
|---|---|---|---|---|---|
| Infant Toddler QOL (ITQOL) (www.healthactchq.com) | Pediatrics (infants and toddlers: 2 months to 5 years) | Proxy | 97 | English for the United States/Y | Infant concepts: physical abilities, growth and development, bodily pain/discomfort, temperament and mood, general behavior perceptions, getting along with others, health perceptions, and change in health. Parent concepts: impact-emotional and time, mental health, general health, and family cohesion |
| KIDSCREEN (KIDSCREEN) (www.kidscreen.org) | Pediatrics, Adolescent | Self, Proxy | KIDSCREEN-52: 52 items, KIDSCREEN-27: 27 items, KIDSCREEN-10 Index: 10 items | Swedish, Spanish, Polish, Hungarian, Greek, German, French, English, Dutch, Czech | Physical well-being, psychological well-being, moods and emotions, self-perceptions, autonomy, paent relations and home life, peers and social support, school environment, bullying, financial support |
| Pediatric Quality of Life Inventory (PedsQL) (www.pedsql.org) | Pediatrics, Adolescent | Self, Proxy | 21–23 | English for the United States | Functioning: physical, social, emotional, school |
| Warwick Child Health and Morbidity Profile (WCHMP) | Pediatrics | Proxy-rated (parent-reported instrument) | 10 | English for the United Kingdom | General health status, acute minor illness status, behavior status, immunization status, chronic illness status, functional health status, HRQL |

### 33.5.2  Existing Studies: HRQOL of Pediatric IF Patients

Early surveys on HRQOL among IF patients reported that most pediatric HPN patients attend school regularly, and participate in sports and activities with their families, but that their nights are frequently disturbed by enuresis and their parenteral nutrition/enteral nutrition pumps [28]. Other authors have speculated that HRQOL of pediatric IF patients may be adversely affected by the fact that HPN is time intensive and relatively invasive, and can be complicated by other issues such as the presence of a stoma, high stool outputs, and unpredictable future health [29].

Currently there are only a limited number of adequately designed published studies concerning HRQOL in pediatric HPN patients. The French, multicenter cross-sectional study by Gottrand et al. [30] is one of the largest HRQOL studies of pediatric HPN/IF patients to date. The investigators mailed age-appropriate surveys to patients and/or their care providers. Three French age-specific surveys were used—the Qualin questionnaire for patients <3 years of age, the AUQUEI questionnaire for children between 3 and 11 years old, and the OK.ado questionnaire for patients ≥12 years old. Seventy-two of 104 eligible patients (70%) responded. HRQOL scores were high across all age groups and did not differ significantly from scores of a healthy reference population. For children aged 3–11 years, overall HRQOL did not differ from healthy children of similar age, although HPN patients did have lower scores than controls on items related to hospitals, health, doctors, medications, and obligations. Overall scores for adolescent patients were higher compared to healthy adolescents. Patient scores were not affected by HPN characteristics such as duration, start of PN in early childhood, number of infusion days per week, or the number of hospitalizations. The only significant factor associated with lower HRQOL was the presence of a stoma. Specifically, adolescents with a stoma reported a lower HRQOL for items related to social life and the future, while children aged 3–11 years with or without a stoma reported no difference in HRQOL.

This study also found that HRQOL scores for siblings did not differ significantly from those of patient scores. HRQOL scores of siblings showed a higher satisfaction level compared to patients only in items related to health and eating. Parents of infants on HPN reported lower scores compared to healthy norms in the categories of health, eating, and speaking. Mothers of patients had lower HRQOL scores compared to reference mothers. The mothers' HRQOL scores were not significantly correlated with their children's scores. Scores of mothers were lower relative to fathers for items related to work, inner life, and freedom. Furthermore, patient HRQOL scores were not significantly different between two-parent and single-parent families. Interestingly, physicians completing the same surveys for their patients reported lower scores compared to parental scores. Variations in scores between health care professionals, family members, and patients highlight the importance of the need to better understand the factors that can account for these differences in HRQOL perception.

### 33.5.3  Existing Studies: HRQOL Following Pediatric Intestinal Transplantation

Despite the fact that children account for a large proportion of ITx recipients, little work has been done on HRQOL for such children and their families. Initial attempts to measure HRQOL following pediatric ITx have centered mostly on growth- and nutrition-related issues, such as the amount of time on total parenteral nutrition (TPN) and tube feeds, the incidence of oral aversion, and linear growth and weight gain post-transplantation [31–33]. These initial descriptive reports represent early efforts at uncovering HRQOL by also reporting the frequency of rehospitalizations, school days missed after transplantation, and other outcomes.

The most meaningful published work to date in the field of HRQOL for pediatric ITx recipients is by Sudan et al. [34] who employed the CHQ questionnaire in a cross-sectional study of 22 families. The mean age of patients was 10.6 years and of parents was 40.8 years. Pediatric patients reported no significant difference in any of the domains compared with healthy norms. In contrast, parent responses revealed the perception of lower function in six domains compared to parents of healthy children. These included physical function, role limitations due to physical problems, general health perception, emotional and time impact on parents, and negative affect on family activities. Parents reported no difference in their child's level of bodily pain, general behavior, mental health, self-esteem, or family cohesion compared to sample norms. Only the lower scores in general health perception and role limitations resulting from physical problems reached statistical significance. In addition, parent scores tended to be lower than child scores.

We recently completed a prospective, cross-sectional, single-center study using both the CHQ and PedsQL4.0 surveys [35]. Thirty-three parents of ITx patients were studied in an outpatient clinic setting. The median ages at transplant and at administration of the questionnaire were 2.2 years and 5.5 years, respectively. Compared to parents of healthy children, parents of ITx patients reported lower scores in eight of 12 domains using the CHQ and lower scores in five of five domains using the PedsQL4.0. When compared with parents of LTx recipients, ITx parents scored lower in four of 12 domains using the CHQ and three of five domains using the PedsQL4.0.

A handful of studies have begun to examine HRQOL outcomes in a closely related field—pediatric LTx. The interested reader is referred to studies by Alonso et al. [36], Bucuvalas et al. [6], Ng and Otley [37], and Taylor et al. [38]. The majority of these studies used CHQ, PedsQL, or ITQOL instruments to measure HRQOL. The most recent multicenter study by Alonso et al. also incorporated family functioning into the study by using the Family Assessment Device, a potentially important tool when studying pediatric HRQOL [26]. These studies have generally found the following: an improvement in HRQOL in LTx recipients compared to their pretransplant status, a trend toward worse HRQOL in comparison with a healthy population, and similar or better HRQOL in LTx recipients than in children with other chronic illnesses. Some of these studies have discovered that specific HRQOL domains are impacted by important demographic factors. Such factors include ethnic minority, single parent, young parental age, lower parental education level, and shorter duration since transplantation [26,38]. The relevance of these findings to patients who have undergone ITx remains to be seen.

Results from the above-mentioned published cross-sectional studies suggest that HPN and ITx positively impact pediatric patient's perceived HRQOL. For the most part, children undergoing these treatments generally perceive their HRQOL similar to normal healthy children. Parents, on the other hand, are more prone to report lower scores in several key categories. These differences suggest that patients and their guardians each process the experience differently. While these studies are important contributions to the field of caring for children with IF, they also highlight the ongoing need to better understand the HRQOL for these children and their families. It will be crucial to not only identify the way in which HRQOL changes over time, but also to identify the specific domains of HRQOL that lead or lag as these changes occur. Longitudinal studies will also provide a better understanding of the predictors of HRQOL and will aid in the comparison of HRQOL in children with IF who can be maintained on HPN versus those who go on to require ITx.

### 33.5.4  ADULT HRQOL INSTRUMENTS

A comprehensive discussion of all the available measurements of HRQOL in adults is beyond the scope of this chapter; the more commonly used adult HRQOL instruments are described in Table 33.2 [39]. Most adult HRQOL studies of IF and ITx patients have used either the Short Form-36 (SF-36) Profile Questionnaire or the EuroQOL Index [40,41]. Both instruments are generic and standardized for patients with chronic medical disorders, but are nonspecific to IF or ITx patients. The SF-36 is composed of eight multiple item scales: physical functioning, role limitations due to physical problems, bodily pain, general health perceptions, vitality, social functioning, role limitations due to emotional problems, and mental health. It also has a single item that addresses patients' perceived change in health. The scales are scored on a 1–100 range with higher scores indicating better well-being. The instrument takes 7–10 min to complete and can be self-administered or administered by an interviewer. Shorter versions (SF-12 and SF-8) have been developed, although

**TABLE 33.2**

**Features of Selected Adult Generic HRQL Instruments**

| Instrument | Administration | No. of Items | Original Language | Objective |
|---|---|---|---|---|
| COOP/WONCA Charts (COOP-C or COOP/WONCA) | Self-administered | 6–8 | English for the United States | To measure the patients' overall functional health |
| Euroqol EQ-5D (EQ-5D) | Proxy-administered Self-administered Telephone-administered | 5 + 1 Visual Analog Scale (VAS) | Dutch English Finnish Norwegian Swedish | To assess health outcome from a wide variety of interventions on a common scale, for the purpose of evaluation, allocation, and monitoring |
| Health Utilities Index (HUI) | Telephone-administered Self-administered Proxy-administered Interviewer-administered Computer-administered Caregiver-administered | Self-administered format: 15, Interviewer-administered format: 40 | English for the United Kingdom English for North America English for Australia | To describe health status, measure within attribute morbidity and HRQOL, and produce utility scores |
| McMaster Health Index Questionnaire (MHIQ) | Self-administered Telephone-administered Interviewer-administered | 59 | English for the United States | To supplement clinical ratings of health status, with QOL measures based on physical, social, and emotional functions |
| Nottingham Health Profile (NHP) | Self-administered | 38 | English for the United Kingdom | To provide a brief indication of a patient's perceived emotional, social, and physical health problems |
| Quality of Life Inventory (QOLI) | Interviewer-administered Self-administered | 36 | English for the United States | To measure life satisfaction and outcome with a single score based on 16 key areas of life, including love, work, and recreation and to show problems in living and strength in each of the 16 areas |

| Instrument | Administration | Items | Language/Country | Purpose |
|---|---|---|---|---|
| Quality of Well-Being scale (QWB) | Telephone-administered<br>Proxy-administered<br>Interviewer-administered | 24 | English for the United States | To measure HRQOL, to monitor the health of populations over time, or to evaluate the efficacy and effectiveness of clinical therapies or practices |
| Quality of Well-Being scale Self-Administered (QWB-SA) | Self-administered<br>Interviewer-administered | 78 | English for the United States | To measure HRQOL, to monitor the health of populations over time, or to evaluate the efficacy and effectiveness of clinical therapies of practices using a preference-weighted self-administered measure |
| SF-12 Health Survey and SF-12v2 Health Survey | Computer-administered<br>Interviewer-administered<br>Self-administered<br>Telephone-administered | 12 | English for the United States | Developed to be a much shorter, yet valid, alternative to the SF-36 for use in large surveys of general and specific populations as well as large longitudinal studies of health outcomes |
| SF-36 Health Survey and SF-36v2 Health Survey | Computer-administered<br>Interviewer-administered<br>Self-administered<br>Telephone-administered | 36 | English for the United States | The SF-36 was developed during the Medical Outcomes Study (MOS) to measure generic health concepts relevant across age, disease, and treatment groups |
| Sickness Impact Profile (SIP) | Self-administered<br>Interviewer-administered | 136 | English for the United States | To provide a descriptive profile of changes in a person's behavior due to sickness |
| World Health Organization Quality of Life assessment instrument (WHOQOL-100 and WHOQOL-BREF) | Self-administered<br>Interviewer-administered | WHOQOL-100: 100 items; WHOQOL-BREF: 26 items | (The WHOQOL was originally developed in Australia, Croatia, France, India, Israel, Japan, The Netherlands, Panama, Russia, Spain, Thailand, the United Kingdom, the United States, Zimbabwe) | To assess individuals' perceptions on the quality of their life |

they may be less reliable. Currently, the SF-36 is available in more than 50 different languages. There have been efforts by Smith et al. [42, 43] to develop HRQOL instruments specific to HPN patients, but to date these have not been widely used.

### 33.5.5   EXISTING STUDIES: HRQOL OF ADULT IF PATIENTS

There has been a steady increase in the number of adult HPN HRQOL studies with approximately seven review articles published over the past 15 years. A 2005 review by Winkler reported that the SF-36 and the QOL Index were the most commonly used surveys at the time [44]. This review identified 24 studies of HPN and HRQOL. The author concluded that HRQOL was worse in HPN patients compared to healthy patients. The technical aspects of HPN administration was also thought to interfere with daily routine activities. Comparison of the different studies was limited because of the variability of instruments, scales, and lifestyle domains. In another review by Baxter et al. [45], the SF-36 was the most common instrument used, with other instruments cited included the EuroQOL, the Sickness Impact Profile, and the Nottingham Health Profile. Eight prospective studies cited in this review found either QOL to be improved or comparable to healthy norms after starting HPN. Differences in the findings from these studies highlight several underlying challenges in investigating HRQOL in HPN patients. First, the majority of the studies are cross sectional with few addressing the longitudinal outcomes for HPN patients. There have been only two studies that suggest that QOL improves over time [46,47]. Ideally, QOL needs to be assessed in patients with IF before, during, and after management with HPN [45]. Second, the diversity of surveys used along with the variations in the methodology and variable timeframes make it difficult to compare the results of one study to another. The field is in great need of a condition-specific instrument that is rigorously developed and validated using recognized psychometric properties.

### 33.5.6   EXISTING STUDIES: HRQOL OF FOLLOWING ADULT ITX

To date many of the described benchmarks of HRQOL following ITx have focused on superficial surrogate measures such as the percentage of patients off PN at 1 month post-ITx and modified Karnofsky performance scores. According to the International Transplant Registry over 80% of recipients who survive the initial period will stop PN and resume their normal activities within 6 months post-ITx [2]. Such reports are superficial and subject to bias as they are reported directly from the transplant centers as opposed to being self-reported by individuals and families.

Several single centers have presented data on HRQOL of adult ITx recipients. The University Hospital, London, Ontario has reported qualitatively that the often protracted ITx postoperative course is followed by frequent setbacks and discomfort [48]. A high incidence of postoperative emotional disorders owing to difficulty in adjustment has also been reported among adult ITx recipients [49]. HRQOL has been studied in a small group of adult patients following ITx at the University of Pittsburgh [50,51]. The Quality of Life Inventory (QOLI) was used to compare HRQOL in 10 ITx recipients and 10 patients on HPN. Change in HRQOL was followed longitudinally over a 2-year period. The QOLI used in the study consists of 125 questions, was designed for adult transplant recipients, and had been previously validated in adult LTx recipients at their center. They found HRQOL to be similar among the two groups, with statistically significant differences noted in only two of the 25 domains.

## 33.6   IMPLEMENTING HRQOL STUDIES

### 33.6.1   IMPORTANT PRACTICAL POINTS

Programs that care for IF patients and/or ITx recipients should strongly consider incorporating HRQOL assessment into their long-term management plan. Several key factors that should be

**TABLE 33.3**

**Practical Consideration in HRQOL Assessment**

- What definition of QOL is most relevant to the current patient population? What domains of QOL are important to include that would fit the chosen QOL definition?
- What are the predominant languages/ethnicities represented at the center? Are these languages available in the survey instrument being considered?
- What is the goal of assessment: research question, to identify potential problems and needs, to identify clinical predictors of HRQOL, to understand changes in HRQOL over time or between different treatment modalities (e.g., pre-TPN, TPN, adaptation, ITx, and LTx) or different patient/family populations (e.g., parents, siblings, ethnicity, and socioeconomic class), and so on.
- What is the age range of the target population? Will both patients and parents/care providers be participating in the survey?
- What is the comprehension level of the patients and parents?
- Where will the surveys be conducted? (e.g., mailed home vs. clinic)?
- Who will complete the surveys? (e.g., patient, one or both parents, siblings, or medical care providers)
- Will this be a cross-sectional or a longitudinal study?

considered in developing a HRQOL assessment program are highlighted in Table 33.3. Understanding the answers to these questions will aid in the selection of the appropriate instrument and the design of the HRQOL study. For pediatric populations we would advocate that investigators consider incorporating concomitant neurodevelopmental and family assessment questionnaires into the study design.

In most published studies using self-administered instruments, surveys are mailed to potential participants. One advantage of mailed surveys is the ease of administration. However, some caution should be taken with this approach. The response rate, while acceptable, may not be as high as surveys completed in the outpatient setting [34,35]. Additionally, most surveys were designed to be completed by one individual, not groups of individuals. With a mailed survey, it may be difficult to monitor if anyone other than the intended parent or patient is completing or assisting in completing the survey. Office administration may address these problems. However, office administration has the potential pitfall of biasing responses due to the fact that they are in a "medical setting." This influence can be minimized by administering the survey prior to beginning any activity associated with the visit including blood work, collecting vital signs, and discussion with any medical or ancillary staff. Of course, these steps may adversely affect the normal flow of an already busy clinic.

Other practical issues to consider prior to embarking on HRQOL studies is that they will likely require informed consent letters and approval from Institutional Review Boards. In addition, in order to be able to provide perspective on the HRQOL of IF and ITx patients, we would recommend that investigators compare their survey results with those of other chronically ill groups of patients. Researchers should also consider collecting a number of demographic, clinical, and developmental variables on their patients in order to assess the influence such independent factors may have in predicting HRQOL.

### 33.6.2 POTENTIAL CHALLENGES AND FUTURE DEVELOPMENTS

Most single centers in the field of IF or ITx face the challenge of inadequate sample size needed to demonstrate meaningful HRQOL findings. In the pediatric HPN literature, even the largest published single-center studies tend to have less than 100 patients and to span two decades or more [52–54]. In 2008, only 185 ITx were performed throughout the United States including both adults and children [1]. Studies performed at any one center may therefore be potentially subject to biases related to variations in disease severity, demographics, and health care delivery; multicenter studies are clearly needed.

In addition to potential barriers such as language and age-appropriateness of the available surveys, another limitation of studying HRQOL in IF and ITx patients is that there are no widely used disease-specific instruments for this medically fragile, understudied population. Despite the relatively very few number of pediatric IF or ITx patients who have participated in HROQL studies, five different instruments have been used [30,34,35]. As more data is gathered one can envision age-appropriate, reliable, and validated disease-specific instruments being used to measure HRQOL for these patients. The transition from childhood to adulthood should also be taken into account as such an instrument is being developed. Whereas the hallmarks of childhood HRQOL may rely on factors such as emotional and cognitive development, and school achievement, measurements of long-term success in adults may include marriage, parenthood, and employment. Moreover, given the continued advances in telemedicine and information technology, HRQOL assessments for research or clinical purposes can occur in a multicenter fashion from satellite locations or even from home. This approach would streamline data collection and analysis, and provide clinicians with more useful real-time measurements.

## 33.7 CONCLUSION

Fortunately, survival rates of IF and ITx patients have improved greatly over the past several decades. Outcomes will ultimately need to be judged by the amount of quality life years restored, a measure which incorporates both survival rate and the quality of the time survived [17]. A handful of reliable and validated generic pediatric and adult instruments exists which can be used to gauge this and related concepts. There is clearly a need to develop age-appropriate and disease-specific instruments that can be used longitudinally to better elucidate HRQOL for IF and ITx patients. Improved understanding of HRQOL findings can be used to better inform patients and families. Such findings can also help medical care teams to advocate for patients in order to continue to improve the quality of health care.

## REFERENCES

1. Fishbein TM. Intestinal transplantation. *NEJM* 2009;361(10):998–1008.
2. Grant D et al. 2003 report of the intestine transplant registry: A new era has dawned. *Annals of Surgery* 2005;241:607–613.
3. World Health Organization. *Constitution of the WHO Basic Document*. Geneva, Switzerland: WHO, 1948.
4. Bradlyn AS et al. Quality of life research in pediatric oncology. Research methods and barriers. *Cancer* 1996;78:1333–1339.
5. Bravata DM et al. Health-related quality of life after liver transplantation: A meta-analysis. *Liver Transplantation and Surgery* 1999;5:318–331.
6. Bucuvalas J et al. Health-related quality of life in pediatric liver transplant recipients: A single-center study. *Liver Transplantation* 2003;9(1):62–71.
7. Barrera M et al. Health-related quality of life of children and adolescents prior to hematopoietic progenitor cell transplantation: Diagnosis and age effects. *Pediatric Blood Cancer* 2006;47(3):320–6.
8. Pais-Ribeiro J. Quality of life is a primary end-point in clinical settings. *Clinical Nutrition* 2004;23:121–130.
9. Cramer J. Quality of life for people with epilepsy. *Neurologic Clinics* 1994;12:1–13.
10. Leidy N et al. Recommendations for evaluating the validity of quality of life claims for labeling and promotion. *Value Health* 1994;2:113–127.
11. Ferrans C et al. Psychometric assessment of the quality of life index. *Research in Nursing & Health* 1992; 15:29–38.
12. Calman K. Quality of life in cancer patients: An hypothesis. *Journal of Medical Ethics* 1984;10:245–251.
13. Orley J and WHOQOL Group. The World Health Organisation (WHO) quality of life project. In: Trimble MR and Dodson WE, editors. *Epilepsy and Quality of Life* New York: Raven Press; 1994. pp. 99–107.
14. Litwin M. Reliability and validity. In: Litwin MS, editor. *How to Assess and Interpret Survey Psychometrics*. 2nd ed. Thousand Oaks: Sage Publications; 2003. pp. 5–41.

15. Hays R and Revicki D. Reliability and validity (including responsiveness). In Fayers P and Hays R, editors *Assessing Quality of Life in Clinical Trials*. 2nd ed. New York: Oxford Press; 2005. pp 25–40.

16. Kaufman S et al. Indications for pediatric intestinal transplantation: A position paper of the American Society of Transplantation. *Pediatric Transplant* 2001;5(2):80–87.

17. Bucuvalas J and Alonso E. Outcome after liver transplantation: More than just survival rates. *Liver Transplantation* 2005;11(1):7–9.

18. Theunissen NC et al. The proxy problem: Child report versus parent report in health-related quality of life research. *Quality Life Research* 1998;7:387–97.

19. Varni J et al. The pedsQL in pediatric cancer. *Cancer* 2002;94:2090–2106.

20. Landgraf J et al. *The CHQ User's Manual*. 1st ed. Boston: The Health Institute, New England Medical Center; 1996.

21. Landgraf JM, Abetz L, Ware JE. *The CHQ: A User's Manual*. 2nd ed. Boston, MA: HealthAct. 1999. http://www.healthact.com/bibliography.php

22. Eiser C. Children's quality of life measures. *Archives of Disease in Childhood* 1997;77:350–354.

23. Raat H et al. *Journal of Clinical Epidemiology* 2002;55:67–76.

24. Varni J et al. PedsQL 4.0: Reliability and validity of the pediatric quality of life inventory version 4.0 generic core scales in healthy and patient populations. *Medical Care* 2001;39:800–812.

25. Varni J et al. The PedsQL™ family impact module: Preliminary reliability and validity. *Health and Quality of Life Outcomes* 2004;2:55.

26. Alonso E et al. Health-related quality of life and family function following pediatric liver transplantation. *Liver Transplantation* 2008;14(4):460–468.

27. Bucuvalas JC and Britto M. Health-related quality of life after liver transplantation: It's not all about the liver. *Journal of Pediatric Gastroenterology and Nutrition* 2003;37(2):106–108.

28. Colomb V. Home parenteral nutrition: The pediatric point of view. *Nutrition* 1999;15(2):172–173.

29. Brook G. Quality of life issues: Parenteral nutrition to small bowel transplantation—A review. *Nutrition* 1998;14(10):813–816.

30. Gottrand F et al. Satisfaction in different life domains in children receiving home parenteral nutrition and their families. *The Journal of Pediatrics* 2005;146(6):793–797.

31. Sudan D et al. Assessment of function, growth and development, and long-term quality of life after small-bowel transplantation. *Transplantation Proceedings* 2000;32:1211–1212.

32. Nucci A et al. Serum growth factors and growth indices pre and post pediatric intestinal transplantation. *Journal of Pediatric Surgery* 2003;38:1043–1047.

33. Nucci A et al. Long-term nutritional outcomes after pediatric intestinal. *Transplantation* 2002;37:460–463.

34. Sudan et al. Quality of life after pediatric intestinal transplantation: The perception of pediatric recipients and their parents. *American Journal of Transplantation* 2004;4:407–413.

35. Ngo KD et al. XIth international small bowel transplant symposium. 2009. Oral presentation. "Quality of life after pediatric intestinal transplantation: Outcomes and predictors," Bologna, Italy. *Oral Abstract #06*.

36. Alonso E et al. Functional outcomes of pediatric liver transplantation. *Journal of Pediatric Gastroenterology and Nutrition* 2003;37(2):155–160.

37. Ng VL and Otley AR. Understanding quality of life for children after liver transplantation: A work in progress. *Liver Transplantation* 2008;14(4):460–468.

38. Taylor R et al. A Critical review of the health-related quality of life of children and adolescents after liver transplantation. *Liver Transplantation* 2005;11(1):51–60.

39. Vetter TR. A Primer on health-related quality of life in chronic pain medicine. *Anesthesia and Analgesia* 2007;104:703–718.

40. Ware, J. *SF 36 Health Survey, Manual and Interpretation Guide, Medical Outcomes, Trust*. Boston, MA; 1993.

41. EurolQoL Group. EuroQoL—A new facility for the measurement of health related quality of life. *Health Policy* 1990;16:199–208.

42. Smith CE et al. Home parenteral nutrition: Does affiliation with a national support and education organization improve patient outcome? *Journal of Parenteral and Enteral Nutrition* 2002;26:159–163.

43. Smith CE et al. Quality of life in long-term TPN patients and their family caregivers. *Journal of Parenteral and Enteral Nutrition* 1993;17:501–506.

44. Winkler M. Quality of life in adult home parenteral nutrition patients. *JPEN* 2005;29:162–170

45. Baxter J et al. A review of the quality of life of adult patients treated with long-term parenteral nutrition. *Clinical Nutrition* 2006;25:543–553.

46. Smith C et al. Clinical trail of interactive and video taped educational interventions reduce infection, reactive depression and re-hospitalisations for sepsis in patients on home parenteral nutrition. *JPEN* 2003;27:137–146.

47. Howard L. Home parenteral nutrition: Survival, cost, and quality of life. *Gastroenterology* 2006;130:S52–S59.

48. Stenn P et al. Psychiatric psychosocial and ethical aspects of small bowel transplantation. *Transplantation Proceedings* 1992;24:1251.

49. DiMartini A et al. Quality of life after small intestinal transplantation and among home parenteral nutrition patients. *Journal of Parenteral and Enteral Nutrition* 1998;22(6):357–62.

50. Rovera GM et al. Quality of life of patients after intestinal transplantation. *Transplantation* 1998;66(9):1141–1145.

51. Rovera GM et al. Quality of life after intestinal transplantation and on total parenteral nutrition. *Transplantation Proceedings* 1998;30:2513–2514.

52. Goulet O et al. Neonatal short bowel syndrome. *Journal of Pediatrics* 1991;119(1 (Pt 1)):18–23.

53. Quirós-Tejeira R et al. Long-term parenteral nutritional support and intestinal adaptation in children with short bowel syndrome: A 25-year experience. *Journal of Pediatrics* 2004;145(2):157–163.

54. Spencer AU et al. Pediatric short bowel syndrome: Redefining predictors of success. *Annals of Surgery* 2005;242(3):403–412.

# 34 Social and Medical Insurance Issues

*Julie Iglesias and Stephanie Petruzzi*

## CONTENTS

## 34.1 INTRODUCTION

Patients with intestinal failure (IF) represent a challenge for any institution because of the complexity of their condition. Due to their unique medical needs, patients are often hospitalized for extended periods of time, thus leaving institutions with the charge of obtaining insurance approvals for lengthy admissions, oftentimes involving out-of-state approvals. In addition to the medical and insurance challenges, many families face additional social and financial hardships in order to be evaluated and treated at facilities that may be far from home. This chapter highlights the intricacies of caring for IF patients and discusses the common social issues that arise during treatment along with insurance roadblocks faced by many families in navigating the approval process.

In discussing best practices, intestinal rehabilitation programs should ultimately be an interdisciplinary group of clinicians and administrative staff that are dedicated to the care of this medically diverse group of patients. A recently published study concluded that a multidisciplinary approach to IF management is associated with improved survival in pediatric short bowel syndrome patients [1].

Ideally, programs should include services that are patient- and diagnosis-focused and can be provided in both the inpatient and outpatient setting. IF rehabilitation programs should be able to care for patients with diagnoses such as necrotizing enterocolitis, gastroschisis, intestinal atresias, volvulus, intestinal pseudo-obstruction, and microvillus inclusion disease. The ultimate goal should be to meet the needs of these complex patients in a holistic manner, encompassing both the patient and the family. Psychosocial support should be provided, often in conjunction with social services. Patients that are followed by programs with a multidisciplinary staff should be made aware of the various team members' availability to them and to understand what each individual provider's role is, in order to optimize the amount of services available.

## 34.2   INSURANCE COVERAGE

As with treating any medical condition, insurance coverage is necessary. Furthermore, given that IF is a complex disease, one often associated with high costs, working with the insurance providers to receive the necessary prior approvals and comprehending specific coverage details can be overwhelming and frustrating for patients, families, as well as the treating provider. Many insurance plans require that the patient have a primary care provider (PCP). If a patient does not have a PCP, the provider can often help the patient or caregivers select one. If the patient already has a PCP, but needs to see a specialist (e.g., a surgeon or gastroenterologist), the PCP must first make a referral for an appointment. In most cases, the patient will need a prior authorization or approval number from their insurance plan; this authorization or approval number is needed by the patient when they call to make an appointment with the specialist. Many insurance plans require the patient pay for a percentage of the charge for a specialist visit or a copayment fee. It is always recommended that the patient or family member gather as much information from the insurance carrier as possible to determine the extent of benefits and what authorizations are needed.

There are several types of health plans available to consumers. Private health care plans are very common and include those offered by employers to their employees. They can also be purchased by an individual. Typically, a health benefit plan is a contract between an employer and a third party (i.e., an insurance company). These contracts vary widely depending on the benefits and coverage levels negotiated by the employer. Oftentimes, the benefits information provided to the patient by the health plan is confusing, leaving the patient unsure of what services will or will not be covered. The benefits booklet given to the patient at the time of enrollment is merely a *summary* of benefits—not actual contract language. The actual policy or contract may need to be examined to determine the plan's coverage and limitations. This can be obtained from the employee's benefits manager. In many cases, it is imperative that this is reviewed *before* the patient receives services.

In 1965, the Social Security Act established both Medicare and Medicaid. Medicaid is government funded health care, typically provided for low-income individuals and families. It is jointly funded by the federal and state governments. Although the federal government establishes national guidelines, each state has the authority to establish its own eligibility standards, determine the type and duration and scope of services, set the rates of payments, and administer the program. Eligibility criteria can be found on the Centers for Medicaid and Medicare Services (CMS) website (Table 34.1). As part of the plan, the state must offer medical assistance for certain basic services to those living beneath the poverty level. For patients over the age of 21, states are not required to provide some services that are available for children. To ascertain the coverage for a specific state, that state's Medicaid agency must be contacted. Medicare is government-funded health care, typically provided for individuals aged 65 and over. Although directed toward a specific age bracket, Medicare plans are also applicable to certain disabled people. Medicare has two major parts: Part A is hospital insurance and is financed through federal taxes, while Part B is supplementary medical insurance and has a monthly premium. Medicare Part A helps cover hospital stays, limited skilled nursing facility care when daily skilled services are needed, home health care, and hospice care. Medicare regulations allow rehabilitation services when significant functional progress is

**TABLE 34.1**

**Contact Information for Federal Programs**

| Program | Website |
|---|---|
| Centers for Medicaid and Medicare Services (CMS) | http://www.cms.hhs.gov/ |
| Consolidated Omnibus Budget Reconciliation Act (COBRA) | http://www.dol.gov/dol/topic/health-plans/cobra.htm |
| Family Medical Leave Act (FLMA) | http://www.dol.gov/whd/fmla/index.htm |
| Medicaid | http://www.cms.hhs.gov/home/medicaid.asp |
| Medicare | http://www.medicare.gov/ |
| Social Security | http://www.ssa.gov/ |
| Special Supplemental Nutrition Program for Women, Infants, and Children (WIC) | http://www.fns.usda.gov/wic/aboutwic/ |

expected and/or maintenance care is needed. Medicare Part B helps cover physician services, outpatient hospital services, rehabilitation agency services, and comprehensive outpatient rehabilitation facility services.

### 34.2.1 THE UNDERINSURED OR UNINSURED PATIENT

Currently in the United Sates, the topic of medical insurance is widely debated. Within the existing health care system, the numerous needs of chronically ill patients are being met but often at a high cost. There are many individuals who are unable to receive optimal health care because they cannot afford a more extensive health care insurance plan or they have no health care coverage at all. Fortunately, there are programs to which patients can apply if they do not have insurance. Such patients are often referred to state-specific Medicaid programs or federal Medicare programs, but these programs have medical or financial guidelines and vary based on age, diagnosis, or state.

### 34.2.2 FEDERAL PROGRAMS

Patients with IF should apply for the most appropriate state Medicaid program. In the case of the elderly adult patients with IF, Medicare should also be researched to determine which program is most appropriate. Since many of these programs frequently change and have specific applications, it recommended that patients access the government websites to obtain the most accurate instructions and information (Table 34.1). Often the website will encourage online applications to start the process as soon as possible, but often this is laborious and overwhelming. It is recommended that patients seek out hospital staff who are well versed on these programs, or patients should contact the programs directly to get the necessary information. If patients do not qualify for these programs or are not using insurance to pay for the visit, they should be advised to call the medical institution at which they wish to be treated to discuss out-of-pocket options that are often costly.

### 34.2.3 ENTITLEMENT PROGRAMS

Entitlement programs can be summarized as those services that are available locally in the patient's community, or federally within the United States, to provide financial or supportive assistance based on the patient's current diagnosis. Entitlement programs ultimately answer the question of what the patient's rights are and what options are available to them. Examples of programs that IF patients often utilize are Social Security Insurance (SSI), Social Security Disability Insurance (SSDI), the Consolidated Omnibus Budget Reconciliation Act (COBRA), and the Family Medical Leave Act (FMLA). There are also other financial services that are income based, such as welfare programs or local food stamp/food pantry programs.

Anyone with a medical disability who has little or no income to sustain one's basic needs of food, clothing, and shelter should apply for SSI/SSDI. If a patient's IF prevents them from holding a job, they should apply for SSI/SSDI assistance; if the patient with IF is under the age of 18, the parent/guardian should apply for SSI on behalf of the child. The criteria used to determine if the patient or family qualifies for SSI is income, previously worked/paid social security taxes, and other cash or medical benefits the patient may be receiving. Social Security Childhood Disability Benefit (CDB) is aimed at helping adults with disabilities whose parents have worked enough to qualify.

The COBRA of 1986 is also commonly utilized by patients or caregivers and is a guaranteed right to buy ongoing insurance coverage from their former employer for at least 18 months or less for up to 3 years after resignation or termination if there was no gross misconduct. This coverage plan extends to state and local government employees and independent contractors and includes qualifying events that impact beneficiaries including the employee, the spouse, or a dependent child. For example, if the patient is employed but is forced or voluntarily terminates or reduces their working hours, then the eligible beneficiary for continued insurance coverage through COBRA would be the patient as the employee. If applicable, the patient's spouse and any dependent children may be covered for up to 18 months. However COBRA does not extend to individual plans, federal employees, certain church-related organizations, and firms with fewer than 20 employees.

The FMLA of 1993 is often utilized by the parents or caretakers of a patient of a chronic illness. This Act states that covered employers must grant an eligible employee up to a total of 12 work-weeks of unpaid leave during any 12-month period for one or more of the following reasons: for the birth and care of the newborn child of the employee; placement with the employee of a son or daughter for adoption or foster care; to care for an immediate family member (spouse, child, or parent) with a serious health condition; or to take a medical leave when the employer is unable to work because of a serious health condition. FMLA applies to all state and local federal employers and public agencies. Private sector employers that employ >50 employees engaged in any activity affecting commerce must also provide FMLA benefits. Furthermore, FMLA is somewhat flexible as it can be used on an intermittent basis allowing the employee to work on a less than full-time schedule. The employee, however, must provide a 30-day advance notice to their employer for anticipated events but the employer can delay the start of FMLA for 30 days if the employee does not provide advance notice, and/or until the employee can provide certification from a medical provider.

### 34.2.4  ADDITIONAL RESOURCES

In addition to the entitlement programs discussed above, it is suggested that patients and health care teams be creative in looking for additional resources that may provide assistance. There are many organizations that provide support to patients with particular diseases; if an IF patient has numerous co-morbid diagnoses, they should apply for any additional programs offered, such as those available through cystic fibrosis, oncology, or liver disease-associated organizations. Furthermore, patients and families should utilize local community and/or religious organizations if applicable.

### 34.2.5  OTHER PROGRAMS

Medical insurance benefits will vary depending on each plan or state Medicaid plan. In some cases, a patient may be eligible to continue to use the primary insurance program they have been using and also apply and utilize a secondary insurance at the same time to maximize benefits. Examples of this would be carrying a policy provided by an employer which would act as the patient's primary insurance but then also applying for state Medicaid if applicable. If the state Medicaid is approved in this scenario, then the Medicaid would become the secondary insurance and the patient would be able to utilize both policies for medical costs.

In most cases, the primary insurance policy will pay standard benefits, although a secondary health plan sometimes may offer a higher level of benefits. A secondary medical plan may pay more of the cost of care, or allow payment for services that are not available through first plan. In these cases, after the primary insurer has paid its standard benefits, the health care provider may bill the secondary health insurer to see if it will cover the remaining costs. Even with secondary health insurance plans, a patient can expect that they may have to pay copayments and deductibles out of their own pocket. It is important that the patient discloses all their health insurance coverage to the insurance company involved; failing to do so can lead to fraud charges. All health care providers must be informed when the patient has secondary health insurance. All claims for health treatment must go to the primary insurer first.

## 34.3  INSTITUTIONAL RESOURCES

Many treating institutions will have departments that can assist patients or caregivers with the myriad of questions that arise during the admission or transfer process. It is important to note that policies and regulations along with insurance plans often change throughout the year. Working with insurance providers can be an arduous task but, with time, patients and families will become more comfortable with the process. They should be encouraged to contact their insurance plan if they have questions about authorization or approval numbers, copayments, or policy coverage. Patients should be advised to ask for a case manager at their insurance company in order to get a more detailed understanding of their insurance plan's coverage.

### 34.3.1  SOCIAL WORK

Typically, a clinical social worker is available to families and patients of the IF clinic to assist the patient and their families in dealing with the broad range of psychosocial issues and stresses related to coping with illnesses and maintaining health. As a member of the multidisciplinary health care team, clinical social workers are trained, licensed professionals who provide a range of psychosocial services to enhance the quality of care for the patient and their families, both within the hospital and the community. In working with families and understanding patient and family concerns, professional social workers join with families to develop options and plans that meet the patient's health, developmental, and emotional needs. Services provided depend on the unique needs of each patient or family and may include counseling and financial assistance. Issues that can be addressed include dealing with chronic illness, coping with diagnosis, illness or hospitalization, the impact of illness on family members, parenting and caregiver concerns, grief, loss or end of life issues, trauma, school or educational concerns, financial difficulties, housing problems, access to community resources, depression, anxiety, and psychiatric concerns.

### 34.3.2  CASE MANAGEMENT

Insurance-based case management (CM) is a thorough review that is typically provided via telephone support to the patient or referral center. In recent years, the importance of CM services has expanded as a fundamental building block to the care management system. Since CM is an intensive service, selection of which cases are to be managed is quite important.

The CM team includes nurses with a variety of backgrounds, many with advanced degrees in specialty areas such as parent–child health, public health, community health, and business administration. Most are care manager certified (CMCs) and participate in local and national professional CM organizations. Many institutions include several liaisons from payer organizations, community health agencies, and government agencies. Program-based CMC provide care coordination services, including discharge planning for post-hospitalization services. As defined by Commission for Case Manager Certification, case management is "a collaborative process that assesses, plans, implements, coordinates, monitors, and evaluates the options and services required to meet an individual's health needs, using communication and available resources to promote quality, cost-effective outcomes."

## 34.4   PLANNING THE INITIAL VISIT/ADMISSION

### 34.4.1   THE INTAKE PROCESS

After insurance coverage or payment options have been initiated, the intake process begins with the patient or an outside institutional contact inquiring about treatment at a specific IF center. Figure 34.1 describes the inpatient intake process used by the Center for Advanced Intestinal Rehabilitation program at Children's Hospital Boston. The medical history is obtained by a nurse practitioner (NP) or a member of the medical staff, during which it is determined if the patient should be seen in the outpatient clinic or be admitted directly to the inpatient floor. Often it is helpful to involve the case manager or staff member who has been in communication with the insurance provider early in the referral process to facilitate and plan the transfer appropriately.

Once the transfer has been approved, it is important to notify the inpatient nursing that will be receiving the patient so that a bed will be available. Depending on the medical plan of care, different services or medical staff may be involved, such as dietitians, pharmacists, NPs, or consult MDs. Patients that do not require an inpatient admission are scheduled to come to an outpatient clinic. In those instances, the patient or caregiver are encouraged to contact their insurance carrier *prior* to the first appointment to ensure the visit is covered in their plan's provider network. If the patient is deemed appropriate for an inpatient admission, insurance approval is also necessary.

### 34.4.2   TRANSPORTATION CONSIDERATIONS

Whenever a patient is admitted directly from another medical institution, transportation is generally the responsibility of the referring facility. The facility works directly with the patient. If appropriate and the patient is clinically stable, the patient may travel by car or commercial airline. If necessary, a medical ambulance or flight may be arranged. If any patient is unable to utilize their insurance policy to cover the cost of traveling to the new medical facility, then local and national agencies should be sought out for assistance. Examples of agencies that can often assist in helping patients travel to medical appointments are Angel Flight, Miracle Flights, and Mercy Flight (Table 34.2). Some of these agencies are specific to providing assistance to pediatric patients under a certain age but it is recommended to research and contact any agency and discuss what the need is to see if they are able to assist. Commercial airlines may also have a medical assistance programs, and should be contacted to see what is available. Airlines and agencies often change their guidelines and can have restrictions on how to access assistance so they should be contacted directly. Other ways to seek help is to consider fundraising on a local level. Families should contact charitable and religious organizations in their community for financial and/or emotional support. Often, local business establishments may also provide financial assistance.

### 34.4.3   TRANSFERRING TO ANOTHER INPATIENT FACILITY

When a patient is transferred from one medical institution directly to another facility's inpatient unit, it is essential to review the medical information prior to transfer and communicate with the receiving medical team on the patient's current medical status. This is extremely important when making decisions such as if a patient needs to be admitted to an intensive care unit versus a regular inpatient unit, and the status of bed availability at the accepting facility at the time of transfer.

Shortly before the patient is transferred to the receiving institution, it is essential that there is communication to all team members regarding the plan of care of the new patient. In many

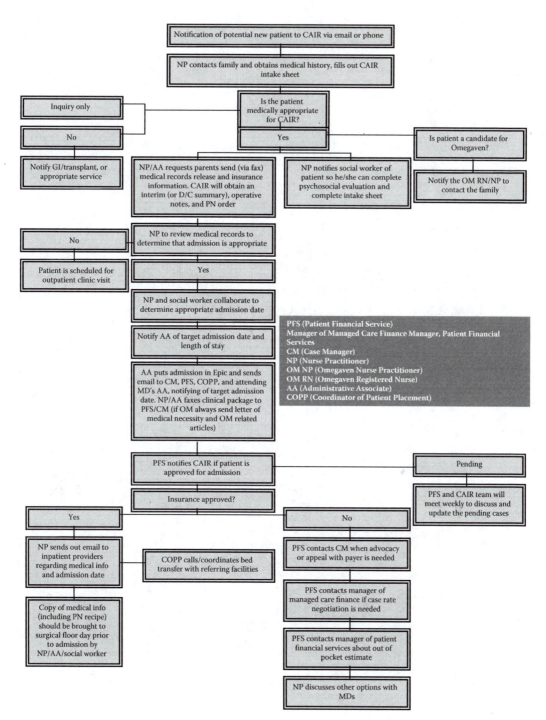

*Referring facility is responsible for transportation to and from CHB.

**FIGURE 34.1**  Example of the intake process. (CAIR = Center for Advanced Intestinal Rehabilitation at Children's Hospital Boston.)

**TABLE 34.2**
**Agencies That Provide Transportation Assistance**

| Flight Resource | Summary | Contact | Website |
|---|---|---|---|
| Angel Flight | Angel Flight provides free air transportation for people that have a medical need for services not found in their local area. Angel Flight serves primarily patients who are traveling from, to, or through the states of Georgia, Alabama, Mississippi, Tennessee, and the Carolinas. | Angel Flight 2000 Airport Road Suite 227 Atlanta, Georgia 30341 1-877-426-2643 Fax: 770-452-7391 | http://www.angelflightsoars.org/ index.htm |
| Wings of Mercy | Wings of Mercy provides free air transportation for people with limited financial means who need treatment at distant medical facilities. Since 1991 the charity has grown to include several chapters in the Midwest. | Wings of Mercy 513 E. 8 th Street, Suite 25 Holland, MI 49423 888.78.MERCY Fax: 616.396.0650 | www.wingsofmercy.org |
| Northwoods AirLifeLine | Northwoods AirLifeLine is a nonprofit organization of volunteer pilots from Michigan's Upper Peninsula and northeast Wisconsin who donate their time and aircraft to help patients and their families with urgent medical needs for services not found locally. | Northwoods AirLifeLine P.O. Box 2973 Kingsford, MI 49802-2973 800.311.1760 | www.northwoodsairlifeline.org |
| Children's Flight of Hope | Children's Flight of Hope was Founded in 1991, This provides free private air transportation to and from distant medical facilities for children with critical medical needs. Flight typically involves flying children from North Carolina to out-of-state treatment facilities or bringing children from out-of-state to facilities in North Carolina. | Children's Flight of Hope, Inc. 113 Edinburgh South, Suite 210 Cary, NC 27511 919.466.8593 Fax: 919.467.5299 | www.childrensflightofhope.org |
| AirLifeLine | AirLifeLine helps people in financial need obtain equal access to health care by coordinating free air transportation. AirLifeLine coordinates free air transportation by matching a person in need with a compassionate AirLifeLine volunteer pilot. All flights are coordinated at NO COST to passengers. | AirLifeLine Operations Center 50 Fullerton Court, Suite 200 Sacramento, CA 95825 877.AIR.LIFE Fax: 916.641.0600 | www.airlifeline.org |
| Miracle Flights for Kids | The mission of Miracle Flights for Kids is to improve access to health care by providing free air transportation to hospitals across America. Miracle Flights for Kids believes that all children have the right to be able to access the best medical care, no matter where the treatment is located, and no matter what the personal or financial situation of their families might be. | Miracle Flights for Kids Headquarters 2756 N. Green Valley Parkway #115 Green Valley, NV 702.261.0494 Fax: 702.261.0497 | www.miracleflights.org |

institutions, this is in the form of an email, detailing the patient's medical background and needs. The nursing staff on the inpatient floor also must be notified of the impending admission so that a bed can be made available along with the appropriate equipment and level of nursing staff specific for that patient's needs.

### 34.4.4   INTERNATIONAL PATIENTS

International patients are often a unique subgroup of patients to work with as they can have varying insurance policies and/or embassy involvement. Ideally, it is most helpful to work with resources that are familiar with international policies and travel regulations. It may take weeks to a month to arrange an international patient's admission. This group of patients can be challenging due to language and cultural differences. They can also be medically demanding since not all medications, supplies, and enteral formulas are available in a patient's country once they return home. Follow-up with physicians in their home country is essential. Also, prior to transfer, it may be difficult to obtain medical information, and to have it all appropriately translated in a timely fashion. Additional services that may be helpful include: interpreter services, medical records transfer and appointment scheduling; liaison services between the patients' primary doctor and the treating institution; financial consultation, including estimates of medical costs and anticipated living expenses; assistance with travel arrangements, including visa applications, US immigrations, and customs clearance.

## 34.5   SPECIAL CONSIDERATIONS

### 34.5.1   COMORBID MEDICAL CONDITIONS

Many patients with IF have other equally as complex medical conditions that require ongoing management. It is imperative to know if the patient has any other medical issues (e.g., patent ductus arteriosus, renal dysfunction, or neurological problems) prior to admission to the receiving institution. The accepting center should communicate with the current inpatient team prior to transfer to determine the need for any consults with other services while the patient is inpatient at the new facility. This information is critical in determining the anticipated length of stay prior to transfer as this is necessary for obtaining insurance approval. Proper planning and communication of the medical plan between both institutions is essential as it will ensure a smooth patient transfer.

### 34.5.2   SOCIAL ISSUES

For optimal treatment, it is best to consider the patient's/family's home situation and the various other life events and stressors that can influence treatment outcomes. This can include concrete issues such as having a suitable living environment, having adequate financial resources, or access to getting to the medical treatment and equipment upon discharge. In the case of treating a pediatric patient, other family members, such as the parents, may have preexisting issues to deal with that will directly impact the child's treatment; these problems cannot be overlooked and must be addressed in tandem with the child's medical care. For example, a 2005 study by Enrione et al. [2] reviewed the psychosocial needs of caregivers of children on home enteral nutrition (HEN) and showed that family interactions involved with providing HEN create increased stress for the caregiver, spouse, and siblings, which may have a negative impact on family functions. As part of a multidisciplinary IF program, it is customary for a social worker or other suitable staff member to meet with the family and/or patient to assess the ongoing problem and provide support or refer to the appropriate resource for the issue.

Often, an ongoing lack of basic resources (i.e., housing, finances, and employment) may impact patient care. The medical team must be kept abreast of any pertinent household issues such as

**464**

Clinical Management of Intestinal Failure

domestic violence and substance abuse that can impact the patient's well-being, as can the lack of basic necessities such as heat, water, electric, and telephone services. Child protection matters within the home, the educational and skill level of family members participating in patient care, and any mental health problems should also be discussed among the health care team. Comorbidities, including mental health issues, are common when treating chronically ill patients. Depression, anxiety, adjustment disorder, or post-traumatic stress disorder are commonly seen diagnoses. At times, the mental health of a patient's family member may interfere with treating the chronically ill IF patient, similar to that seen in infants born to mothers with post-partum depression. This important health matter should not be overlooked by the medical team as it can have a direct impact on the overall well-being of the patient. Referrals within the medical institution or to a community resource are essential for proper treatment of mental health issues.

Like others with chronic illnesses, IF patients come from a variety of socioeconomic backgrounds. Financial limitations can adversely impact treatment as patients may have difficulty getting to medical appointments, paying any out-of-pocket medical expenses, and may eventually become noncompliant if they are unable to get the correct medication or equipment. Simply taking time off from work too frequently can be damaging to the family unit and result in a loss of wages.

It is important to assess the patient's emotional resources, including other family members involved in treatment, friends, and/or support groups. The presence of a support system should be at least discussed as it will affect treatment outcomes. It may offer respite for caregivers or patients or provide needed emotional support to the patient or caregiver around the many stressors [3]. Chapter 38, discusses in detail the role of support groups in the IF patient.

## 34.6 DISCHARGE PLANNING

Given their complex needs, IF patients require many services and supports. Many will require PN at home, necessitating the need for infusion pumps and weekly delivery of solutions in addition to homecare nursing (see Chapter 32). Ideally, discharge teaching and discussion should begin at the time of admission to ensure a smooth and less stressful transition home. Parents and caregivers are taught, by the inpatient and homecare nursing staff, all facets of care and are encouraged to participate in treatment throughout the admission to become comfortable with each technique and ask any questions as they arise. At Children's Hospital Boston, prior to the day of discharge, parents are required to complete and independently demonstrate all skills necessary to care for their child at home. Typical skills that the patient or caregivers should be proficient at include all aspects of central venous catheter care, infection control issues, ostomy care, feeding tube care, medication administration, and wound care.

Regardless of financial means, medical teams often see a variety of patients with diverse learning styles that may enhance or impede their ability to comprehend the complexities involved in the care of the IF patient. Educational materials should be provided both orally and in written form to the patient and family. Often a "readback–feedback" approach is best where the skill is shown to the caregiver and demonstrated back to the nurse. At least two caregivers should be trained in complete patient care prior to discharge. It is also important that the family receives training prior to leaving the hospital of all devices such as infusion pumps and nebulizers that will be used at home as they can vary from those used in a hospital setting; this training is completed by the home care companies that will supply the equipment. In most cases, a homecare nurse would review the use of these devices with the family on their first day home.

Homecare is not inexpensive. The cost associated with the care of this group of patients can be sizeable. A study performed by Spencer et al. in 2008 [4] found that the cost of home care for children continued to rise over time. The rise in cost of care occurred despite the predicted improvement for many of the children for the same time period. The authors suggest that although there are numerous benefits for patients to receive homecare, the cost for such services remain a substantial financial burden to the patient's families and insurance providers. Just as discharge education begins at time of arrival, so too is the importance of reviewing the patient's insurance policy while they are still an inpatient in order to determine what will be covered in the outpatient setting. Not all insurance policies provide home nursing coverage or particular treatments and equipment. It is important to contact the insurance provider and get any prior approvals needed prior to admission. The hospital's financial department or a case manager should be able to assist the patient in this process. If the insurance provider does deny any medication, equipment, or home services, the patient may need to work with the insurance company to appeal the denial or provide documentation of justification of treatment. In some cases, the team may need to consider therapeutic alternatives to the denied therapy. Also, prior to discharge, interdisciplinary team meetings/conference calls should be scheduled. Direct contact should be made to outside agencies (Visiting Nurses Association, early intervention, physical therapy, etc.), including the primary care physician or specialist, to provide seamless patient care across the continuum.

## 34.7   HOME ISSUES

As a patient leaves the hospital, it is important that the patient and their caregivers feel comfortable about going home. Discharge to home can be extremely overwhelming. Prior to discharge, the patient and family should be provided with phone triage information detailing how to manage common issues such as hydration status, feeding tube care, ostomy care, feeding intolerance, infection control, lab results, new medications, and prescription refills. Plans for follow-up outpatient appointments with the IF outpatient program should be made while the patient is still in hospital. Initially, patients should be seen frequently, on a weekly basis by either the IF team or in concert with their local health care provider, who can provide weight checks, well-care visits, and immunizations in addition to routine health maintenance.

## 34.8   CONCLUSION

Treating patients with IF requires a dedicated group of clinicians willing to care for such medically complex patients. During each visit, known barriers and/or stressors should be addressed so that appropriate referrals for assistance can be made. Having the medical team acknowledge that having IF can create stressors and can be a financial burden to the patient and family demonstrates that the team has an understanding of the situation and is empathetic to the patient's plight, thereby creating a stronger alliance between the health care providers and the patient. Typically, this group of patients can be very challenging to manage, as they are often readmitted to the hospital and receive expensive therapies, such as PN, for prolonged periods of time. As with any population of chronically ill patients, there are social and family issues that further complicate care. Due to their multiple needs, IF patients have access to federal and local programs that should be able to provide some assistance. Despite these hurdles, care by a dedicated group of clinicians will make it possible to meet their medical and emotional needs in a safe and cost-effective manner.

## REFERENCES

1. Modi BP, Langer M, Ching YA et al. Improved survival in a multidisciplinary short bowel syndrome program. *J Pediatr Surg* 2008;43:20–24.
2. Enrione EB, Thomlison B, and Rubin A. Medical and psychosocial experiences of family caregivers with children fed enterally at home. *JPEN* 2005;29:413–419.
3. Howard LJ. Length of life and quality of life on home parenteral nutrition. *JPEN* 2002;26:S55–S59.
4. Spencer AU, Kovacevich D, McKinney-Barnett M et al. Pediatric short-bowel syndrome: The cost of comprehensive care. *Am J Clin Nutr* 2008;88:1552–1559.

# 35 Oral Aversion

*Virginie Colomb*

## CONTENTS

In children with intestinal failure (IF), optimal postoperative and long-term nutritional management is essential to optimize the function of the gut toward the acquisition of intestinal autonomy in the first year of life, and to ensure normal growth [1–3]. In children with short bowel syndrome (SBS), oral and more generally enteral nutrition have been shown to contribute to gut development and adaptation [4,5]. After weaning from parenteral nutrition (PN), enteral and, if possible, oral feeding should allow the child normal growth. Hyperphagia is often seen as part of the adaptative compensatory features in adult patients with SBS [6] but data on this topic in children are scarce. Normal or hyperphagic feeding behavior in children can be threatened or delayed by the accumulation of endogenous and exogenous events that contribute to early and profound oral aversion. Despite the constraints related to the disease and its treatments, some errors may be avoided, some simple preventive measures can be taken early, if all professionals involved in infant and children's care are convinced that prevention of oral aversion is both feasible and critical for optimal outcomes.

## 35.1 PHYSIOLOGY OF NUTRIENT INTAKE

### 35.1.1 ONTOGENY OF THE ORAL CAVITY

The oral cavity belongs to the gastrointestinal (GI) tract; the nose and mouth originate from the same embryological ectodermal tissue, whereas the rest of the GI tract is a derivative of the endoderm [7]. Beside the role of salivary secretions, reflexes initiated during the oral phase of feeding contribute to the regulation of gastric and intestinal functions. The oral cavity appears and develops over the first two months of gestation. Sucking begins around the 10th week, swallowing starts between the 12th and 15th weeks, and then the fetus sucks his fingers and toes and swallows amniotic fluid. Coordinated sucking movements usually appear after 33 weeks of gestation [8]. Sucking and swallowing develop rapidly after 34 weeks of gestation and further in the first weeks of life. In the neonate, coupling of sucking and swallowing, which implies integrity of all the motor nuclei of cerebral trunk, is a criteria of maturity. Suction is a reflex stimulated by sensory stimuli of the lips, oral mucosa, and tongue, as well as by hunger. Intraoral stimulation can stimulate both nutritive and nonnutritive sucking. It was demonstrated that a thick rubber breast shield reduced milk intake by more than 50% as compared to sucking normally at breast, whereas a thinner shield reduced milk intake by less than 30% [9]. Early in the neonatal period, the taste of fluid, as well as the nutrient content, affects the efficiency of nutritive sucking. Sucking activities increase with the concentration of glucose, fructose, sucrose, and lactose in the fluid [10,11]. Over the first 3 months of life, breathing during breast-feeding occurs exclusively through the nose, because the lips are tightly closed around the nipple or the teat. Odor and visual stimuli can also affect sucking. Among internal factors which might influence sucking, it has been demonstrated that in sucking babies with tracheoesophageal fistulas and gastrostomies, real or sham feedings or the state of gastric distention do not affect nonnutritive sucking [12].

After the fourth month, feeding behavior involves the cerebral cortex. Learning to feed from a spoon involves both eyesight and the voluntary control of swallowing. In newborns, the spoon or food placed onto the anterior part of the mouth induces an extrusion reflex by movements of the lips and the tongue. By the second half-year of life, the reflexes change, and food deposited in the anterior part of the tongue is normally moved back and swallowed. Rhythmic mastication movements (cutting, crushing, and grinding) appear by 7–9 months of age. The movements of the tongue from the front to the back are associated with vertical movements. Swallowing is divided into three phases: the oral, the pharyngeal, and the esophageal, of which the first two are under voluntary control [8].

### 35.1.2 DEVELOPMENT OF FEEDING BEHAVIOR

The development of feeding behavior is influenced both by inborn and acquired factors. Inborn preferences for sweetness, as well as bitter rejection, account for specific face answers that occur from birth, according to the type of flavor stimulation: indifference or preference for salty flavor, satisfaction for sweetness and umami [13], and grimace for bitterness. The mucosa of the tongue detects temperature, pain, pressure, and taste. Taste and olfactory cues both contribute to the feeding preferences. Olfactory cues seem to yield strong and early preferences [14].

### 35.1.3 CENTRAL REGULATION OF APPETITE

The hypothalamus plays a key role in appetite signaling (Figure 35.1), as it integrates peripheral signals such as adiposity, energy intake, or afferent signals from the gut and in turn regulates pathways within the central nervous system, which modulates food intake and energy expenditure. The hypothalamus is subdivided into interconnecting nuclei: the arcuate nucleus (ARC), paraventricular nucleus, ventromedial nucleus, dorsomedial nucleus, and lateral hypothalamic area. The ARC is a key nucleus in the regulation of appetite, with two major neuronal populations out of which one is orexigenic and coexpresses neuropeptide Y (NPY) and agouti-related protein (AgRP) and the other is anorexigenic and coexpresses cocaine and amphetamine-related transcript (CART) and pro-opiomelanocortin (POMC).

### 35.1.4 ROLE OF THE GI TRACT IN THE REGULATION OF FOOD INTAKE

The GI tract is a richly innervated secretory and absorptive organ. Its neural and humoral signals to central regulatory centers participate in the regulation of food intake. Under physiologic conditions, gastric contractions are thought to influence food intake [15]. Oropharyngeal receptors and gastric repletion also act in appetite control. In experimental studies, dogs fitted with esophageal fistulas had more prolonged eating time and shorter intervals between meals than controls, which suggests that oropharyngeal receptors have a certain but limited satiety signal [16]. In the same animals,

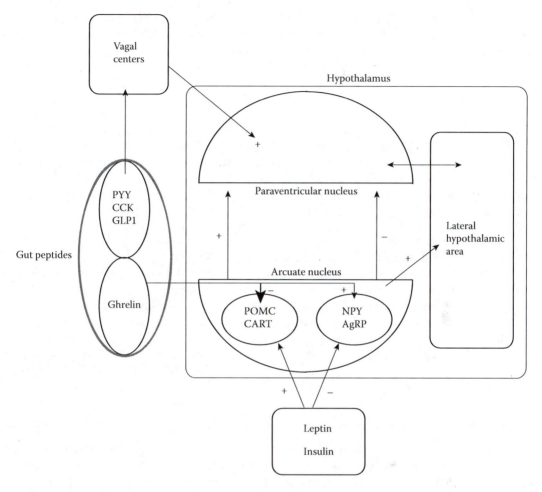

**FIGURE 35.1** Central regulation of appetite. Pathways are shown between gut peptides: ghrelin, peptide YY (PYY), cholecystokinin (CCK), glucagon-like peptide 1 (GLP-1), and the hypothalamic nuclei, and also between insulin, leptin, and the hypothalamic nuclei. The ARC includes two major neuronal populations involved in the regulation of appetite. The orexigenic neuronal population coexpresses neuropeptide Y (NPY) and agouti-related protein (AgRP), while the other one, which inhibits food intake, coexpresses cocaine and amphetamine-related transcript (CART) and pro-opiomelanocortin (POMC). These two neuronal populations communicate with the other areas of the hypothalamus involved in appetite control.

introduction of food (or water balloon) in the stomach during sham-feeding reduce the duration of sham-feeding [16,17]. The fact that noncaloric bulk has the same effect as a meal supports the hypothesis that gastric distension acts as a major satiety signal. Once absorbed, nutrients contribute to appetite control through the energy intake and the postprandial insulinemic response [18]. The qualitative aspects of nutrients also play a role in appetite control. Different dietary proteins, inducing different blood amino acid profiles, have different effects on appetite ratings [19].

### 35.1.5 Gut Hormones, Leptin, and Route of Nutrient Delivery

The manner of delivery of the so-called artificial nutrition, delivered either enterally or parenterally, can be continuous, intermittent, or both. The metabolic benefits of intermittent or cyclic PN compared to continuous PN have been demonstrated, with a switch from net lipogenesis to net lipolysis during cyclic PN, mimicking the physiological pattern of oral feeding [20]. However, the role and manner of nutrition delivery on the secretion of circulating satiety peptide levels and therefore in the regulation of appetite has long been a matter of debate. Ghrelin, derived from endocrine cells in the stomach, has short-term, early orexigenic effects, whereas peptide YY (PYY) released by gut cells into the circulation following a meal, reduces appetite (Figure 35.1). Circulating ghrelin concentrations are regulated by fasting (up) and refeeding (down), whatever the route of nutrient delivery, and not by the presence or absence of food in the upper digestive tract [21]. Glucose or mixed glucose-amino acid infusion has been shown to decrease ghrelin levels in rats [21] and humans [22]. Lipid infusion decreases PYY levels in adults with IF [22]. However, in patients with SBS and adaptive hyperphagia, fasting plasma ghrelin and PYY have not been found to be related to energy intake or absorption [23]. Leptin, a satiety hormone that belongs to the adipokine family secreted by the adipose tissue, crosses the blood brain barrier and activates anorectic POMC neurons and inhibit orexigenic AgRP/NPY neurons (Figure 35.1). Leptin secretion seems to be equally stimulated by oral, enteral, or parenteral feeding in rodents, which suggests that it is unlikely that satiety factors secreted by the gut play a significant role in the control of leptin secretion [24]. In humans studied before and after surgical stress on PN, no significant changes of plasma leptin concentration were found, but leptin concentrations were significantly correlated with insulin concentrations [25]. In adults with SBS, leptin plasma concentrations have been found to correlate positively with age, body mass index (BMI), fat mass, rate of glucose infusion, and insulin level, whereas no correlations have been found between leptin concentration and the presence of hyperphagia [26,27]. Few studies have been performed in children. In preterm infants on PN within the first week of life, plasma concentrations of leptin were correlated with body weight and BMI, but not with serum insulin [28]. Finally, according to these data, cyclic PN may be considered as a way to stimulate oral intake by creating a "fasting period." However, few data exist regarding the effect of cyclic versus continuous PN on food intake in animals and human. One animal study showed that cyclic PN did not increase food intake as compared to continuous PN [29].

### 35.1.6 EFFECT OF BOWEL REST AND PN ON β-CELL MATURATION AND GLUCOSE TOLERANCE

A pediatric study showed that metabolic conditions associated with long-term PN could impair insulin release with an alteration of the first phase of insulin release [30]. The decrease in glucagon-like peptide 1 (GLP-1) release observed in these children could be involved in such disorder, since the implication of GLP-1 in enhancing insulin release and hepatic glucose captation has been reported [30,31]. GLP-1 has also been implicated in the postnatal maturation and trophicity of β-cells, in animal models [32]. In patients who have no or low oral/enteral caloric intake, GLP-1 secretion is poorly stimulated, irrespective of the nature of the underlying disease, the nutritional condition, or length of the residual small bowel [30]. In children with congenital IF, one can hypothesize that GLP-1 secretion has not been stimulated from birth because of intestinal resection or mucosal dysfunction, or because of the lack of oral intake. Taken as a whole, PN and bowel rest are conditions that might impair insulin secretion, through the decrease in GLP-1 secretion in children with IF.

### 35.1.7 INFLAMMATION

Inflammation is a known anorexic condition. Cytokines, such as interleukin 1 (IL-1) and tumor necrotic factor-α (TNF-α) administered peripherally or in the central nervous system reduce food intake, suggesting that these are involved in anorexia during infections or inflammatory diseases. Cytokines produced in the periphery inhibit appetite through neural and humoral pathways. Cytokines may act directly on the central nervous system as demonstrated for IL-1β through increasing central melanocortin signaling, a key pathway in the regulation of energy homeostasis [33]. It has been demonstrated in rodents that IL-1 and bacterial lipopolysaccharide (LPS) induce anorexia by distinct signaling pathways [34,35]. The central up-regulation of the microsomal prostaglandin E (PGE) synthase-1, an enzyme involved in prostaglandin E2 biosynthesis, has been demonstrated to be an essential mediator for immune-induced anorexia [36]. The increase in leptin expression by cytokines and LPS also contribute to their anorexic effect [37]. Inflammation-related molecules such as Toll-like receptors and interferon (IFN) receptors are present in taste buds, a process which may contribute to taste disorders [38]. A model of intestinal infection in the mice has shown that upregulation of duodenal cholecystokinin (CCK) is associated with an increase in plasma CCK concentrations and a decrease in food intake under the control of CD4+ T lymphocytes [39]. Taken together, these studies suggest that bacterial and immune intestinal inflammation might contribute to oral aversion in IF patients.

## 35.2 RISK FACTORS FOR ORAL AVERSION IN CHILDREN WITH IF

### 35.2.1 Post-Traumatic Anorexia and Motility Disorders in Children with IF

The mouth is the location of breathing, feeding, and speaking which are all crucial functions for both quantity and quality of life in human. The establishment of taste patterns during fetal and neonatal life is threatened by diseases and conditions that either disturb normal feeding over the first days of life or induce painful experiences at the time of oral feeding. Feeding disorders and oral aversion originate in different kinds of organic diseases that disturb or limit oral feeding within the first days or weeks of life, or induce painful experiences associated with the digestive tract, whether or not they are provoked by oral/enteral feeding. These feeding disorders may be considered "post-traumatic anorexia."

More than any other children with chronic disease, children with IF are at risk for oral aversion and chronic feeding problems [40,41]. Among identified risk factors, children with IF often undergo a combination of events (Table 35.1), such as prolonged neonatal care and airway intubation, multiple painful conditions including gastroesophageal reflux (GER), with vomiting and esophagitis and painful procedures, including endoscopy and multiple surgeries. Oral feeding is often delayed or interrupted in infants who present with congenital digestive disease, and nonnutritive sucking is not always encouraged. The taste of infant formula (often hydrolyzed or elemental) is very different from the taste of human milk [42].

Some data also suggest that children with oral aversion may present with motility disorders of the upper GI tract which might be attributable to hypoxic damage of the enteric nerves. Gastric fundoplication, which is sometimes performed early in children with severe IF, may contribute to oral aversion by decreasing the gastric volume threshold for retching, by decreasing gastric compliance and also by

## TABLE 35.1
## Combination of Risk Factors for Oral Aversion in Children with Congenital IF

| Risk factors for Oral Aversion in Children | Visceral Pain | Pain Within the Face and Mouth Area | GER | Retching and Nausea | Exclusion of Oral Feeding | Continuous PN/EN |
|---|---|---|---|---|---|---|
| Neonatal surgery | + | + | + | + | + | + |
| Intensive care | + | + | + | + | + | + |
| NGT | + | + | + | + | + | + (EN) |
| Fundoplication | + | | | + | | |
| Motility disorders | + | | + | + | + | |

Note: EN: enteral nutrition; GER: gastroesophageal reflux; IF: intestinal failure; NGT: nasogastric tube; PN: parenteral nutrition. The cross indicates the association of two events that may be considered as risk factors for oral aversion.

delaying esophageal emptying. Repeated painful or abnormal sensations in the early infancy are also thought to contribute to the pathogenesis of the so-called visceral hyperalgesia [43–45].

## 35.3 PSYCHOLOGICAL CONSEQUENCES OF ORAL AVERSION AND IMPACT ON QUALITY OF LIFE

Premature infants are especially at risk of feeding disorders including oral aversion. In addition, many children, even with organic disease, have a significant behavioral component to their feeding disorder [40]. Congenital malformations or diseases disrupt the normal process of eating and can lead the child and his caregivers to develop abnormal behavioral patterns. The importance attached to oral feeding by parents, which is known to be increased by the presence of physical problems, is probably increased among parents of children with IF, since the importance of the GI tract for PN weaning is so widely acknowledged.

The use of gastrostomy tubes (G-tubes) in children with chronic diseases has increased substantially over the past two decades [46,47]. G-tube feedings are often necessary to accelerate weaning of PN in children with IF, especially in the case of SBS, when oral feedings may not meet energy and nutrient requirements. However, establishing or improving normal eating behavior in children who have required early or prolonged G-tube feedings can be challenging, since G-tube feedings may reduce the hunger drive to eat and may lead caregivers to decrease oral stimulations [21]. Our approach has been to continue to emphasize oral sucking and swallowing skills while using the G-tube for increasing amounts of enteral nutrition, gradually increasing the volume of oral feeds as well.

Oral aversion is not only a complication of IF that delays the acquisition of intestinal autonomy and weaning of PN, but is also one of the more obvious sign of the disease in the daily child's and family's life. Mealtime for families of sick children can offer a brief respite from the burdens of chronic illness, unless mealtime itself is a reminder of the disease process, especially when enteral feeding is such an important therapeutic goal. In children who have undergone intestinal transplantation, protracted oral aversion can lead to prolonged dependence on enteral G-tube feeding [48] and delays the expected feeling of "recovery" symbolized by total digestive autonomy and normal oral eating. Therefore, the feeding behavior of the sick child becomes a major component of the quality of life for the child and family [49,50]. Oral aversion is also a "public symptom" of IF, especially in settings such as school, eating out at a restaurant, or eating in the presence of extended family members.

## 35.4 PREVENTION AND TREATMENT OF ORAL AVERSION

The prevention of oral aversion in children with IF should start immediately after birth, by identification of children at risk of developing feeding disorders.

Nonnutritive sucking (teat or pacifier, eventually with sugar taste) should be encouraged even when the patient is NPO. In children with neonatal SBS and other congenital causes of IF, minimal oral feeding (breast or bottle) should be initiated as soon and frequently as possible, with maximal parental' involvement. In children who undergo abdominal surgery, feeding should take place as soon as the postoperative ileus resolves. True indications for prolonged bowel rest are exceptional, even in congenital/neonatal diseases of the GI tract.

GER and other peptic diseases should be treated aggressively [51]. If possible, the use of nasogastric tubes, for either feeding or gastric decompression, should be minimized. A feeding gastrostomy should be created, either at the time of the first surgical procedure, especially in children with SBS, or later, in children with other causes of IF.

Cyclic PN should be used as soon as possible, with oral or enteral feedings given while PN is not administered. In fact, PN-induced increase in gastric acid hypersecretion [52] may be associated with a poor tolerance of enteral infusion. During progressive bowel adaptation, nocturnal enteral feeding can progressively replace PN, as soon as the clinical and metabolic tolerance of one night without PN has been demonstrated [53].

Aggressive attempts at introducing oral nutrition should be avoided since these can produce negative experiences and in fact worsen oral aversion. Psychologists, physiotherapists, and speech and language therapists [51] can advise caregivers in helping the child enjoy positive sensations from his body and progressively accept oral stimuli, using a variety of techniques:

1. Lip stimulation, games with the mouth (e.g., kiss, fish mouth, noises produced with the mouth, and others), with the tongue (e.g., lick, stick out the tongue, and others), with breath (e.g., blowing, making bubbles, and others).
2. Games which help to identify smells.
3. Games when the child can handle foods of different colors, temperatures, textures, and discover the noises associated to foods (e.g., crisp, crunchy).
4. Having the child handle utensils and other eating equipment.

When the child starts to eat, recommendations should be given to the parents and caregivers to

1. Give meals in a calm atmosphere, without force-feeding, without games or television which disturbs child's attention, and without blackmail.
2. Avoid prolonged meals (over half an hour).
3. Do not fill the plates completely.
4. Favor mouth occlusion at each mouthful.
5. Optimize head and body positioning during meals.

The food texture and type, seating arrangement, eating equipment (cup, spoon, bottle, teat, etc.) and the level of caregiver assistance should be tailored to the individual patient's needs. At the same time, dietetic and nutritional adjustments should be considered, including the duration of PN or enteral nutrition infusion. We recommend giving enteral tube feeding immediately after oral meals, decreasing caloric and fluid intake in order to stimulate appetite, and increasing energy density of enteral feeding. These steps can be difficult to perform simultaneously and the response of the child to changes in PN and enteral nutrition should be monitored closely with clinical, nutritional, and biochemical parameters. One group has proposed a family-focused short-term intensive behavioral feeding program and showed an improvement in oral intake and a significant decrease in gastrostomy intake in patients receiving gastrostomy feedings [21].

Children with IF have numerous risk factors for oral aversion, a finding that has significant physical and psychological effects and may affects ultimate prognosis. An intensive, prolonged behaviorally oriented feeding plan needs to be undertaken in many IF patients, individualized to the specific clinical scenario. The patient should be strongly encouraged for all efforts, since progress can be slow and painstaking. As with the general medical care of IF patients, a multidisciplinary approach should be undertaken since cross-disciplinary communication and collaboration are critical [54]. The final transition from parenteral to enteral to oral nutrition is among the most rewarding aspects of the medical care of these patients.

# REFERENCES

1. Goulet O, Ruemmele F, Lacaille F, Colomb V. Irreversible intestinal failure. *J Pediatr Gastroenterol Nutr* 2004;38:250–69.
2. Quiros-Tejeira RE, Ament ME, Reyen L et al. Long-term parenteral nutritional support and intestinal adaptation in children with short bowel syndrome: A 25-year experience. *J Pediatr* 2004;145:157–63.
3. Goulet O, Baglin-Gobet S, Talbotec C et al. Outcome and long-term growth after extensive small bowel resection in the neonatal period: A survey of 87 children. *Eur J Pediatr Surg* 2005;15:95–101.
4. Castillo RO, Fenq JJ, Stevenson DK, Kwong LK. Maturation of jejunoileal gradients in rat intestine: The role of intraluminal nutrients. *Biol Neonate* 1992;62:351–62.

5. Tappenden KA. Mechanisms of enteral nutrient-enhanced intestinal adaptation. *Gastroenterology* 2006;130:S93–9.
6. Crenn P, Morin MC, Joly F, Penven S, Thuillier F, Messing B. Net digestive absorption and adaptative hyperphagia in adult short bowel patients. *Gut* 2004;53:1279–86.
7. Liebow C. Ontogeny of the oral cavity and its relationship to ontogeny of the gastrointestinal tract. In: Lebenthal E, editor. *Human Gastrointestinal Development*. Ch. 9. New York: Raven Press; 1989. pp. 209–27.
8. Herbst JJ. Development of suck and swallow. In Lebenthal E, editor. *Human Gastrointestinal Development*, Ch. 10. New York: Raven Press; 1989. pp. 229–39.
9. Woolridge MW, Baum JD, Drewett RF. Effect of a traditional and of a new nipple shield on sucking patterns and milk flow. *Early Hum Dev* 1980;4:357–64.
10. Dubingnon J, Campbell D. Discrimination between nutrients in the human neonate. *Psychonomic Sci* 1969;16:186–7.
11. Desor JA, Maller O, Turner R. Taste in acceptance of sugars by human infants. *J Comp Physiol Psychol* 1973;84:496–501.
12. Wolff PH. The interaction of state and non-nutritive sucking. In: Bosma JF, editors. *Third symposium on oral sensation and perception*. Springfield, IL: Charles C. Thomas; 1972. pp. 293–310.
13. Beauchamp GK. Sensory and receptor responses to umami: An overview of pioneering work. *Am J Clin Nutr* 2009;90:723S–7S.
14. Beauchamp GK, Mennella JA. Early flavor learning and its impact on later feeding behavior. *J Pediatr Gastroenterol Nutr* 2009;48(Suppl 1):S25–30.
15. Janowitz HD. Role of the gastrointestinal tract in the regulation of food intake. In: *Handbook of Physiology. Volume I—Control of food and Water Intake*. Section 6: Alimentary canal. Ch. 16. Washington DC: American Physiological Society; 1967. pp. 219–24.
16. Janowitz HD, Grossman MI. Some factors affecting the food intake of normal dogs and dogs with esophagostomy and gastric fistula. *Am J Physiol* 1949;159:143–8.
17. Share I, Martiniuk E, Grossman MI. Effect of prolonged intragastric feeding on oral food intake in dogs. *Am J Physiol* 1952;169:229–35.
18. Flint A, Moller BK, Raben A et al. Glycemic and insulinemic responses as determinants of appetite in humans. *Am J Clin Nutr* 2006;84:1365–73.
19. Veldhorst MA, Nieuwenhuizen AG, Hochstenbach-Waelen A et al. Dose-dependent satiating effect of whey relative to casein or soy. *Physiol Behav* 2009;96:675–82.
20. Just B, Messing B, Darmaun D, Rongier M, Camillo E. Comparison of substrate utilization by indirect calorimetry during cyclic and continuous total parenteral nutrition. *Am J Clin Nutr* 1990;51:107–11.
21. Qader SS, Salehi A, Hakanson R, Lundquist I, Ekelund M. Long-tem infusion of nutrients (total parenteral nutrition) suppresses circulating ghrelin in food-deprived rats. *Regul Pept* 2005;131:82–8.
22. Murray CD, Le Roux CW, Gouveia C et al. The effect of different macronutrient infusions on appetite, ghrelin and peptide YY in parenterally fed patients. *Clin Nutr* 2006;25:626–33.
23. Compher CW, Kinosian BP, Metz DC. Ghrelin does not predict adaptative hyperphagia in patients with short bowel syndrome. *JPEN* 2009;33:428–32.
24. Levy JR, LeGall-Salmon E, Santos M, Pandak WM, Stevens W. Effect of enteral versus parenteral nutrition on leptin gene expression and release into the circulation. *Bioch Biophys Res Commun* 1997;237:98–102.
25. Hernandez C, Simo R, Chacon P et al. Influence of surgical stress and parenteral nutrition on serum leptin concentration. *Clin Nutr* 2000;19:61–4.
26. Molina A, Pita A, Farriol M, Virgili N, Soler J, Gomez JM. Serum leptin concentration in patients with short bowel syndrome. *Clin Nutr* 2000;19:333–8.
27. Rifai K, Bischoff SC, Widjaja A, Brabant G, MannsMP, Ockenga J. Leptin and insulin response to long-term parenteral nutrition depends on body fat mass. *Clin Nutr* 2006;25:773–9.
28. Park MJ, Namgung R, Kim JN, Kim DH. Serum leptin, IGF-I and insulin levels in preterm infants receiving parenteral nutrition during the first week of life. *J Pediatr Endocrinol Metab* 2001;14:429–33.
29. Yang ZJ, Bodoky G, Meguid MM. Nocturnal cyclic total parenteral nutrition: Food intake and feeding pattern in rats. *Physiol Behav* 1992;51:431–5.
30. Beltrand J, Colomb V, Marinier E et al. Lower insulin secretory response to glucose induced by artificial nutrition in children: Prolonged and total parenteral nutrition. *Pediatr Res* 2007;62:1–6.
31. Thorens B, Waeber G. Glucagon-like peptide-I and the control of insulin secretion in the normal state and in NIDDM. *Diabetes* 1993;42:1219–25.

32. Hardikar AA, Wang XY, Williams LJ et al. Functional maturation of fetal porcine beta-cell by glucagon-like peptide-I and cholecystokinin. *Endocrinology* 2002;143:3505–14.

33. Scarlett JM, Jobst EE, Enriori PJ et al. Regulation of central melanocortin signaling by interleukin-1 beta. *Endocrinology* 2007;148:4217–25.

34. Ogimoto K, Harris MK Jr, Wisse BE. MyD88 is a key mediator of anorexia, but not weight loss, induced by lipopolysaccharide and interleukin-1 beta. *Endocrinology* 2006;147:4445–53.

35. Elander L, Engström L, Hallbeck M, Blomqvist A. IL-1 beta and LPS induce anorexia by distinct mechanisms differentially dependent on microsomal prostaglandin E synthase-1. *Am J Physiol Regul Integr Comp Physiol* 2007;292:R258–67.

36. Pecchi E, Dallaporta M, Thirion S et al. Involvement of central microsomal prostaglandin E synthase-1 in IL-1 beta induced anorexia. *Physiol Genomics* 2006;25:485–92.

37. Sachot C, Poole S, Luheshi GN. Circulating leptin mediates lipopolysaccharide -induced anorexia and fever in rats. *J Physiol* 2004;561:263–72.

38. Wang H, Zhou M, Brand J, Huang L. Inflammation and taste disorders: Mechanisms in taste buds. *Ann N Y Acad Sci* 2009;1170:596–603.

39. Mc Dermott JR, Leslie FC, D'Amato M, Thompson DG, Grencis RK, McLaughlin JT. Immune control of food intake: Enteroendocrine cells are regulated by CD4+ T lymphocytes during small intestinal inflammation. *Gut* 2006;55:492–7.

40. Burklow KA, Phelps AN, Schultz JR, McConnell K, Rudolph C. Classifying complex pediatric feeding disorders. *J Pediatr Gastroenterol Nutr* 1998;27:143–7.

41. Byars KC, Burklow KA, Ferguson K, O'Flaherty T, Santoro K, Kaul A. A multicomponent behavioral program for oral aversion in children dependent on gastrostomy feeding. *J Pediatr Gastroenterol Nutr* 2003;37:473–80.

42. Mennella JA, Forestell CA, Morgan LK, Beauchamp GK. Early milk feeding influences taste acceptance and liking during infancy. *Am J Clin Nutr* 2009;90:S780–8.

43. Fitzgerald M, McIntosh N. Pain and analgesia in the newborn. *Arch Dis Child* 1989;64:441–3.

44. Zangen T, Ciarla C, Zangen S et al. Gastrointestinal motility and sensory abnormalities may contribute to food refusal in medically fragile toddlers. *J Pediatr Gastroenterol Nutr* 2003;37:287–93.

45. Miranda A. Early life events and the development of visceral hyperalgesia. *J Pediatr Gastroenterol Nutr* 2008;47:682–4.

46. Avitsland TL, Kristensen C, Emblem R, Veenstra M, Mala T, Bjornland K. Percutaneous endoscopic gastrostomy in children: a safe technique with major symptom relief and high parental satisfaction. *J Pediatr Gastroenterol Nutr* 2006;43:624–8.

47. Daveluy W, Guimber D, Uhlen S et al. Dramatic changes in home-based enteral nutrition practices in children during an 11-year period. *J Pediatr Gastroenterol Nutr* 2006;43:240–4.

48. Lacaille F, Vass N, Sauvat F et al. Long-term outcome, growth and digestive function in children 2 to 18 years after intestinal transplantation. *Gut* 2008;57:455–61.

49. Engström I, Björnestam B, Finkel Y. Psychological distress associated with home parenteral nutrition in Swedish children, adolescents, and their parents: Preliminary results. *J Pediatr Gastroenterol Nutr* 2003;37:246–51.

50. Gottrand F, Staszewski P, Colomb V et al. Satisfaction in different life domains in children receiving home parenteral nutrition and their families. *J Pediatr* 2005;146:793–7.

51. Strudwick S. Gastro-oesophageal reflux and feeding: The speech and language therapist's perspective. *Int J Pediatr Otorhinolaryngol* 2003;67(Suppl):S101–2.

52. Levine GM, Mullen JL, O'Neill F. Effect of total parenteral nutrition on gastric acid secretion. *Dig Dis Sci* 1980;25:284–8.

53. François B, Colomb V, Bonnefont JP et al. Tolerance to starvation in children on long-term total parenteral nutrition. *Clin Nutr* 1997;16:113–7.

54. Ayoob KT, Barresi I. Feeding disorders in children: Taking an interdisciplinary approach. *Pediatr Ann* 2007;36:478–83.

# 36 A Patient's Perspective

*Jonathan Lockwood*

My life changed abruptly on December 16, 1980. I was only 15 years old and had been experiencing severe lower abdominal pains over the course of 2 days until my stomach became board like, and it was impossible for me to stand up straight. During emergency surgery, the doctors disclosed that their initial incision of the abdomen revealed ruptured and gangrenous intestines that emitted a necrotic odor. The surgeons were prompted to perform an anastomosis upon witnessing pink tissue. It was communicated to my parents upon viewing previous x-rays that the malrotation of the intestines occurred because I was missing the ligament of Treitz that they understood to be a birth defect. I was left with a portion of small bowel and a third of descending colon, estimated to be 14 inches. My family and I wondered how I could subsist with minimal intestines. Now 43 years old, I am thankful my relationship with Boston Children's Hospital which began later that same day.

Needless to say, I was scared. Boston Children's Hospital became my home for 8 weeks while I recovered from surgery and learned how to engage my nightly infusions of home total parenteral nutrition (TPN). I started learning to adapt to my new way of life on intravenous (IV) nutrition. Appreciatively, the nurses and medical professionals made my adjustment very manageable. Their persistence enabled me to transition fairly smoothly into the TPN world. These individuals deserve much recognition! I received something even better: a new lease on life, a home away from home, and a 29-year (and counting) relationship with these accomplished people.

It was a very emotional departure for me and the people I had become attached to. I was very distressed to hear that my doctors' believed I would not be able to take food orally ever again; for fear of chronic diarrhea, acid reflux, and general bowel discomfort. Being an adult one would have acknowledged the gravity of this sentence. But as a persistent 15 year old I did not. On the way home from the hospital I insisted on drinking a frozen chocolate frappe. My parents obliged, and it was delectable going down. But with 14 in. of intestines, the transit time was almost immediate.

Becoming so comfortable in a hospital setting made it bittersweet to go back home. I was unsure of how friends and acquaintances would view me. It was difficult dragging an IV pole with two large glass bottles of TPN around the house. Time and again I would drag the pole up over a threshold and the wheels would catch causing a loud crash and a detonation of sticky solution all over the floor. I took some time before going back to school but gradually I managed. My friends saw me as no different (perhaps a little skinnier). And accepted me into whatever it was they were doing. With only a catheter under a shirt there was nothing else to advertise my issues (Picture 36.1).

My mother and I attended pharmaceutical courses. We purchased a sterile hood and although we were going to make 1 week worth of hyperal together, my mother ultimately concocted the solutions herself. That was many years ago. I now receive bimonthly shipments of TPN from a pharmacy. As an adolescent trying to adjust and cope with my chronic condition, I more often than not became rebellious and partook in some foolish notions. I will not list them all. Although, one comes to mind regarding a very bad fungal infection I contracted while swimming in a fresh water lake. The 2-week duration of burning antibiotics and the cost of a brand new catheter was a hard lesson. I now swim only in chlorinated swimming pools. I finished high school with a medical excuse stamped on my diploma. I was not ready to enter college, but was very satisfied with my work as a land surveyor's assistant for 12 years.

In 1984 my cousin Gary and I traveled cross country by van (Picture 36.2). In 1988 I bought 24 acres and built a log cabin (Picture 36.3).

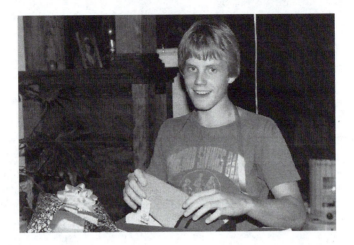

**PICTURE 36.1**   Jon as a teen.

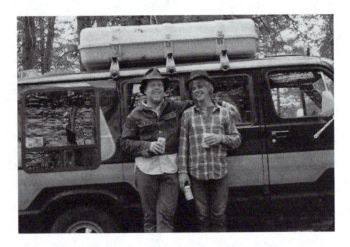

**PICTURE 36.2**   Jon and his cousin's cross country trip by van.

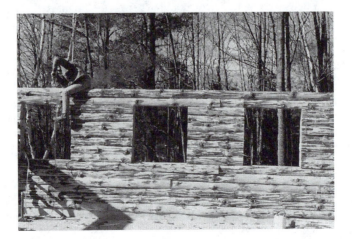

**PICTURE 36.3**   Jon building a cabin.

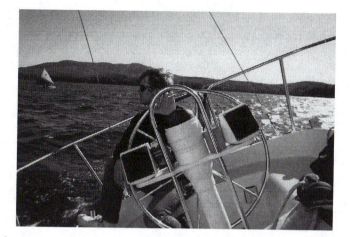

**PICTURE 36.4**   Jon with a sailboat.

I loved racing my 28′ sailboat each summer on a local lake (Picture 36.4). My wife Jennifer and I were married in 1992 (Picture 36.5). We feel very blessed to have two children: Sam and Sadie (Picture 36.6). In 2001, I opened my own retail store and fishing guide business (Picture 36.7).

My work and my family keep me very busy. Many years have gone by now and sometimes I wonder how long I can keep going this way. I hear that I am reaching the outer limits of TPN duration. Not necessarily a termination but no one really has been infusing much beyond 20–25 years without complications. I am not sure I like the idea of being a pioneer.

My overall health is good. I do have issues with long-term TPN, liver problems, and bone density concerns as well. I am, however, being monitored with the best of care. And for that reason, I turned down the idea of transplantation as long as things are functioning somewhat properly. Medical science moves forward at a rapid rate and I may be fortunate someday to receive a new bowel. I feel no different physically now at 43 than I did at 33. Some days are better than others. I have days where I lose a tremendous amount of body fluid which I cannot get back until I hook up at night. I can weigh in at 180 pounds in the morning and by the end of the day weigh 175 pounds. I do get it all back though. Now I know what a wilted flower feels like.

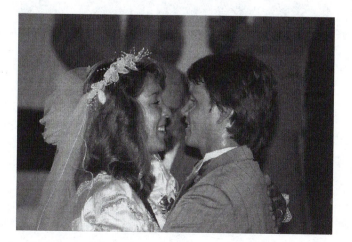

**PICTURE 36.5**   Jon and Jennifer's wedding.

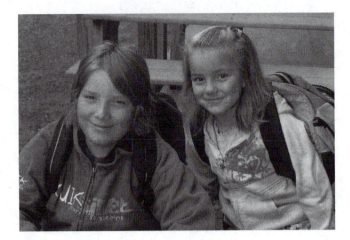

**PICTURE 36.6**   Kids Sam and Sadie.

My normal diet consists of anything I want. Even though my stomach is hungry and growling when I wake up, I typically do not eat breakfast or lunch. It is alright if a bathroom is nearby. I do eat a very substantial meal in the evening; meat and potatoes seem to settle the best. Over the years my stomach has expanded to allow in more food. My stool content resembles what a blender would churn up; no consistency, but I can honestly say my stomach and short gut does better with food in it than without. In 29 years, I have had three catheters; one of which has been under my skin for the last 17 years, one fungal and four staph infection (Picture 36.8).

I have "hooked up" in the middle of nowhere and "unhooked" on a boat 20 miles out at sea. The biggest stunt I have pulled so far was a fly in caribou hunt to Ungava Bay, Canada, 1300 miles away from home or doctors. If anything was to go wrong I would have been packed in ice with the meat for the trip home. The six of us had to travel extra light so that my eight bags of TPN could be stuffed on the float plane. No refrigeration. I left the bags out on the front porch at night. I packed out hundreds

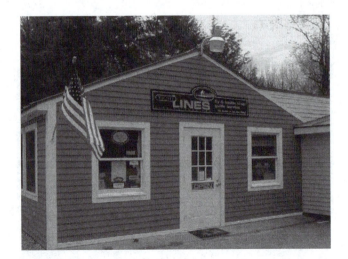

**PICTURE 36.7**   Jon's business.

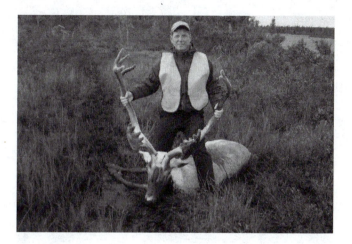

**PICTURE 36.8**  Jon with caribou.

of pounds of caribou meat to our camp for six straight days. At night we washed from a pan of heated water on top of the woodstove (Picture 36.8).

I work as a fishing and hunting guide (Picture 36.9). This job typically translates into very early mornings and long days. Meeting clients at 3 o'clock in the morning with the remainder of my TPN stuffed into a fanny pack. How my TPN pumps have evolved in the last 25 years is great!

As I am getting older I seem to think more about my own mortality. This could be normal for a 43 year old. I am afflicted with the usual maladies of growing up: my eyes need glasses, my right ear is deaf (probably from hunting without ear plugs), and my heart needs blood pressure pills. Who is complaining? I was not sure I could make it this far. I have been a very fortunate individual. It all boils down to what you really want to accomplish.

My parents, Bonnie and Stan, and my sister, Jane (Picture 36.10). Without the tremendous amounts of love and support from my wife and children, my parents, my sister and her husband Jay, my extended family and friends, and my nutritional and surgical team, I know I would not be here

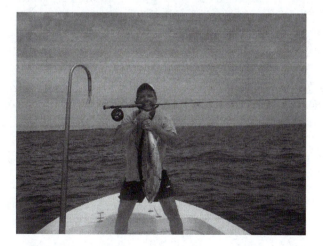

**PICTURE 36.9**  Jon with fish and rod in teeth.

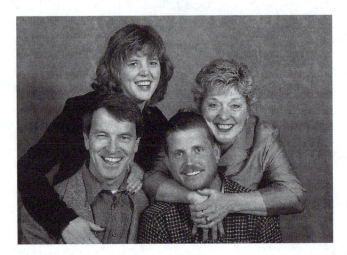

**PICTURE 36.10**   Jon with his sister and parents.

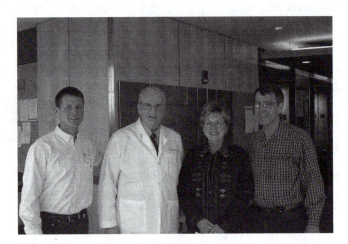

**PICTURE 36.11**   Jon with Dr. Folkman and parents.

today. I am not sure about the next 29 years; however, medical progress has never moved faster. I am most thankful for the person who decided to throw some life giving ingredients into a bottle and call it total parenteral nutrition.

This perspective is dedicated to Judah Folkman, MD (Picture 36.11).

# 37 Ethical Issues in Patient Care

*Daniel S. Kamin*

## CONTENTS

## 37.1 INTRODUCTION

Tremendous advancement in the medical and surgical care of patients with severe intestinal disorders has transformed many diagnoses that were once fatal diseases into chronic illnesses. Before parenteral nutrition (PN) became available for home use in the early 1970s, long-term survival for patients with significant short bowel syndrome (SBS) was impossible. Currently, patients with the most difficult diagnoses such as extreme SBS and pseudo-obstruction can not only survive long-term, but also enjoy a good quality of life at home.[1–5] For patients failing PN, intestinal transplantation offers the hope of life without PN. Whereas durable intestine graft function was unsuccessful in 1970s and 1980s,[6] many transplant centers have now reported[7,8] long-term graft survival rates and quality of life that compare favorably to that achieved for more traditional solid organ transplants.

Indeed, intestinal transplantation intended as "a last ditch effort" to prolong the lives of hospitalized patients has now become standard of care in specialized centers throughout the world. Patients with intestinal transplants are at home, return to work or school, and interact with outpatient nursing, physician, and rehabilitation communities. The focus on improving survival has expanded to include quality of life, neurocognitive development, and optimal growth;[9–11] multidisciplinary programs have become compulsory in meeting the needs of this unique population.

This evolution has brought with it a complex ethical terrain. Whereas decision-making may have once been isolated to the challenges of end-of-life care, current ethics concerns range from the optimal approach to adolescents on PN to debate over nonmedical criteria for transplant candidacy. The primacy of physician authority is waning, comparing outcomes among treatment options is increasingly complex, financial considerations are looming, and patient communities are heterogeneous in thought, race, religion, and values. The intestinal failure literature includes few examples of how to grapple with these concerns. This chapter examines critical ethical questions and tensions in intestinal failure and transplantation. It will first introduce basic concepts in bioethics, followed by an overview of ethical problems encountered in pediatrics, intestinal failure, and intestinal transplantation. Case examples are used throughout the chapter to strengthen readers' understanding of the important concepts set forth here.

## 37.2   CONCEPTS IN BIOETHICS

Ethics refers to the study or process of delineating moral norms that inform evaluations of how to conduct oneself or ourselves, and why. Moral norms are shared notions of right and wrong, which are powerful enough to constitute a stable social agreement among members of a social group. Moral stakeholders are individuals or groups of individuals for whom an ethical dilemma or concern matters. When approaching any ethical issue, it is crucial to identify the stakeholders. In the following, the core bioethical principles are described, and short examples are given that exemplify each principle "in action."

### 37.2.1   AUTONOMY

Respect for autonomy has become a very familiar theme in bioethics because of the focus on informed consent in health care and medical research in the last several years. Beauchamp and Childress define autonomy this way:

> Personal autonomy encompasses, at a minimum, self-rule that is free from both controlling interference by others and from certain limitations such as an inadequate understanding that prevents meaningful choice (p. 99).[12]

Being at liberty to make a choice and having the capacity to make it are equal partners engendering autonomy.

> A competent adult, having suffered a vascular accident and lost the entirety of her small intestine, may decline PN and therefore succumb to malnutrition. Her doctors may encourage her, ask her to speak with psychiatry, but in many countries including the United States, we respect her autonomy even though it will result in her own death.

Respect for autonomy has obvious limits, including when persons' autonomous choices adversely impact others, or when individuals (such as infants and children) lack the capacity to make a meaningful choice.

### 37.2.2   NONMALEFICENCE

This concept is defined well by the Latin maxim *Primum non nocere*: "first, do no harm." The most memorable sentence in the Hippocratic oath includes the promise of never harming patients. Generally speaking, obligations not to harm are quite stringent, and violations usually lead to formal censure, loss of professional licensure, or even criminal indictment.

Two months after an isolated intestinal transplant because of recurrent central venous catheter infections and thromboses, a young woman with a history of superior mesenteric artery thrombosis, SBS and Lupus-associated thrombophilia wants to have her allograft ileostomy reversed. Her medical team notes that she has already had one bout of acute rejection, and the team is convinced she will have a major thrombotic event, even with maximal anticoagulation in the postoperative period. Motivated by the principle of nonmaleficence, her transplant team cannot comply with her request because of the harm they believe they will cause.

Unchecked nonmaleficence could promote "aggressive" inaction in the face of disease, for fear of causing harm. However, balanced against the basic ethical principles therein, we instead iteratively consider harms and benefits of any treatment(s), in the context of honoring patients' autonomous choices.

## 37.2.3 BENEFICENCE

Indeed, the world would seem unjust if moral action only included the avoidance of causing harm. Often we act to promote the welfare of others. From professional codes of conduct to unwritten societal mores, obligations that specify how to promote the good of others derive from the principle of beneficence. Nonmaleficent and beneficent action overlap, but the latter is distinguished by an obligation for positive action. Beauchamp and Childress state this distinction in this way: "we are obligated to act nonmaleficently toward all persons at all times, but it is generally not possible to act beneficently toward all persons."[12]

Paternalism is a concept that derives from beneficence overtaking patient autonomy. A physician may believe that a given treatment will promote the good of a patient, and yet a patient may not want this treatment. Unbridled paternalism would have the result be that the treatment occurs anyway, by coercion, or the omission of treatment options in discussion. The tension can be acute in pediatrics, when parents' beliefs collide with the medical establishment.

A transplant team may conclude that the best treatment for a child with intestinal failure and severe liver disease is a liver/intestine transplant. The parents may not agree. The team believes they have an obligation to act beneficently: they believe that the child will on balance substantially benefit from the procedure, and feel obligated to compel the team to expend abundant time and creativity convincing the family that this is the best course of action to save the child's life.

Differential perceptions of risk and benefit are commonplace; honoring such differences (i.e., not compelling or requiring transplantation in this patient) legitimizes the concomitant allegiance to the other fundamental ethical principles of nonmaleficence and respect for autonomy.

## 37.2.4 JUSTICE

Perhaps the most complex and philosophically rich concept in ethics, justice refers to fairness: finding a fair way to distribute a good, offer a service, or resolve a problem. Most modern societies strive for fairness. Most simply, fairness is achieved when equals are treated equally, and when unequals are treated unequally. Many difficult problems in ethics stem from competing approaches to the definition and scope of fairness. Violations of this principle can be the most difficult problems to resolve in medical ethics, because of the complexity underlying the theory and application of Justice.

An undocumented foreigner in the United States has developed decompensated cirrhosis presumably from undiagnosed long-standing autoimmune liver disease, and is hospitalized in the ICU because of deteriorating mental status consistent with worsening hepatic encephalopathy. She needs a transplant to survive. Is it just to offer her access to the transplant waiting list, because she is "in need" in equal fashion to anyone else in the United States in liver failure? Or, is she "unequal" because she is not a citizen and does not yet have financial resources or insurance to support her posttransplantation?

This provocative question does not map to one answer, and this would be the case because of varying conceptions of the nature and role of Justice in society.

## 37.3 GENERAL ETHICAL CONCERNS

There are important ethical issues that are generally applicable to both intestinal failure and transplantation. Review and clarification here will inform the discussion of specific topics below.

### 37.3.1 ADULTS, CHILDREN, AND THE INCOMPETENT

Out of respect for patients' autonomous choices, clinicians obtain informed consent from competent adult patients before medical interventions and procedures, a process that has been well established and codified. However, patients who cannot make decisions for themselves rely on others to do so. Standards for decision-making on behalf of other persons include "substituted judgment" or "best interests." Substituted judgment is usually reserved for once competent adult patients, and asks a surrogate decision-maker "what would the patient have wanted in these circumstances?" Even in the best of circumstances, surrogates can have difficulty making decisions in line with loved-ones' wishes.[13]

Properly executed living wills and advanced directives serve to guide or "direct" surrogates and health care staff when previously competent adults are faced with serious illness or important medical decisions. The exact force of these documents will depend on state law, and becomes a matter for lawyers and courts when conflicts arise between document specifications and the wishes of the legal surrogate.[14]

For children who could never have been competent, incompetent adults that have never previously been competent, and once competent adults suddenly incapacitated and whose wishes are entirely unknown, surrogate decision-makers must rely on the standard of "best interests." Parents are widely presumed to know best what is "best" for their own children, and thus serve as the legally and morally sanctioned decision-makers for their own children. In other contexts, the legal surrogate decision-maker depends on statute, but is typically the next of kin.[15]

The American Academy of Pediatrics[16] stipulates that parents do not give "consent," but instead "permit" medical staff to perform procedures on their children. The distinction is important because, while we presume parents are the best decision-makers for their own infants and children, parental prerogative is not unlimited. Clinicians, hospitals, and governments also have obligations to protect and promote the best interests of children. In this way, "permission" implies greater collaboration, such that parents and clinicians consider a range of reasonable options. Options outside this range, choices that might be acceptable for an adult that provides autonomous consent, ought to be morally unjustifiable for children (see Section 37.3.3).

Controversy emerges when what constitutes *reasonable treatment* evolves asynchronously over time among health care institutions and individual health care workers. For instance, decisions may be judged neglectful, abusive, or motivated by self-interest when medical staff or other morally relevant parties (such as nonguardian family members) significantly disagree with parents or surrogates. The involvement of Ethics committee could help clarify the morally relevant arguments on both sides and/or provide mediation. A legal review may be necessary if disagreement involves accusations of neglect or endangerment (see Section 37.3.6).

### 37.3.2 OLDER CHILDREN AND DECISION-MAKING

Older children ought to participate in decision-making about their own care, "to the degree commensurate to their abilities" (p. 138).[1] Doing so promotes the autonomy of minor patients who will soon be competent adults. This process of assent assesses a child's understanding of her/his problem, relays expectations of proposed tests or treatments, seeks to understand a child's reasoning, and solicits a child's willingness to accept the proposed treatment. While it is occasionally necessary to provide care despite a child's objections, assent ensures that doing so occurs without deception, and with adequate medical justification. In parallel, an informed permission process occurs with parents.[16]

Special situations exist where minors are empowered legally to make decisions independently from their parents or legal guardians. Certain medical and social conditions have come to be understood as "definitional" of adulthood (parenthood, financial independence, serving in the armed forces, and pregnancy) while some mental and medical conditions may be effectively impossible to treat if parental oversight were required (e.g., substance abuse and sexually transmitted diseases). In these cases, statute deems "emancipated minors" empowered to make independent medical decisions, provided they have the capacity to do so. A "mature minor" is a related concept, which provides that an older child may benefit (or conversely, may suffer if not granted) from the capacity to make independent medical decisions in particular circumstances. A "mature minor" is context specific, and the status usually must be granted by a court. Both concepts are defined by State law, and thus there can be important differences in this regard depending on the state of residence.[18]

### 37.3.3 Decisions When Outcomes Are Uncertain, and Benefits and Burdens Are Extreme

It is a common problem in clinical medicine that the benefits and harms of different treatment options have comparable weight, so that no single option is clearly best. The best choice will depend on that particular patient's values and preferences, on input or counsel from medical staff, and on discussion with family members or friends. For minors or incompetent patients, parents or legal guardians decide, as discussed above (see Sections 37.3.1 and 37.3.2). In this context, decision-making with deference to parent/guardian autonomy is well supported by ethical analysis and opinion (see Table 37.1).[19]

The model relies on an intact capacity to understand, weigh benefits and burdens, and choose among treatment options. However, when information is complex, required decisions are swiftly sought, benefits or burdens are extreme, and decision-makers are experiencing intense negative emotions, it is unreasonable to suppose that all competent individuals or surrogates can make informed decisions. Moreover, a medical system that supposes this to be the case arguably lacks compassion and caring for the well-being of imperiled patients. The opposite pole is no solution either: an approach that capitalizes on beneficent action by limiting options according to what

### TABLE 37.1
### Treatment Options in Relation to Patient or Surrogate's Preference

| Clinical Assessment of Treatment Options | Parents Wish to Accept or Continue Treatment | Parents Wish to Forego or Withhold Treatment |
|---|---|---|
| One is clearly beneficial | Provide treatment | Provide treatment with review |
| Ambiguous or uncertain which option is best | Provide treatment | Forego treatment |
| Treatment is harmful | Forego or withdraw treatment with review | Forego treatment |

*Source:*    Adapted from President's Commission, 1983, p. 218. (Abram MB. Deciding to forego life-sustaining treatment. In: President O., editor. Washington, DC: U.S. Government Printing Office; 1983.)

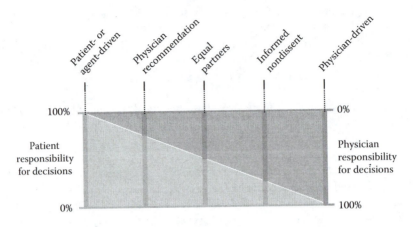

**FIGURE 37.1**    The shared decision-making continuum. (From Kon AA. *JAMA* 2010;304: 903–4. With permission.)

physicians deem best for overwhelmed patients/surrogates could justifiably be criticized for being unacceptably paternalistic.

The "shared decision-making" model offers the most compelling solution to this problem. Best viewed as a shared decision-making "continuum" (Figure 37.1),[20] medical staff offer information, opinion, guidance, reassurance, and/or directives that match particular decision-makers' cognitive and emotional needs. This kind of decision-making can be successful only when a multidisciplinary group of physicians, nurses, social workers, and mental health providers offer responsive, often time-consuming forums for discussion and deliberation. Multidisciplinary intestinal rehabilitation teams are a good example of such groups. An individualized, decision-specific approach is substantiated by qualitative research demonstrating that decision-making in difficult circumstances worked best when physicians convey painful, uncertain, or preliminary information according to the particular emotional and cognitive context of individual patients/ families.[21–23]

### 37.3.4    CONFIDENTIALITY AND PRIVACY IN THE DIGITAL AGE

Adolescents and parents of young children with chronic health problems are increasingly writing about their experiences online, under the auspices of dedicated medical web sites (such as CarePages. com or CaringBridge.org), more general web sites such as MySpace, or web sites developed personally. CarePages.com has more than 4 million registered visitors and 150,000 individual patient web pages, while approximately 700 hospitals/medical care facilities receive their services.[24] Such "blogs" have important benefits for patients and families. Self-expression promotes improved coping and acceptance of ongoing medical treatments through "cathartic narration," while enhanced ability to communicate with friends and family strengthens a patient or family's community of support.[25]

There is concern, however, that the proliferation of online expression and communication has outstripped the development of policy and cultural mores that protect against invasions of privacy, unintended breaches of confidentiality, and challenges to professionalism. Unintended consequences may occur when a patient or family posts information online but fails to appreciate the implications of public information.

For instance, the family of an organ donor could contact a recipient who has posted information describing the surgery on a particular date. Families or patients may want to discuss their experience in the hospital, and may post identifying information or pictures of other patients without appreciating the importance of asking for consent. Medical staff may learn disturbing information about patients not shared in real time, or further, become inflamed by misstated facts or derogatory comments. Even if staff are invited to read patient or parent blogs, staff must question their motivation to read: is the act for the benefit of the patient, or more out of self-interest to verify that the family "likes" them?

Many hospitals are developing staff, patient, and family educational tools to address these problems.[26] Discussion should be upfront regarding whether and when staff will read blogs, how privacy and confidentiality will be respected, and assurances that conflicts/disagreements will handled quickly, honestly, and respectfully.[25]

### 37.3.5   INTESTINAL FAILURE

Ethical concerns in the care of patients with intestinal failure have evolved significantly in the last 20 years. As noted above, before the widespread use of PN, many diseases now considered chronic were fatal in the neonatal or early infant period. Adults that acquired SBS or prolonged severe intestinal disease (e.g., radiation enteritis) would uniformly die of inanition. Thus, ethical concerns have, in the past, largely been focused on tensions between and among family, patient, and staff regarding the nature and care of the dying patient.

These kinds of concerns still exist, but now that intestinal failure is a chronic disease supportable in the community, the variety and depth of ethical concerns have expanded. The exploration below addresses critical issues specific to intestinal failure; the reader should look to other resources for particular ethical analysis and background regarding provision or withholding medically administered hydration and nutrition,[27,28] caring for the chronically ill adolescent,[29] and managing suspicion for Munchausen syndrome by proxy.[30]

### 37.3.6   CONTROVERSIAL INITIATION AND/OR CONTINUATION OF PN

Treatment ought to be started or stopped will not present as an ethical dilemma when patients, decision-makers, and/or medical staff are reasonably aligned with respect to the goals of care. However, what are the circumstances, particular ethical tensions, and best-principled resolution to situations where this is not the case? Six general situations can be resolved (Table 37.2), depending on the capacity of the patient, whether a parent is involved, whether the decision will hasten death, and the magnitude of harm perceived by interested parties.

A. *The adult patient refuses to initiate or wishes to discontinue PN when medical staff or family believes it would be best to use PN.* This situation is perhaps the least controversial. As discussed above, the primacy of patient self-determination—to freely make informed decisions about what treatments one does and does not want—justifies decisions even if this means the decision-maker's life will be shortened. Staff and family are obliged to verify that the adult has capacity, that the decision is truly informed, and that the decision is not being made under duress or in hast.

An adult dependent on PN for 5 years because of a car accident which led to near complete enterectomy has requested that her central line be removed and that she be allowed to die peacefully at home. She has had frequent line infections, and has been hospitalized frequently. She is not depressed, but it seems she made this decision without much notice. Her medical providers wonder if it is morally right to comply with her request.

If indeed this is an informed decision, clinicians ought to comply with her request. Beneficence would require that clinicians be convinced that the decision is fully informed, and, should a clinician be unable to comply because of his/her own conscience, most would claim a persistent duty to find a clinician who could.

**TABLE 37.2**

**Controversial PN**

| Scenario | Patient Child | Patient Adult | Decision-Maker | Patient Wish[a] | Medical Opinion | Major Harm | Comment |
|---|---|---|---|---|---|---|---|
| A | | √ | Self | No | Yes | Unwanted treatment | Assure adequate IC |
| B | | √ | Self | Yes | No | Death | Unless frankly harmful, best to favor offering PN |
| C | | √ | Surrogate | Yes | No | Death | Legal review if cannot agree |
| D | | √ | Surrogate | No | Yes | Unwanted treatment | Assure trustworthy surrogate; review living will |
| E | √ | | Parent | No | Yes | Unwanted treatment | Stronger moral claim to override parent if choice is "unreasonable" |
| F | √ | | Parent | Yes | No | Death | Most troubling situation; cannot force clinician to cause harm; legal review helpful |

*Note:* IC: informed consent.

[a] Surrogate or parents in the context of an incapacitated adult or child, respectively.

B. *The adult desires PN or wishes PN to be continued while medical staff believe that PN would not be beneficial.* This situation ought to be rare. The dominant ethical tension would be between medical staff's obligation to do no harm while at the same time honoring the adult patient's self-determination in knowing what treatment options are best for himself or herself, even if risks are substantial. If reasonable medical opinion holds that PN would be *frankly harmful*, staff have no obligation to offer such a treatment. However, if there is disagreement about the nature and/or magnitude of benefit derived from PN, and the patient has capacity to consider such factors, deference in most cases ought to favor a patient's interpretation of benefit and assessment of risk.

For an adult with incurable cancer, radiation enteritis requiring PN, and a prior history of renal failure requiring dialysis three times per week, medical staff may reasonably conclude that home PN is on balance not beneficial, or even "not indicated." However, the patient may have a strong desire to be at home and derive benefit from the potential extra weeks/months of life on PN, and may already be quite accustomed to outpatient dialysis.

In this situation, modern patient-centered ethics would favor supporting the patient in his/her decision to initiate or continue PN. (See Section 37.3.8 for further consideration of this case.)

C. *The decision-maker for the incapacitated patient believes PN will be beneficial while medical staff do not.* This structure shares many elements with situation B. However, because the conflict is with a surrogate, not the patient himself or herself, respecting autonomy would translate to assurances that the surrogate's judgment is in keeping with the incapacitated patient's wishes. Living wills are powerful tools for specifying direction of care when situations are characterized by discord. If, for instance, the will stipulates that the incapacitated patient wanted life-prolonging therapy until and unless she had a life-ending heart attack or stroke, it would seem reasonable, indeed, medical staff would be obliged to accommodate a request for PN, unless, as above, medical staff believe PN to be frankly harmful.

A greater burden must be overcome when a disputed decision hastens death; nonmaleficence often includes proscriptions against actions that hasten death. Without specific knowledge of a patient's values or wishes, the presumption is that most people would prefer being alive to being dead; in the absence of good information to the contrary, presuming that life-prolonging therapy is best ought to be generally appropriate.

D. *The decision-maker for the incapacitated patient believes PN will not be beneficial, while medical staff believe it will be.* As we have discussed, fully informed patients ought not be subject to medical intervention or technologies they do not desire, even if this means life will be shortened or suffering will be greater. When the decision-maker is a surrogate, the same concerns pertain from C, with heightened scrutiny. Because the surrogate's decision will most likely hasten death, interested parties must well believe that decisions closely align with what the incapacitated patient would have wanted for himself or herself, and/or with what is stipulated in a living will. An ethics consultation should be obtained followed by a legal review if disagreements cannot be remediated.

E. *Parents do not think continuing or initiating PN will be beneficial, while medical staff believe it will be.* As discussed above (see Section 37.3.1), parents judge what is best for their children, within a range of acceptable or reasonable choices; indeed, medical staff may not agree that a particular choice is best. Moral authority of parents ought to be questioned when decisions reflect neglectful or self-interested attitudes. However, distinguishing neglectful from well-intentioned yet difficult-to-accept decisions may not always be straightforward.

An infant who develops midgut volvulus and loses her entire jejunum, ileum, and right colon will arguably require lifelong PN without a transplant. The parents, upon hearing this news, do not want PN started and would like to pursue comfort care until their daughter dies. Medical staff sensitively discuss the benefits and burdens of alternative approaches, but, the parents continue to be resolute in their decision. Modern medical ethics would support honoring the parents' wishes to initiate comfort care, in a situation where no alternative is clearly most beneficial.

However, it is now possible to support such patients on home PN for months and possibly years. Medical staff might conclude that this counts as being "clearly beneficial" (see Table 37.1). Could denying PN for this infant constitute neglect? Determining whether achieving a life with permanent intestinal failure is "clearly beneficial" depends on evaluating the quality of such a life. Such a determination is subjective, and depends on a patient or family's valuing of the benefits and burdens of multiple factors. The central concern is whether medical staff think that foregoing treatment unreasonably denies the infant a chance at enjoying a life where its benefits clearly outweigh its burdens. While there is little literature to guide consideration of this particular topic,[31] other diseases such as severe congenital heart disease have grappled with similar dilemmas,[32,33] and might serve as a useful model for developing an organized multidisciplinary approach to this question.

F. *Parents believe initiating or continuing PN is beneficial, when medical/staff believe the treatment will not be beneficial.* As with situations B and C, if medical staff believe that the PN will be frankly harmful (see Table 37.1), such a therapy ought not be offered or continued on the basis of nonmaleficence.[34] However, not honoring a parent's request to initiate or continue even "futile" PN has serious ethical ramifications: hastening the death of a child against the wishes of a loving parent pits autonomy against nonmaleficence, in starkest relief.

A child with prolonged irreversible intestinal failure and loss of all traditional central venous access points also has worsening liver disease and coagulopathy. A transplant team concludes that the child is not a candidate for transplantation. The parents are requesting that interventional radiology attempt securing a line using sharp cannulation of a recently thrombosed subclavian vein, so that PN can continue to be delivered at home, which is what the family would like. The IR team is greatly concerned about causing life-threatening bleeding or lung injury during the procedure, and does not want to attempt it. Without central access, the child cannot leave the hospital.

Underlying emotional, religious, or social concerns could be influencing the parents thinking, and would need to be explored carefully. If the parents are unflagging in their wishes, medical staff are ought not to comply only if staff remained convinced that the acute harms of the procedure, coupled with an arguably limited amount of benefit from home PN, more than reasonably outweighed the burdens of continued hospitalization, presumably until death. For intractable disagreements, legal review may be necessary to distinguish between what is ambiguous, clearly beneficial, or clearly harmful (see Table 37.1). Alternatively, efforts could be made to find a team or hospital that might consider the treatment differently.[35]

### 37.3.7  USING PN IN PATIENTS WITH NEUROLOGICAL INJURY OR SEVERE NEUROLOGICAL DIAGNOSES

From a modern ethical standpoint, adults and children with acquired or congenital neurological disease ought not to be considered prima facie less worthy of receiving PN.[36] However, particular issues must be examined:

- Is informed consent with the patient possible along with consideration of alternatives including palliative care?
- If the patient is or becomes incompetent, were her/his wishes known, and to whom?
- If the neurologic disease is progressive, how will family and medical staff come to decide when PN is, on balance, more harmful than beneficial?

At base, vigilance is required to make sure that PN, as well as any other treatment, is administered to benefit the patient, and not a loved one. If a patient is, or, is expected to be, unable to derive pleasure or benefit from living (e.g., a person in a persistent vegetative state and thus with no hope for regaining consciousness), one can advance a reasonable ethical argument that PN is at best without benefit and at worst harmful, providing justification for the view that PN ought not be offered or continued in this context. If there are disagreements, they should fall into the categories discussed above.

### 37.3.8  RESOURCE ALLOCATION, JUSTICE CONSIDERATIONS, AND THE USE OF PN

The perennial tension between advancing the care of the individual while also promoting the health of the community indelibly marks any discussion of high-cost technologies. PN is expensive, and its near universal financing through insurance companies or government forms the basis for asking a formidable question: ought an expensive therapy such as PN be used with some regard to the relationship between cost and benefit?

The decision-making model familiar to most in the United States includes only the patient and her/his physician: if the decision is that a therapy ought to be tried, then that is what is best/just/good. This model might have been reasonable when the range of medical and surgical therapies was more limited. Now, with the ever-increasing number of expensive therapies and technologies, doing whatever is possible is unsustainable from an economic perspective. There is broad agreement that this is true; major controversies begin when deciding who gets to make limiting decisions and what particular policies will be used to differentiate groups of patients.[37]

Consider the example above of the adult with cancer on dialysis and home PN (see Section 37.3.6). Would it be reasonable to restrict PN on the basis of an unfavorable cost–benefit analysis for this man who is expected to die of incurable cancer in the next 6 months? One supposes that in the context of extreme resource shortages, it would indeed be reasonable to first use the PN to support the life of individuals expected to live for many years to come. But this is rarely the context. Currently in the United States, having or getting medical insurance determines if you can obtain home PN. Moving to a practice of access based on cost–benefit ratio would be unfamiliar and morally objectionable to many in the United States.[38] Nevertheless, in a time of exponentially growing costs, and lack of attention to the most basic of health care needs for large swaths of society, it may come to pass that a just, if unhappy, result is that a man who desires life for 6 more months may have to pay for the opportunity to do so.

### 37.3.9  PN Nonadherence and Obligation to Continue Prescribing PN

Home PN is a life-sustaining medically and technically complex treatment with parallels to outpatient dialysis and chemotherapy. When patients do not adhere to lab schedules, do not show up to clinical appointments to monitor weight and review catheter care, refuse or decline visiting nurses, or there is suspicion or documentation of risky behaviors such as intravenous drug use, what are our obligations with regard to the provision of PN?

There are no published resources to guide prescribers of PN in this regard. Basic principles can provide a context for approaching nonadherent patients. On the basis of nonmaleficence, physicians and health care workers ought not to prescribe PN if they have strong suspicion that the PN will cause life-threatening injury.

> An argumentative adult with intestinal failure from superior mesenteric artery thrombosis and mild renal insufficiency from long-standing atherosclerosis and diabetes is determined to give her PN over 5 h instead of 12 h, even though the prescribing physician and staff are convinced this will cause dangerous hyperkalemia.

On the basis of nonmaleficence, PN ought not be prescribed, potentially against the patient's wishes. However, on the basis of beneficence, the PN team would have a robust duty to promote the welfare of this difficult PN patient, using a creative, sensitive, conscientious, flexible approach. Could the PN be made potassium-free, and any necessary potassium supplements taken throughout the day orally? Could a compromise be fashioned, and safety monitored, by administering over 8 h? Does the team have a social worker or psychologist who can help understand the nature of the patient's intransigence?

Respect for her autonomy ought to compel PN staff to avoid using threats of abandonment or coercive inducements to subdue her appeals to deliver the PN over 5 h. She may have a particularly good understanding or sense of what her body can "handle," and some weight ought be given to the position that a competent, fully informed individual should be able to make decisions for herself, even against the best advice of her PN team.

From a justice perspective, we could consider the impact her care has on other patients. A morally objectionable result could occur if resources—durable goods and staff time—are not available to other patients because of the sheer amount of time taken by trying to take care of this patient. For example, if her behavior in the clinic were disturbing or intimidating to other patients or staff, and no accommodations exist to see her in an alternative setting, justification could be afforded an approach that ultimately invites her to be seen in another center.

For pediatric patients, respect of autonomy may be less compelling than appeals for beneficent action. Imagine the case scenario if a parent wanted to administer PN over 5 h instead of 12 h, even though hyperkalemia would most likely ensue. Absent a logical argument for abundant medical benefit to the child, the moral justification for allowing such a treatment to proceed might be far weaker than the view that such a request is tantamount to medical abuse; medical staff could have broad ethical support to pursue legal means to prevent this outcome.

## 37.4   INTESTINAL TRANSPLANTATION

Much has been written about the ethics of organ transplantation. Donor identification,[39,40] recipient candidacy (particularly nonmedical unsuitability),[41] the matching of donors and recipients,[42] living donation,[43,44] and financial considerations[45,46] are broad topics deeply shot through with ethical considerations. The reader can refer to the texts and reviews that cover these topics in detail. The following discussion will concern itself with emerging topics that are particularly germane to the field of intestinal transplantation.

### 37.4.1   QUALITY OF LIFE AND DECISION TO PERFORM AN INTESTINAL TRANSPLANT

The concept of transplant "candidacy" suggests that there are medical and nonmedical criteria that ought, or must, to be met before one can be placed on an organ waitlist. The legitimacy of such determinations rests on the just and efficient distribution of scarce resources, and the protection of patients from unjustifiable harm. Particularly for intestinal transplantation, where long-term graft and patient survival are still considered to be suboptimal,[47] guidelines and policy support its application only for those at high risk of otherwise dying from intestinal failure or complications of its therapy.[48]

Many patients on long-term PN do not qualify for consideration based on these standards. Nevertheless, their lives may be so undermined by poor quality of life that some would prefer death to continued home PN.

> A thirty-year-old woman has been on PN for 2 years, after having suffered mesenteric thrombosis during a severe episode of pancreatitis, resulting in loss of nearly all of her small intestine. She has been admitted to hospital since her initial discharge once for an easily treated central venous line infection, but has been mostly at home unable to work because of pain and frequent need for IV infusions. She wants an intestinal transplant, and is well educated about the risks and benefits.

Indeed, some authorities in the intestinal transplant field have argued that posttransplant outcomes are "good enough" to consider intestinal transplantation for quality of life.[48,49] Ethical considerations that inform a decision to transplant for poor quality of life divide themselves between those applicable to the individual doctor–patient relationship and those informing transplant program and public policy.

From the individual perspective, examination reveals tensions between fundamental ethical principles. Respect for patient autonomy would offer the competent adult patient a chance at intestinal transplantation after an extensive informed consent process. Nevertheless, if a physician were convinced transplant will, on balance, be frankly harmful (see Table 37.1 if the patient were a child), the duty for not harming patients would compel a physician to decline honoring this patient's request. And yet again, professional virtues, such as the duty not to abandon patients and to be compassionate, might be jeopardized when a competent patient construes the hesitancy as "refusal" to help.

Transplant programs often evaluate whether patients ought to be candidates for transplant, even before developing personal relationships with individual patients. Programs ought to consider stakeholders as well in this discussion, because acceptance of a patient may impact other patients on the program waitlist, and could also draw from limited monetary and service resources at the program. In this context, ought the program ask if it is appropriate to offer intestinal transplantation to those whose need is not as great as others?

Such a justice consideration would mirror the concerns of regional and national regulatory bodies whose duty it is to optimize the efficient and just distribution of scarce transplantable organs. Policies need to balance the duty of prioritizing organs to those in greatest need with the sometimes opposing good that maximizes the life of transplanted organs (e.g., efficiency).[50] If a consensus were attained that intestinal transplantation for poor quality of life were ethically justifiable, regulation at the national level would be valuable for ensuring that the treatment be available widely, according to standardized, publically vetted criteria.

## 37.4.2 UNSUITABILITY FOR TRANSPLANTATION IN RELATION TO TRANSPLANT OUTCOME

When diseases are irreversible and/or progressive, patients may be, or become, "unsuitable" for transplantation. Generally agreed-upon medical contraindications for transplantation include active malignancy, untreated serious infections, and untreatable disease in other organ systems likely to jeopardize successful transplantation in the near future. Nonmedical criteria for unsuitability typically include homelessness, prolonged history of nonadherence, untreated severe psychiatric disease, and significant neurological disability, although there are no published guidelines in this regard. Children specifically may be considered unsuitable if the family unit is seriously unstable, or if the child is a ward of the state but without an identified family or adoptive parent interested and able to care for the child post-transplantation. Individual transplant programs are responsible for setting criteria for unsuitability, so long as the criteria are free of bias on the basis of race, age, class, or ethnicity.[50]

Important ethical problem arises when the stringency of nonmedical criteria is correlated with the chance of long-term success.

Joe is 8 months old and has advanced PN-associated liver disease and SBS from gastroschisis and midgut volvulus. He has been in hospital for 3 months, and has just returned from the ICU after a septic episode. He has four other siblings. Mother is in her early 20s, did not finish high school, has two jobs, and lives in temporary housing. She wants Joe to have "every chance to live." The transplant team is concerned that the social circumstances will assuredly cause unacceptable nonadherence, and do not want to go ahead with listing on this basis. When asked to clarify the reason for their hesitation, the team believes that outcomes are not good enough to risk taking on this patient.

The team's ethical argument could be compelling. Without malice, they may believe that the care for Joe will be so complex, and mother utterly unable to follow through, that the duty not to harm (the sure burdens of a liver/intestine transplant operation, the complications and toxicities related to nonadherence) outweighs the duty to benefit, which in the team's view, is already qualified by the success of only 50% at >5 years.

Nevertheless, substantial ethical concerns burden Joe's disqualification on this basis. Long-term success is only one measure of benefit; shorter-term outcomes are substantially better than 50%, and even 1–2 years of significantly improved life would have substantial value. Further, inaction will surely result in death soon (failed beneficence), while the certainty of his poor posttransplant outcome is arguably less clear. The disqualification based on social circumstances could be interpreted as class bias, which, even if not outwardly intended, could still leave the decision open to scrutiny from a justice perspective.

Nonmedical criteria in transplantation are legitimate. But each transplant program should think carefully about its criteria in the context of the community they serve. Best practice[50] would include multidisciplinary development of such protocols, with input from relevant community members, and transparency for transplant candidates with respect to how these criteria are applied.

## 37.4.3 THE MORAL LIABILITY OF PERFORMING TRANSPLANTS AT SMALLER CENTERS

Clinical intestinal transplantation beyond single cases began in 1989, offered in select locations in the United States and in two locations in Europe.[11] At that time, intestinal transplantation was an innovative approach to saving the lives of patients who would soon die from complications of intestinal failure. Individuals with the financial, social, and education capacity to travel to these centers were able to benefit. With the 2001 Medicare approval for patients failing standard treatment for intestinal failure, the number of programs began to increase; intestinal transplantation is now being performed at approximately 18 centers in the United States.[51]

Long-term (>5 year) organ and patient survival has not improved since 2000, based on the latest data from the Intestinal Transplant Registry (ITR).[52] Among few other factors, transplant center volume has been a consistent positive predictor of survival in the 2005, 2007, and 2009 ITR reports. While the four largest centers in the United States performed approximately 80% of the intestinal transplants in 2008,[47] about half of active centers in the United States perform 0–3 transplants per year,[51] The already limited number of intestinal transplants performed per year may be falling,[52] suggesting that smaller centers may have even fewer opportunities for maintaining experience and expertise in intestinal transplantation.

What are the moral concerns associated with small transplant centers performing intestinal transplants? If indeed it is true that smaller centers have poorer outcomes, and that poorer outcomes are related to inexperience performing and caring for intestinal transplant patients, a strong ethical claim could be made that unnecessary harm ought to be minimized by referring patients to centers with higher volumes. A mirror image, but distinct duty for beneficent action, would compel physicians and medical staff to refer patients to centers where positive outcomes are most apt to occur. Professional obligations to improve medical practice would consist of supporting the notion that unusual and high-risk treatments are apt to improve faster when performed in fewer centers.

Ethical justification for broad availability of intestinal transplantation would also engage autonomy. Some patients and families would choose to have complex and ongoing care at centers they trust, and which might be geographically close to home and work, providing ongoing security and access to social supports. Even knowing that outcomes may not be optimal, patients or families arguably ought to have the opportunity to make this decision. Justice claims include the inability of many families without significant financial means to successfully travel and reside near large transplant centers. Geography is an unfair arbiter of access to intestinal transplantation and thus survival, especially if it were feasible to rectify this injustice by the availability of reliable, dedicated local transplant teams.

United network for organ sharing (UNOS) has been grappling with some of these concerns in ongoing discussion regarding the licensing of intestinal transplant centers and physicians, without clear resolution. The transplant literature is mixed regarding whether a volume-outcome relationship exists for heart,[53] lung,[54] and liver[55] transplantation; implications are uncertain for UNOS or center for medicare and medicaid services (CMS) policy. UNOS policy does favor autonomy[56] in its bylaws requiring transplant centers to share comparative center-specific survival statistics, and all potential transplant recipients must be informed that they are free to visit (but with no assurance that insurance will support) and be listed at more than one transplant center.

## 37.5  CONCLUSIONS

Clinical care of patients with intestinal failure is complex. Beyond medical or surgical decisions, discussion often represents moral deliberation. The intent here has been to introduce a vocabulary of moral deliberation, demonstrate how basic concepts work through example, and then survey the field shedding light on important and unique ethical concerns. Increased awareness and discussion of these and other ethical controversies in our field will not only optimize outcomes, but also enhance communication and discussion in an actively evolving field.

## REFERENCES

1. Colomb V, Dabbas-Tyan M, Taupin P et al. Long-term outcome of children receiving home parenteral nutrition: A 20-year single-center experience in 302 patients. *J Pediatr Gastroenterol Nutr* 2007;44:347–53.
2. Amiot A, Joly F, Alves A, Panis Y, Bouhnik Y, Messing B. Long-term outcome of chronic intestinal pseudo-obstruction adult patients requiring home parenteral nutrition. *Am J Gastroenterol* 2009;104:1262–70.

3. Gottrand F, Staszewski P, Colomb V et al. Satisfaction in different life domains in children receiving home parenteral nutrition and their families. *J Pediatr* 2005;146:793–7.
4. Chambers A, Powell-Tuck J. Determinants of quality of life in home parenteral nutrition. *Curr Opin Clin Nutr Metab Care* 2007;10:318–23.
5. Bonifacio R, Alfonsi L, Santarpia L et al. Clinical outcome of long-term home parenteral nutrition in non-oncological patients: A report from two specialised centres. *Intern Emerg Med* 2007;2:188–95.
6. DeLegge M, Alsolaiman MM, Barbour E, Bassas S, Siddiqi MF, Moore NM. Short bowel syndrome: Parenteral nutrition versus intestinal transplantation. Where are we today? *Dig Dis Sci* 2007;52:876–92.
7. Abu-Elmagd KM, Costa G, Bond GJ et al. Five hundred intestinal and multivisceral transplantations at a single center: Major advances with new challenges. *Ann Surg* 2009 Oct;250(4):567–81.
8. Lao OB, Healey PJ, Perkins JD, Reyes JD, Goldin AB. Outcomes in children with intestinal failure following listing for intestinal transplant. *Pediatrics* 2010 Mar;125(3):e550–8. Epub 2010 Feb 8.
9. Sudan D. Long-term outcomes and quality of life after intestine transplantation. *Curr Opin Organ Transplant* 2010 Jun;15(3):357–60.
10. Golfieri L, Lauro A, Tossani E et al. Psychological adaptation and quality of life of adult intestinal transplant recipients: University of Bologna experience. *Transplant Proc* 2010 Jan–Feb;42(1):42–4.
11. Nayyar N, Mazariegos G, Ranganathan S et al. Pediatric small bowel transplantation. *Semin Pediatr Surg* 2010 Feb;19(1):68–77.
12. Beauchamp T, Childress J. *Principles of Biomedical Ethics*. 6th ed. New York: Oxford University Press; 2009.
13. Fried TR, Bradley EH, Towle VR. Valuing the outcomes of treatment: Do patients and their caregivers agree? *Arch Intern Med* 2003;163:2073–8.
14. Down Your States Advanced Directives. 2007. (Accessed September 13, 2010, at http://www.caringinfo.org/PlanningAhead/AdvanceDirectives/Stateaddownload.htm.).
15. Surrogate Decision Making. 1999. (Accessed September 13, 2010, at http://www.ama-assn.org/ama/upload/mm/369/report_119.pdf.).
16. Informed consent, parental permission, and assent in pediatric practice. Committee on Bioethics, American Academy of Pediatrics. *Pediatrics* 1995;95:314–7.
17. Opinion 5.055—Confidential Care for Minors. American Medical Association, 1994. (Accessed March 25, 2010, at http://www.ama-assn.org/ama/pub/physician-resources/medical-ethics/code-medical-ethics/opinion5055.shtml.).
18. An Overview of Minors' Consent Law. GUTTMACHER INSTITUTE, 2010. (Accessed September 13, 2010, at http://www.guttmacher.org/statecenter/spibs/spib_OMCL.pdf.).
19. Abram MB. Deciding to forego life-sustaining treatment. In: President O., editor. *Foregoing Life-Sustaining Treatment*. Washington, DC: U.S. Government Printing Office; 1983.
20. Kon AA. The shared decision-making continuum. *JAMA* 2010; 304:903–4.
21. Evans LR, Boyd EA, Malvar G et al. Surrogate decision-makers' perspectives on discussing prognosis in the face of uncertainty. *Am J Respir Crit Care Med* 2009;179:48–53.
22. Rodriguez-Osorio CA, Dominguez-Cherit G. Medical decision making: Paternalism versus patient-centered (autonomous) care. *Curr Opin Crit Care* 2008;14:708–13.
23. Truog RD, Meyer EC, Burns JP. Toward interventions to improve end-of-life care in the pediatric intensive care unit. *Crit Care Med* 2006;34:S373–9.
24. CarePages INC. (Accessed October 25, 2009, at http://www.carepagesinc.com/index.html.).
25. Tunick R, Mednick L. Commentary: Electronic communication in the pediatric setting–dilemmas associated with patient blogs. *J Pediatr Psychol* 2009;34:585–7.
26. Greysen SR, Kind T, Chretien KC. Online Professionalism and the Mirror of Social Media. *J Gen Intern Med* 2010 Nov;25(11):1227–9. Epub 2010 Jul 15.
27. Diekema DS, Botkin JR. Clinical report–Forgoing medically provided nutrition and hydration in children. *Pediatrics* 2009;124:813–22.
28. Geppert CM, Andrews MR, Druyan ME. Ethical issues in artificial nutrition and hydration: A review. *JPEN* 2010 Jan–Feb;34(1):79–88. Epub 2009 Nov 6.
29. Michaud PA, Suris JC, Viner R. The adolescent with a chronic condition. Part II: Healthcare provision. *Arch Dis Child* 2004;89:943–9.
30. Squires JE, Squires RH, Jr. Munchausen syndrome by proxy: Ongoing clinical challenges. *J Pediatr Gastroenterol Nutr* 2010 Sep;51(3):248–53.
31. Severijnen R, Hulstijn-Dirkmaat I, Gordijn B, Bakker L, Bongaerts G. Acute loss of the small bowel in a school-age boy. Difficult choices: To sustain life or to stop treatment? *Eur J Pediatr* 2003;162:794–8.

32. Kon AA. Healthcare providers must offer palliative treatment to parents of neonates with hypoplastic left heart syndrome. *Arch Pediatr Adolesc Med* 2008;162:844–8.
33. Kon AA. Ethics of cardiac transplantation in hypoplastic left heart syndrome. *Pediatr Cardiol* 2009;30:725–8.
34. Paris JJ, Crone RK, Reardon F. Physicians' refusal of requested treatment. The case of Baby L. *N Engl J Med* 1990;322:1012–5.
35. Guidelines on forgoing life-sustaining medical treatment. *Pediatrics* 1994;93:532–36.
36. Panocchia N, Bossola M, Vivanti G. Transplantation and mental retardation: What is the meaning of a discrimination? *Am J Transplant* 2010 Apr;10(4):727–30.
37. Truog RD. Screening mammography and the "r" word. *N Engl J Med* 2009;361:2501–3.
38. Mariner WK. Rationing health care and the need for credible scarcity: Why Americans can't say no. *Am J Public Health* 1995;85:1439–45.
39. Hippen B, Matas A. Incentives for organ donation in the United States: Feasible alternative or forthcoming apocalypse? *Curr Opin Organ Transplant* 2009;14:140–6.
40. Miller FG, Truog RD, Brock DW. The dead donor rule: Can it withstand critical scrutiny? *J Med Philos*;35:299–312.
41. Veatch RM. A general theory of allocation. In: *Transplantation Ethics*. Washington DC: Georgetown University Press; 2000. pp. 287–310.
42. Stegall MD. Developing a new kidney allocation policy: The rationale for including life years from transplant. *Am J Transplant* 2009;9:1528–32.
43. Ventura KA. Ethical considerations in live liver donation to children. *Prog Transplant* 2010 Jun;20(2):186–90.
44. Cynowiec J, Kim J, Qazi YA. Incentivizing living organ donation. *Curr Opin Organ Transplant* 2009;14:201–5.
45. Laurentine KA, Bramstedt KA. Too poor for transplant: Finance and insurance issues in transplant ethics. *Prog Transplant* 2010 Jun;20(2):178–85.
46. Daniels N. Comment: Ability to pay and access to transplantation. In: Caplan A, Coelho DH, editors. *The Ethics of Organ Transplants*. Amherst, MA: Prometheus Books; 1998. p. 242.49.
47. Mazariegos GV, Steffick DE, Horslen S et al. Intestine transplantation in the United States, 1999–2008. *Am J Transplant* 2010;10:1020–34.
48. Fishbein TM. Intestinal transplantation. *N Engl J Med* 2009;361:998–1008.
49. Abu-Elmagd KM. Intestinal transplantation for short bowel syndrome and gastrointestinal failure: Current consensus, rewarding outcomes, and practical guidelines. *Gastroenterology* 2006;130:S132–7.
50. OPTN/UNOS Ethics Committee Report to the Board of Directors. 2009. (Accessed September 13, 2010, at http://optn.transplant.hrsa.gov/CommitteeReports/board_main_EthicsCommittee_2_18_2009_16_14.pdf.).
51. Organ Procurement and Transplantation Network. 2010. (Accessed May 25, 2010, at http://optn.transplant.hrsa.gov/.).
52. Grant D. Intestinal Transplant Registry, 2009. Personal communication.
53. Weiss ES, Meguid RA, Patel ND et al. Increased mortality at low-volume orthotopic heart transplantation centers: Should current standards change? *Ann Thorac Surg* 2008;86:1250–9; discussion 9–60.
54. Weiss ES, Allen JG, Meguid RA et al. The impact of center volume on survival in lung transplantation: An analysis of more than 10,000 cases. *Ann Thorac Surg* 2009;88:1062–70.
55. Northup PG, Pruett TL, Stukenborg GJ, Berg CL. Survival after adult liver transplantation does not correlate with transplant center case volume in the MELD era. *Am J Transplant* 2006;6:2455–62.
56. Organ Distribution: Organ Procurement, Distribution and Allocation. 2009. (Accessed May 25, 2010, at http://optn.transplant.hrsa.gov/PoliciesandBylaws2/policies/pdfs/policy_6.pdf.)

# 38 Support Groups

*Lisa Crosby Metzger, Joan Bishop, and Lyn Howard*

## CONTENTS

Individuals coalesce into a support group because of life-altering circumstances, such as chronic illness, dependency, or grief. For those who come to the Oley Foundation, the circumstance is severe bowel dysfunction that has led to the need for home parenteral and/or enteral nutrition (HPEN). For many of them, HPEN has been life saving. However, they are aware that potentially life-threatening complications come hand in hand with HPEN's life-saving properties, and that both HPEN and the illnesses that lead to HPEN can come with psychosocial side effects [1–5]. The HPEN consumer or caregiver has his or her hands full with care issues, and then often faces grieving, depression, and feelings of isolation and bewilderment as well [6–9]. Financial stress, too, often accompanies chronic illness and expensive therapies such as HPEN [10,11].

One such organization is the Oley Foundation. Oley offers HPEN consumers learning opportunities to make day-to-day living safer, more manageable, and more satisfying; and networking and social opportunities to combat the isolation and provide consumers with hope. In addition, the Oley Foundation gives HPEN consumers an opportunity to be heard, both by other consumers and by a larger audience. In this way, Oley can help bridge the gap between the consumer's medical and personal worlds.

The Oley Foundation, and other support groups, can help HPEN consumers live life to the fullest, as independently as possible—and complement the goals of the medical professionals on whom the consumers rely. An Oley member who is fed enterally says, "One of the first things you learn when you have to live with being tube fed or living with other complications dealing with your health is that the more you learn about your condition, the better you can cope with it." Further, the more the consumer knows about HPEN, from how to reduce episodes of sepsis to how to incorporate it into their lives, the safer, healthier, and happier he or she will be.

## 38.1   ROLE OF A SUPPORT GROUP

There are thousands of support groups in the United States that focus on health issues, from the large and well-known (e.g., the American Cancer Society), to the smaller, more obscure (e.g., the Organic Acidemia Association). They may be local or national, and moderated by a professional or peer-to-peer based; they may meet weekly, monthly, irregularly, or be organized around the Internet or the telephone; and they may combine any or all of these elements. Different support groups have different goals, and they can be successful on a variety of levels.

Support groups offer people opportunities to talk to others who share a common experience; give and receive emotional support; share problems, concerns, and coping skills; and gather information and learn [12,13]. They can also represent their members in the public arena, giving an organized voice to members' concerns (consider lobbying efforts by the American Lung Association or the public awareness campaigns by the March of Dimes). Support groups generate understanding and compassion by sharing members' stories (e.g., in 2009 the Jerry Lewis Muscular Dystrophy Association telethon, in its 44th year, spotlighted seven families [14]). Such understanding can help reduce any stigma that may be attached to illness or "otherness." These groups also often fund or otherwise support research on their particular health problem.

## 38.2   BENEFIT OF PARTICIPATION

The relationship between better patient outcomes and better quality of life (QoL), and support group participation, has been demonstrated by numerous studies in a wide range of chronic health disorders. Cancer support groups are perhaps the most widely studied. Pertinent to our concerns—whether participation in a support group is beneficial to people with intestinal failure, and particularly those on HPEN—are the studies by Dr. Carol Smith and her team at the School of Nursing, University of Kansas Medical Center.

In 2002, Dr. Smith and colleagues published the results of a study focused specifically on the relationship between affiliation with a national support group (the Oley Foundation) and home parenteral nutrition (HPN) patient outcomes [15]. The study looked at two groups of HPN patients: group 1 was comprised of 52 patients from large academic center medical programs and group 2 was comprised of 43 patients who were supervised by a physician in private practice. Patients were separated out in this way because many of those in group 1 had access to a nutrition support team through the center that provided their care, and this support might have reduced what these individuals gained from a national organization.

Twenty-four of the participants in group 1 were affiliated with the Oley Foundation and 28 matched case controls were not; 21 of the participants in group 2 were affiliated with Oley and 22 matched controls were not. The matched case controls had similar primary diagnoses, duration on HPN, sex, and age distribution. All these factors are known to independently influence clinical outcome. Participants each filled out the 35-question Quality of Life Index (QLI) and a 20-question reactive depression questionnaire. "This study," Dr. Smith writes, "showed that patients affiliated with a national organization have a better outcome, regardless of HPN program size. Specifically, affiliated patients, compared with nonaffiliated case-matched controls, experienced a significantly higher quality of life, less reactive depression, and a lower incidence of catheter-related sepsis" [15, p. 162].

Dr. Smith has also reported favorable results in a peer support program initiated at the University of Kansas Medical Center in the late 1990s [16]. In this program, patients who were identified as successfully managing their own HPN underwent training to become preceptors. Their instruction included reinforcement exercises to: (1) develop listening skills; (2) appropriately respond to concerns reported by patients; and (3) avoid providing medical advice (Carol Smith, 4 November 2009, pers. comm.). They were subsequently paired with more recently diagnosed HPN patients. In the results published in 2001, Dr. Smith notes "new patients' post-preceptor interaction depression scores decreased, whereas confidence to master home HPN increased .... Also, each patient and their peer preceptor rated the interactions as helpful" [16, p. 176].

Also relevant to our concerns is a study by Dr. Mary Trainor based on the "helper therapy principle" [17,18]. In this study, 318 members of the United Ostomy Association (UOA) completed a 50-statement scale designed to measure their ostomy acceptance level. Respondents were also asked to provide personal information, including whether they had participated in visitor programs sponsored by local UOA chapters. Fifty-four percent of the participants indicated they had visited other ostomates ("visitors"); the remaining 46% had not visited other ostomates ("nonvisitors"). Dr. Trainor concluded, "visitors had a greater acceptance of their ostomy than nonvisitors .... Results support Riessman's theory (1965) that persons benefit from helping others" [17, p. 105, 18].

## 38.3   OLEY FOUNDATION HISTORY

The Oley Foundation is a nonprofit, independent organization that provides education, emotional support, and clinical outcome information for HPEN consumers, their families, and supporting professionals. The foundation was initiated in 1983 by Dr. Lyn Howard, then Director of the Clinical Nutrition HPEN program, Albany Medical Center, Albany, New York, and her patient, Clarence Oldenburg (nicknamed "Oley"). Dr. Howard strongly believes that HPEN consumers benefit from talking to one another, but she recognized that at that time very few had such an opportunity. HPEN are complicated therapies. Further, HPN was relatively new in the early 1980s; information about it was difficult to come by and patients were widely dispersed. The Oley Foundation was established to fill this void. It currently has over 11,500 members across the United States and in Canada, Australia, Europe, and India. Membership is almost equally divided between HPEN consumers or caregivers (63% in 2011) and HPEN professionals (37% in 2011).

Don Young, who has been on HPN since 1975, has been part of Oley since its inception. "I had eight years' experience [on HPN] prior to Oley," he says. "I think we were unique in our area in that we had a physician who drew us all in together. We used to have clinic on the same day and we always planned to get together after our appointments, so we had that support group right from day one. When I started there was only one other patient in the Albany program, and he soon died. It took a year until we got to the grand total of four. But we still were a group, and we did see each other, and we talked to each other on the phone. So we had kind of a mini Oley Foundation going before the foundation actually started."

In 1978, Marshall and Lee Koonin had begun a patient group in Sharon, Massachusetts. When Lee began HPN in 1977, she remembers that it was considered an experimental therapy "that was not even allowed in some hospitals" [19]. Lee felt very alone and Marshall was determined to find others who were using HPN, both to bring them together and to let others know the therapy worked and maybe shouldn't be considered experimental. The Koonins' Lifeline Foundation grew to about 600 members. They published a newsletter, organized picnics, and started a network of consumers who were willing to talk to other consumers. It was, however, a huge commitment of the Koonins' time and money, and after reassuring themselves that the Oley Foundation would continue the work they had begun, in 1984 the Koonins were relieved to hand the Lifeline Foundation over to the newly established Oley Foundation.

## 38.4   MAKING CONNECTIONS

It is now over 25 years since the Oley Foundation was founded, but it is often still difficult for HPEN consumers to connect with one another or for new HPEN consumers to learn about the Oley Foundation or other HPEN support groups (see list of support groups at end of chapter). Many health care providers and hospital discharge planners do not know about these groups; and those who do may initially have little success introducing them to new consumers, who are so preoccupied with the medical issues surrounding HPEN—such as maintaining sterile technique or avoiding infection—that they cannot think about future needs.

One HPEN consumer says, "You're just so busy dealing with the day-to-day in the beginning that you don't even think about the long term or whether you're going to be secure in the long term." On the other hand, the mother of a child born with intestinal dysfunction remembers: "When they gave us a diagnosis, I said, 'I want a way to figure out how we're going to get her home, and I need to have support. Find me another child someplace in this world with this diagnosis. At the time we were told there wasn't anybody because it was such a rare disorder.'" She learned of Oley, and did find another child with the same diagnosis, through one of the intensive care nurses, who had read about a child with this diagnosis in an Oley newsletter.

Sometimes patients who receive information about the Oley Foundation while in the hospital read the literature they received much later, when they are able to process that information or when they are looking for answers to specific questions. Consumers or caregivers often turn to the Internet for information on HPEN. The Internet has been a tremendous source of growth for the Oley Foundation, with the Web site (www.oley.org) averaging 8757 hits/day in July 2011. Sometimes consumers learn about the Oley Foundation through their home care companies; some companies, however, are reluctant to encourage this kind of networking between consumers for fear of losing customers or receiving demands for different/better equipment, supplies, or services that another company offers.

However, reluctant people or companies may be to refer HPEN consumers to Oley, patient and family connections are important. Steve Swensen, who served as president of the Oley board of trustees, likens the Oley Foundation to a mosaic: "I feel as though all the 'catheter people' I've met through the Oley Foundation—those who have them or care for them, who place them or make them or manage them clinically—all of these individuals have a tile or two to add to a larger mosaic that depicts how to live with central lines. You can't see much by looking at just your own tiles, you have to step back and see what others have added to get the [big] picture" [1, p. 38].

## 38.5   OLEY FOUNDATION PROGRAMS

Oley Foundation membership and all of the programs the group offers are free to HPEN consumers and their families or caregivers. Any program that brings consumers together offers both learning and networking opportunities.

Why is networking so important? One long-term HPEN consumer says, "I've talked to an awful lot of people who just got out of the hospital or have been home for a few months, and they're telling me the same things that I've heard for 35 years: they talk about feeling like they're the only one, of being isolated, that it's very difficult to explain [about HPEN to other] people. That after five minutes of explaining, it doesn't seem worth talking any longer ... It's unrealistic to expect [friends, family, and acquaintances to] just grasp it all."

In the following dialog, three mothers, all Oley members who manage HPEN-dependent children, echo this sentiment:

L.M.: I think that for the first couple of years, I really wanted somebody outside my immediate family to "get it." And I really invested in that .... People said, "Oh, you're home? You don't work? Can you babysit my kids?" After about the sixteenth person said, "Oh, you're so lucky. Can you babysit?" I realized they aren't going to get it. And I finally stopped trying to make them understand our life. Because ... unless somebody lives with you—and even then it's iffy—they're never going to get it. And just because they don't get it, doesn't mean they don't love you .... S.K., I remember your approach from our [online] support group helped me as well. You said that when family members were less than understanding during a crisis, it helped when someone close to you said, "Why are you expecting a normal response? They are incapable."

S.K.: Yes, [this was when my daughter] perforated her bowel .... It pushed me off the edge. But once I came to that understanding, I've been able to deal with it.

L.M.: I think the second I let that go I was much better emotionally. I do not need anyone to get it because I can go to Oley and they get it, and that's all I need.

A.W.: But if you don't have that there's a need. I can clearly remember thinking I had to tell everybody the whole story and try to make them understand. And I reached the point where I didn't explain things and then situations cropped up when I realized, Oh yeah, I suppose you really need to know. Because honestly, if you look at ... many of the kids, you would have no clue...that they have anything going on.

[When our son was] about 18 months old ... we went to visit [my mother-in-law. We] sent the supplies ahead. One of the first nights we were there she told us, "You could try your best to explain everything to me, but when the supplies came to my house—three boxes full—and I started putting stuff in the refrigerator and started putting stuff away and seeing all the stuff, I had to sit down and cry. Because it just overwhelmed me. What you deal with. You couldn't have told me."

"The general population as a whole," says one of these mothers, "doesn't grasp the nature of a chronic condition. They don't grasp the fact that it is up and down. I certainly experience it at work. Many people just expect your kid to be sick and then you move on and life is fine. And you learn that it's not like that. I remember early on one of the social workers talking to us in the NICU about chronic conditions. We grieve and re-grieve all the time. You never heal because the condition never goes away. We certainly celebrated the time that [our son] came off HPN. Being on tube feeds for many people would not be considered a happy life, but for us it was phenomenal. Then to go back [on HPN] and have this bumpy road that we've had for the past two years—we long for just tube feeds. Stability is nice. With a chronic condition the best you can hope for is stability."

## 38.5.1 CONFERENCES

At the large annual Oley Foundation consumer/clinician conference and the smaller, regional conferences Oley sponsors, consumers and their families, clinicians, and industry representatives meet in large and small groups and one-on-one, in both educational and social settings.

The mother of a 14 year old tells how her daughter was more comfortable with her HPEN after attending an Oley Foundation conference: "[My daughter's] perspective started to change a little bit when we started meeting more people .... What really did it for her was when we went to [the Oley conference in] Cape Cod .... At the time she had gone through a stage where she didn't want to be seen in public infusing. [She was] body conscious ... And I remember, a couple of weeks [after the conference] she says, 'I've decided I'm going to go out in public.' I said, 'Well, why is that?' And she [told me how another teen] was infusing the entire evening that [the two of them] were together ... And she didn't realize it until 45 minutes before the end of the evening. She said, 'Mom, I keep thinking people see it. I should have noticed it and if I didn't notice it ...'"

Another mother of an HPEN-dependent child tells this story about attending an Oley Foundation conference soon after her son had his first central line placed (at age three) because of short bowel due to infarction from malrotation. Previously she and her husband had been told that their son probably would not survive:

For forty days our son had fevers at night. We were brand spanking new, so we didn't know what to do. We stood over our son, who was vomiting and had a temperature of 105, and I remember my husband saying, "We might need to bury our child. He might die.".. .

Then we were in the hospital and in walked [a health care provider who had] overheard me talking to the social worker. She said, "You *need* to contact Oley." I was too overwhelmed, but my mom contacted our local [Oley regional] coordinator, who said, "We just happen to have the annual conference right near you in June." So for the seventh time in four months our son was discharged. He was then readmitted with another fever. This time he grew out a bacterial line infection. It was also fungal. They pulled the line. Everything was going on, including the Oley conference. On the first day we gathered family and friends and split up to cover as many presentations as possible. Later we met in "headquarters" upstairs in the hotel room, and everybody starts looking at each other saying, "You know what? You can live on HPN. Our doctor and nurses said you die on HPN! They said he'd never eat. He can eat. You know what? We're not being sterile with the line, and you're not supposed to have a cap with lipid crud coming out the top.". . .We actually met a man who had been on HPN for twenty years!

Later, I went downstairs and met a woman who said, "The two best things I've ever done in my life were to go to a different home care company and switch to Dr. [so and so at the other hospital]." So I went to the home care company booth, which was at the conference . . . . I told them how our first seven months on HPN had been. One of the representative said to his colleagues, "Come over here and listen to this story." I remember thinking, "What do you mean *listen* to me? Nobody listens to me. I'm the crazy mom!"

After the Oley sessions were over, we took [our son] out of the hospital on a day pass to go ride the rides at Knott's Berry Farm with other Oley families at the Oley picnic. Our son saw the other [HPEN] kids, all his cousins saw the other kids, and everybody was so excited. We were like, "Oh my gosh, I think he's going to live."

And that was when we switched to [another hospital] . . . . [Our son] had been inpatient seventy days, with probably six line infections, none of which grew out because the nurses kept pulling what should have been the culture and throwing it out as "waste." That was the last time we were in the hospital, pretty much . . . . Because we were able to attend the Oley conference, we talked to the HPN pharmacist, took notes, switched home care companies, switched doctors. It's been really stable ever since . . . . In our first seven months the hospital days were seventy and now there have been seven in-patient days in eight years . . . . His central line is now over seven years old! The Oley conference saved his life, there is no question. And it changed our lives because all the new people we met didn't look at us like we were crazy.

About the learning opportunities at an Oley conference, one member writes, "I underwent a subtotal gastrectomy for an abdominal tumor in 1995. Along with numerous other complications, I developed gastroparesis. I struggled for ten years, depending on oral nutrition, motility meds, and little amounts of food. I became very malnourished, which led to severe neurological symptoms. In 2006, I went on HPN via a PICC line. I had amazing results, but developed too many infections and went through five [lines] in one year. I went to my first Oley conference in June 2006. I learned so much, that by that August, I had a jejunostomy button inserted by a physician I learned of at Oley. I am now living the best quality of life [I have had] in fourteen years."

## 38.5.2 Regional Coordinator Program and Toll-Free Phone Lines

The Oley Foundation also supports networking with an extensive Regional Coordinator (RC) program. Over 60 HPEN consumers and/or caregivers have volunteered to represent the foundation in their regions. These volunteers answer phone calls and e-mails, make visits, reach out through the Oley online forum, and generally support other members. Some of them have established support groups that meet regularly in their areas (e.g., there are groups in Clearwater, Florida; Toledo, Ohio; Chicago, Illinois; and Northfield, New Jersey; a list of groups and meeting schedules can be found at www.oley.org). The foundation also maintains three toll-free phone lines that are staffed by different consumers and/or caregivers each month (in addition to a toll-free line to the foundation offices).

The toll-free numbers and RC network are valuable for one-on-one, peer-to-peer support. An Oley RC, talking to another RC, tells how important it is for her to be able to communicate with a peer (both of these RCs have HPEN-dependent children): "There are things that are difficult to say out loud to other people. Other people won't grasp it. If I share my fears with you, I know that you know how heavy they make my heart. People just don't comprehend or grasp that. It's just nice to know there are people out there who understand what I say." Further, she adds, "When I say to you, 'Four liters of output,' you understand the magnitude. I get these blank looks from people at work. I say, 'You know the two-liter pop bottles? Two of them. Two of them in three hours!'"

For online networking, the Oley Foundation started a forum in 2008. The community of users grew quickly. One forum user writes, "This forum has been like a lifeline for me—who knew there were others out there like me? I thought I was a medical mystery." For those who are unable to attend a conference for health or financial reasons, the forum provides a good alternative. The forum can be accessed through the Oley Foundation website (http://www.oley.org).

### 38.5.3 NEWSLETTER

The bimonthly newsletter features a medical article and a personal consumer/caregiver coping or biographical article. It also regularly carries a column with practical tips for home enteral nutrition (HEN) consumers; information about major HPEN and/or intestinal management centers; pertinent clinical trials; and any new research or information deemed of interest to HPEN consumers/caregivers/clinicians. For many members, the newsletter is the Oley Foundation's most conspicuous program.

An article about how to write an effective insurance appeal letter is an example of a typical "coping" article. After reading the article, a member wrote, "I was inspired to start the appeal process with Medicare. Medicare was refusing to pay for my hydration and supplies (I have short bowel). It took four appeals, but I finally received a favorable decision .... With the well-needed letter from my doctor ... and Medicare rights' knowledge ... I had [my home care company] reimbursed for great work and care: $12,000."

### 38.5.4 INFORMATION CLEARINGHOUSE

Since its inception, the Oley Foundation has collected, compiled, and distributed the most current information available about HPEN and related issues. Foundation staff answer hundreds of information requests each month via e-mail and phone calls. When needed, staff refer members' questions to medical advisors. The information clearinghouse also includes educational videos and DVDs, which members may borrow. Many of the DVDs cover educational sessions from Oley conferences, allowing more members to benefit from the knowledge imparted by the expert speakers.

The newest educational tool being developed by the foundation is *MY HPN*, an online program where members can learn more about managing their parenteral nutrition (PN) in the comfort of their home at a time that is convenient to them. Topics range from becoming a more active health care partner, to understanding the nutritional content of a PN solution, to avoiding HPN-related complications.

### 38.5.5 RESEARCH

The Oley Foundation is well known for the North American Home Parenteral and Enteral Nutrition Patient Registry (1987–1994), which is the largest registry of HPEN consumers to date and which allowed researchers to assess outcome on HPEN for different underlying diseases and different age groups. Outcome was measured by mortality on therapy, duration on therapy, complications on therapy, and QoL on therapy [20].

More recently, the Oley Foundation supported the research workshop at the American Society of Parenteral and Enteral Nutrition's 2009 meeting (Clinical Nutrition Week), titled "Micronutrients in Parenteral Nutrition: Too Little or Too Much?" "In 1979, and again in the mid-1980s, the American Medical Association established guidelines regarding micronutrients in PN. Concerned that these guidelines and the resulting Federal Drug Administration recommendations are outdated, Dr. Howard and Dr. Alan Buchman located funding for the workshop and invited specialists from around the world to present the most up-to-date research on several micronutrients where new data or controversy exists" [21, p. 4]. The research proceedings have been published as a supplement to *Gastroenterology* [22]. "'We hope,' said Dr. Howard, 'this research workshop will lead to an FDA multi-trace element reformulation and the availability of safer commercial products'" [21, p. 4].

Currently, the foundation is coordinating the US portion of a large international HPN QoL study in conjunction with the Home Artificial Nutrition workgroup of the European Society for Parenteral and Enteral Nutrition. Among other things, this research will provide a valuable tool in assessing QoL on HPEN versus QoL after intestinal transplant.

The Oley Foundation also has a research committee that reviews research protocols pertinent to HPEN consumers. If the committee deems it appropriate, these protocols are briefly described in the Oley Foundation newsletter and on the Web site so consumers can find out more about these studies and decide whether they'd like to participate.

### 38.5.6    EQUIPMENT-SUPPLY EXCHANGE

The Oley Foundation maintains a database of equipment and supplies that consumers no longer need and wish to donate for someone's use. The foundation facilitates contact between the donor and recipient, who arrange for the delivery of the equipment or supplies. This program is especially popular with HEN consumers, and as a whole, saves participants thousands of dollars each year in out-of-pocket expenses.

## 38.6    CONSUMERS' NEEDS CHANGE OVER TIME

The amount of experience an HPEN consumer has with his or her therapy affects their relationship to the Oley Foundation as a support group and as a source of information, as evidenced in this dialog between three long-term HPEN consumers:

A.D.: The role of Oley has changed for me through the years. In the beginning it was ... just awesome, like kids say, both in terms of learning about real basic stuff, like a new portable pump, and [losing the sense of isolation]. [Dr. H.] has been a wonderful physician and she took care of ... me for many years, but you're sitting with [her] once every three or four months if you're stable, and she takes a lot of time, but how much information can she convey? There's just so much that you learn at the Oley conferences that's amazingly empowering. That was one part of it. And the other part was losing the sense of isolation— talking to other people about how they cope with a lot of the basics, and just knowing that there were other people like you out there. Both of those were amazing, at least for me, in the early stages of my relationship with Oley.

  Now my relationship with Oley is ... the newsletter, in terms of what I get out of it .... Every once in a while I get an in-depth article that's really relevant to me, [in a for-mat] where I can sit and digest it and really get a lot out of it—probably in some ways even more than I can if I go to a conference where ... it's hard to absorb it all.

L.T.: I think that's true. [My home care company] people actually got me to Oley in 1989, and ... it was really nice to see other people who were on HPN. That was really wonderful. Plus learning all the new information and everything .... [Now], I think [it has become] more a case of wanting to give back and help other people who are in the situation that I was in all those years ago. But also, I find that when I come to a conference I always learn at least one thing that has changed, or that's new, or something that I didn't know yet.

D.Y.: Absolutely. The Oley Foundation started in '83 ... We're a ways down the road now, and... I guess what ... I really get—ham that I am—is a great deal of satisfaction when people I don't know come up to me at the conference, after I've spoken, and say you've been a real inspiration to me. L., you just said you're kind of coming to the point where you're giving back. And that element is very important now .... But I find, especially now that [my physician] is retired, that the information I get, the technical information, either comes from Oley, or if I [go] to a Crohn's and Colitis meeting and hear somebody speak.

## 38.7 CONCLUSION

It is well documented that dependency on HPEN affects the consumer's QoL. Yet many of the issues that influence a consumer's QoL often fall outside the scope of services clinicians and/or intestinal rehabilitation centers can—or have time to—provide. The support and information available from peers and independent support groups can be invaluable. As Smith notes, "Any intervention that can improve the patient's quality of life and ability to manage at home and reduce expensive complications offers significant benefit to patients, payers, and health care professionals" [15, p. 159].

"I think not knowing—anything, whether it's dealing with HPN or even things outside of that realm—I think typically people's imagination is much worse than reality," says a long-term HPN consumer. "You know the old saying, knowledge is power? That's absolutely true. But also, ... in any situation where people are dealing with life-threatening illnesses, they feel the sense of isolation. It isn't coincidental that there are cancer survivor or cancer support groups all around the world .... There are all kinds of support groups out there. There's a reason these things develop, and that's because there's a need .... It's very important to me that Oley survive and thrive because of what it did for me [and] knowing that other people are going to continue to need it."

Between them, D.Y., L.T., and A.D. estimate they have over 75 years' experience on HPEN. At the end of an Oley teleconference, D.Y. concluded: "Here L.T., A.D., and I have just spent a nice [hour] talking on the phone, chatting. It was a really great conversation. Wouldn't it be nice if that person just coming out of the hospital, one week with a catheter heading home, could realize that this is what your future could be. That twenty, or thirty, or thirty-five years from now you could be sitting around talking to friends that you met. And yeah, you've been through a lot. But here we are."

## OTHER GROUPS

Other organizations that might be of interest to HPEN consumers include:

Association of Gastrointestinal Motility Disorders, Inc. (AGMD) (www.agmd-gimotility.org)
Caring Bridge (www.CaringBridge.org)
Crohn's and Colitis Foundation of America (CCFA) (www.ccfa.org)
International Foundation for Functional Gastrointestinal Disorders (IFFGD) (www.iffgd.org)
MitoAction (www.mitoaction.org)
MUMS National Parent-to-Parent Network (www.netnet.net/mums)
National Family Caregiver Association (NFCA) (www.nfcacares.org)
PINNT (organization for HPEN consumers in the UK) (www.pinnt.org)
PN-DU (organization for HPN consumers in Australia and New Zealand) (http://parenteral-nutrition-down-under.webs.com/#)
United Ostomy Associations of America (www.uoaa.org)
Yahoo! group, TPN Support (http://health.groups.yahoo.com/group/tpnsupport) or Short Bowel Support (http://health.groups.yahoo.com/group/SBS_Support)

(See www.oley.org/links.html for the most up-to-date listing of Web sites considered of interest to Oley members.)

## SUGGESTED READING

Jeejeebhoy, Shireen. *Lifeliner, The Judy Taylor Story.* New York: iUniverse, Inc., 2007.

## REFERENCES

1. Swensen S. Coming to terms with a central line. *JVAD.* 2001;6(1):36–38.
2. Howard L. Length of life and quality of life on home parenteral nutrition. *J Parenter Enteral Nutr.* 2002;26(5):S55–S59.

3. Kindle R. Life with Fred: 12 years of home parenteral nutrition. *Nutr Clin Pract.* 2003;18:235–7.

4. Huisman-de Waal G, Schoonhoven L, Jansen J, Wanten G, van Achterberg T. The impact of home parenteral nutrition on daily life—A review. *Clin Nutr.* 2007;26:275–88.doi:10.1016/j.clnu.2006.10.002

5. Drossman D, Chang L, Schneck S, Blackman C, Norton W, Norton N. A focus group assessment of patient perspectives on irritable bowel syndrome and illness severity. *Dig Dis Sci.* 2009;54:1532–41.

6. Winkler M. Quality of life in adult home parenteral nutrition patients. *J Parenter Enteral Nutr.* 2005;29(3):162–70.

7. Malone, M. Longitudinal assessment of outcome, health status, and changes in lifestyle associated with long-term home parenteral and enteral nutrition. *J Parenter Enteral Nutr.* 2002;26(3):164–8.

8. Richards D, Carlson G. Quality of life assessment and cost-effectiveness. In: Nightingale J, editor. *Intestinal failure.* Cambridge: Greenwich Medical Media, Ltd. 2001. pp. 447–57.

9. Casati J, Toner B, De Rooy E, Drossman D, Maunder R. Concerns of patients with inflammatory bowel disease. *Dig Dis Sci.* 2000;45(1):26–31.

10. Hoffman K. Psychosocial concerns of home nutrition therapy consumers. *Nutr Clin Pract.* 1989 Apr;4:51–56.

11. Ehrenpreis B, Hilf A. Home parenteral nutrition: The consumer's perspective. *LifelineLetter.* 1998 Nov/Dec;19(6):1–7.

12. Johnson J, Lane C. Role of support groups in cancer care. *Support Care Cancer.* 1993; 1:52–56.

13. Marlow B, Cartmill T, Cieplucha H, Lowrie, S. An interactive process model of psychosocial support needs for women living with breast cancer. *Psychooncology.* 2003;12:319–30. doi:10.1002/pon.645.

14. Muscular Dystrophy Association. Telethon. Internet: http://www.mda.org/telethon/families.html (accessed 1 November 2009).

15. Smith C, Curtas S, Werkowitch M, Kleinbeck S, Howard L. Home parenteral nutrition: Does affiliation with a national support and educational organization improve patient outcomes? *J Parenter Enteral Nutr.* 2002;26(3):159–63.

16. Smith C, Curtas S, Robinson J. Case study of patients helping patients program. *Nutrition.* 2001; 17:175–6.

17. Trainor MA. Acceptance of ostomy and the visitor role in a self-help group for ostomy patients. *Nurs Res.* 1982 Mar–Apr;31(2):102–6.

18. Riessman F. The "helper" therapy principle. *Soc Work.* 1965 Apr;10:27–32.

19. The Oley Foundation. LifelineLetter. Koonin, L & M. How it all began. Internet: http://oley.org/lifeline/history.html (accessed November 1, 2009).

20. North American Home Parenteral and Enteral Nutrition Patient Registry (1987–1994). Annual reports, 1985–1992. Oley Foundation, Albany, New York.

21. Metzger L. Information exchange at clinical nutrition week. *Lifeline Letter.* 2009 Mar/Apr;30(2):4–5.

22. Supplement to Gastroenterology, Micronutricants in Parenteral Nutrition: Too Little or Too Much? Proceedings from the American Society for Parenteral and Enteral Nutrition 2009 Research workshop.

# Index